Oesophagus and Stomach

GASTROINTESTINAL SURGERY LIBRARY

Abdominal Trauma, Peritoneum, and Retroperitoneum
Aditya Nanavati and Sanjay Nagral

Appendix, Colon, and Rectum
Parul J. Shukla, Jeffrey Milsom, and Kota Momose

Duodenum and Small Bowel
John A. Windsor, Sanjay Pandanaboyana, and Anil K. Agarwal

Liver, Gall Bladder, and Bile Ducts
Mohamed Rela and Pierre-Alain Clavien

Oesophagus and Stomach
Matthias Reeh and Jakob R. Izbicki

Pancreas
Shailesh V. Shrikhande and Markus W. Büchler

Oesophagus and Stomach

EDITED BY

Matthias Reeh
Senior Consultant, Department of General, Visceral and Thoracic Surgery, University Hospital Hamburg-Eppendorf, Hamburg, Germany

Jakob R. Izbicki
Chairman, Department of General, Visceral and Thoracic Surgery, University Hospital Hamburg-Eppendorf, Hamburg, Germany

SERIES EDITORS

Samiran Nundy
Emeritus Consultant, Sir Ganga Ram Hospital, New Delhi, India

Dirk J. Gouma
Emeritus Professor of Surgery, Amsterdam University Medical Centre, Amsterdam, The Netherlands

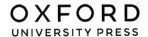

OXFORD
UNIVERSITY PRESS

Great Clarendon Street, Oxford, OX2 6DP,
United Kingdom

Oxford University Press is a department of the University of Oxford.
It furthers the University's objective of excellence in research, scholarship,
and education by publishing worldwide. Oxford is a registered trade mark of
Oxford University Press in the UK and in certain other countries

© Oxford University Press 2023

The moral rights of the authors have been asserted

First Edition published in 2023

All rights reserved. No part of this publication may be reproduced, stored in
a retrieval system, or transmitted, in any form or by any means, without the
prior permission in writing of Oxford University Press, or as expressly permitted
by law, by licence or under terms agreed with the appropriate reprographics
rights organization. Enquiries concerning reproduction outside the scope of the
above should be sent to the Rights Department, Oxford University Press, at the
address above

You must not circulate this work in any other form
and you must impose this same condition on any acquirer

Published in the United States of America by Oxford University Press
198 Madison Avenue, New York, NY 10016, United States of America

British Library Cataloguing in Publication Data
Data available

Library of Congress Control Number: 2022952042

ISBN 978–0–19–286359–1

DOI: 10.1093/med/9780192863591.001.0001

Printed and bound by
CPI Group (UK) Ltd, Croydon, CR0 4YY

Oxford University Press makes no representation, express or implied, that the
drug dosages in this book are correct. Readers must therefore always check
the product information and clinical procedures with the most up-to-date
published product information and data sheets provided by the manufacturers
and the most recent codes of conduct and safety regulations. The authors and
the publishers do not accept responsibility or legal liability for any errors in the
text or for the misuse or misapplication of material in this work. Except where
otherwise stated, drug dosages and recommendations are for the non-pregnant
adult who is not breast-feeding

Links to third party websites are provided by Oxford in good faith and
for information only. Oxford disclaims any responsibility for the materials
contained in any third party website referenced in this work.

Foreword to the Gastrointestinal Surgery Library

We are currently led to believe that textbooks are déclassé. Information is no longer gathered other than online through PubMed or Google and their equivalents. This is not so. First, much of the world, especially in low- and middle-income countries, still derives scholarly information from textbooks; and second, we ignore the obvious, where does the online information come from? Certainly, for a narrow, topic-specific search we can immediately reach for PubMed, but where does generic broad disease-based topic information come from? Is it possible to educate our current and future surgeons on Wikipedia alone? Truth is hard to find, truth in surgery even harder. We surgeons, like the rest of the world, find it easy to fall back on the confirmation biases of our already held beliefs. We all still struggle with 'We do this this way, because that is the way we have always done so'. Only in recent decades have surgeons moved from numerator doctors remembering the energizing success and the damaging failure to provide denominators for our actions. How to find the truth or even the facts is a great challenge in our information-overloaded society. Clinical trials in the discipline of surgery are hard to do, and even harder where equipoise does not exist. Our best recourse is to begin with those leading their respective fields, often in academic environments where challenge and controversy are healthy endeavours. A culture where the student becomes the conscience of the professor is what academia should be about.

Where can we go to look for the most current validated information? Where can our trainees go beyond their immediate environment? Nowhere is this more important as we become a global surgical society. The low- and middle-income countries look to the high-income countries for leadership and guidance, but is that correct? What we do in tertiary institutions may well not serve our colleagues in resource-poor countries. This should be a two-way street; what can we in tertiary centres learn from less privileged but equally demanding societies? We embrace technology for technology's sake, we think little of value but only of perceived benefit. What an opportunity to embrace excellence and define the greater benefit for the greatest number.

The *Gastrointestinal Surgery Library* series has taken on this Herculean task.

The lead editors Professor Samiran Nundy from New Delhi and Professor Dirk J. Gouma from Amsterdam have the stature and fortitude to lead this challenge. A mammoth text focused on a global readership in print, eBook, and online editions. To do this they have assembled a cadre of volume editors from six countries. The volume editors have then recruited leaders within the gastrointestinal surgical fraternity from several more countries to address global problems in gastrointestinal surgery, from oesophagus to anus and all tissues and viscera that surround the alimentary tract. Together, they provide a comprehensive umbrella that most will find weatherproof, but not impermeable.

Sir Murray F. Brennan
Memorial Sloan Kettering Cancer Center
New York, USA

Introduction from the Series Editors

Gastrointestinal (GI) surgery is performed for a range of benign and malignant diseases, in both the elective and emergency settings. Although there are many textbooks related to GI surgery, most of them are addressed to a predominantly Western readership or deal with individual organs or organ systems.

We have strived to create a comprehensive *Gastrointestinal Surgery Library* in which each of the six books deals with a specific organ and is edited by internationally recognized experts from both the developed as well as the developing countries. We thus have 14 editors and 350 contributors from 24 different countries from as far afield as Argentina and New Zealand.

The *Gastrointestinal Surgery Library* will, we hope, serve as reference manuals on this important subject and will cater to a global audience. The inclusion of experts across the world to edit the individual volumes and contribute to the chapters will also result in the description of effective management protocols which are relevant to both economically developed and developing nations.

Samiran Nundy
Dirk J. Gouma

Introduction from the Volume Editors

In bringing forth this volume, our goal was to create a detailed, comprehensive, and educational tool focusing on the oesophagus and the stomach. This textbook should not only be for surgeons or residents in surgery dealing with upper gastrointestinal (GI) surgery, but also to provide detailed information to every medical student, junior medical doctor, or even senior doctors on medical or surgical treatment. Since the early 1990s, diagnostics, staging, and especially medical as well as surgical treatment approaches concerning diseases of the oesophagus and the stomach have changed and improved extensively. Thus, this textbook provides detailed and up-to-date knowledge to the reader about every aspect of diseases of the oesophagus and the stomach. The first part of the textbook deals with basic topics such as anatomy and physiology as well as general and specific diagnostics of upper GI diseases. In the rest of the chapters in Part 1, benign diseases of the oesophagus and the stomach are presented in detail. The last 12 chapters of the volume provide comprehensive knowledge of malignant tumours of the oesophagus (Part 2) and the stomach (Part 3). All chapters are written by worldwide experts in the specific field of upper GI diseases.

In the past, a surgeon had to treat diseases from the head to the toe. This concept has changed and specialization has been included in nearly every medical and surgical department worldwide. For this specialization, a profound knowledge of anatomy, pathophysiology, adequate diagnostics, as well as individualized multimodal treatment approaches remain the foundation of high-quality treatment of diseases of the oesophagus and the stomach.

In summary, we hope that every reader will benefit from this huge effort by combing the work and up-to-date knowledge of many experts in their fields of treatment of diseases of the oesophagus and the stomach.

Matthias Reeh
Jakob R. Izbicki

About the Series Editors

Samiran Nundy was a medical undergraduate at Cambridge University and Guy's Hospital, London, UK and then trained, first in medicine at Hammersmith Hospital, London, and later in surgery at Guy's Hospital, Addenbrooke's Hospital, Hammersmith Hospital, and the Massachusetts General Hospital in Boston, USA. He taught at Cambridge University, University of London, and Harvard University, and returned to the All India Institute of Medical Sciences (AIIMS) in 1975 where he eventually became Professor and Head of the Department of Gastrointestinal Surgery. He left AIIMS in 1996 to start the Surgical Gastroenterology and Liver Transplantation Department in the Sir Ganga Ram Hospital, New Delhi, India. His clinical and research interests are in the management of complicated diseases of the liver, bowel, and pancreas, the quality of Indian medical research and publications, and health information on the web. He has written or edited 37 books and authored or co-authored over 230 research papers. He has been Editor of the *National Medical Journal of India*, *Tropical Gastroenterology*, the *Indian Journal of Medical Ethics*, and the website DrRaxa.com and has served on 24 journal Editorial Boards including the *British Medical Journal*. He is Emeritus Editor of *Current Medicine Research and Practice*, on the Board of Trustees of Sir Ganga Ram Hospital, and President of the AIIMS, Rishikesh.

Dirk J. Gouma is Emeritus Professor of Surgery at the Academic Medical Center Amsterdam, The Netherlands. He served as Chairman of the Department of Surgery and Chairman of the Division of Surgical Specialities at the AMC. During his surgical training he worked as a Fellow at Maastricht University and thereafter as Associate Professor. He conducted his PhD research programme at Maastricht; Hammersmith Hospital, London, UK; Massachusetts General Hospital, Boston, USA; and Hermann Hospital, Houston, USA. His clinical and research efforts concentrated on the outcome of treatment of hepatobiliary and pancreatic disease as well as evaluation of diagnostic strategies and pathophysiology of obstructive jaundice and biliary drainage. More recently, aspects of patient safety programmes and quality control such as centralization and development and implementation of checklists are included. He has served as Chairman of the Scientific Committee of the European Surgical Association (ESA), Council member of the United European Gastroenterology (UEG), President of the European-African Hepato-Pancreatico-Biliary Association (E-AHPBA), Secretary General of the IHPBA, and Chairman of the European Digestive Surgery (EDS). He was a member of the National Health Council, The Netherlands, Chairman of the Concilium Chirurgicum (the Dutch advisory board of surgical education training), and member of the Editorial Board of several medical journals. He was the supervisor of more than 50 PhD fellows and is author/co-author of over 660 publications in peer-reviewed journals (H-index 95) and more than 150 non peer-reviewed papers and/or book chapters.

About the Volume Editors

Matthias Reeh was a medical undergraduate at Kiel University until 2008 and then trained, first in surgery, at University Hospital Hamburg-Eppendorf, Germany, from 2009. In 2016, he became Associate Professor of Surgery and an attending surgeon. In 2018, he became Senior Attending Surgeon at the University Hospital Hamburg-Eppendorf, Germany. His clinical and research interests are in the field of tumour biology and surgical oncology, and in special oesophageal cancer and upper gastrointestinal surgery. He has written several book chapters and authored or co-authored over 70 research papers. Dr Reeh has received several academic research prizes, such as 'Dr. Martinipreis', and has been named as a Fellow of the European Board of Surgeons with honours.

Jakob R. Izbicki was a medical undergraduate at Bonn University, Germany. He trained in surgery at University Hospital Hannover, and the University of Cologne, Germany, following a Senior Residency and Postdoctoral Fellowship at the Ludwig-Maximilians-University of Munich, Germany. In Munich, he became Associate Professor of Surgery and an attending surgeon. In 1992, he went to the University Hospital Hamburg-Eppendorf, Germany, and became Senior Attending Surgeon and Professor of Surgery. In 1998, he became Surgeon-in-Chief, and in 2002 Chairman of the Department of General, Visceral and Thoracic Surgery. He has written or edited over 20 books and authored or co-authored over 700 research papers. Professor Izbicki has received several academic honours such as Honorary Fellowship of the American College of Surgeons; Honorary Fellowship of the Royal College of Surgeons Edinburgh; Honorary Doctorate at the University of Cluj Napoca, Romania; and Honorary Professor at the University of Skopje, Macedonia.

Contents

Abbreviations xvii
Contributors xix

PART 1
Anatomy, physiology, diagnostics, and benign diseases

1. **Anatomy and physiology** 3
   Rainer Grotelüschen, Tarik Ghadban, Kai Bachmann, and Jakob R. Izbicki

2. **Diagnostic tests and principal investigations: endoscopy, manometry and contrast studies** 13
   Yuki B. Werner

3. **Motility disorders of the oesophagus** 25
   Michaela Müller, Stefan Niebisch, and Ines Gockel

4. **Oesophageal diverticula** 39
   Joshua Kapp, Philip Müller, and Christian A. Gutschow

5. **Benign diseases of the stomach: focus on dyspepsia** 45
   Kuniaki Aridome

6. **Gastro-oesophageal reflux disease** 49
   Björn-Ole Stüben, Anna Duprée, and Oliver Mann

7. **Upper gastrointestinal bleeding: non-surgical and surgical management** 65
   Zaheer Nabi and D. Nageshwar Reddy

8. **Upper gastrointestinal perforation: non-surgical and surgical management** 79
   Alexander Hendricks, Mark Ellrichmann, and Clemens Schafmayer

9. **Obesity: non-surgical treatment and bariatric surgery** 89
   Rishabh Shah, Lisandro Montorfano, Emanuele Lo Menzo, Samuel Szomstein, and Raul J. Rosenthal

PART 2
Oesophageal cancer

10. **Oesophageal cancer: epidemiology, symptoms, diagnostics, and staging** 99
    Andrew Tang, Thomas Rice, and Usman Ahmad

11. **Oesophageal cancer: multimodal treatment** 105
    Ben M. Eyck, Berend J. van der Wilk, Maurice J.C. van der Sangen, Ate van der Gaast, and J. Jan B. van Lanschot

12. **Oesophageal cancer: endoscopic treatment** 129
    Thomas Rösch

13. **Oesophageal cancer: surgery** 137
    Björn-Ole Stüben, Karl-Frederick Karstens, Michael Nentwich, Jakob R. Izbicki, and Matthias Reeh

14. **Oesophageal cancer: minimally invasive surgery and robotic surgery** 155
    Gijsbert van Boxel, Pieter C. van der Sluis, Peter P. Grimminger, and Richard van Hillegersberg

15. **Oesophageal cancer: future aspects of treatment** 169
    Thorsten Oliver Goetze and Salah-Eddin Al-Batran

PART 3
Gastric cancer

16. **Gastric cancer: epidemiology, symptoms, diagnosis, and staging** 177
    Takaaki Arigami and Shoji Natsugoe

17. **Gastric cancer: multimodal treatment** 187
    Mickael Chevallay, Thorsten Oliver Goetze, Salah-Eddin Al-Batran, and Stefan Mönig

18. **Gastric cancer: endoscopic treatment** 199
    Chang Seok Bang

19. **Gastric cancer: surgery** 209
   Matthias Biebl, Dino Kröll, Sascha Chopra, and Johann Pratschke

20. **Gastric cancer: minimally invasive surgery and robotic surgery** 217
   Makoto Hikage and Masanori Terashima

21. **Gastric cancer: future aspects of treatment** 231
   Alexander B.J. Borgstein, Suzanne S. Gisbertz, and Mark I. van Berge Henegouwen

Index 241

Abbreviations

5-FU	5-fluorouracil	GI	gastrointestinal
AET	acid exposure time	GLP-1	glucagon-like peptide 1
AGC	advanced gastric cancer	GOJ	gastro-oesophageal junction
AJCC	American Joint Commission on Cancer	GORD	gastro-oesophageal reflux disease
AOG	adenocarcinoma of the oesophagogastric junction	HER2	human epidermal growth factor receptor 2
APC	argon plasma coagulation	HIPEC	hyperthermic intraperitoneal chemotherapy
ASCO	American Society of Clinical Oncology	HR	hazard ratio
BO	Barrett's oesophagus	HRIM	high-resolution impedance manometry
BoTox	botulinum toxin	HRM	high-resolution manometry
BPDDS	biliopancreatic diversion with duodenal switch	ICG	indocyanine green
BRTO	balloon-occluded retrograde transvenous obliteration	IM	intestinal metaplasia
		IRP	integrated relaxation pressure
CI	confidence interval	IV	intravenous
CO_2	carbon dioxide	JCOG	Japan Clinical Oncology Group
COX	cyclooxygenase	LDG	laparoscopic distal gastrectomy
CPS	combined positive score	LG	laparoscopic gastrectomy
CROSS	ChemoRadiotherapy for Oesophageal cancer followed by Surgery Study	LHM	laparoscopic Heller myotomy
		LNM	lymph node metastasis
CT	computed tomography	LOS	lower oesophageal sphincter
C-WLI	conventional white light imaging	LPG	laparoscopic proximal gastrectomy
DCF	docetaxel, cisplatin, and fluorouracil	LTG	laparoscopic total gastrectomy
DCI	distal contractile integral	LVI	lymphovascular invasion
DEP	Doppler endoscopic probe	MAGIC	Medical Research Council Adjuvant Gastric Infusional Chemotherapy
DOS	distal oesophageal spasm		
DVSS	da Vinci Surgical System	MIO	minimally invasive oesophagectomy
EBL	endoscopic band ligation	MITG	minimally invasive total gastrectomy
EBV	Epstein–Barr virus	M-NBI	magnifying narrow-band imaging
ECF	epirubicin, cisplatin, and fluorouracil	NEWS	non-exposed wall-inversion surgery
ECX	epirubicin, cisplatin, and capecitabine	NSAID	non-steroidal anti-inflammatory drug
EFTR	endoscopic full-thickness resection	NSBB	non-selective beta blocker
EGC	early gastric cancer	NVUGIB	non-variceal upper gastrointestinal bleeding
EGC-DH	early gastric cancer with undifferentiated-type histology	OAGB	one-anastomosis gastric bypass
		ODG	open distal gastrectomy
EGC-MH	early gastric cancer with mixed-type histology	OG	open gastrectomy
EGC-UH	early gastric cancer with differentiated-type histology	OGD	oesophagogastroduodenoscopy
		OGJ	oesophagogastric junction
EGFR	epithelial growth factor receptor	OO	open oesophagectomy
EMR	endoscopic mucosal resection	OS	overall survival
EPS	epigastric pain syndrome	OTG	open total gastrectomy
ESD	endoscopic submucosal dissection	OTSC	over-the-scope clip
EUS	endoscopic ultrasound	PAC	papillary adenocarcinoma
FD	functional dyspepsia	PD	pneumatic dilatation
FDA	Food and Drug Administration	PD-1	programmed cell death protein 1
FDG	fluorodeoxyglucose	PD-L1	programmed cell death protein 1 ligand
FLOT	fluorouracil, leucovorin, oxaliplatin, and docetaxel	PDS	postprandial distress syndrome
FPG	function-preserving gastrectomy	PET	positron emission tomography

Abbreviations

PET-CT	positron emission tomography with computed tomography	SG	sleeve gastrectomy
POEM	peroral endoscopic myotomy	SN	sentinel node
PPG	pylorus-preserving gastrectomy	SRC	signet ring cell carcinoma
PPI	proton pump inhibitor	TAE	transcatheter arterial embolization
PUD	peptic ulcer disease	TBE	timed barium oesophagogram
RAMIO	robot-assisted minimally invasive oesophagectomy	TIPSS	transjugular intrahepatic portosystemic shunt
RDG	robot-assisted distal gastrectomy	TNM	tumour, node, and metastasis
RFS	relapse-free survival	TTO	transthoracic oesophagectomy
RG	robotic gastrectomy	TTSC	through-the-scope clip
RHM	robotic Heller myotomy	UGI-XR	upper gastrointestinal barium X-ray radiography
RNYGB	Roux-en-Y gastric bypass	VEGF	vascular endothelial growth factor
RTOG	Radiation Therapy Oncology Group	VS	vessel plus surface
SADI	single-anastomosis duodeno-ileal bypass	VUGIB	variceal upper gastrointestinal bleeding
SCC	squamous cell carcinoma	WECC	Worldwide Esophageal Cancer Collaborative

Contributors

Usman Ahmad Department of Thoracic and Cardiovascular Surgery, Heart, Vascular & Thoracic Institute, Cleveland Clinic, Cleveland, Ohio, USA; Transplant Institute, Cleveland Clinic, Cleveland, Ohio, USA

Salah-Eddin Al-Batran Institute of Clinical Cancer Research, Krankenhaus Nordwest, UCT-University Cancer Center, Frankfurt, Germany; IKF Institut für Klinische Krebsforschung GmbH am Krankenhaus Nordwest, Frankfurt, Germany

Kuniaki Aridome Department of Surgery, Social Welfare Organization Saiseikai Imperial Gift Foundation, Inc, Saiseikai Sendai Hospital, Satsumasendai City, Kagoshima, Japan

Takaaki Arigami Department of Digestive Surgery, Breast and Thyroid Surgery, Kagoshima University Graduate School of Medical and Dental Sciences, Kagoshima, Japan

Kai Bachmann Department of General, Visceral and Thoracic Surgery, University Medical Center Hamburg-Eppendorf, Hamburg, Germany

Chang Seok Bang Department of Internal Medicine, Hallym University College of Medicine, Chuncheon, South Korea; Institute for Liver and Digestive Diseases, Hallym University, Chuncheon, South Korea; Institute of New Frontier Research, Hallym University College of Medicine, Chuncheon, South Korea

Matthias Biebl Department of Surgery, Ordensklinikum Linz, Linz, Austria

Alexander B.J. Borgstein Department of Surgery, Amsterdam UMC, University of Amsterdam, Cancer Center Amsterdam, the Netherlands

Mickael Chevallay Department of Visceral Surgery, Geneva University Hospital, Geneva, Switzerland

Sascha Chopra Department of General and Visceral Surgery, Klinikum am Friedrichshain, Berlin, Germany

Anna Duprée Department of General, Visceral and Thoracic Surgery, University Medical Center Hamburg-Eppendorf, Hamburg, Germany

Mark Ellrichmann Department of General, Visceral, Thoracic, Transplantation and Pediatric Surgery, University Hospital Schleswig-Holstein Campus Kiel, Kiel, Germany

Ben M. Eyck Department of Surgery, Erasmus University Medical Centre, Rotterdam, the Netherlands

Tarik Ghadban Department of General, Visceral and Thoracic Surgery, University Medical Center Hamburg-Eppendorf, Hamburg, Germany

Suzanne S. Gisbertz Department of Surgery, Amsterdam UMC, University of Amsterdam, Cancer Center Amsterdam, the Netherlands

Ines Gockel Department of Visceral, Transplant, Thoracic and Vascular Surgery, University Hospital of Leipzig, Leipzig, Germany

Thorsten Oliver Goetze Institute of Clinical Cancer Research, University Cancer Centre Frankfurt, Krankenhaus Nordwest, Frankfurt, Germany

Peter P. Grimminger Department of General, Visceral and Transplant Surgery, University Medical Center of the Johannes Gutenberg University, Mainz, Germany

Rainer Grotelüschen Department of General, Visceral and Thoracic Surgery, University Medical Center Hamburg-Eppendorf, Hamburg, Germany

Christian A. Gutschow Department of Visceral and Transplant Surgery, University Hospital Zurich, Zurich, Switzerland

Alexander Hendricks Department of General, Visceral, Thoracic, Transplantation and Pediatric Surgery, University Hospital Schleswig-Holstein Campus Kiel, Kiel, Germany

Makoto Hikage Division of Gastric Surgery, Shizuoka Cancer Center, Shizuoka, Japan

Jakob R. Izbicki Department of General, Visceral and Thoracic Surgery, University Medical Center Hamburg-Eppendorf, Hamburg, Germany

Joshua Kapp Department of Visceral and Transplant Surgery, University Hospital Zurich, Zurich, Switzerland

Karl-Frederick Karstens Department of General, Visceral and Thoracic Surgery, University Medical Center Hamburg-Eppendorf, Hamburg, Germany

Dino Kröll Department of Visceral Surgery and Medicine, Inselspital, Bauchzentrum Bern, Bern, Switzerland

Emanuele Lo Menzo The Bariatric and Metabolic Institute, Cleveland Clinic Florida, Weston, Florida, USA

Oliver Mann Department of General, Visceral and Thoracic Surgery, University Medical Center Hamburg-Eppendorf, Hamburg, Germany

Stefan Mönig Department of Visceral Surgery, Geneva University Hospital, Geneva, Switzerland

Lisandro Montorfano The Bariatric and Metabolic Institute, Cleveland Clinic Florida, Weston, Florida, USA

Michaela Müller Department of Gastroenterology, University Hospital of Marburg, Marburg, Germany

Philip Müller Department of Visceral and Transplant Surgery, University Hospital Zurich, Zurich, Switzerland

Zaheer Nabi Asian Institute of Gastroenterology, Hyderabad, India

Shoji Natsugoe Department of Digestive Surgery, Kajiki Onsen Hospital, Kagoshima, Japan

Michael Nentwich Department of General, Visceral and Thoracic Surgery, University Medical Center Hamburg-Eppendorf, Hamburg, Germany

Stefan Niebisch Department of Visceral, Transplant, Thoracic and Vascular Surgery, University Hospital of Leipzig, Leipzig, Germany

Johann Pratschke Department of Surgery, Charité University Medicine Berlin, Berlin, Germany

D. Nageshwar Reddy Asian Institute of Gastroenterology, Hyderabad, India

Matthias Reeh Department of General, Visceral and Thoracic Surgery, University Medical Center Hamburg-Eppendorf, Hamburg, Germany

Thomas Rice Department of Thoracic and Cardiovascular Surgery, Cleveland Clinic, Cleveland, Ohio, USA

Thomas Rösch Department of Interdisciplinary Endoscopy, University Hospital Hamburg-Eppendorf, Hamburg, Germany

Raul J. Rosenthal The Bariatric and Metabolic Institute, Cleveland Clinic Florida, Weston, Florida, USA

Clemens Schafmayer Department of General, Visceral, Thoracic, Transplantation and Pediatric Surgery, University Hospital Schleswig-Holstein Campus Kiel, Kiel, Germany

Rishabh Shah The Bariatric and Metabolic Institute, Cleveland Clinic Florida, Weston, Florida, USA

Contributors

Björn-Ole Stüben Department of General, Visceral and Thoracic Surgery, University Medical Center Hamburg-Eppendorf, Hamburg, Germany

Samuel Szomstein The Bariatric and Metabolic Institute, Cleveland Clinic Florida, Weston, Florida, USA

Andrew Tang Department of Thoracic and Cardiovascular Surgery, Cleveland Clinic, Cleveland, Ohio, USA

Masanori Terashima Division of Gastric Surgery, Shizuoka Cancer Center, Shizuoka, Japan

Mark I. van Berge Henegouwen Department of Surgery, Amsterdam UMC, University of Amsterdam, Cancer Center Amsterdam, the Netherlands

Gijsbert van Boxel Department of Surgery, University Medical Center Utrecht, Utrecht, the Netherlands; and Department of General Surgery, Portsmouth Hospitals University NHS Trust, Portsmouth, UK

Ate van der Gaast Department of Medical Oncology, Erasmus University Medical Centre, Rotterdam, the Netherlands

Maurice J.C. van der Sangen Department of Radiation Oncology, Catharina Hospital, Eindhoven, the Netherlands

Pieter C. van der Sluis Department of General, Visceral and Transplant Surgery, University Medical Center of the Johannes Gutenberg University, Mainz, Germany; Department of Oncologic and Gastrointestinal Surgery, Erasmus University Medical Centre, Rotterdam, the Netherlands

Berend J. van der Wilk Department of Surgery, Erasmus University Medical Centre, Rotterdam, the Netherlands

Richard van Hillegersberg Department of Surgery, University Medical Center Utrecht, Utrecht, the Netherlands

J. Jan B. van Lanschot Department of Surgery, Erasmus University Medical Centre, Rotterdam, the Netherlands

Yuki B. Werner Department of Interdisciplinary Endoscopy, University Medical Center Hamburg-Eppendorf, Hamburg, Germany

PART 1
Anatomy, physiology, diagnostics, and benign diseases

1. Anatomy and physiology 3
   Rainer Grotelüschen, Tarik Ghadban, Kai Bachmann, and Jakob R. Izbicki

2. Diagnostic tests and principal investigations: endoscopy, manometry and contrast studies 13
   Yuki B. Werner

3. Motility disorders of the oesophagus 25
   Michaela Müller, Stefan Niebisch, and Ines Gockel

4. Oesophageal diverticula 39
   Joshua Kapp, Philip Müller, and Christian A. Gutschow

5. Benign diseases of the stomach: focus on dyspepsia 45
   Kuniaki Aridome

6. Gastro-oesophageal reflux disease 49
   Björn-Ole Stüben, Anna Duprée, and Oliver Mann

7. Upper gastrointestinal bleeding: non-surgical and surgical management 65
   Zaheer Nabi and D. Nageshwar Reddy

8. Upper gastrointestinal perforation: non-surgical and surgical management 79
   Alexander Hendricks, Mark Ellrichmann, and Clemens Schafmayer

9. Obesity: non-surgical treatment and bariatric surgery 89
   Rishabh Shah, Lisandro Montorfano, Emanuele Lo Menzo, Samuel Szomstein, and Raul J. Rosenthal

1

Anatomy and physiology

Rainer Grotelüschen, Tarik Ghadban, Kai Bachmann, and Jakob R. Izbicki

The oesophagus

Anatomy

Macroanatomy

The oesophagus is a tubular, elongated organ which connects the pharynx to the stomach. It is a fibromuscular tube about 23–25 cm long in adults that carries food and fluids into the stomach with the help of peristaltic movements.

The oesophagus originates at the inferior border of the cricoid cartilage (C6) and extends to the cardiac orifice of the stomach (T11). It goes through the neck, lies at the back of the mediastinum behind the trachea and heart and ventral to the spine, continues to move caudally through the diaphragm, and finally ends in the cardia of the stomach (Figure 1.1).

The prevertebral fascia connects the oesophagus to the bodies of the sixth to eighth cervical vertebra posteriorly. The thoracic duct, which drains the majority of the body's lymph, passes behind the oesophagus and drains into the systemic blood circulation at the junction of the left subclavian and internal jugular vein. The carotid sheath and the lower poles of the lateral thyroid gland can be found lateral to the oesophagus in the lower part of the neck.

Distally, the oesophagus passes behind the aortic arch at the level of the T4/T5 intervertebral discs and enters the posterior mediastinum, where it runs behind the heart and curves in front of the thoracic aorta (Figure 1.2). The oesophagus also lies in front of parts of the hemiazygos veins and the intercostal veins on

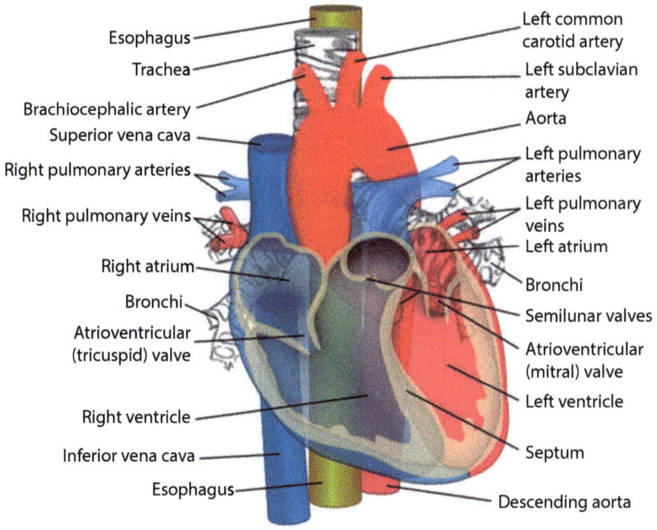

Figure 1.1 The oesophagus (yellow) passes behind the trachea and the heart.
Mikael Hikael Iloand ZooFari. Reproduced under a Creative Commons Attribution-Share Alike 3.0 Unported license (https://creativecommons.org/licenses/by-sa/3.0/deed.en). Available at: https://commons.wikimedia.org/wiki/File:Relations_of_the_aorta,_trachea,_esophagus_and_other_heart_structures.svg

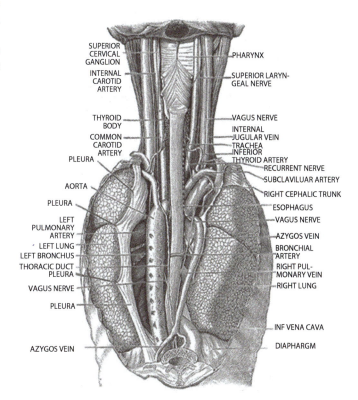

Figure 1.2 The position and relation of the oesophagus in the cervical region and in the posterior mediastinum. Seen from behind.
Reproduced from P. Poirier. and A. Charpy. (eds). *A Treatise of Human Anatomy*. Archibald Constable & Co.: Westminster, 1903.

the right side. The vagus nerve divides and covers the oesophagus in a plexus.[1]

From the bifurcation of the trachea downwards, the oesophagus passes behind the right pulmonary artery, left main bronchus, and left atrium. At this point it passes through the diaphragm.[1]

Sections of the oesophagus

The oesophagus is subdivided into the cervical, the thoracic, and the abdominal segments.

- *Pars cervicalis*: begins at the cricopharyngeus, runs ventral to the cervical spine, and terminates at the suprasternal notch behind the trachea.
- *Pars thoracica*: the longest part, runs in the superior mediastinum dorsal to the trachea, and becomes, after passing through the hiatus oesophagus of the diaphragm, the pars abdominalis.
- *Pars abdominalis*: which runs a short course of 1–3 cm in the gastric cardia. This segment descends and passes through the right crus of the diaphragm at the level of the tenth thoracic vertebra and into the cardia of the stomach at the 11th thoracic vertebra level.

Gastro-oesophageal junction

The gastro-oesophageal junction is between the oesophagus and the stomach.[2] The pink colour of the oesophageal mucosa contrasts with the deeper red of the gastric mucosa, and the mucosal transition can be seen as an irregular zig-zag line, which is called the z-line.[3-5] There is an abrupt transition histologically between the stratified squamous epithelium of the oesophagus and the simple columnar epithelium of the stomach.[6] Normally, the cardia of the stomach is immediately distal to the z-line and the z-line coincides with the upper limit of the gastric folds of the cardia.[7,8] The lower oesophageal sphincter is generally located about 3 cm below the z-line.[3]

Sphincters

The upper and lower oesophageal sphincters are zones with increased muscle tone, which close the oesophagus to the mouth and the stomach. These muscular rings are functional but not anatomical sphincters, meaning that they act as sphincters but do not have any specific sphincteric muscle.[9] The upper and lower oesophageal sphincters allow for the single-direction passage of food into the oesophagus and into the stomach.[10-12]

Upper oesophageal sphincter The upper oesophageal sphincter consists exclusively of striated skeletal muscle but is not under voluntary control. Its functional unit includes the caudal parts of the musculus constrictor pharyngis inferior, as well as parts of the upper oesophageal musculature. The sphincter is innervated by the glossopharyngeal nerve and the vagus nerve. This upper oesophageal occlusion provides a barrier to reflux and prevents aerophagia. Opening is triggered by the swallowing reflex.

Lower oesophageal sphincter The anatomical correlate of the lower oesophageal sphincter is the thickening and overlapping of the internal muscles of the oesophagus below the diaphragm at the junction between the oesophagus and the stomach.[13] Different mechanisms interfere with each other and form a functional unit that ultimately allows the occlusion of the oesophagus. Inadequate occlusion of the lower sphincter leads to reflux of gastric contents.

The following mechanisms form the functional closure unit of the lower sphincter:

- Wringing mechanism: the smooth muscles in the tunica muscularis spiral inward at the caudal end of the oesophagus.
- His angle and phrenico-oesophageal ligament: the oesophagus opens at a sharp angle into the cardia, which prevents a backflow of gastric juice.
- Effect of the diaphragm: the lower crura of the diaphragm help the sphincteric action.[9,14]
- Venous plexus: extensive venous plexus in the lamina propria mucosae and submucosa.

Constrictions of the oesophagus

Adjacent anatomical structures lead to three constrictions in the course of the oesophagus (Figure 1.3):

- *Constrictio cricoidea* (the cricoid constriction): where the laryngopharynx joins the oesophagus. Arises at the cricoid cartilage and is closed by the upper oesophageal sphincter.
- *Constrictio partis thoracicae*: arises from the proximity to the aortic arch and the left main bronchus.
- *Constrictio diaphragmatica*: arises through the hiatus oesophagus of the diaphragm in the posterior mediastinum.

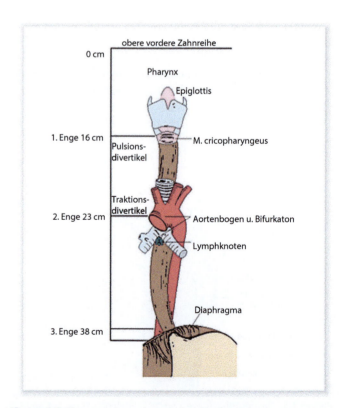

Figure 1.3 The oesophagus is constricted in three places.
Reproduced with permission from Reiche, Dagmar; Hoffmann-La-Roche-Aktiengesellschaft (Grenzach-Wyhlen), *Roche-Lexikon Medizin* 5e, Urban & Fischer, 2003.

Blood supply

The three sections of the oesophagus are supplied by different arteries.

- *Pars cervicalis*: from the inferior thyroid artery (from the truncus thyrocervicalis).
- *Pars thoracalis*: from the bronchial arteries and branches from the aorta and the intercostal arteries.
- *Pars abdominalis*: from the left gastric artery and the left inferior phrenic artery.[3,15]

The upper and middle parts of the oesophagus drain via the small oesophageal vessels into the azygos and hemiazygos veins into the superior vena cava.

The abdominal part of the oesophagus has a mixed venous drainage into the portal circulation via the left gastric vein and into the azygos vein.[3]

Lymphatics

The lymphatic vessels generally follow the course of the arteries. Correspondingly, lymphatic drainage takes place in different lymph node stations depending on the oesophageal section.

The pars cervicalis drains into the truncus jugularis via the deep cervical lymph nodes (nodi lymphatici (nll.) cervicales profundi).

The upper part of the thoracic oesophagus leads via the mediastinal lymph nodes (nll. paratracheales, nll. tracheobronchiales superiores et inferiores) into the truncus bronchomediastinalis, while the lower thoracic part and the pars abdominalis drain via the nll. gastrici sinistri et coeliaci into the left gastric and coeliac lymph nodes.

This leads into the cisterna chyli from which the lymph finally flows in the thoracic duct into the left subclavian vein.[3]

Innervation

Like other parts of the digestive system, the oesophagus is controlled by the autonomic enteric nervous system, modified by the sympathetic and parasympathetic nerves.

Sympathetic innervation occurs via postganglionic sympathetic fibres:

- The stellate ganglion.
- Thoracic ganglia II–V whose postganglionic fibres radiate into the plexus oesophagus.

Activation leads to inhibition of secretion of the oesophageal glands.

Parasympathetic innervation of the upper oesophagus runs via the recurrent laryngeal nerve; the lower part of the oesophagus is supplied by the vagus nerve. Below the tracheal bifurcation, the left and right vagal trunks unite to form the plexus oesophagus, from which the vagal trunks emerge further distally. Activation of the parasympathetic nervous system leads to an increase in gland secretion and peristalsis.

Sensory innervation Afferent fibres containing the viscerosensitive information on pain and strain run from the oesophagus via the nervus laryngeus recurrens and the nervus vagus.

Microanatomy

The wall of the oesophagus from the lumen outwards consists of the mucosa, submucosa, connective tissue, layers of muscle fibres between layers of fibrous tissue, and an outer layer of connective tissue (Figures 1.4 and 1.5). The mucosa is a stratified squamous epithelium of around three layers of squamous cells, which contrasts with the single layer of columnar cells of the stomach. The transition between these two types of epithelia is visible as a zig-zag line (Figure 1.6).

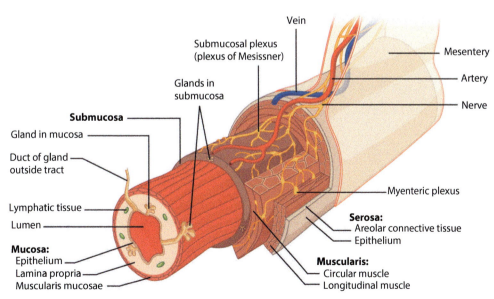

Figure 1.4 Layers of the alimentary canal.
OpenStax College, Rice University. Reproduced under a Creative Commons Attribution-Share Alike 4.0 Unported license (https://creativecommons.org/licenses/by/4.0/). Available at: https://cnx.org/contents/IPvBytyq@15/Overview-of-the-Digestive-System#fig-ch24_01_02

1 Anatomy and physiology

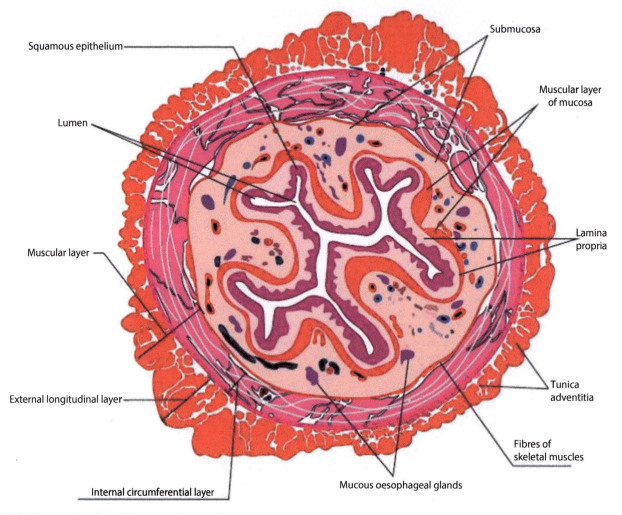

Figure 1.5 Cross-section through the oesophagus wall.
Reproduced with permission from Vasanthan, K.S., Srinivasan, V., Mathur, V. et al. 3D Bioprinting for esophageal tissue regeneration: A review. *Journal of Materials Research* 37, 88–113 (2022).

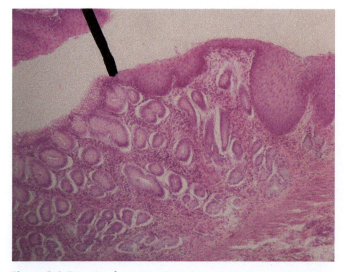

Figure 1.6 Transition from oesophageal to gastric mucosa: ora serrata.
Jpogi. Public domain. Available at: https://commons.wikimedia.org/wiki/File:Gastro-esophageal_jxn.JPG?uselang=de.

Tunica mucosa:

- *Lamina epithelialis mucosae*: the innermost layer consists of multi-layered non-keratinized stratified squamous epithelium.
- *Lamina propria mucosae*: loose connective tissue with an extensive venous plexus.
- *Lamina muscularis mucosae*: smooth muscle cells and submucosal Meissner's plexus.

Tela submucosa:

- *Mucous glandulae oesophageales*.
- *Plexus submucosus*.
- *Extensive venous plexus*.

Tunica muscularis:

- *Stratum longitudinale*: outer longitudinal muscle layer.
- *Stratum circulare*: inner circular muscle layer.

The proximal third of the oesophagus is primarily composed of skeletal muscle while the distal two-thirds are composed of smooth muscle. The muscle fibres of the oesophagus are bidirectional, with the external layer running longitudinally and the internal layer comprising circular fibres. The internal muscle layer allows for the peristaltic contractions that move boluses of food down the oesophagus and is thicker than the external layer. Between the ring and longitudinal muscles is a part of the enteric nervous system—the Auerbach plexus (myenteric plexus). This controls the motility and peristalsis of the oesophagus and the opening of the lower oesophageal sphincter.

Tunica adventitia:

- The outer connective tissue layer, which ensures the free movement of the oesophagus during swallowing. Includes:
  - The large supplying vessels.
  - Lymphatic vessels.
  - Nerve fibre bundles of the vagal trunks and the oesophageal plexus.

Function
Swallowing

The ingestion of food is made possible by a very elastic but well-fixed oesophagus by the surrounding tissue. The swallowing act is under both voluntary and involuntary control. When we swallow a food bolus, it touches the base of the tongue or the posterior pharyngeal wall and afferent fibres in the glossopharyngeal and vagus nerves cause the mechanical stimulus to the swallowing centre in the medulla oblongata. The upper oesophageal sphincter normally remains closed in a contracted position. During swallowing, the muscles relax temporarily and allow the passage of food into the oesophagus. The epiglottis tilts backwards to prevent food from going down the larynx and lungs. This process is adapted to the bolus properties. Thus, information about the smell, taste, texture, and size of the bolus is constantly forwarded to the brain. Through peristaltic movements of the oesophageal musculature the food is moved towards the stomach. The lower oesophageal sphincter is about 3 cm proximal to the stomach. Similar to the upper sphincter, the lower sphincter is normally contracted and prevents stomach contents from entering the oesophagus.

The lower oesophageal sphincter is controlled involuntarily and is triggered to open during oesophageal peristalsis.

Liquids lead to hardly any peristaltic movements of the oesophagus. The upper and lower oesophageal sphincters are opened briefly and the floor of the mouth and tongue push the fluid into the stomach.

Oesophageal peristalsis

Primary, swallow-induced oesophageal peristalsis refers to the contractile waves of the oesophageal musculature and secondary oesophageal peristalsis is created by the extension of the food bolus to the oesophageal wall.

The relaxation of the lower sphincter is a reflex action via the myenteric plexus. After food enters the cardia, the oesophageal sphincter closes again. The passage of a fixed bite lasts between 5 and 25 seconds.

The stomach

Anatomy
Macroanatomy

The stomach is located in the left upper abdomen in the epigastric region and in the left hypochondrium. While the position of most sections of the oesophagus is very variable, there are two consistent sections of the stomach: the gastric cardia, fixed by the lower oesophageal sphincter, and the pylorus, which passes into the retroperitoneum. Two sphincters keep the contents of the stomach contained: the lower oesophageal sphincter and the pyloric sphincter at the junction with the duodenum. In adults, the stomach has a relaxed, near-empty volume of about 75 mL.[16] Because it is a distensible organ, it normally expands to hold about 1 L of food with a maximum volume between 2 and 4 L.[3,15,17]

In addition, the stomach can be divided into four sections (Figure 1.7):

- *Pars cardiaca*: transition of the oesophagus into the stomach, which is closed by a functional sphincter.[13]

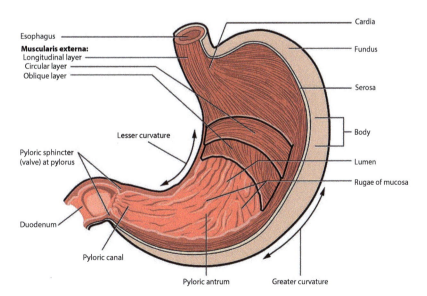

Figure 1.7 The anatomy of the stomach.
OpenStax College, Rice University. Reproduced under a Creative Commons Attribution-Share Alike 4.0 Unported license (https://creativecommons.org/licenses/by/4.0/). Available at: https://openstax.org/books/anatomy-and-physiology/pages/23-4-the-stomach

- *Fundus gastricus*: separated from the cardia by the incisura cardiaca.
- *Corpus gastricus*: main section of the stomach from fundus gastricus to pars pylorica.
- *Pars pylorica*: transition of the wide antrum into the narrow pyloric canal. This consists of a thick muscular ring and thus forms the sphincter pylori muscle as a border to the duodenum.

The external shape of the stomach is very variable and depends on various factors such as the state of filling, gastric motility, and physique.

Sphincters

There are two sphincters of the stomach, the *lower oesophageal sphincter* and the *pyloric sphincter* which control the passage of food.

Lower oesophageal sphincter After passing through the diaphragm via the oesophageal hiatus, the inferior oesophageal sphincter is at located at the level of the T11 vertebra. It allows food to pass through the cardiac orifice and into the stomach.

Pyloric sphincter The pyloric sphincter controls the exit of chyme from the stomach. In contrast to the inferior oesophageal sphincter it is an 'anatomical' sphincter.

Emptying of the stomach occurs intermittently when intragastric pressure overcomes the resistance of the pylorus. The pylorus is normally contracted so that the orifice is small and food can stay in the stomach for a suitable period. Gastric peristalsis pushes the chyme through the pyloric canal into the duodenum.

Greater and lesser omenta

The greater omentum is a duplication of the peritoneum, rich in fatty tissue, which arises during embryonic development through the fusion of the two leaves of the dorsal mesogastrium. It hangs like an apron down the intestines from the greater curvature of the stomach and is attached to the transverse colon. It may adhere to inflamed areas, therefore playing a key role in limiting the spread of intraperitoneal infection.

Furthermore, the following ligaments are part of the greater omentum:

- *Ligamentum gastrophrenicum*: between large curvature of the stomach and underside of the diaphragm.
- *Ligamentum gastrosplenicum*: between stomach and spleen, contains the splenic artery with the gastric artery breves.
- *Ligamentum gastrocolicum*: between great curvature and colon transversum, contains the arteriae gastroomentales dextra et sinistra.

The lesser omentum arises at the lesser curvature and ascends to the liver. It can be divided into the ligamentum hepatogastricum and the ligamentum hepatoduodenale, which contains the portal triad. The main function of the lesser omentum is to attach the stomach and duodenum to the liver.

Blood supply

The coeliac trunk, the first unpaired branch of the abdominal aorta, provides the main arterial blood supply for the stomach (**Figure 1.8**). It usually delivers three arteries: the common hepatic artery, the left gastric artery, and the splenic artery. The left gastric artery forms a vascular arcade at the lesser curve of the stomach (curvatura minor) through the anastomosis with the right gastric artery from the proper hepatic artery, which originates from the common hepatic artery. At the greater curve, anastomoses of the arteria gastroomentalis dextra from the gastroduodenal artery (originating from the common hepatic artery) and the arteria gastroomentalis sinistra from the splenic artery forming another vascular arcade. Furthermore, the splenic artery supplies the gastric fundus via the arteriae gastricae breves as well as the posterior wall of the stomach via the posterior gastric artery.

The veins of the stomach run parallel to the arteries and drain into the portal vein, whereby the venae gastricae dextra et sinistra flow directly into the portal vein, while the left gastro-omental vein drains via the splenic vein and the right gastro-omental vein via the superior mesenteric vein.

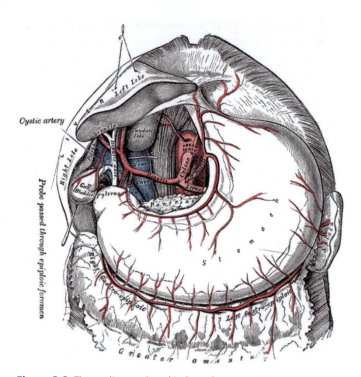

Figure 1.8 The coeliac trunk and its branches.
Reproduced from Gray, Henry. *Anatomy of the Human Body*. Philadelphia: Lea & Febiger, 1918; Public domain. Available at: https://commons.wikimedia.org/wiki/File:Gray532.png

Lymphatics

The outflow of lymph happens via lymph node stations along the supplying arteries. Their size varies greatly between individuals.

Lymph in the area of the lesser curvature is channelled via lymph nodes that lie along the lesser curvature of the cardia. The draining lymph vessels run along the left gastric artery to the nodi lymphatici coeliaci. The lymph along the gastro-omental vessels flows into the spleen lymph nodes, the nll. pylorici and the nll. coeliaci. From the nll. coeliaci the lymph flows further into the intestinal tract and from there into the cisterna chyli and the thoracic duct, which opens into the left vein angle.

In addition, there are connections to the para-aortic, mesenteric, and mediastinal lymph node stations as well as to those of the liver, the pancreas, and the small intestine.

Areas of the stomach which drain into regional lymph nodes:

- *Cardia and proximal lesser curvature* drain into the left gastric lymph nodes, then into coeliac nodes.
- *Pylorus and distal lesser curvature* drain into the right gastric lymph nodes.
- *Proximal part of the greater curvature* drains into the pancreatico-splenic nodes in the splenic hilum.
- *Distal part of greater curvature* drains into the right gastroepiploic nodes and the pyloric nodes at the head of the pancreas.

The following classification has been established from a surgical point of view (Figure 1.9):

- *D1*: regional lymph nodes including the perigastric along the lesser curvature and the proximal and distal greater curvature, the right and left pericardiac, and the supra- and infrapyloric lymph nodes.
- *D2*: regional lymph nodes along the coeliac trunk, the left gastric artery, the common hepatic artery and the hepatoduodenal ligament, the splenic artery, and the splenic hilum.
- *D3*: extra-regional lymph nodes, for example, posterior to the duodenum and pancreas head, mesocolic, and para-aortic lymph nodes.

Innervation

The stomach receives innervation from the autonomic nervous system:

- *The parasympathetic nerve supply* arises from the anterior and posterior vagal trunks, derived from the vagus nerve.
- *The sympathetic nerve supply* arises from the spinal cord segments T6–T9 and passes to the coeliac plexus via the greater splanchnic nerve. It also carries some pain transmitting fibres.

Microanatomy

In the stomach we find the typical structure of the entire gastrointestinal tract (Figures 1.10 and 1.11):

- Tunica mucosa.
- Tela submucosa.
- Tunica muscularis.
- Tunica serosa.

The *tunica mucosa* consists of the:

- *Lamina epithelialis* with a single-layered high-prismatic epithelium (columnar epithelium), which is sharply delineated at the ora serrata (z-line) against the stratified squamous epithelium of the oesophagus.
- *Lamina propria*, composed of loose connective tissue, with a thin layer of smooth muscle.
- *Muscularis mucosae*, separating it from the submucosa.

The *submucosa* consists of fibrous connective tissue and contains Meissner's plexus.

While the *tunica muscularis* in the remaining intestine consists of a stratum longitudinale and a stratum circulare, in the stomach a third innermost muscle layer of oblique fibres, the fibrae obliquae, is present which aids in performance of complex

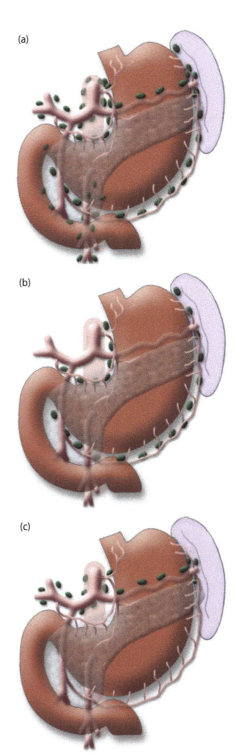

Figure 1.9 (a) All gastric lymph node stations, (b) D1 level, and (c) D2 level.
Reproduced with permission from MySurgery e-learning. Available at: https://www.mysurgery.de/viszeralchirurgie/oberer-gi-trakt/magen-ca/

motions. The Auerbach's plexus is found between the outer longitudinal and the middle circular layer and is responsible for the motor innervation.

The stomach is also covered by a *serosa*, consisting of layers of connective tissue continuous with the peritoneum.

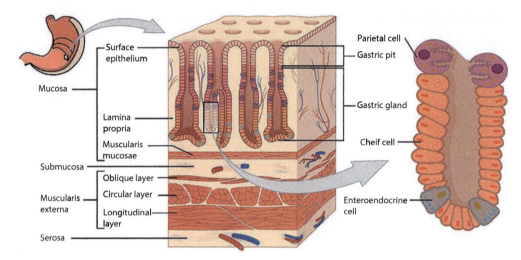

Figure 1.10 The microanatomy of the gastric wall.
OpenStax College, Rice University. Reproduced under a Creative Commons Attribution-Share Alike 4.0 Unported license (https://creativecommons.org/licenses/by/4.0/). Available at: https://openstax.org/books/anatomy-and-physiology-2e/pages/23-4-the-stomach

Gastric glands

At the stomach entrance the wide-lobed, branched glandulae cardiales are located, which produce mucus. The glandulae pyloricae of the pars pylorica also produce mucus. In addition, there are gastrin-producing G cells, which stimulate the parietal cells. The largest part of the mucous membrane is occupied by the gastricae propriae glands, which are in the fundus and corpus. They consist of the following cells:

- *Chief cells*: secrete pepsin, a proteolytic enzyme.
- *Parietal cells*: secrete hydrochloric acid and intrinsic factor (necessary for vitamin B_{12} absorption in the terminal ileum).[8]
- *Mucous cells*: secrete an alkaline mucus that protects the epithelium against shear stress and acid.
- *G cells*: secrete the hormone gastrin.[18]

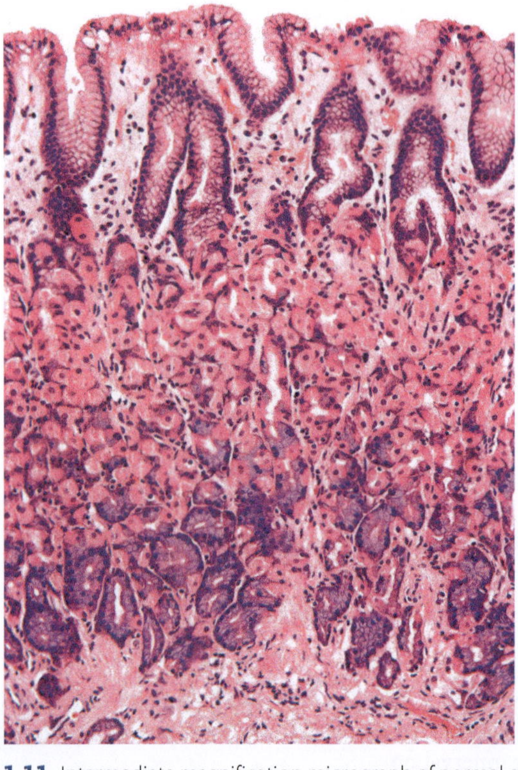

Function

The stomach has a reservoir function and starts the partial chemical digestion of food. The cardia, body, and fundus relax as food enters and the lower stomach contracts rhythmically to support digestion by mixing it with stomach juices. Contractions every 15–20 seconds carry small quantities of liquefied chyme to the pyloric sphincter and allow transfer into the duodenum.

Digestion already begun in the oral cavity is continued here with the gastric digestive enzymes. The inactive precursor *pepsinogen* is activated by contact with gastric acid to pepsin, which splits protein compounds and thus contributes to the pre-digestion of the proteins. Pepsinogen is produced by the chief cells and hydrochloric acid by the parietal cells of the fundus. The *parietal cells* also produce intrinsic factor, that allows for the absorption of vitamin B_{12} (cobalamin) later in the small intestine. Even though the essential function of the stomach is the preparation of the chyme for the further digestive process, liquid and various substances such as some water-soluble vitamins or ethanol and caffeine are absorbed here.[19,20] In addition, the stomach acts as an immunological barrier through the acidic environment that is lethal to many types of bacteria and other microorganisms.[12,21–23]

Digestive hormones regulate the gastric digestive process. *Gastrin* is produced in G cells of the gastric antrum and in the duodenal mucosa. It stimulates acid production by parietal cells and pepsinogen production by chief cells, strengthens contraction waves in the antrum, and increases cardiac sphincter tone.

Cholecystokinin is produced by enteroendocrine cells in the duodenum, jejunum, and upper ileum. It causes satiety, and attenuates

Figure 1.11 Intermediate magnification micrograph of normal gastric mucosa (i.e. inner most layer of the stomach).
Nefron. Reproduced under a Creative Commons Attribution-Share Alike 3.0 Unported license (https://creativecommons.org/licenses/by-sa/3.0/deed.en). Available at: https://commons.wikimedia.org/wiki/File:Normal_gastric_mucosa_intermed_mag.jpg

the postprandial increase in blood sugar levels by affecting gastric emptying through a direct endocrine effect.

The release of *secretin* from duodenal cells is stimulated by pH values below 4.5; it increases bicarbonate secretion in the pancreas, gall bladder, and small intestine, inhibits gastrin secretion in the stomach, increases mucin production in the stomach, and stimulates the secretion of somatostatin and insulin.

Glucagon is released when blood sugar levels drop, leading to glycogenolysis, gluconeogenesis of amino acids and activation of lipases. Glucagon-like peptides promote satiety, slow down gastric emptying, and stimulate intestinal growth.

REFERENCES

1. Drake RL, Vogl W, Mitchell AWM. *Gray's Anatomy for Students*. 1st ed. Tibbitts RM, Richardson P, illustrators. Philadelphia, PA: Elsevier/Churchill Livingstone; 2005:192–194.
2. Dirckx JH, ed. (1997). *Stedman's Concise Medical and Allied Health Dictionary*. 3rd ed. Baltimore, MD: Williams and Wilkins; 1997.
3. Kuo B, Urma D. Esophagus—anatomy and development. In: Goyal RK, Shaker R, eds. *Goyal and Shaker's GI Motility Online*. Nature Publishing Group; 2006. https://www.nature.com/gimo/contents/pt1/full/gimo6.html
4. DiMarino A Jr, Benjamin SB, eds. *Gastrointestinal Disease: An Endoscopic Approach*. 2nd ed. Thorofare, NJ: Slack; 2002.
5. Gore RM, Levine MS, eds. *High-Yield Imaging*. 1st ed. Philadelphia, PA: Saunders/Elsevier; 2010.
6. Moore KL, Agur AMR. *Essential Clinical Anatomy*. 2nd ed. Baltimore, MD: Lippincott Williams & Wilkins; 2002.
7. Barrett KE. Esophageal motility. In: *Gastrointestinal Physiology*. 2nd ed. New York: McGraw Hill; 2014:130–146.
8. Long RG, Scott BB, eds. Upper gastrointestinal disease Philadelphia, PA. In: Specialist Training in: Gastroenterology and Liver Disease. Elsevier Mosby, 2005; 14–58.
9. Mu L, Wang J, Su H, Sanders I. Adult human upper esophageal sphincter contains specialized muscle fibers expressing unusual myosin heavy chain isoforms. *J Histochem Cytochem*. 2007;55:199–207.
10. Goizueta AA, Bordoni B. *Anatomy, Thorax, Lung Pleura and Mediastinum*. Treasure Island, FL: StatPearls Publishing; 2019.
11. Bardo DME, Biyyam DR, Patel MC, Wong K, van Tassel D, Robison RK. Magnetic resonance imaging of the pediatric mediastinum. *Pediatr Radiol*. 2018;48:1209–1222.
12. Ilahi M, Ilahi TB. *Anatomy, Thorax, Thoracic Duct*. Treasure Island, FL: StatPearls Publishing; 2018.
13. Hall AC, Guyton JE. Secretory Functions of the Alimentary Tract In: *Textbook of Medical Physiology*. 11th ed. Philadelphia. Saunders/Elsevier. 2005;776–777.
14. Mittal K. Neuromuscular anatomy of esophagus and lower esophageal sphincter. In: *Motor Function of the Pharynx, Esophagus, and its Sphincters*. Morgan & Claypool Life Sciences; 2011. https://www.ncbi.nlm.nih.gov/books/NBK54283/
15. Patti MG, Gantert W, Way LW. Surgery of the esophagus. Anatomy and physiology. *Surg Clin North Am*. 1997;77:959–970.
16. Palmer KR, Penman ID. Alimentary tract and pancreatic disease. In: *Davidson's Principles and Practice of Medicine*. 21st ed. Colledge NR, Walker BR, Ralston SH, eds. 2010; 838–844.
17. Drake RL, Vogl W, Mitchell AWM. *Gray's Anatomy for Students*. 2nd ed. Tibbitts RM, Richardson P, illustrators. Philadelphia, PA: Elsevier/Churchill Livingstone; 2009.
18. Ross M, Pawlina W. Digestive System II: Esophagus and Gastrointestinal Tract. In: *Histology: A Text and Atlas. 6th ed*. Baltimore, MD. Lippincott Williams & Wilkins. 2011;583.
19. Albert D. *Dorland's Illustrated Medical Dictionary*. 32nd ed. Philadelphia, PA: Saunders/Elsevier; 2012.
20. Purves D. *Neuroscience*. 5th ed. Sunderland, MA: Sinauer; 2011.
21. Fischer NJ, Morreau J, Sugunesegran R, Taghavi K, Mirjalili SA. A reappraisal of pediatric thoracic surface anatomy. *Clin Anat*. 2017;30:788–794.
22. Bradley PJ. Symptoms and signs, staging and co-morbidity of hypopharyngeal cancer. *Adv Otorhinolaryngol*. 2019;83:15–26.
23. Sanghi V, Thota PN. Barrett's esophagus: novel strategies for screening and surveillance. *Ther Adv Chronic Dis*. 2019;10:2040622319837851.

2

Diagnostic tests and principal investigations
Endoscopy, manometry and contrast studies

Yuki B. Werner

Endoscopy

Diagnostic upper endoscopy is a routine procedure and usually the first study in diagnostic evaluation when abdominal symptoms appear, for prevention of progress and for clarification of imaging and laboratory findings. It allows a direct visual examination of the mucosa and tissue sampling in areas of interest. Endoscopic ultrasound (EUS) can image the deeper tissue layers of the oesophagus and stomach, and evaluate submucosal lesions, perioesophageal structures, and lymph nodes; in addition, using an EUS-guided fine-needle aspiration leads to a higher diagnostic yield. The main symptoms which indicate a diagnostic upper endoscopy are dysphagia, heartburn, regurgitation, epigastric or retrosternal pain, dyspepsia, melaena, a family history of cancer, and anaemia (Figure 2.1).

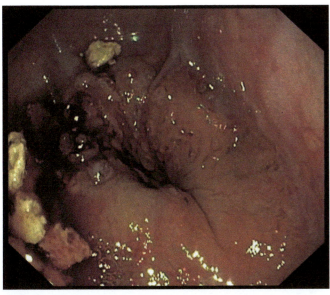

Figure 2.1 Diagnostic endoscopy in a 47-year-old man with a short history of dysphagia. Tissue samples confirmed a distal oesophageal squamous cell carcinoma.

In a routine endoscopic procedure, anatomical landmarks include the site of the upper oesophageal sphincter, the proximal and distal oesophagus, the squamocolumnar junction (or Z-line), the oesophagogastric junction (OGJ) or upper end of the gastric folds, and the diaphragmatic indentation during evaluation of the entire oesophagus. The most important anatomical landmarks when evaluating the stomach are the cardia and fundus in a retroflexed view, angulus (incisura), antrum, pylorus, and thereafter the superior duodenal angle, major papilla, and the duodenum. When reporting a gastric abnormality, its localization in relation to the four walls of the stomach (lesser or greater curvature, superior or posterior wall) should also be included. Accurate photo documentation of all normal anatomical landmarks and all abnormal findings mentioned in the report is recommended.[1]

Patients with dysphagia caused by structural or motility oesophageal abnormalities are at higher risk for aspiration and for iatrogenic perforation during endoscopy. Scoping without a clear view of the correct lumen also increases the risk of perforation. Therefore, the gastroscope should be inserted with caution in patients with a suspected Zenker's diverticulum, where the intubation of the oesophageal lumen may be difficult, or in patients with suspected proximal oesophageal strictures. A distal transparent attachment cap placed on the end of the endoscope facilitates the view by maintaining a constant distance between endoscope and mucosa or a switch to a paediatric gastroscope with a smaller diameter may be useful.

Classification

Several validated and clinically relevant classification systems for benign oesophageal diseases have been developed and are in use, including the Paris classification for superficial neoplastic lesions in the gastrointestinal tract,[2,3] the tumour, node, and metastasis (TNM) classification in general,[4] and the Siewert classification system for adenocarcinoma at the OGJ.[5]

A detailed morphological description of any visible superficial neoplastic lesion in the oesophagus and stomach should be a part of the standardized endoscopic terminology and is provided by the Paris classification.[2,3] Neoplastic superficial lesions in the oesophagus and stomach are limited to the mucosa and defined as type 0, therefore the Paris classification is more often used for the evaluation of an endoscopic resection. The superficial morphology (type 0) can be divided into polypoid (type 0-I) and non-polypoid (type 0-IIa–c and type 0-III) types. Type 0-II (a: flat and elevated; b: completely flat; c: superficially depressed) tumours are predominately found in the oesophagus and stomach. Type 0-III (excavated form) tumours are rare but more frequently found in the oesophageal part of the gastrointestinal tract. The endoscopic resectability in lesions of type 0-III (excavated form) remains difficult as there is a higher risk of deep infiltration and lymph node metastases in these and a surgical procedure as the alternative primary approach has to be considered.

The Siewert classification system[5] describes topographically three subtypes of adenocarcinomas of the OGJ (AOG types I–III) depending on the localization of the tumour's epicentre while the oesophageal versus gastric extent entails different surgical strategies, and provides a practical overview. A tumour with its epicentre 1–5 cm above the OGT is classified as AOG type I (e.g. a distal oesophageal adenocarcinoma, Barrett's carcinoma). Its distal margin may also extent into the OGJ. AOG type II arises from the gastric cardiac epithelium with its epicentre within 1 cm above and 2 cm below the OGJ, while tumours with epicentres located 2–5 cm below the OGJ are classified as AOG type III. Endoscopically, the upper and lower border measurements of the tumour margin, its epicentre, and the localization of the OGJ are described as their distance from the incisors. The latest TNM classification[4] has incorporated the tumour's epicentre location and stages Siewert AOG types I/II as oesophageal cancers while AOG type III is staged as a gastric cancer.

Erosive reflux oesophagitis is endoscopically classified into four grades (A–D) by the Los Angeles (LA) group describing the appearance of erosive lesions and mucosal breaks in the distal oesophagus[6] (Table 2.1). The LA classification is well established since its introduction in 1996 due to its ease of use and minor interobserver variability assessment. Recently, the evidence-based Lyon consensus related to gastro-oesophageal reflux disease (GORD) considered high-grade oesophagitis (LA grade C/D) as confirmatory evidence for chronic GORD.[7] Milder forms of endoscopic reflux oesophagitis (LA grade A/B) provide adequate evidence for initiating medical treatment.

The Prague C&M classification has been regarded as the standard for measuring the length of Barrett's oesophagus.[8] The length of the columnar epithelium in the oesophagus is measured by its circumferential (C) and maximal (M) extent from the OGJ (the upper end of the gastric folds) and any separate island proximal to the maximal extent. Of note is that the maximal extent describes the longest Barrett's segment. The C&M classification is clinically relevant especially as long-segment Barrett's oesophagus (≥3 cm) has an increased risk of dysplasia compared to short-segment (≥1 to <3 cm) or ultrashort-segment (<1 cm) Barrett's oesophagus. A study of 1017 patients with newly diagnosed T1 oesophageal carcinoma evaluated the annual cancer transition rates for patients with long, short, and ultrashort Barrett's oesophagus, as 0.22%, 0.03%, and 0.01%, respectively.[9] Different endoscopic surveillance strategies are recommended based on the extent of Barrett's oesophagus.

Oesophageal varices can be classified into three different grades (I–III) by the Paquet classification with higher grades indicating an increased risk of bleeding.[10] Grade I varices extend just above the mucosal level and are completely compressed by air insufflation while grade III varices extend for more than 50% of the luminal diameter or touch each other. The appearance of red wale marks or cherry spots on the surface of a varix are further risk signs for an increased risk of bleeding, independent of its grade, and prophylactic endoscopic treatment is therefore indicated.

The Forrest classification is a widely used classification system for ulcer-related upper gastrointestinal bleeding introduced in 1974 to estimate the risk of persistent bleeding, re-bleeding, and mortality.[11,12] It differentiates between acute haemorrhage (Forrest Ia or Ib), signs of recent haemorrhage (Forrest IIa–c), and lesions without active bleeding (Forrest III) in non-variceal upper gastrointestinal bleeding (Table 2.2). Patients with Forrest Ia or Ib lesions and those with signs of recent bleeding (Forrest IIa–c) showed a tenfold greater risk of recurrence of haemorrhage than those with a clean ulcer base.[12]

Table 2.1 Los Angeles classification of erosive oesophagitis

Grade	Endoscopic characterization
A	One or more mucosal breaks of 5 mm in length or less
B	One or more mucosal breaks of longer than 5 mm
C	Mucosal breaks that extend between two or more mucosal folds (but involve <75% of the circumference of the oesophagus)
D	Mucosal breaks that involve ≥75% of the luminal circumference

Adapted with permission from Armstrong D, Bennett JR, Blum AL, et al. The endoscopic assessment of esophagitis: a progress report on observer agreement. *Gastroenterology*. 1996;111:85–92.

Table 2.2 Forrest classification of non-variceal upper gastrointestinal bleeding

Classification	Endoscopic characterization
Acute haemorrhage	
Ia	Active spurter
Ib	Active oozing
Signs of recent haemorrhage	
IIa	Non-bleeding visible vessel
IIb	Adherent clot
IIc	Flat pigmented spot
No sign of recent or active bleeding	
III	Clean-based ulcer

Source: data from Forrest JA, Finlayson N, Shearman DJ. Endoscopy in gastrointestinal bleeding. *Lancet*. 1974;2:394–397; and Guglielmi, A, Ruzzenente, A, Sandri, M, et al. Risk assessment and prediction of rebleeding in bleeding gastroduodenal ulcer. *Endoscopy*. 2002;34:778–786.

Chromoendoscopy

Further development of high-definition scopes and virtual chromoendoscopy techniques as technical imaging systems (e.g. narrow-band imaging, multiband imaging or Fujinon Intelligent Chromo Endoscopy (FICE), and i-scan imaging) are continuously improving the visualization and detection of mucosal irregularities. For example, virtual chromoendoscopy is routinely applied for screening and surveillance in Barrett's oesophagus.[13] The narrow-band imaging filter system easily detects gastric intestinal metaplasia which is sharply demarcated from the normal gastric mucosa.[14] Currently, the application of machine learning techniques is a focus of research interest and a promising tool to be used in the future, especially in the diagnosis and surveillance of Barrett's oesophagitis.[15] In real-time chromoendoscopy, the topical application of stains directly onto the mucosal surface enhances the tissue pattern or contrast and improves the evaluation of irregularities, dysplasia, or early cancer. Lugol's solution and acetic acid are widely used in the oesophagus and stomach.[16,17] A 1% Lugol's solution contains an iodine component which immediately reacts with glycogen present in normal squamous oesophageal mucosa. After spraying Lugol's solution onto the oesophageal surface under visual control, the normal mucosa stains dark brown. Suspected areas, such as inflammatory or dysplastic lesions, do not stain as they lack glycogen and appear yellowish (Figure 2.2). Targeted tissue samplings of unstained lesions are easily taken. Therefore, Lugol's solution is used in the oesophagus for the detection of squamous cell cancer and its precursors in addition to imaging systems and it is also used to visualize the lateral margins of a lesion to determine its extent (e.g. for planning endoscopic resection).

Acetic acid chromoendoscopy is based on the initial whitening reaction when dilute acetic acid (1.5% solution) is applied to the mucosal surface. Acetic acid leads to a reversible denaturation of intracellular proteins resulting in a contrast enhancement of the mucosal surface and different mucosal pit patterns can be well described. This effect lasts only 2 or 3 minutes. Especially in Barrett's oesophagus, but also in gastric lesions, acetic acid improves the detection of mucosal irregularities and dysplasia. A further improvement for detecting irregularities occurs if magnification endoscopy is also used.

Tissue sampling

Multiple endoscopic tissue samples should be taken for a specific diagnosis of mucosal changes or inflammatory areas, irregularities, ulcers, and tumours. Furthermore, validated systematic endoscopic biopsy protocols improve the benefit of surveillance programmes, such as in patients with Barrett's oesophagus or atrophic gastritis.

The differential diagnosis of eosinophilic oesophagitis in a medical work-up for dysphagia has to be clarified by two to four biopsies each from the proximal and the distal oesophagus even if the mucosa appears normal[18] (Figure 2.3). The distal oesophageal biopsies must be accompanied by proximal biopsies to exclude a reflux oesophagitis as a cause of intraepithelial eosinophilia. Native biopsy samples in suspected infectious or uncertain oesophagitis should be taken additional for viral polymerase chain reaction techniques that are more sensitive than histopathology alone.

The Seattle protocol is recommended and the current gold standard for tissue sampling in Barrett's oesophagus includes obtaining biopsies from lesions and four-quadrant biopsies at intervals of every 1–2 cm throughout the columnar-lined oesophagus separately.[19] These systematic biopsies improve the detection rates of dysplasia and early neoplasia in Barrett's oesophagus.[20]

The diagnostic yield of random biopsies to evaluate for *Helicobacter pylori*-associated gastritis and gastric intestinal metaplasia increases following the Sydney protocol,[21,22] where biopsies from the greater and lesser curvature in the antrum, and biopsies from the greater and lesser curvature in the corpus are taken separately. Biopsies from the incisura angularis can be included in the surveillance endoscopy of patients with atrophic gastritis. The Sydney protocol is recommended in several current guidelines for precancerous conditions.[23,24]

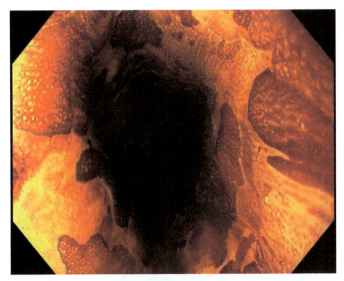

Figure 2.2 Chromoendoscopy with Lugol's solution for the evaluation of oesophageal squamous cell lesions. Notable areas have reduced or absent iodine staining (yellowish instead of brown appearance). In this case, tissue samplings should follow.

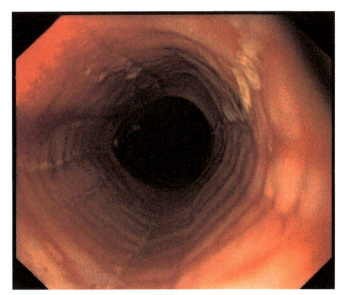

Figure 2.3 An example of eosinophilic oesophagitis with circular rings, linear furrows, and whitish exudates in the oesophagus (not to be confused with reflux oesophagitis!).

Endoscopic resection techniques, such as endoscopic mucosal resection and endoscopic submucosal dissection, are mainly used for treatment but they can also provide more detailed diagnostic information or be used as staging tools.[25] The introduction of the peroral endoscopic myotomy technique into clinical practice[26] has allowed safe endoscopic access to the submucosal space, creating more diagnostic and therapeutic possibilities.[27]

Endoscopic ultrasound

EUS is used for imaging the deeper tissue layers of the oesophagus and stomach and for evaluating lymph nodes and other surrounding structures. Its diagnostic accuracy can be improved by the addition of fine-needle aspiration. There are two types of EUS scope systems. The radial scan scope with a 360° view gives an improved overview of the gastrointestinal tract wall and its adjacent structures; it is often used for staging of oesophageal cancer or evaluating submucosal or mediastinal tumours and its image is similar to that of a computed tomography scan. The curved linear array endoscope with a limited view has the advantage of passing a needle through a working channel for performing fine-needle aspiration under direct visualization.

EUS is recommended in current guidelines for patients with oesophageal cancer,[28,29] but the accuracy of EUS is operator dependent. Correct T-staging by an expert endoscopist was observed in 34 out of 37 patients (91.9%) in contrast to correct T-staging by a non-expert endoscopist in 26 out of 36 patients (72.2%; $p = 0.035$).[30]

Diagnosis of functional gut disorders

Major functional disorders of the oesophagus are confirmed by the assessment of its function including high-resolution manometry (HRM), long-term oesophageal pH measurement with multichannel intraluminal impedance monitoring, and measurement of the distensibility (endoluminal functional lumen imaging probe (EndoFLIP)). The findings help in predicting the response to therapy in some diseases.

Oesophageal manometry

Dysphagia and non-cardiac chest pain with negative endoscopic results are the commonest symptoms suggestive of a motility disorder. The gold standard to diagnose oesophageal motility disorders is HRM. In addition, patients with refractory reflux symptoms—especially before antireflux surgery—should pass through a manometric examination to exclude major motility disorders of the oesophagus. The HRM catheter consists of 36 pressure transducers each 1 cm apart. Therefore, pressure and peristaltic conditions can be measured simultaneously along the entire length of the oesophagus. This procedure is superior to conventional manometry regarding the achievement of the correct diagnosis and its technical practicability.[31] In a randomized trial of 245 patients with dysphagia, who underwent HRM ($n = 123$) or conventional manometry ($n = 122$), Roman et al.[31] found that achalasia was significantly more often diagnosed by HRM than by conventional manometry (26% vs 12%; $p <0.01$). After insertion of a HRM catheter through the nose into the stomach, a standard protocol is performed consisting of ten swallows of 5 mL of water in the supine position. Each swallow is analysed regarding the morphology and relaxation response at the OGJ and the contractile pattern in the body of the oesophagus. The OGJ is determined by the lower oesophageal sphincter and the crural diaphragm and the presence of a hiatal hernia can be easily detected by HRM. The integrated relaxation pressure is an essential diagnostic metric that evaluates the relaxation response of the OGJ. The integrated relaxation pressure represents the mean of the lowest pressure that can be measured within a period of 4 seconds after initiating the swallow. The manometric pattern of an intact swallow is shown in Figure 2.4. The peristaltic nature of

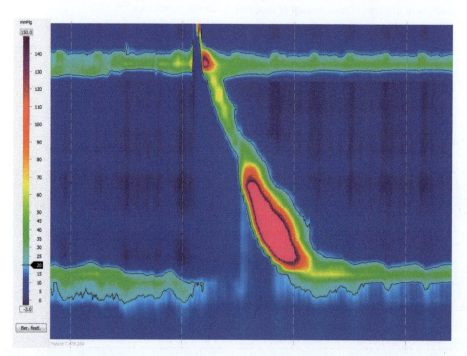

Figure 2.4 A regular, normal swallow evaluated by HRM. Note the relaxation phase (blue) at the OGJ directly following the initial swallow and the propulsive peristaltic wave within the oesophageal body.

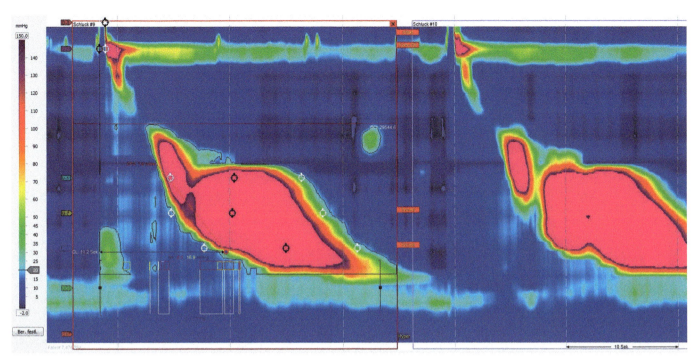

Figure 2.5 Two hypercontractile swallows evaluated by HRM. The distal contractile integral is greater than 29,000 mmHg/s/cm in both swallows, integrated relaxation pressure is normal (<15 mmHg).

the contractions in the tubular oesophagus may be lost and replaced by failed, weak, or abnormal contractions. Premature contractions as associated in distal oesophageal spasm and type III achalasia are evaluated by the distal contractile latency. The distal contractile integral (DCI) is a parameter describing the vigour of the contraction. Roman et al.[32] reviewed 72 healthy volunteers and 2000 consecutive HRM studies. They identified 40 patients out of the 2000 studies with normal contractile propagation and normal distal contractile latency but with an extreme phenotype of hypercontractility defined by the occurrence of at least a single contraction with DCI greater than 8000 mmHg/s/cm, usually accompanied with dysphagia. This was in contrast to the control group where the highest value of DCI was 7732 mmHg/s/cm. An example is shown in Figure 2.5. Based on the standard swallow protocol, major and minor oesophageal motor disorders are classified by the Chicago Classification scheme (Table 2.3).[33] Additionally, manometric examination can predict the therapeutic response in some diseases. Pandolfino et al.[34] studied 99 patients with newly diagnosed achalasia. They showed that therapeutic response was most successful in patients with type II achalasia (83%, vs 44% in type I and 9% in type III achalasia). These results were confirmed by a post hoc analysis of the data from the European Achalasia Trial in 2011.[35] Figure 2.6 shows a manometric example of achalasia type II. Further improvements of swallow protocols, such as additional multiple swallow testing or solid test meal, increase the diagnostic yield of HRM.[36,37] Wang et al.[36] prospectively evaluated 57 symptomatic and 12 asymptomatic patients following antireflux surgery with standard swallow protocol plus multiple swallow testing and a solid test meal. Clinically relevant findings were seen with the solid test meal in 33 of 57 symptomatic patients (58%) in contrast to 11 of 57 symptomatic patients (19%) with the standard swallow protocol (p <0.001), whereas findings were unremarkable in the asymptomatic control.

Combined oesophageal pH and multichannel intraluminal impedance monitoring

Combined oesophageal pH/impedance monitoring detects reflux events due to pH measurements and bolus movements within

Table 2.3 Chicago Classification of oesophageal motility disorders by HRM

Classification	HRM characterization
Major disorders	
Achalasia subtype I	IRP >15 mmHg, 100% failed peristalsis
Achalasia subtype II	IRP >15 mmHg, panoesophageal pressurization with ≥20% of swallows
Achalasia subtype III	IRP >15 mmHg, premature spastic contractions with ≥20% of swallows
OGJ outflow obstruction	IRP >15 mmHg, evidence of peristalsis
Hypercontractile oesophagus, jackhammer oesophagus	≥2 swallows with DCI >8000 mmHg/s/cm
Distal oesophageal spasm	IRP normal, premature spastic contractions with ≥20% of swallows
Absent contractility	IRP normal, 100% failed peristalsis
Minor disorders	
Ineffective oesophageal motility	≥50% of ineffective swallows
Fragmented peristalsis	≥50% fragmented contractions with DCI >450 mmHg/s/cm
Normal motility	Not fulfilling any of the above classifications

IRP, integrated relaxation pressure.
Adapted with permission from Kahrilas PJ, Breedenoord AJ, Fox M, et al. The Chicago classification of esophageal motility disorders, v3.0. *Neurogastroenterol Motil*. 2015;27:160–174.

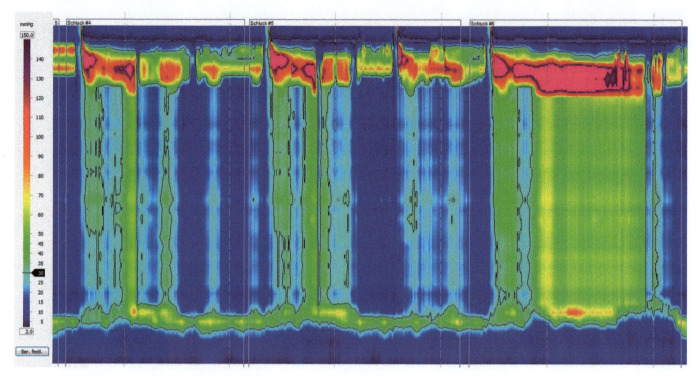

Figure 2.6 Achalasia subtype II according to the Chicago Classification. The HRM detected an impaired integrated relaxation pressure of 28 mmHg and showed oesophageal pressurization in more than 20% of all swallows.

the oesophageal lumen. Guidelines recommend combined 24-hour pH/impedance monitoring on proton pump inhibitor (PPI) therapy over pH monitoring alone to diagnose persisting GORD in adults with typical oesophageal reflux symptoms and previous confirmatory evidence of GORD and in patients with inconclusive evidence of GORD on PPI therapy.[7,38] The pH/impedance catheter is positioned with the oesophageal pH sensor 5 cm proximal to the lower oesophageal sphincter, ideally identified using HRM. The catheter also contains multiple (commonly six to eight) segmental ring electrodes for impedance measurements in varied intervals spanning the length of the oesophagus. The catheter is placed transnasally and connected to a mobile recorder. As for oesophageal pH monitoring alone, the acid exposure time (AET) is the primary outcome of the recording (Figure 2.7). The AET is calculated as the percentage of time the pH is less than 4 at the distal oesophageal pH sensor within 24 hours. A severe acid exposure (AET >6%) confirms the diagnosis of GORD. The existence of GORD is also confirmed by borderline values (AET between 4% and 6%) that are supported by a pathological increased number of reflux episodes on impedance monitoring (>80 episodes per 24 hours) or by additional HRM data (detected hiatal hernia or ineffective oesophageal motility).[7] Patel et al.[39] showed that an abnormal AET predicts symptom improvement from antireflux therapy including surgery when prospectively followed up in $n = 187$ patients undergoing pH/impedance monitoring off PPI therapy. pH/impedance monitoring on PPI therapy allows selection of a group of patients who might improve from surgical antireflux therapy as recently shown in a randomized controlled trial.[40] In that trial, the selected patients were identified by the detection of an abnormal acid reflux and/or a positive symptom association probability despite omeprazole intake, 20 mg twice daily. The symptom association probability evaluates the association between heartburn (assessed by the patient) and reflux episodes (acid, non-acid, or all by impedance monitoring) using complex statistical analysis.[41] It is positive when the symptom association probability value is greater than 95%, indicating a significant observed association. Symptom reports during the recording are further considered by the symptom index. The symptom index is the percentage of symptom events that are related to the reflux episodes. The symptom index is assumed as positive when the value is 50% or greater. These indices have been validated but their use is limited.[42] Non-GORD diseases, such as reflux hypersensitivity or functional heartburn, are based on their results in patients monitored off PPI therapy by pH/impedance. Reflux hypersensitivity is defined as a positive reflux–symptom association in patients with normal AET and/or normal number of reflux episodes. Patients with reflux symptoms but without objective evidence are diagnosed as having functional heartburn. In patients with a persistent cough suspected to be due to GORD, pH/impedance monitoring assists in selecting patients who may improve from antireflux surgery Johnson et al.[42] performed pH/impedance monitoring in 50 patients on acid suppressive therapy (PPI twice daily with/without nocturnal histamine-2 receptor antagonist), evaluating the association between cough and non-acid reflux episodes. In six of 13 symptom index-positive patients, a laparoscopic Nissen fundoplication was performed with a treatment success rate in five out of six patients (83%) after a median follow-up of 17 months.

The advantage of combined pH/impedance monitoring over oesophageal pH monitoring alone is the detection of non-acid reflux episodes causing complaints and its informative value in patients on PPI therapy. Oesophageal pH monitoring is still preferred to

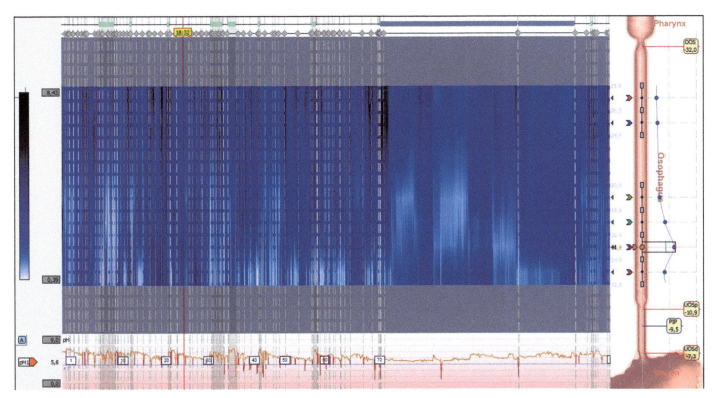

Figure 2.7 An example of combined intraluminal impedance monitoring and pH monitoring that detected a non-erosive reflux disease. Results show a normal AET (2.4%) but 118 reflux episodes within 24 hours. The symptom association probability was positive (98%).

quantify GORD in straightforward cases regarding clinical practicability and costs. Traditionally, the DeMeester score is used to categorize patients for GORD (yes/no) and has been considered to be the gold standard test. This score is composed of six metrics including the total AET.[42] However, the clinical utility of composite scores has not yet been clearly demonstrated.[43,44]

Wireless pH monitoring via a telemetry capsule has been validated as an alternative to catheter-based monitoring systems. Pandolfino et al. showed a successful recording of the oesophageal acid exposure over 24 hours in 82 (96%) of 41 patients with GORD and 44 healthy subjects.[45] It provides a tolerable method for patients in whom catheter-based pH monitoring has previously failed due to intolerance and discomfort to assist the definite diagnosis of GORD in this group.[46]

Endoluminal functional imaging

The functional lumen imaging probe (FLIP) allows assessment of the distensibility of the lower oesophageal sphincter, the oesophageal lumen, and the gastric pylorus.[47] The ratio of the area across the inside and the intraluminal pressure, which are simultaneously measured between 17 electrodes, is calculated and represents the distensibility or compliance. The distensibility index is a main metric. This technique is promising and may complement results by HRM, but further studies are needed to determine its use in clinical practice.[48] One potential advantage is its feasibility during real-time diagnostic endoscopy or therapeutical procedures. Figure 2.8 shows an example of measurement before peroral endoscopic myotomy.

Contrast studies

Fluoroscopic contrast studies still have clinical importance regarding the diagnosis and prognosis of oesophageal diseases. Barium studies of the oesophagus are performed to evaluate morphology and function, providing better contrast images. Contrast-enhanced studies in patients with a suspected or possible oesophageal perforation (e.g. following interventional procedures) have to be performed using water-soluble agents.

Several modifications to the protocol of the barium swallow oesophagogram are available. It can simply provide information in patients with dysphagia and/or regurgitation with a normal endoscopy. Typically, a small Zenker's diverticulum or epiphrenic or traction oesophageal diverticula are detected, or a narrowing of the oesophagus or signs of an external compression may be seen (Figure 2.9). In contrast to HRM, fluoroscopic assessment is inferior as a screening examination for the detection of oesophageal dysmotility.[49] The timed barium oesophagogram (TBE) provides validated information about oesophageal emptying and anatomical configuration in patients with suspected or diagnosed achalasia. An example is shown in Figure 2.10. Patients ingest a low-density barium sulphate suspension to the amount they could tolerate without regurgitation or aspiration (100–250 mL). The oesophageal emptying is assessed in an upright, slightly left posterior oblique position. Radiographs are taken at 1, 2, and 5 minutes after barium intake. The height and width of the barium column are measured and compared on 1- and 5-minute films. The barium height is measured as the distance from the distal oesophagus to the top of the distinct barium column.[50] A barium height greater than 2 cm

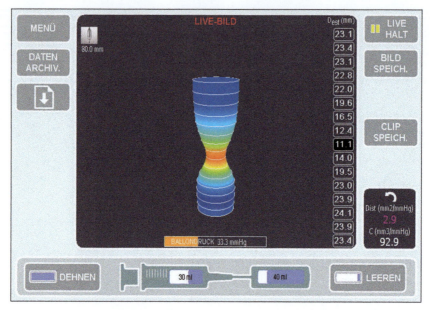

Figure 2.8 Impaired distensibility of the distal oesophageal sphincter is measured by a FLIP in a patient with achalasia type II before peroral endoscopic myotomy. The distensibility index is 2.9 mm²/mmHg at the narrowest diameter (11.1 mm), the intraluminal pressure is 33.3 mmHg.

at 5 minutes may be used as a cut-off point for identifying an achalasia. A sensitivity of 85% and a specificity of 86% has been shown for this value in 117 patients with untreated achalasia compared to patients with OGJ outflow obstruction or no-achalasia dysphagia.[51] In a study of 41 patients with a long-standing and asymptomatic achalasia, 26 had oesophageal stasis greater than 5 cm on TBE and seven patients had an elevated lower oesophageal sphincter pressure on oesophageal manometry (>10 mmHg) at baseline. During a follow-up of 10 years, 25 out of 41 patients were regarded as therapeutic failures. Of these 25 recurrent patients, 22 (88%) initially had oesophageal stasis in comparison to five (20%) with an elevated pressure at baseline. In contrast to an elevated lower oesophageal sphincter pressure, an oesophageal stasis greater than 5 cm in TBE is a more reliable predictor for achalasia recurrence in patients with long-standing achalasia.[52]

Solid boluses (e.g. a barium tablet (13 mm) or toast dipped into barium paste) can add more information regarding radiological evaluation, especially in patients with non-achalasia dysphagia.[49,51,53] Out of 132 (32%) patients with non-achalasia dysphagia, 42 showed normal TBE results for liquid barium but retained a 13 mm barium

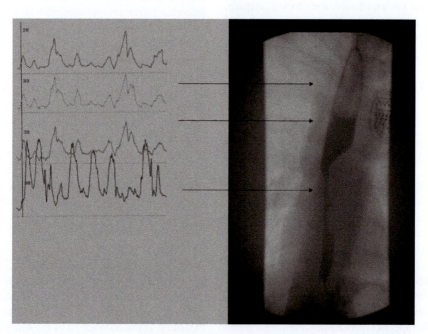

Figure 2.9 An example of a barium swallow in a patient with dysphagia caused by a rapidly developing tumour compression. An upper endoscopy was unremarkable 3 months previously.

Contrast studies

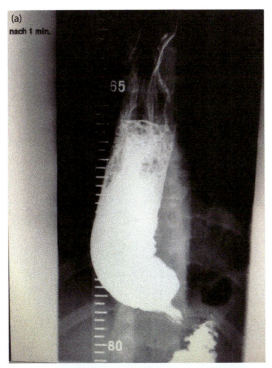

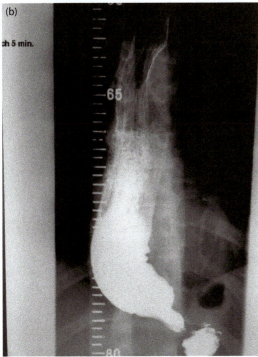

Figure 2.10 TBE performed in a symptomatic patient with achalasia treated by balloon dilation 2 years previously. At 5 minutes after ingestion of barium suspension (b) the barium column's height was marginally lower than at 1 minute (a).

tablet in the oesophagus.[51] Marked contractions of the oesophagus in the barium studies reveal a corkscrew appearance suggestive of the presence of a diffuse oesophageal spasm or a hypercontractile oesophagus (Figure 2.11).

International guidelines recommend to perform a barium swallow in patients suspected to have a hiatal hernia or a short oesophagus

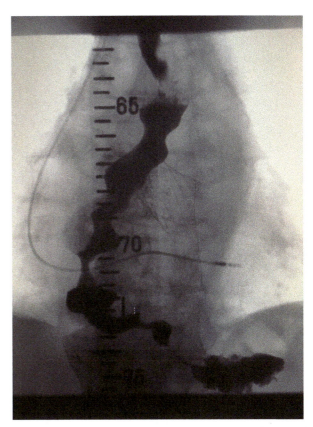

Figure 2.11 A patient with dysphagia caused by a spastic disorder of the oesophagus. Typically, a corkscrew oesophagus can be seen in a barium swallow.

prior to antireflux surgery.[54,55] Patients ingest barium in the prone right anterior oblique position. When the patient is upright, small sliding hiatal hernias are often reduced. In contrast, large hiatal hernias that persist in the upright position may indicate a fixed longitudinal oesophageal shortening. Less frequently, barium studies may reveal paraoesophageal hernias.[56]

REFERENCES

1. Bisschops R, Area M, Coron E, et al. Performance measures for upper gastrointestinal endoscopy: a European Society of Gastrointestinal Endoscopy (ESGE) quality improvement initiative. *Endoscopy*. 2016;**48**:843–864.
2. Participants in the Paris workshop. The Paris endoscopic classification of superficial neoplastic lesions: esophagus, stomach, and colon. *Gastrointest Endosc*. 2003;**58**(Suppl 6):S3–S43.
3. Endoscopic Classification Review Group. Update on the Paris classification of superficial neoplastic lesions in the digestive tract. *Endoscopy*. 2005;**37**:570–578.
4. Rice TW, Patil DT, Blackstone EH. 8th edition AJCC/UICC staging of cancers of the esophagus and esophagogastric junction: application to clinical practice. *Ann Cardiothorac Surg*. 2017;**6**:119–130.
5. Siewert JR, Hölscher AH, Becker K, Gössner W. Cardia cancer: attempt at a therapeutically relevant classification. *Chirurg*. 1987;**58**:25–32.

6. Armstrong D, Bennett JR, Blum AL, et al. The endoscopic assessment of esophagitis: a progress report on observer agreement. *Gastroenterology*. 1996;**111**:85–92.
7. Gyawali CP, Kahrilas PJ, Savarino E, et al. Modern diagnosis of GERD: the Lyon consensus. *Gut*. 2018;**67**:1351–1362.
8. Sharma P, Dent J, Armstrong D, et al. The development and validation of an endoscopic grading system for Barrett's esophagus: the Prague C & M criteria. *Gastroenterology*. 2006;**131**:1392–1399.
9. Pohl H, Pech O, Arash H, et al. Length of Barrett's oesophagus and cancer risk: implications from a large sample of patients with early oesophageal adenocarcinoma. *Gut*. 2016;**65**:196–201.
10. Paquet KJ. Prophylactic endoscopic sclerosing treatment of the esophageal wall in varices—a prospective controlled randomized trial. *Endoscopy*. 1982;**14**:4–5.
11. Forrest JA, Finlayson N, Shearman DJ. Endoscopy in gastrointestinal bleeding. *Lancet*. 1974;**2**:394–397.
12. Guglielmi A, Ruzzenente A, Sandri M, et al. Risk assessment and prediction of rebleeding in bleeding gastroduodenal ulcer. *Endoscopy*. 2002;**34**:778–786.
13. Kara MA, Bergman JJ. Autofluorescence imaging and narrow-band imaging for the detection of early neoplasia in patients with Barrett's esophagus. *Endoscopy*. 2006;**48**:627–631.
14. Pimentel-Nunes P, Libanio D, Lage J, et al. A multicenter prospective study of the real-time use of narrow-band imaging in the diagnosis of premalignant gastric conditions and lesions *Endoscopy*. 2016;**48**:723–730.
15. de Groof AJ, Struyvenberg MR, van der Putten J, et al. Deep-learning system detects neoplasia in patients with Barrett's esophagus with higher accuracy than endoscopists in a multi-step training and validation study with benchmarking. *Gastroenterology*. 2020;**158**:915–929.
16. Sugimachi K, Kitamura K, Baba K, et al. Endoscopic diagnosis of early carcinoma of the esophagus using Lugol's solution. *Gastrointes Endosc*. 1992;**38**:657–661.
17. Guelrud M, Herrera I, Essenfeld H, Castro J. Enhanced magnification endoscopy: a new technique to identify specialized intestinal metaplasia in Barrett's esophagus. *Gastrointest Endosc*. 2001;**53**:559–565.
18. Nielsen JA, Lager DJ, Lewin M, Rendon G, Roberts CA. The optimal number of biopsy fragments to establish a morphologic diagnosis of eosinophilic esophagitis. *Am J Gastroenterol*. 2014;**109**:515–520.
19. Levine DS, Blount PL, Rudolph RE, Reid BJ. Safety of a systematic biopsy protocol in patients with Barrett's esophagus. *Am J Gastroenterol*. 2000;**95**:1152–1157.
20. Abrams JA, Kapel RC, Lindberg GM, et al. Adherence to biopsy guidelines for Barrett's esophagus surveillance in the community setting in the United States. *Clin Gastroenterol Hepatol*. 2009;**7**:736–742.
21. Dixon MF, Genta RM, Yardley JH, Correa P. Classification and grading of gastritis: the updated Sydney system. *Am J Surg Pathol*. 1996;**20**:1161–1181.
22. Lash JG, Genta RM. Adherence to the Sydney System guidelines increases the detection of Helicobacter gastritis and intestinal metaplasia in 400 738 sets of gastric biopsies. *Aliment Pharmacol Ther*. 2013;**38**:424–431.
23. Pimentel-Nunes P, Libânio D, Marcos-Pinto R, et al. Management of epithelial precancerous conditions and lesions in the stomach (MAPS II). *Endoscopy*. 2019;**51**:365–388.
24. Banks M, Graham D, Jansen M, et al. British Society of Gastroenterology guidelines on the diagnosis and management of patients at risk for gastric adenocarcinoma. *Gut*. 2019;**68**:1545–1575.
25. Mino-Kenudson M, Hull MJ, Brown I, et al. EMR for Barrett's esophagus-related superficial neoplasms offer better diagnostic reproducibility than mucosal biopsy. *Gastrointest Endosc*. 2007;**66**:660–666.
26. Inoue H, Minami H, Kobayashi Y, et al. Peroral endoscopic myotomy (POEM) for esophageal achalasia. *Endoscopy*. 2010;**42**:265–271.
27. Inoue H, Ikeda H, Hosoya T. Submucosal endoscopic tumor resection (SET) for subepithelial tumors in the esophagus and cardia. *Endoscopy*. 2012;**44**:225–230.
28. Porsche R, Fischbach W, Gockel I, et al. S3-Leitlinie Diagnostik und Therapie der Plattenepithelkarzinome und Adenokarzinome des Ösophagus. *Z Gastroenterol*. 2019;**57**:336–418.
29. Dumonceau JM, Deprez PH, Jenssen C, et al. Indications, results, and clinical impact of endoscopic ultrasound (EUS)-guided sampling in gastroenterology: European Society of Gastrointestinal Endoscopy (ESGE) clinical guideline—updated January 2017. *Endoscopy*. 2017;**49**:695–714.
30. Lee WC, Lee TH, Jang JY, et al. Staging accuracy of endoscopic ultrasound performed by nonexpert endosonographers in patients with resectable esophageal squamous cell carcinoma: is it possible? *Dis Esophagus*. 2015;**28**:574–578.
31. Roman S, Huot L, Zerbib F, et al. High-resolution manometry improves the diagnosis of esophageal motility disorders in patients with dysphagia: a randomized multicenter study. *Am J Gastroenterol*. 2016;**111**:372–380.
32. Roman S, Pandolfino JE, Chen J, Boris L, Luger D, Kahrilas PJ. Phenotypes and clinical context of hypercontractility in high-resolution esophageal pressure topography (EPT). *Am J Gastroenterol*. 2012;**107**:37–45.
33. Kahrilas PJ, Breedenoord AJ, Fox M, et al. The Chicago classification of esophageal motility disorders, v3.0. *Neurogastroenterol Motil*. 2015;**27**:160–174.
34. Pandolfino JE, Kwiatek MA, Nealis T, Bulsiewicz W, Post J, Kahrilas PJ. Achalasia: a new clinically relevant classification by high-resolution manometry. *Gastroenterology*. 2008;**135**:1526–1533.
35. Rohof WO, Salvador R, Annese V, et al. Outcomes of treatment for achalasia depend on manometric subtype. *Gastroenterology*. 2013;**144**:718–725.
36. Wang YT, Tai LF, Yazaki E, et al. Investigation of dysphagia after antireflux surgery by high-resolution manometry: impact of multiple water swallows and a solid test meal on diagnosis, management, and clinical outcome. *Clin Gastroenterol Hepatol*. 2015;**13**:1575–1583.
37. Ang D, Misselwitz B, Hollenstein M, et al. Diagnostic yield of high-resolution manometry with a solid test meal for clinically relevant, symptomatic oesophageal motility disorders: serial diagnostic study. *Lancet Gastroenterol Hepatol*. 2017;**2**:654–661.
38. Gyawali CP, Carlson DA, Chen JW, Patel A, Wong RJ, Yadlapati RH. ACG clinical guidelines: clinical use of esophageal physiologic testing. *Am J Gastroenterol*. 2020;**115**:1412–1428.
39. Patel A, Sayuk GS, Gyawali CP. Parameters on esophageal pH–impedance monitoring that predict outcomes of patients with gastroesophageal reflux disease. *Clin Gastroenterol Hepatol*. 2015;**13**:884–891.
40. Spechler SJ, Hunter JG, Jones KM, et al. Randomized trial of medical versus surgical treatment for refractory heartburn. *N Engl J Med*. 2019;**381**:1513–1523.

41. Taghavi SA, Ghasedi M, Saberi-Firoozi M, et al. Symptom association probability and symptom sensitivity index: preferable but still suboptimal predictors of response to high dose omeprazole. *Gut*. 2005;**54**:1067–1071.
42. Johnson LF, DeMeester TR. Development of the 24-hour intraoesophageal pH monitoring composite scoring system. *J Clin Gastroenterol*. 1986;**8**(Suppl):52–68.
43. Roman S, Gyawali CP, Savarino E, et al. Ambulatory reflux monitoring for diagnosis of gastro-esophageal reflux disease: update of the Porto consensus and recommendations from an international consensus group. *Neurogastroenterol Motil*. 2017;**29**:1–15.
44. Neto RML, Herbella FAM, Schlottmann F, Patti MG. Does DeMeester score still define GERD? *Dis Esophagus*. 2019;**32**:doy118.
45. Pandolfino JE, Richter JE, Ours T, Guardino JM, Chapman J, Kahrilas PJ. Ambulatory esophageal pH monitoring using a wireless system. *Am J Gastroenterol*. 2003;**98**:740–749.
46. Sweis R, Fox M, Anggiansah R, et al. Patient acceptance and clinical impact of Bravo monitoring in patients with previous failed catheter-based studies. *Aliment Pharmacol Ther*. 2009;**29**:669–676.
47. Kwiatek MA, Pandolfino JE, Hirano I, Kahrilas PJ. Esophagogastric junction distensibility assessed with an endoscopic functional luminal imaging probe (EndoFlip). *Gastrointest Endosco*. 2010;**72**:272–278.
48. Desprez C, Roman S, Leroi AM, Gourcerol G. The use of impedance planimetry (Endoscopic Functional Lumen Imaging Probe, EndoFlip) in the gastrointestinal tract. A systematic review. *Neurogastroenterol Motil*. 2020;**32**:e13980.
49. O'Rourke AK, Lazar A, Castell DO, Martin-Harris B. Utility of esophagogram versus high-resolution manometry in the detection of esophageal dysmotility. *Otolaryngol Head Neck Surg*. 2016;**154**:888–891.
50. de Olivereira JM, Birgisson S, Doinoff C, et al. Timed barium swallow: a simple technique for evaluating esophageal emptying in patients with achalasia. *AJR Am J Roentgenol*. 1997;**169**:473–479.
51. Blonski W, Kumar A, Feldman J, Richter JE. Timed barium swallow: diagnostic role and predictive value in untreated achalasia, esophagogastric junction outflow obstruction, and non-achalasia dysphagia. *Am J Gastroenterol*. 2018;**113**:196–203.
52. Rohof WO, Lei A, Boeckxstaens GE. Esophageal stasis on a timed barium esophagogram predicts recurrent symptoms on patients with long-standing achalasia. *Am J Gastroenterol*. 2013;**108**:49–55.
53. Van Westen D, Ekberg O. Solid bolus swallowing in the radiologic evaluation of dysphagia. *Acta Radiol*. 1993;**34**:372–375.
54. Pauwels A, Boecxstaens V, Andrews CN, et al. How to select patients for antireflux surgery? The ICARUS guidelines (international consensus regarding preoperative examinations and clinical characteristics assessment to select adult patients for antireflux surgery). *Gut*. 2019;**68**:1928–1941.
55. Jobe BA, Richter JE, Hoppo T, et al. Preoperative diagnostic workup before antireflux surgery: an evidence and experience-based consensus of the esophageal diagnostic advisory panel. *J Am Coll Surg*. 2013;**217**:586–597.
56. Levine MS, Carucci LR, DiSanits DJ, et al. Consensus statement of society of abdominal radiology disease-focused panel on barium esophagography in gastroesophageal reflux disease. *AJR Am J Roentgenol*. 2016;**207**:1009–1015.

3

Motility disorders of the oesophagus

Michaela Müller, Stefan Niebisch, and Ines Gockel

Introduction

Innervation of the oesophagus

The motor innervation of the oesophagus is provided by the vagus nerve via the myenteric plexus (or Meissner plexus) as shown in **Figure 3.1**.

The nerve supply differs significantly in the proximal and the distal oesophagus. The striated musculature in the upper third is innervated by somatic efferent fibres of the vagus nerve, which arises from the nucleus ambiguus and terminates in the motor end-plates, as illustrated in **Figure 3.2**.[1,2] By contrast, the striated musculature of the lower third of the oesophagus is innervated by vagal preganglionic fibres, whose cell bodies are located within the dorsal nucleus of the vagus nerve.[3] Preganglionic fibres initially innervate the myenteric plexus via their cholinergic branches. The oesophageal wall and the lower oesophageal sphincter (LOS) are successively supplied by postganglionic neurons, which also consist of excitatory and inhibitory neurons. Excitatory activity of the neurons stimulates contraction of the smooth muscle cells (comparable to closure of the LOS), which is, again, cholinergic (i.e. acetylcholine mediated). Inhibitory activity, controlled by the messenger substances nitric oxide (NO) and vasoactive intestinal polypeptide, causes the LOS to relax and open.[4,5]

Classification of oesophageal motility disorders

Motility disorders of the oesophagus comprise a group characterized by malfunction of the swallowing act.[6] Overall, these are rare diseases, the aetiopathogenesis of which is often unclear. Oesophageal manometry represents the gold standard to diagnose motility disorders of the oesophagus which have been defined in the Chicago

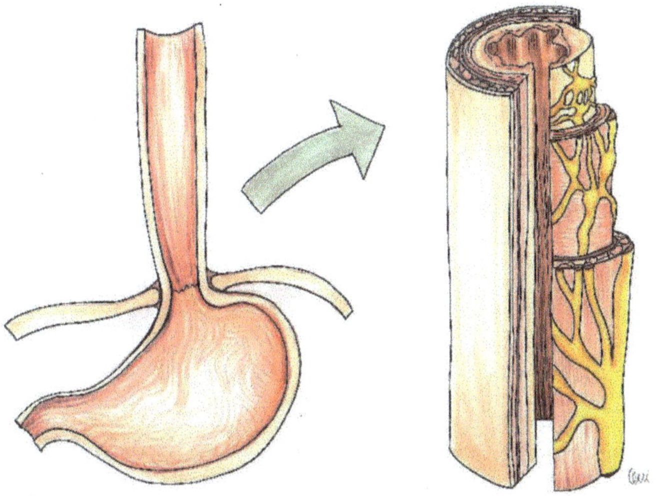

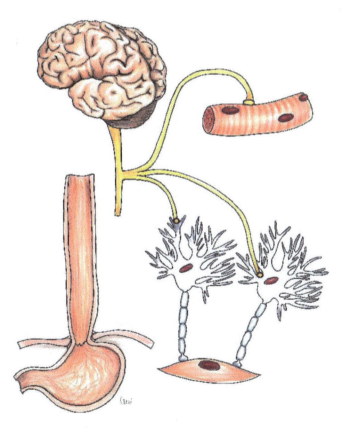

Figure 3.2 The striated musculature in the upper third of the oesophagus is innervated by somatic efferent fibres of the vagus nerve which arises from the nucleus ambiguous and binds to cholinergic receptors at the motor end-plate.

Figure 3.1 Motor innervation of the oesophagus is provided by the vagus nerve via the myenteric plexus or the Meissner plexus.

3 Motility disorders of the oesophagus

Table 3.1 Diseases associated with secondary motility disorders of the oesophagus

Organic oesophageal disorders	Corrosive disorders of the oesophagus Eosinophilic oesophagitis Gastro-oesophageal reflux disease Oesophageal diverticula Radiation injuries
Neuromuscular disorders	Diseases of the central nervous system (e.g. multiple sclerosis, stroke, Parkinson's disease) Diseases of the peripheral nervous system Muscular diseases (e.g. myasthenia gravis, inclusion body myositis, muscular dystrophy)
Collagenoses	Lupus erythematosus Mixed connective tissue disease (Sharp's syndrome) Polymyositis, dermatomyositis Sjögren's syndrome Systemic sclerosis
Metabolic disorders	Diabetes mellitus Hyper- or hypothyreosis

Classification since the introduction of high-resolution impedance manometry (HRIM).[7,8]

The most recent update of the Chicago Classification, version 4.0, characterizes in addition to achalasia—currently most distinguished and most relevant functional disorder of the oesophagus in gastroenterology and surgery—oesophagogastric junction (OGJ) outflow obstruction and disorders of the peristalsis such as distal oesophageal spasm (DOS), hypercontractile oesophagus (jackhammer), ineffective oesophageal motility, and absent contractility.[9]

This classification is relevant as a guide to therapy and surgical procedures. As illustrated in Table 3.1, in principle, a distinction is made between primary and secondary motility disorders, the latter being associated with other underlying diseases.[10] In addition to the cardinal symptoms of dysphagia and retrosternal cramps/pain, regurgitation with associated aspiration and pulmonary symptoms as well as weight loss have been described. Odynophagia (painful swallowing) and heartburn are frequent accompanying symptoms. Diagnosis is usually made by oesophageal manometry, although endoscopy and radiology are essential for the exclusion of inflammatory or neoplastic changes.

A specific therapy for primary functional disturbances that is based on aetiology does not exist and all therapeutic approaches therefore serve to alleviate the symptoms and to improve the patient's quality of life. New treatment concepts for achalasia have been developed in the recent past.

Conditions leading to secondary motility disorders are very heterogeneous and include—in addition to organic disorders of the oesophagus—collagenoses, as well as neuromuscular and metabolic disorders. The therapy for these disorders focuses on the treatment of the underlying disease.

Achalasia

Definition and aetiopathogenesis

The term achalasia derives from the Greek (αχαλασία = lack of relaxation) and was coined by Sir Arthur Hurst in 1927.[11] Achalasia is a functional disorder of the smooth muscle segment of the oesophagus. It is characterized by an absent or insufficient swallow-induced LOS relaxation, as well as by a lack of propulsive peristalsis of the tubular oesophagus. Achalasia represents a neurodegenerative oesophageal disorder whose aetiology and pathogenesis are still largely unknown. The permanent spasm of the LOS is due to malfunction or the complete loss of inhibitory nerve cells of the myenteric plexus with predominance of excitatory innervation.[12] Recent investigations have suggested that an initial insult, such as a viral infection (varicella zoster, measles, or human papillomavirus) may cause inflammation of the myenteric plexus (Auerbach's plexus). In genetically predisposed individuals, this results in the formation of anti-myenteric antibodies, which cause the destruction or (irreversible) function loss of the oesophageal nerve cells, which leads to the development of achalasia.[13–15] The extremely high frequency of simultaneous autoimmune disorders in patients with achalasia emphasizes the autoimmune genesis of the disease. *Chagas disease* is an infectious and parasitic disorder caused by *Trypanosoma cruzii*, which occurs predominantly in South America and closely resembles the phenotype of achalasia. A monogenetic cause which, however, affects less than 1% of all achalasia patients is the Allgrove syndrome (synonym: *triple A syndrome*). This is an autosomal recessive disorder characterized by achalasia, alacrima, as well as by (generally adrenocorticotropic hormone-resistant) adrenal insufficiency and neurological abnormalities. Mutations have recently been identified in the triple A syndrome gene (*AAAS*), a type II keratin gene with a locus on chromosome 12q13, which encodes the ALADIN protein.[16]

Epidemiology

Idiopathic achalasia is a rare disorder with an incidence of approximately 2–3:100,000 and occurs at the same frequency in both men and women. A lifetime prevalence of 10–15:100,000 has been indicated. It may manifest at any age, although it is generally diagnosed between 25 and 60 years of age.[17,18]

Clinical symptoms

The clinical picture of achalasia is very heterogeneous due to the slowly progressing development of the disorder. The most prominent clinical symptoms are dysphagia and regurgitation. Swallowing difficulties are initially manifest for solid food and later also for liquids, and may lead to significant weight loss. Patients report their quality of life as being adversely affected due to the presence of retrosternal pain and cramps, caused by uncoordinated contractions of the oesophagus and concomitant hypertension of the LOS. Clinical practice has shown the Eckardt score described in Table 3.2 to be practical and pragmatic in the evaluation of symptom

Table 3.2 Eckardt score for the clinical evaluation of achalasia severity

Symptoms	None	Occasional/weekly	Daily	At each meal
Dysphagia	0	1	2	3
Regurgitation	0	1	2	3
Chest pain	0	1	2	3
Weight loss (recent)	None = 0	<5 kg = 1	5–10 kg = 2	>10 kg = 3

Adapted with permission from Eckardt VF, Aignherr C, Bernhard G. Predictors of outcome in patients with achalasia treated by pneumatic dilation. *Gastroenterology*. 1992;103(6):1732–1738.

severity not only at the time of the initial diagnosis, but also in the course after therapy. The intensity of the four cardinal symptoms ranging from 0 (= no symptoms) to 3 (= most pronounced) can thus be both rated and summed up. The Eckardt score can thus range from a minimum of 0 points (= no symptoms) to a maximum of 12 points (most pronounced), depending on the intensity of the individual symptoms.[19]

Possible complications include recurrent aspiration pneumonia and carcinomatous degeneration which may develop in patients over the long term. Gastric stasis of food and lactic acid fermentation processes are frequent causes of subjective reflux, which has to be differentiated from gastro-oesophageal reflux disease and does not respond to acid-blocking medications.[20]

Diagnosis

In establishing the correct diagnosis, endoscopy and barium swallow are useful in only 33% and 66% of patients, respectively.[21] Endoscopy of the upper gastrointestinal tract is nevertheless essential in establishing the primary diagnosis, in particular with a view to the exclusion of a malignant process. The X-ray barium swallow may show a 'bird's beak' sign or a 'champagne flute'-shaped configuration of the gastro-oesophageal junction (Figure 3.3). The timed barium swallow is useful in obtaining initial functional information on oesophageal clearance or the speed of oesophageal emptying. However, a sensitivity of 98% renders HRIM clearly superior to endoscopic and radiological diagnostics with regard to the relaxation pattern of the LOS.[22] This technique is currently viewed as the gold standard in the diagnosis of achalasia, as well as in the differential diagnosis of other oesophageal functional disorders. Further differential diagnoses include both hypercontractile and hypocontractile oesophageal motility disorders. On the basis of HRIM, the Chicago Classification differentiates between three types of achalasia: type I, with complete aperistalsis of the tubular oesophagus; type II, with panoesophageal compressions; and type III, with spastic oesophageal contractions, as illustrated in Figure 3.4.[9]

The division into the described subtypes is of assistance both in making a prognostic assessment and in developing a treatment plan. Patients with type II achalasia are associated with the most favourable treatment success rates, while patients with type III achalasia have the poorest outcomes, independent of the therapy. Patients with type II achalasia generally respond favourably to pneumatic dilation (PD) and surgery, while surgical or peroral endoscopic myotomy (POEM) constitutes a better therapy option in patients with type III achalasia, since the spastic contractions affect the entire oesophagus in these patients.[23]

Therapy

The first description of a therapy for achalasia by means of oesophageal dilatation using a whalebone was published by Sir Thomas Willis as early as 1874. Currently available therapeutic options are aimed at both an improvement in the passage of food via the gastro-oesophageal junction and the prevention of progression to megaoesophagus. The three main approaches to the therapy of achalasia today include (1) *oral medication* (smooth muscle relaxation by calcium antagonists, nitrates, or phosphodiesterase inhibitors); (2) *endoscopic* botulinum toxin (BoTox) injection into the LOS, PD, and POEM; and (3) *surgery* (Heller's cardiomyotomy is generally carried out laparoscopically (LHM) and increasingly also with the DaVinci robot (RHM))—an open approach is rarely used today (e.g. in cases of recurrent achalasia requiring revision surgery). Subtotal esophagectomy with gastric pull-up is indicated in end-stage achalasia with advanced megaoesophagus (>6 cm in diameter), sigma-shaped configuration of the oesophagus, and the failure of less invasive therapies (LHM/RHM, POEM).[24] If the stomach is no longer suitable for this procedure due to repeated surgical interventions in the region of the OGJ, reconstruction of the intestinal passage by means of colonic interposition should be considered.

The choice of the therapeutic procedure is dependent upon the type of achalasia according to the Chicago Classification as well as on patient age, comorbidity, surgical risk, prior surgical interventions to the OGJ, as well as the preferences of the patient, and will be further discussed below. Interdisciplinary guidelines for achalasia therapy are currently not available for Germany and reference is therefore made to the guidelines of the International Society for Diseases of the Esophagus ('I-GOAL') published in 2018, as well as to the European guidelines of the United European Gastroenterologists and the European Society of Neurogastroenterology and Motility guidelines.[18,25]

Oral drug therapy

Currently, there is no convincing evidence that calcium antagonists, nitrates, or phosphodiesterase inhibitors represent an efficient therapy in adult patients with achalasia.[18]

In view of the short duration of action, tachyphylaxis, and a wide spectrum of adverse effects, the described drugs are currently used at most for 'bridging', or for the initiation of further therapy options.

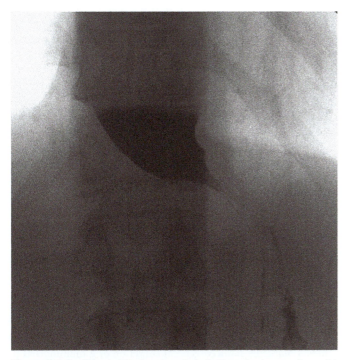

Figure 3.3 Radiological findings in achalasia: X-ray barium swallow with dilated oesophageal body and beak-shaped ('birdhageal') constricted cardia, as well as a stagnant contrast medium column.

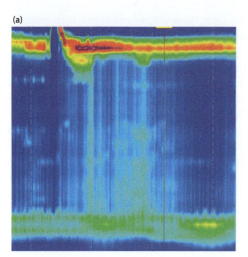 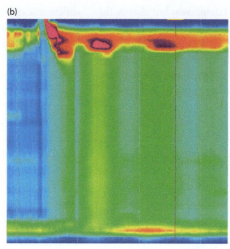 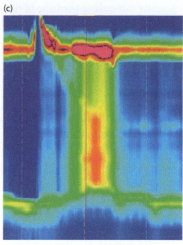

Figure 3.4 Achalasia subtypes on high-resolution oesophageal manometry. (a) Type I: normal reflexive swallow-induced opening of the upper oesophageal sphincter; the LOS is characterized by elevated resting pressure without swallow-induced relaxation; no pressures are measured in the lower two-thirds of the oesophagus, indicating the absence of tubular peristalsis. (b) Type II: continuous increase in LOS resting pressure and absence of swallow-induced relaxation at a simultaneous pressure increase and absent propulsive peristalsis of the tubular oesophagus. (c) Type III: the LOS is characterized by incomplete swallow-induced relaxation; the tubular oesophagus is marked by the absence of normal peristaltic propulsion at increased and extended contractions in the distal oesophagus.

Endoscopic therapy

Injection of BoTox

The injection of BoTox into the LOS represents one of the endoscopic treatment options for achalasia. It constitutes a pharmacological therapy, where BoTox type A, a neurotoxin that inhibits the release of acetylcholine at the nerve endings in the myenteric plexus and thus counteracts the contraction of the LOS, which is controlled by cholinergic excitatory nerves. This causes a reduction in the resting pressure of the LOS of up to 50% and leads to improved oesophageal emptying. The initial therapy success rate is approximately 75% and the most pronounced symptom improvement is found in elderly patients.[26] The outcome is not improved by an increase in the dose. Two injections of 100 IU BoTox (25 IU per quadrant), each at an interval of 30 days, were found to be most effective.[27] In the long term, the effectiveness of the therapy was noted to be markedly poorer and more costly compared to PD and cardiomyotomy.[28] BoTox injection represents a therapeutic option primarily for patients with high comorbidities, who are at a high risk for more invasive procedures, or for the diagnosis of cases with inconclusive manometric findings.[29] The indications for BoTox applications are limited in patients in good general health who are less than 50 years of age.[18]

PD

POEM and PD represent the most effective non-surgical therapeutic options for achalasia. There is currently no general consensus on the optimum technique for the performance of PD in patients with achalasia.[30,31] Furthermore, for various balloon systems, a wide range of different procedures regarding balloon size, time of inflation, inflation pressure, and frequency of dilatations in the course of an intervention, as well as the type and frequency during re-dilation have been described. The concept of graded dilation, that is, stepwise PD at increasing balloon diameters (30, 35, and 40 mm) has been recommended with a view to reduction of the perforation risk and increased efficiency.[18]

The procedure is performed with standard sedation. After a Jagwire or Savary guidewire is placed in the stomach and the OGJ has been safely identified, a balloon is inserted under radiological or endoscopic guidance via this wire and placed directly in the LOS area. This is followed by complete dilation up to the disappearance of the balloon waist (~7–10 psi). Rapid filling of the balloon with air leads to at least partial tearing of the LOS muscle fibres. The balloon is then emptied completely and can be removed together with the guidewire. This is followed by the endoscopically controlled exclusion of possible complications such as perforations, bleeding, or haematoma. At several centres, an additional radiological examination of the oesophagus using a water-soluble contrast medium is carried out that may be dispensed with, if the post-interventional endoscopic examination was clinically unremarkable and there were no patient complaints in the hours after the intervention.

The perforation rates reported in the literature vary markedly, ranging from 0% to 5%, with a statistical mean of approximately 2%.[32] The perforation site is generally located on the left, slightly above the cardia along the oesophagus, which constitutes an anatomically weak point. Large perforations with fluid leakage into the mediastinum and the threat of mediastinitis require immediate surgical intervention and, depending on the specific clinic, smaller defects can be treated with endoscopic treatments (e.g. with use of the EndoVac-system). Advanced patient age, the presence of oesophageal diverticula, a twisted oesophagus, pressures greater than 10–11 psi, and a large balloon diameter constitute risk factors for a perforation.[33] With a view to consideration of the different therapeutic options, mention should be made that approximately 20–30% of patients develop gastro-oesophageal reflux after PD because—in contrast to surgical therapy—no antireflux measures are performed with this procedure. These patients generally respond favourably to proton pump inhibitors.[34] Relevant contraindications for PD include a markedly reduced general condition or a multimorbid patient for whom it would be too risky to undergo emergency surgery for perforation repair.[35] While the initial success rates reported for PD are approximately 85%, long-term remission after a single PD is only approximately 10 years in 40% of cases, and in more than half of the patients, repeated dilation is required.[36] Performance of the surgical procedure described below is recommended in cases with insufficient symptom improvement after at least three PD procedures.[37] Patients older than 40 years of age appear to respond more favourably than younger ones to the procedure. In contrast, patients with type III achalasia and megaoesophagus do not respond well to PD. The best predictor for a successful long-term result is a postinterventional decrease in the initial LOS resting pressure of more than 50%.[38]

POEM

POEM—the newest of all available methods for the therapy of achalasia—constitutes a long sectional endoluminal myotomy using a flexible standard endoscope, which is inserted into the mucosal gateway in the proximal oesophagus. POEM was first described in Japan by Inoue et al. in 2010.[39] Myotomy is performed in the submucosa along the oral–aboral axis and extended beyond the cardia into the proximal stomach with the use of endoscopic submucosal dissection, as illustrated in Figure 3.5. In the next step, and again in an antegrade direction, myotomy of the accessible musculature is carried out, although—in contrast to surgical myotomy—the inner annular muscles are generally split using either a needle-tip knife with a triangular tip (TT) or a hybrid needle-tip knife with integrated water jet function. While the longitudinal outer muscle layer may be left intact, serving as an 'overcoat', some authors favour a full-wall myotomy, although this procedure is associated with increased postinterventional reflux rates. In the last step, the proximal mucosal 'entry' is closed using clips. POEM may therefore be described as a natural orifice transluminal endoscopic surgery (known as 'NOTES') procedure. The intervention is usually performed under general anaesthesia by gastroenterologists or surgeons. Whether POEM of the anterior or the posterior wall of the oesophagus is more efficient can only be evaluated after the results of future long-term studies become available.

Complications associated with this procedure include oesophageal perforation, mediastinitis, mediastinal emphysema, aortic and tracheal injuries, as well as vagus nerve lesions. The occurrence of significant gastro-oesophageal reflux has been reported and was thought it was because these patients do not undergo antireflux repair.[40] Short-term results obtained by recently published large case series and studies show success rates for POEM of greater than 90%. In particular, patients with type III achalasia benefit from a very long sectional myotomy.[41]

Surgical therapy

LHM/RHM

The 'extramucosal cardioplasty for chronic cardiospasm'[42] was described by Ernst Heller as early as in 1913, and in 1923, a modified version of this technique was published by Zaaijer,[43] which consists of cutting the high-pressure zone of the LOS and the simultaneous establishment of a partial fundus wrap to protect against reflux. Myotomy of the longitudinal and circular muscle layers of the distal oesophagus begins at the oesophagocardiac junction, continues over a distance of 6–7 cm upwards on the distal oesophagus, and extends 2–3 cm onto the proximal gastric fundus, as shown in Figure 3.6. The preferred antireflux procedures consist of a 180° anterior semifundoplication according to Dor/Thal, illustrated in Figure 3.7, or of a dorsal partial 270° wrap according to Toupet. The 360° Nissen fundoplication is not indicated in patients with achalasia. Good long-term results and low complication rates have made LHM the first-line therapy for achalasia, in particular in younger patients (<40 years). Favourable results have further been reported for LHM when used as a 'rescue' procedure for patients with prior unsuccessful PD, BoTox therapy, or POEM.[37]

LHM is particularly suitable for the therapy of patients with type I or type II achalasia.[44] LHM should also be considered for first-line therapy in patients with a sigmoid-shaped megaoesophagus. A mortality rate of 0.1% makes LHM one of the safest laparoscopic procedures applied in visceral surgery. Mucosal leak from the oesophagus or the gastric fundus has been reported in approximately 5–7% of cases; however, only 0.7% are of clinical significance, as

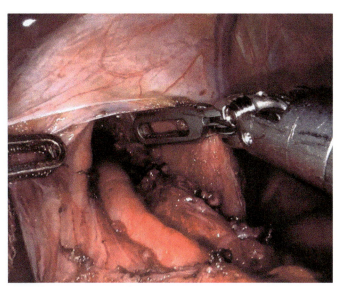

Figure 3.6 Robotic myotomy of the longitudinal and circular muscle layers of the distal oesophagus is carried out during LHM; beginning at the oesophagocardiac junction the procedure is continued over a distance of 6–7 cm upwards on the distal oesophagus and extended 2–3 cm onto the proximal gastric fundus. RHM, Robotic Heller Myotomy.

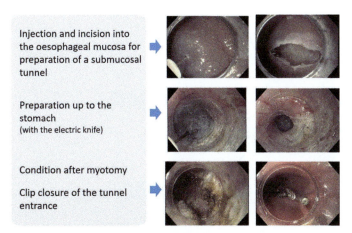

Figure 3.5 POEM is performed along the oral–aboral axis and extended beyond the cardia into the submucosa with the use of endoscopic submucosal dissection.

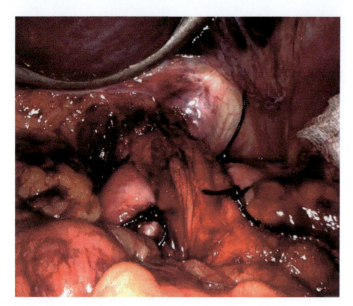

Figure 3.7 Antireflux plasty during RHM: partial dorsal 270° fundoplication according to Toupet.

they are frequently identified during LHM and can generally be oversewn during the operation.[45] The minimally invasive Heller cardiomyotomy is currently increasingly performed robotically. Among the described advantages of the procedure is the angulation of the surgical instruments, which provides a more favourable angle for the performance of the myotomy, as well as a possible lower rate of intraoperative mucosal leaks, and improved visualization of the oesophageal high-pressure zone. Reports of long-term data or the availability of results of prospective randomized studies on robotic myotomy are still pending.[46]

Comparison of treatment methods

The choice of an adequate therapy for achalasia is complex and needs to be adjusted to the needs of the individual patient. A possible interdisciplinary algorithm (expert consensus decision) is shown in Figure 3.8. Furthermore, according to patient age and a better response to LHM/RHM on the part of younger patients, the preoperative diagnosis by means of HRIM plays a crucial role in the establishment of the described algorithm.[44] Patients with type I and type II achalasia especially respond very favourably to LHM/RHM while, conversely, type III achalasia represent a particular therapeutic challenge: an extended myotomy (POEM or LHM) comprising the entire spastic segment of the distal part as well as a segment of the middle part of the oesophagus is indicated. Due to the individually adjusted length of the procedure, HRIM-based myotomy offers the optimum conditions for a tailored approach, that is, a therapy for achalasia individually suited to a specific HRIM high-pressure zone. The described procedure thus enables the long-term success of achalasia therapy.[47]

A prospective European multicentre study did not report a significant difference between PD with repeat dilations and LHM, although the results of the dilation appear to be distorted, as some of the patients with perforation after PD were excluded and the study protocol was changed over the course of the study. Similar success rates have been reported for both types of therapy after a minimum follow-up of 5 years, and there were no differences in oesophageal function and emptying.[48] However, after a 2-year follow-up POEM appears to be superior to PD despite a higher gastro-oesophageal reflux rate.[49] Results of a prospective randomized study comparing LHM plus Dor versus POEM were recently published. After 2 years, POEM was not inferior to LHM with regard to symptom control, although it was associated with gastro-oesophageal reflux.[50]

Of prime importance is the interdisciplinary, stage-related management of achalasia in close consultation between interventional gastroenterology and surgery. Depending on the patient's age, general condition, and pretreatment, as well as the patient's wishes, surgery is always available as a 'rescue' procedure, also in cases of other unsuccessful interventional procedures. A redo myotomy may also be promising, if scarring of the initial myotomy develops or adhesions with repeat fusion of the muscle fibres occurs. Under these conditions, a redo myotomy will have to be a conventional open procedure that is carried out contralaterally to the initial intervention (i.e. in the dorsal region of the oesophagus). The described procedure is not only technically complex, but it also carries the risk of vagal nerve injury. However, both PD and POEM are effective available procedures in cases of achalasia recurrence after prior LHM. In these instances, the selected site of the surgery should be at the greatest possible distance from the site of the initial intervention and the possibility of an increased risk of perforation needs to be considered.[51]

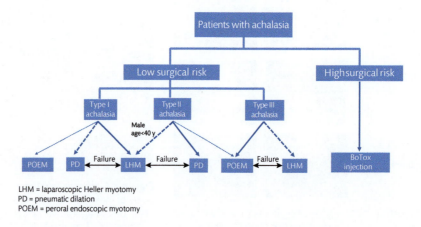

Figure 3.8 Interdisciplinary treatment algorithm for achalasia (exclusively expert consensus decision).

Oesophagogastric junction outflow obstruction

Definition and aetiopathogenesis

In addition to the different types of achalasia, disturbed swallow-induced LOS relaxation at complete or partially maintained propulsive peristalsis in the oesophagus is observed in some patients, as described in Table 3.3 and Figure 3.9. Analogous to patients with a known mechanic obstruction, the presence of elevated intrabolus pressure has been noted in patients with OGJ outflow obstruction.[52] OGJ outflow obstruction may therefore be a variant of achalasia.[9,53] However, OGJ obstruction has been described for both benign and malignant disorders with infiltrative pathology of the distal oesophagus or the OGJ, and endosonography or computed tomography are therefore recommended imaging procedures for the exclusion of the presence of a malignancy.

Since the primary dysfunction constitutes an impaired swallow-induced relaxation of the LOS in both achalasia and OGJ outflow obstruction, the appropriate treatments are frequently also similar. Nevertheless, since the appropriate therapy for OGJ outflow obstruction is nearly always pharmacological or via interventional endoscopy, the indication for surgery is comparatively rare in these patients.

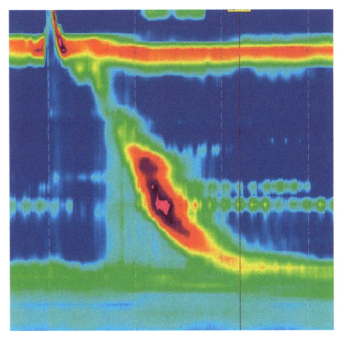

Figure 3.9 OGJ outflow obstruction with normal propulsive peristalsis of the tubular oesophagus and inadequate swallow-induced relaxation of the LOS (integrated relaxation pressure 28 mmHg) visualized on high-resolution oesophageal manometry.

Table 3.3 Classification of oesophageal motility disorders according to the Chicago Classification version 4.0

Motility disorders	Criteria
Disorders of OGJ outflow (IRP ≥15 mmHg)	
Type I achalasia	100% failed peristalsis
Type II achalasia	100% failed peristalsis ≥20% swallows with panoesophageal pressurization
Type III achalasia	≥20% swallows with premature/spastic contractions No evidence of peristalsis
OGJ outflow obstruction	Abnormal median IRP (supine and upright) ≥20% elevated intrabolus pressure (supine) Not meeting criteria for achalasia Symptoms (dysphagia and/or pain) Complementary testing to confirm diagnosis
Disorders of peristalsis	
Distal oesophageal spasm	Normal median IRP ≥20% swallows with premature/spastic contractions Symptoms (dysphagia, and/or pain)
Hypercontractile oesophagus	Normal median IRP ≥20% hypercontractile swallows Symptoms (dysphagia and/or pain)
Absent contractility	Normal median IRP 100% failed peristalsis
Ineffective oesophageal motility	Normal median IRP >70% ineffective swallows or ≥50% failed peristalsis

Source: data from Yadlapati R, Kahrilas PJ, Fox MR, et al. Esophageal motility disorders on high-resolution manometry: Chicago classification version 4.0©. *Neurogastroenterol Motil.* 2021;33:e14058. doi:10.1111/nmo.14058.

Disorders of peristalsis

Oesophageal hypermotility disorders

Definition and aetiopathogenesis

Oesophageal hypermotility disorders (DOS, hypercontractile oesophagus) are characterized by one or more measures of contractile activity that exceed the upper limit of normal. They can be a cause of recurrent dysphagia to solid and liquid foods and a cause of non-cardiac chest pain.[54] Barium swallow can show changes with non-peristaltic contractions (corkscrew oesophagus and tertiary contractions) as shown in Figure 3.10 up to normal findings and it is therefore not sufficiently sensitive for an accurate diagnosis. This is why oesophagus manometry is essential.

The pathogenesis remains elusive, although among other findings the increased incidence of spastic oesophageal motility disorders under opioid administration could be observed. Opioids inhibit neuronal excitability, which leads to the secretion of inhibitory neurotransmitters, such as NO and vasoactive intestinal peptide, and, thus, induces neural inhibition.[55]

Distal oesophagus spasm

Definition and aetiopathogenesis

The symptoms of DOS were first described by Dr Osgood in 1889.[56] The definition of the described motility disorder was repeatedly changed over time and most recently following the introduction of HRIM.[57,58] The current version of the Chicago Classification, version 4.0, bases the diagnosis of DOS on the presence of spastic or premature (distal latency <4.5 seconds) contractions in at least 20% of ten wet swallows in the setting of a distal contractile integral

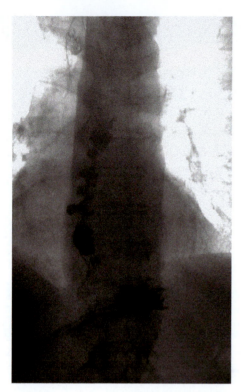

Figure 3.10 X-ray examination of the oesophagus with barium swallow shows a so-called corkscrew oesophagus as a sign for tertiary contractions, indicative of a hypercontractile oesophageal motility disorder.

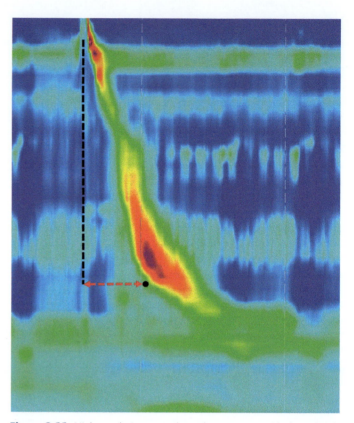

Figure 3.11 High-resolution oesophageal manometry with short distal latency (<4.5 seconds) in DOS.

(DCI) greater than 450 mmHg/cm/s and a normal LOS swallow response, as illustrated in Figure 3.11. Furthermore[7], the presence of relevant clinical symptoms such as dysphagia and/or chest pain is required.[9]

As the described changes occur primarily in the distal oesophagus, the name 'diffuse oesophagus spasm' was changed to 'distal oesophageal spasm'.[59]

As mentioned above, the aetiology of DOS has not yet been unambiguously elucidated. There are indications of the presence of NO deficiency, which, in turn, induces an impairment of neuronal inhibition. While coexistent gastro-oesophageal reflux disease is frequently diagnosed, its role in the pathogenesis of the disorder has not been conclusively identified,[60] and the frequent finding of the disorder in psychiatric patients with DOS[61] is also still open to question. In some patients, DOS may progress to achalasia over the course of the disease.[62,63]

Epidemiology

With an incidence of approximately 0.1:100,000, DOS is a very rare disorder and generally occurs in older patients (generally from 60 years old). It is diagnosed slightly more often in women. The lifetime prevalence in symptomatic patients ranges from 3% to 9%.[59,64]

Clinical symptoms

The clinical presentation is very heterogeneous in patients with DOS. Frequently described symptoms include dysphagia and/or thoracic pain, but regurgitation, heartburn, and weight loss are also reported.[65]

Diagnosis

The diagnosis of DOS is based chiefly on oesophageal manometry; the definition is shown in Table 3.3. However, an unremarkable oesophageal manometry result does not preclude the presence of DOS due to the intermittent character of the disorder.[66] In cases with the clinical suspicion of DOS but normal manometry findings, HRIM should be repeated over the course of the disorder. An endoscopic examination should always be performed for the exclusion of malignant or inflammatory changes. Radiological changes, such as corkscrew or rosary bead oesophagus, may indicate the presence of DOS, although these findings are non-specific. The performance of a 24-hour pH-metry test should be considered to enable the exclusion of a reflux disorder as a possible cause of DOS. In patients presenting with retrosternal chest pain, a diagnostic work-up should always be considered to enable the exclusion of coronary heart disease.[67]

Hypercontractile (jackhammer) oesophagus

Definition and aetiopathogenesis

The jackhammer oesophagus is a hypercontractile motility disorder and was first described by Benjamin et al. in 1979.[68] It is characterized by pathological oesophageal motility with maintained propulsive peristalsis and the development of abnormally high contraction amplitudes, as well as by prolonged contraction times of the distal oesophagus. Since the Chicago Classification version 3.0, only the jackhammer oesophagus with extremely high DCI values of greater than 8000 mmHg/s/cm in at least 20% of ten wet swallows (illustrated in Figure 3.12) is considered pathological, because this

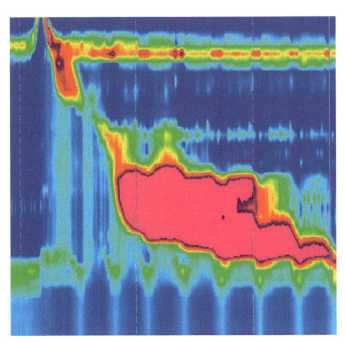

Figure 3.12 High-resolution oesophageal manometry with propulsive hypertensive peristalsis (DCI >8000 mmHg/s/cm) and normal propagation velocity in jackhammer oesophagus.

constellation has thus far not been demonstrated in healthy control subjects, whereas DCI values of 5000 mmHg/s/cm (nutcracker oesophagus) are found in 5% of the normal population.[69] However, it has been shown that the frequency of dysphagia and thoracic pain is the same as that of patients with a jackhammer oesophagus, so the nutcracker oesophagus should also be considered pathological in symptomatic patients.[70]

The Chicago Classification version 4.0 also requires the clinically relevant symptoms of dysphagia and/or chest pain as well as the occurrence of hypercontractile swallows in the supine position and upright position for diagnosis. Furthermore, the diagnosis should only be made if criteria of achalasia or DOS are not met and mechanical obstruction could be ruled out.[9]

The pathogenesis has not been conclusively established and the hypercontractile oesophagus can be primary or secondary (e.g. as the result of an acid-induced gastric irritation). Asynchronicity between the circular and longitudinal muscles during the propulsive contraction has been visualized on intraluminal ultrasound. It has further been shown that the condition might be triggered as the result of a hypercholinergic state, which can be normalized with anticholinergics such as atropine.[71] An OGJ outflow obstruction has been diagnosed in a number of patients. It has further been hypothesized that the described hypercontractility may be a mechanism to overcome an outflow obstruction at the gastro-oesophageal junction.[72] A possible connection between jackhammer oesophagus and eosinophilic oesophagitis has also been described.[73] In some patients, achalasia reportedly developed in the course of the disease.[74] A possible link between hypercontractile oesophagus and negative postoperative results after laparoscopic antireflux surgery has also been suggested.[75]

Epidemiology

The nutcracker oesophagus is a very rare disease and occurs predominantly during the sixth decade of life.

Clinical symptoms

A leading symptom of the hypercontractile oesophagus in addition to dysphagia is chest pain that often resembles angina pectoris and may radiate to the angle of the mandible and the shoulders.[68]

Diagnosis

The diagnosis is exclusively made by oesophageal manometry. Radiological and endoscopic findings are usually normal, in some cases a corkscrew-shaped oesophagus can be observed on barium swallow.

Therapy of oesophageal hypermotility disorders

Despite the differences in the pathophysiology of spastic motility disorders of the oesophagus, the therapeutic procedures are similar for all entities.[69] The therapeutic regimen is oriented to the specific symptoms; it is not standardized and may have to be tailored to individual patient requirements.

Oral medical therapy

Proton pump inhibitors should initially be used in the therapy of patients with gastro-oesophageal reflux disease. NO is known to play an important role in the pathogenesis of hypercontractile oesophageal function disorders. Medications suitable for therapy are those known to increase NO concentrations such as nitrites (e.g. isosorbide dinitrate 5–10 mg sublingual, 5–10 minutes before meals, if dysphagia is the leading symptom; if chest pain is in the forefront, 'on-demand' administration of the medication is recommended), as well as phosphodiesterase-5 inhibitors (e.g. sildenafil 50 mg/day). Also used with varying degrees of therapeutic success are calcium antagonists (e.g. diltiazem 180–240 mg/day), which promote smooth muscle relaxation, as well as antidepressants (e.g. imipramine 20–25 mg/nights for chest pain therapy).[64,76,77]

Endoscopic therapy

Injection of BoTox BoTox injection represents one of the endoscopic treatment options. However, in contrast to the therapy for achalasia, the technique is not standardized and injections both in the distal oesophagus and in the OGJ have been described. A significant improvement of clinical symptoms after BoTox injection has thus far been reported in individual cases only. A prospective placebo-controlled study reported a significant improvement of symptoms for dysphagia that was, however, not found in patients with thoracic pain.[78] The short duration of action described for the therapy (~6 months) as well as the loss of effectiveness of BoTox injection over the long term constitute limiting factors.

PD The application of PD for the therapy of hypercontractile motility disorders with dysphagia has resulted in only a slight improvement of symptoms.[69]

POEM POEM has been established as a successful treatment for achalasia. The endoluminal and therefore only minimally invasive possibility of cutting the longitudinal muscles of the tubular oesophagus has recently emerged as a promising treatment option in patients with spastic oesophageal motility disorders. The rare occurrence of achalasia may, among other reasons, account for the scarcity of available results published by only a small number of multicentre studies to date. POEM has also been shown to be effective in the therapy of non-achalasia oesophageal motility disorders, albeit with somewhat less success than in the treatment of achalasia.[79–81] Because POEM continues to be carried out by experts at highly specialized medical centres only, it is not consistently available nationwide.

Surgical therapy

While LHM and RHM are well-established effective treatments for achalasia, the procedures have been less successful in the therapy of hypercontractile oesophageal functional disorders. Improved results have been reported for the upper thoracic myotomy.[82] A high thoracic myotomy to the middle oesophagus is, however, more readily achieved endoscopically than with the use of a surgical abdominal procedure. A viable alternative in these cases is the thoracic approach, although this procedure is associated with higher morbidity due to the need for double-lumen intubation and compression of the (right) lung. LHM or RHM therefore constitute viable therapeutic options in cases where pharmaceutical therapy is not successful and POEM does not represent an option.[83] As in the treatment for achalasia, the advantage of a surgical procedure is the option of the simultaneous performance of an antireflux procedure (e.g. partial fundoplication) to reduce the risk of postinterventional gastro-oesophageal reflux disorder.

Absent contractility

Definition and aetiopathogenesis

Absent peristalsis is defined as 100% of swallows with a DCI less than 100 mmHg/s/cm with a normal LOS swallow-induced relaxation (integrated relaxation pressure (IRP) <15 mmHg), as shown in Figure 3.13. Due to the lack of tubular peristalsis, symptoms such as dysphagia or heartburn occur.[9]

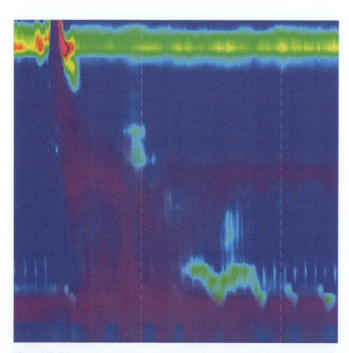

Figure 3.13 High-resolution oesophageal manometry contour plot demonstrating absent peristalsis in the tubular oesophagus in ineffective oesophageal motility disorders.

Results of various studies have shown that some patients with aperistalsis and normal IRP have amnestic, radiological, and endoscopic criteria associated with those of type I achalasia.[84] The aperistalsis is usually distinguished from achalasia type I using HRM based on normal or elevated IRP values.[9] However, the diagnostic algorithm of the described differentiation is based on a single quantitative measurement of swallow-induced LOS relaxation, the IRP. It is known that manometric IRP measurements may be associated with measurement errors. The decision regarding therapeutic management is therefore based on the relevant distinction between absent peristalsis and type I achalasia. Type I achalasia is treated with PD, BoTox, POEM, or Heller myotomy.[85] However, such treatment would be contraindicated in patients with absent peristalsis and false high IRP values. In contrast, achalasia type I patients with a false 'normal' IRP might not receive the appropriate treatment and, thus, be denied an improvement in their quality of life. The diagnostic uncertainty due to the exclusive use of the IRP value as the basis for the differentiation between aperistalsis and type I achalasia requires additional testing in some of the patients.

It has been hypothesized that distinctive responses to pharmacological provocation using amyl nitrite and cholecystokinin could reliably distinguish between patients with absent peristalsis and type I achalasia. For this purpose, Babaei et al. administered the rapid drink challenge test with administration of both pharmacological substances in two patient cohorts.[86] The IRP values did not permit an accurate separation between aperistalsis and type I achalasia. The authors were nevertheless able to identify manometric criteria for oesophageal responses to both of the above substances that permitted the correct classification of both patient cohorts. The authors concluded that nearly a quarter of the patients are misdiagnosed based on manometric IRP criteria alone. The drug provocation test has the potential to facilitate the correct diagnosis in these complex patients.

The aetiology of aperistalsis is often unclear, in a small proportion of patients an underlying disease such as collagenosis may be the reason for the peristaltic disorder.

Since anticholinergic drugs lead to ineffective oesophageal motility, it is assumed that pathophysiologically there is a reduction in cholinergic activity, as this leads to a reduction in contraction force as well as frequency.[86,87]

Epidemiology

No valid epidemiological data exist.

Clinical symptoms

The clinical presentation is heterogeneous with dysphagia, heartburn, and regurgitation.

Diagnosis

The diagnosis of failed peristalsis is based on oesophageal manometry; the definition is shown in Table 3.3.

Therapy

If no cause is known, the treatment focuses mainly on controlling the presence of gastro-oesophageal reflux symptoms with proton pump inhibitors and changing eating habits, such as soft and liquid food and eating in an upright position, and possibly the use of prokinetics.

Ineffective oesophageal motility

Definition and aetiopathogenesis

According to the Chicago Classification version 4.0, ineffective oesophageal motility is defined as at least 70% ineffective peristalsis (DCI <450 mmHg/s/cm) and/or fragmented peristalsis (a peristaltic break >5 cm at DCI >450 mmHg/s/cm) or at least 50% of swallows with failed peristalsis (DCI <100 mmHg/s/cm) combined with regular swallow-induced LOS relaxation (IRP <15 mmHg).

The changes in peristalsis can lead to ineffective bolus clearance[9] and approximately a third of the affected patients complain of relevant dysphagia (Figure 3.14).

Hypotensive oesophageal motility disorders may be idiopathic or occur secondary to a number of disorders such as gastrooesophageal reflux disease, collagenoses including scleroderma, and infiltrative disorders, like amyloidosis.[88] Hypotensive disorders have further been reported for patients with eosinophilic oesophagitis.[89,90]

For the surgeon, the hypomotile disorders are ultimately only relevant in the context of reflux surgery.

Currently, no effective pharmacotherapy exists and the primary aim of therapy therefore consists of symptom control. There is an ongoing discussion regarding whether hiatal procedures with (partial) fundoplication are associated with worsening of symptoms in patients with hypomotile oesophagus. Under the described conditions, a clinical provocation manoeuvre with multiple rapid swallows can be performed during HRIM. If the described manoeuvre leads to stimulation of the smooth musculature, this serves as an indication of the presence of a contraction reserve which, in turn, speaks in favour of a better prognosis and permits the performance of an antireflux procedure as a possible therapeutic option.[91]

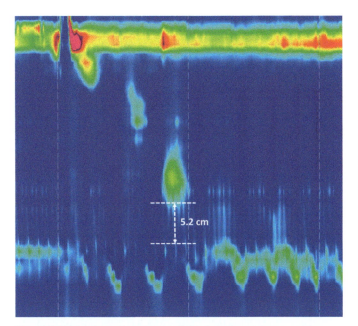

Figure 3.14 High-resolution oesophageal manometry presentation of fragmented oesophageal peristalsis with propulsive peristalsis in the tubular oesophagus, showing an extended peristaltic break (>5 cm) and low contraction amplitude as well as normal swallow-induced LOS relaxation.

REFERENCES

1. Goyal RK, Chaudhury A. Physiology of normal esophageal motility. *J Clin Gastroenterol*. 2008;**42**:610–619.
2. Park H, Conklin JL. Neuromuscular control of esophageal peristalsis. *Curr Gastroenterol Rep*. 1999;**1**:186–197.
3. Diamant NE, El-Sharkawy TY. Neural control of esophageal peristalsis. A conceptual analysis. *Gastroenterology*. 1977;**72**:546–556.
4. Goyal RK, Rattan S. Nature of the vagal inhibitory innervation to the lower esophageal sphincter. *J Clin Invest*. 1975;**55**:1119–1126.
5. Boeckxstaens GE. The lower esophageal sphincter. *Neurogastroenterol Motil*. 2005;**17**:13–21.
6. Müller M, Gockel I. Motilitätsstörungen des Ösophagus. *Internist (Berl)*. 2015;**56**:615–620.
7. Bredenoord AJ, Fox M, Kahrilas PJ, Pandolfino JE, Schwizer W, Smout AJPM. Chicago classification criteria of esophageal motility disorders defined in high resolution esophageal pressure topography. *Neurogastroenterol Motil*. 2012;**24**(Suppl 1):57–65.
8. Pandolfino JE, Kwiatek MA, Nealis T, Bulsiewicz W, Post J, Kahrilas PJ. Achalasia: a new clinically relevant classification by high-resolution manometry. *Gastroenterology*. 2008;**135**:1526–1533.
9. Yadlapati R, Kahrilas PJ, Fox MR, et al. Esophageal motility disorders on high-resolution manometry: Chicago classification version 4.0©. *Neurogastroenterol Motil*. 2021;**33**:e14058.
10. Koop I. *Gastroenterologie Compact: Sekundäre Motilitätsstörungen*. 3rd ed. Stuttgart: Thieme; 2013.
11. Hurst AF, Rowlands RP. Case of achalasia of the cardia relieved by operation. *Proc R Soc Med*. 1924;**17**:45–46.
12. Ates F, Vaezi MF. The pathogenesis and management of achalasia: current status and future directions. *Gut Liver*. 2015;**9**:449–463.
13. Clark SB, Rice TW, Tubbs RR, Richter JE, Goldblum JR. The nature of the myenteric infiltrate in achalasia: an immunohistochemical analysis. *Am J Surg Pathol*. 2000;**24**:1153–1158.
14. Gockel I, Becker J, Wouters MM, et al. Common variants in the HLA-DQ region confer susceptibility to idiopathic achalasia. *Nat Genet*. 2014;**46**:901–904.
15. Wouters MM, Lambrechts D, Becker J, et al. Genetic variation in the lymphotoxin-α (LTA)/tumour necrosis factor-α (TNFα) locus as a risk factor for idiopathic achalasia. *Gut*. 2014;**63**:1401–1409.
16. Allgrove J, Clayden GS, Grant DB, Macaulay JC. Familial glucocorticoid deficiency with achalasia of the cardia and deficient tear production. *Lancet*. 1978;**1**:1284–1286.
17. Francis DL, Katzka DA. Achalasia: update on the disease and its treatment. *Gastroenterology*. 2010;**139**:369–374.
18. Zaninotto G, Bennett C, Boeckxstaens G, et al. The 2018 ISDE achalasia guidelines. *Dis Esophagus*. 2018;**31**:doy071.
19. Eckardt VF, Aignherr C, Bernhard G. Predictors of outcome in patients with achalasia treated by pneumatic dilation. *Gastroenterology*. 1992;**103**:1732–1738.
20. Jung DH, Park H. Is gastroesophageal reflux disease and achalasia coincident or not? *J Neurogastroenterol Motil*. 2017;**23**:5–8.
21. Gockel I, Rabe SM, Niebisch S. Before and after esophageal surgery: which information is needed from the functional laboratory? *Visc Med*. 2018;**34**:116–121.
22. Ghosh SK, Pandolfino JE, Rice J, Clarke JO, Kwiatek M, Kahrilas PJ. Impaired deglutitive EGJ relaxation in clinical esophageal manometry: a quantitative analysis of 400 patients

and 75 controls. *Am J Physiol Gastrointest Liver Physiol*. 2007;**293**:G878–G885.
23. Kahrilas PJ, Pandolfino JE. Treatments for achalasia in 2017: how to choose among them. *Curr Opin Gastroenterol*. 2017;**33**:270–276.
24. Orringer MB, Stirling MC. Esophageal resection for achalasia: indications and results. *Ann Thorac Surg*. 1989;**47**:340–345.
25. Nijhuis RO, Zaninotto G, Roman S. European guideline on achalasia—UEG and ESNM recommendations. *United European Gastroenterol J*. 2020;**8**:13–34.
26. Pasricha PJ, Rai R, Ravich WJ, Hendrix TR, Kalloo AN. Botulinum toxin for achalasia: long-term outcome and predictors of response. *Gastroenterology*. 1996;**110**:1410–1415.
27. Annese V, Bassotti G, Coccia G, et al. A multicentre randomised study of intrasphincteric botulinum toxin in patients with oesophageal achalasia. GISMAD Achalasia Study Group. *Gut*. 2000;**46**:597–600.
28. Uppal DS, Wang AY. Update on the endoscopic treatments for achalasia. *World J Gastroenterol*. 2016;**22**:8670–8683.
29. Katzka DA, Castell DO. Use of botulinum toxin as a diagnostic/therapeutic trial to help clarify an indication for definitive therapy in patients with achalasia. *Am J Gastroenterol*. 1999;**94**:637–642.
30. Müller M, Keck C, Eckardt AJ, et al. Outcomes of pneumatic dilation in achalasia: extended follow-up of more than 25 years with a focus on manometric subtypes. *J Gastroenterol Hepatol*. 2018;**33**:1067–1074.
31. Eckardt AJ, Eckardt VF. Treatment and surveillance strategies in achalasia: an update. *Nat Rev Gastroenterol Hepatol*. 2011;**8**:311–319.
32. Katzka DA, Castell DO. Review article: an analysis of the efficacy, perforation rates and methods used in pneumatic dilation for achalasia. *Aliment Pharmacol Ther*. 2011;**34**:832–839.
33. Nair LA, Reynolds JC, Parkman HP, et al. Complications during pneumatic dilation for achalasia or diffuse esophageal spasm. Analysis of risk factors, early clinical characteristics, and outcome. *Dig Dis Sci*. 1993;**38**:1893–1904.
34. Min YW, Lee JH, Min B-H, Lee JH, Kim JJ, Rhee PL. Association between gastroesophageal reflux disease after pneumatic balloon dilatation and clinical course in patients with achalasia. *J Neurogastroenterol Motil*. 2014;**20**:212–218.
35. Moonen A, Boeckxstaens G. Finding the right treatment for achalasia treatment: risks, efficacy, complications. *Curr Treat Options Gastroenterol*. 2016;**14**:420–428.
36. Eckardt VF, Gockel I, Bernhard G. Pneumatic dilation for achalasia: late results of a prospective follow up investigation. *Gut*. 2004;**53**:629–633.
37. Gockel I, Junginger T, Bernhard G, Eckardt VF. Heller myotomy for failed pneumatic dilation in achalasia: how effective is it? *Ann Surg*. 2004;**239**:371–377.
38. Ghoshal UC, Rangan M. A review of factors predicting outcome of pneumatic dilation in patients with achalasia cardia. *J Neurogastroenterol Motil*. 2011;**17**:9–13.
39. Inoue H, Minami H, Kobayashi Y, et al. Peroral endoscopic myotomy (POEM) for esophageal achalasia. *Endoscopy*. 2010;**42**:265–271.
40. Familiari M, Greco S, Gigante G, et al. Gastroesophageal reflux disease after peroral endoscopic myotomy: analysis of clinical, procedural and functional factors, associated with gastroesophageal reflux disease and esophagitis. *Dig Endosc*. 2016;**28**:33–41.
41. Shiwaku H, Inoue H, Sato H, et al. Peroral endoscopic myotomy for achalasia: a prospective multicenter study in Japan. *Gastrointest Endosc*. 2020;**91**:1037–1044.
42. Heller E. Extramuköse Kardioplastik beim chronischen Kardiospasmus mit Dilatation des Oesophagus. *Mitt Grenzgeb Med Chir*. 1913;**27**:141–149.
43. Zaaijer JH. Cardiospasm in the aged. *Ann Surg*. 1923;**77**:615–617.
44. Rohof WO, Salvador R, Annese V, et al. Outcomes of treatment for achalasia depend on manometric subtype. *Gastroenterology*. 2013;**144**:718–725.
45. Salvador R, Spadotto L, Capovilla G, et al. Mucosal perforation during laparoscopic heller myotomy has no influence on final treatment outcome. *J Gastrointest Surg*. 2016;**20**:1923–1930.
46. Afaneh C, Finnerty B, Abelson JS, Zarnegar R. Robotic-assisted Heller myotomy: a modern technique and review of outcomes. *V J Robot Surg*. 2015;**9**:101–108.
47. Triantafyllou T, Theodoropoulos C, Georgiou G, et al. Long-term outcome of myotomy and fundoplication based on intraoperative real-time high-resolution manometry in achalasia patients. *Ann Gastroenterol*. 2019; **32**:46–51.
48. Boeckxstaens GE, Annese V, Des Varannes SB, et al. Pneumatic dilation versus laparoscopic Heller's myotomy for idiopathic achalasia. *N Engl J Med*. 2011;**364**:1807–1816.
49. Ponds FA, Fockens P, Lei A. Effect of peroral endoscopic myotomy vs pneumatic dilation on symptom severity and treatment outcomes among treatment-naive patients with achalasia: a randomized clinical trial. *JAMA*. 2019;**322**:134–144.
50. Werner YB, Hakanson B, Martinek J. Endoscopic or surgical myotomy in patients with idiopathic achalasia. *N Engl J Med*. 2019;**381**:2219–2229.
51. Fernandez-Ananin S, Fernandez AF, Balaque C. What to do when Heller's myotomy fails? Pneumatic dilatation, laparoscopic remyotomy or peroral endoscopic myotomy: a systematic review. *J Minim Access Surg*. 2018;**14**:177–184.
52. Van Hoeij FB, Smout AJPM, Bredenoord AJ. Characterization of idiopathic esophagogastric junction outflow obstruction. *Neurogastroenterol Motil*. 2015;**27**:1310–1316.
53. Scherer JR, Kwiatek MA, Soper NJ, Pandolfino JE, Kahrilas PJ. Functional esophagogastric junction obstruction with intact peristalsis: a heterogeneous syndrome sometimes akin to achalasia. *J Gastrointest Surg*. 2009;**13**:2219–2225.
54. Clouse RE. Spastic disorders of the esophagus. *Gastroenterologist*. 1997;**5**:112–127.
55. Ratuapli SK, Crowell MD, DiBaise JK et al. Opioid-induced esophageal dysfunction (OIED) in patients on chronic opioids. *Am J Gastroenterol*. 2015;**110**:979–984.
56. Osgood H. A peculiar form of esophagismus. *Boston Med Surg J*. 1889;**120**:401–403.
57. Gorti H, Samo S, Shahnavaz N, Qayed E. Distal esophageal spasm: update on diagnosis and management in the era of high-resolution manometry. *World J Clin Cases*. 2020;**8**:1026–1032.
58. Bredenoord AJ, Fox M, Kahrilas PJ, Pandolfino JE, Schwizer W, Smout AJ. International High Resolution Manometry Working Group. Chicago classification criteria of esophageal motility disorders defined in high resolution esophageal pressure topography. *Neurogastroenterol Motil*. 2012;**24**:57–65.
59. Sperandio M, Tutuian R, Gideon RM, et al. Diffuse esophageal spasm: not diffuse but distal esophageal spasm (DES). *Dig Dis Sci*. 2003;**48**:1380–1384.
60. Achem SR, Gerson LB. Distal esophageal spasm: an update. *Curr Gastroenterol Rep*. 2013;**15**:325.

61. Clouse RE. Psychiatric disorders in patients with esophageal disease. *Med Clin North Am.* 1991;**75**:1081–1096.
62. Müller M, Eckardt AJ, Göpel B, Eckardt VF. Clinical and manometric course of nonspecific esophageal motility disorders. *Dig Dis Sci.* 2012;**57**:683–689.
63. De Schepper HU, Smout AJ, Bredenoord AJ. Distal esophageal spasm evolving to achalasia in high resolution. *Clin Gastroenterol Hepatol.* 2014;**12**:A25–A26.
64. Khalaf M, Chowdhary S, Elias PS, Castell D. Distal esophageal spasm: a review. *Am J Med.* 2018;**131**:1034–1040.
65. Almansa C, Heckman MG, DeVault KR, Bouras E, Achem SR. Esophageal spasm: demographic, clinical, radiographic, and manometric features in 108 patients. *Dis Esophagus.* 2012;**25**:214–221.
66. Tsuboi K, Mittal SK. Diffuse esophageal spasm: has the term lost its relevance? Analysis of 217 cases. *Dis Esophagus.* 2011;**24**:354–359.
67. Tutuian R, Castell DO. Review article: oesophageal spasm—diagnosis and management. *Aliment Pharmacol Ther.* 2006;**23**:1393–1402.
68. Benjamin SB, Gerhardt DC, Castell DO. High amplitude, peristaltic esophageal contractions associated with chest pain and/or dysphagia. *Gastroenterology.* 1979;**77**:478–483.
69. Roman S, Kahrilas PJ. Management of spastic disorders of the esophagus. *Gastroenterol Clin North Am.* 2013;**42**:27–43.
70. Al-Qaisi MT, Siddiki HA, Crowell MD, et al. The clinical significance of hypercontractile peristalsis: comparison of high-resolution manometric features, demographics, symptom presentation, and response to therapy in patients with jackhammer esophagus versus nutcracker esophagus. *Dis Esophagus.* 2017;**30**:1–7.
71. Korsapati H, Bhargava V, Mittal RK. Reversal of asynchrony between circular and longitudinal muscle contraction in nutcracker esophagus by atropine. *Gastroenterology.* 2008;**135**:796–802.
72. Jia Y, Arenas J, Hejazi RA, et al. Frequency of jackhammer esophagus as the extreme phenotypes of esophageal hypercontractility based on the new Chicago classification. *J Clin Gastroenterol.* 2016;**50**:615–618.
73. Clément M, Zhu WJ, Neshkova E, Bouin M. Jackhammer esophagus: from manometric diagnosis to clinical presentation. *Can J Gastroenterol Hepatol.* 2019;**2019**:5036160.
74. Abdallah J, Fass R. Progression of jackhammer esophagus to type II achalasia. *J Neurogastroenterol Motil.* 2016;**22**:153–156.
75. Winslow ER, Clouse RE, Desai KM, et al. Influence of spastic motor disorders of the esophageal body on outcomes from laparoscopic antireflux surgery. *Surg Endosc.* 2003;**17**:738–745.
76. Gockel I, Lord RV, Bremner CG, et al. The hypertensive lower esophageal sphincter: a motility disorder with manometric features of outflow obstruction. *J Gastrointest Surg.* 2003;**7**:692–700.
77. Miller DR, Averbukh LD, Kwon SY, Farrell J, Bhargava S, Horrigan J, Tadros M. Phosphodiesterase inhibitors are viable options for treating esophageal motility disorders: a case report and literature review. *J Dig Dis.* 2019;**20**:495–499.
78. Vanuytsel T, Bisschops R, Farré R, et al. Botulinum toxin reduces dysphagia in patients with nonachalasia primary esophageal motility disorders. *Clin Gastroenterol Hepatol.* 2013;**11**:1115–1121.
79. Shiwaku H, Inoue H, Beppu R, et al. Successful treatment of diffuse esophageal spasm by peroral endoscopic myotomy. *Gastrointest Endosc.* 2013;**77**:149–159.
80. Khashab MA, Familiari P, Draganov PV, et al. Peroral endoscopic myotomy is effective and safe in non-achalasia esophageal motility disorders: an international multicenter study. *Endosc Int Open.* 2018;**6**:E1031–E1036.
81. Sharata AM, Dunst CM, Pescarus R, et al. Peroral endoscopic myotomy (POEM) for esophageal primary motility disorders: analysis of 100 consecutive patients. *J Gastrointest Surg.* 2015;**19**:161–170.
82. Leconte M, Douard R, Gaudric M, Dumontier I, Chaussade S, Dousset B. Functional results after extended myotomy for diffuse oesophageal spasm. *Br J Surg.* 2007;**94**:1113–1118.
83. Gorti H, Samo S, Shahnavaz N, Qayed E. Distal esophageal spasm: update on diagnosis and management in the era of high-resolution manometry. *World J Clin Cases.* 2020;**8**:1026–1032.
84. Sanagapalli S, Roman S, Hastier A, et al. Achalasia diagnosed despite normal integrated relaxation pressure responds favorably to therapy. *Neurogastroenterol Motil.* 2019;**31**:e13586.
85. Pandolfino JE, Gawron AJ. Achalasia: a systematic review. *JAMA.* 2015;**313**:1841–1852.
86. Leite LP, Johnston BT, Barrett J, Castell JA, Castell DO. Ineffective esophageal motility (IEM): the primary finding in patients with nonspecific esophageal motility disorder. *Dig Dis Sci.* 1997;**42**:1859–1865.
87. Tutuian R, Castell DO. Clarification of the esophageal function defect in patients with manometric ineffective esophageal motility: studies using combined impedance-manometry. *Clin Gastroenterol Hepatol.* 2004;**2**:230–236.
88. Babaei A, Shad S, Massey BT. Diagnostic differences in the pharmacologic response to cholecystokinin and amyl nitrite in patients with absent contractility vs type I achalasia. *Neurogastroenterol Motil.* 2020;**32**:e13857.
89. Mercado U, Arroyo de Anda R, Avendano L, et al. Metoclopramide response in patients with early diffuse systemic sclerosis. Effects on esophageal motility abnormalities. *Clin Exp Rheumatol.* 2005;**23**:685–688.
90. Weiss AH, Iorio N, Schey R. Esophageal motility in eosinophilic esophagitis. *Rev Gastroenterol Mex.* 2015;**80**:205–213.
91. Gyawali CP, Sifrim D, Carlson DA. Ineffective esophageal motility: concepts, future directions, and conclusions from the Stanford 2018 symposium. *Neurogastroenterol Motil.* 2019;**31**:e13584.

4

Oesophageal diverticula

Joshua Kapp, Philip Müller, and Christian A. Gutschow

Introduction

An oesophageal diverticulum is a rare entity with a prevalence between 0.06% and 0.2% in radiological and endoscopic series.[1-3] As most patients with diverticula are asymptomatic or express only minimal symptoms, the rate of diverticula requiring therapy is considerably lower.[1] The incidence increases with age and culminates in the seventh to eighth decade of life.[4]

The pharyngo-oesophageal junction is the most frequent location of foregut diverticula (>80%). In contrast, epiphrenic diverticula (localized up to 10 cm above the oesophagogastric junction) or diverticula of the oesophageal middle third are observed more rarely[4] (Figure 4.1). Of note, oesophageal pseudodiverticulosis—caused by a dilatation of submucosal glands within the oesophageal wall—will not be dealt with in this chapter, since it represents an aetiologically separate entity.[5]

Aetiology and pathophysiology

The basic pathophysiological mechanism involved in the formation of oesophageal diverticula is an imbalance between the intra-oesophageal pressure and the local stability of the oesophageal wall. Mild intraluminal pressure peaks occur during the normal act of swallowing (intrabolus pressure) but may be extreme in certain motility disorders (jackhammer oesophagus). Typically, oesophageal diverticula develop within preformed or acquired weak spots of the oesophageal muscle coat. The wall of the outpouchings consists of mucosa and submucosa, and they are called 'pulsion' or 'false' diverticula.

Most diverticula arise in the oesophageal sphincter regions. In epiphrenic diverticula, an oesophageal motility disorder can typically be diagnosed with manometric or radiological evaluation. Conversely, the pathogenesis of pharyngo-oesophageal diverticula is less well defined, because motility disorders of the upper oesophageal sphincter are difficult to diagnose by manometry. Another important point is that pharyngo-oesophageal diverticula typically arise in Killian's triangle as a preformed muscular *locus minoris resistentiae*.

Infrequent causes of oesophageal pulsion diverticula are general (e.g. Ehlers–Danlos syndrome) or local tissue weaknesses that may occur following iatrogenic damage of the oesophageal wall after myotomies or tumour enucleations (Figure 4.2a). In addition, pulsion diverticula may develop as a result of distal mechanical obstructions (antireflux surgery, tumours) (Figure 4.2b).

By contrast, so-called traction diverticula (or true diverticula) occur because of external tensile stress, most often in the context of inflammatory adhesions caused by granulomatous diseases such as tuberculosis or sarcoidosis. These 'true' diverticula typically form in the middle third of the oesophagus with close relationship to the tracheobronchial system and are formed by the entire oesophageal wall. Owing to the low prevalence of pulmonary tuberculosis in recent times, traction diverticula have become very rare.[4] Another, extremely rare form of 'true' oesophageal diverticula occurs congenitally as a result of embryonic malformation.[6]

Symptoms and diagnostic work-up

Typical symptoms range from mild or occasional dysphagia to complete aphagia with the need for acute medical care. Another typical symptom is the regurgitation of undigested food components and saliva, which can lead to aspiration with coughing attacks,

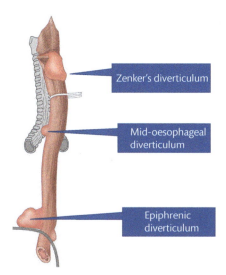

Figure 4.1 Topographic anatomy of the oesophagus with typical localization of oesophageal diverticula.

4 Oesophageal diverticula

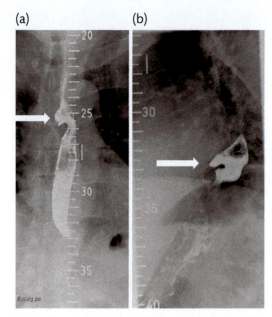

Figure 4.2 Contrast visualization of (a) a mid-oesophageal diverticulum (arrow) occurring after thoracoscopic enucleation of oesophageal leiomyoma, and (b) of an epiphrenic diverticulum (arrow) occurring after laparoscopic fundoplication.

hoarseness, and recurrent pneumonia. Not infrequently, refractory bad breath or disturbing gurgling noises while drinking are reported. Large phreno-oesophageal diverticula may occasionally present as a local swelling of the left side of the neck. Regurgitation of bloody components may be the sign of a tumorous mass in the diverticulum. However, carcinomatous degeneration is extremely rare with a reported incidence of 0.3–0.7%. Only about 60 such cases have been published in the literature.[1,7]

The diagnostic algorithm entails a careful history and an endoscopic, radiographic, manometric, and pH-metric work-up. These diagnostic investigations serve to determine location and size and may help to identify motility disorders or gastro-oesophageal reflux disease. In addition, malignant changes of the oesophagus and the diverticulum lumen should be excluded before therapy.[8,9] The classical radiological contrast study usually allows the size and position of the diverticulum to be determined. In addition, Zenker's diverticulum can be categorized according to Brombart's classification[10] (Table 4.1). In case of unclear findings, a video cinematography may provide further information by dynamic observation of the swallowing act. By contrast, the diagnostic value of flexible video-endoscopy is based on the exclusion of other causes of dysphagia and the possibility of histological identification of mucosal irregularities. Clinical experience shows that small diverticula are detected endoscopically less frequently than by radiological procedures. Rigid endoscopy in the context of diagnostic clarification has become obsolete because of the considerable expenditure on equipment, the increased risk for perforation, the need for anaesthesia, and because of the limited additional benefit. In contrast, high-resolution manometry has gained increasing importance for planning diagnosis and therapy. This is especially true for the treatment of epiphrenic diverticula, as these patients have a high prevalence of specific and unspecific oesophageal motility disorders.[11,12]

Pharyngo-oesophageal diverticulum

Since its first description by Ludlow in 1769[13] and the pathophysiological classification of the disease by von Zenker in 1877,[14] a wide range of therapeutic options has been developed. Zenker's diverticulum arises in Killian's triangle, a muscle-weak area between the thyropharyngeal muscle and the oblique part of the cricopharyngeus (Figure 4.3). As the cricopharyngeal muscle anatomically represents the oesophageal inlet, Zenker's diverticulum in its true sense represents a hypopharyngeal rather than an oesophageal diverticulum. Another (oesophageal) localization of pharyngo-oesophageal diverticula is the so-called Killian–Jamieson gap, which is situated laterally below the cricopharyngeal muscle[15] (Figure 4.3). Pharyngo-oesophageal diverticula are rare with a prevalence of about 0.1%, and most commonly occur between 60 and 80 years of age, with men being affected more frequently than women.[16]

By contrast, cricopharyngeal bars are characterized by hypertrophy and loss of function of the cricopharyngeal muscle without formation of a diverticular sac (Figure 4.4).[17] The prevalence of cricopharyngeal bars (up to 19%) is significantly higher than that of pharyngo-oesophageal diverticula, but symptoms are generally milder and only rarely require therapy.[18]

Aetiology and pathophysiology

The pathogenesis of pharyngo-oesophageal diverticula is still not fully understood and is probably multifactorial. The English surgeon Belsey[19] was the first to point out that increased pharyngeal bolus pressure during swallowing—conditioned by a reduced compliance

Table 4.1 Classification of Zenker's diverticulum according to Brombart

Stage I	2–3 mm, 'rose thorn'-shaped
Stage II	7–8 mm, club-shaped, perpendicular to the oesophagus
Stage III	>10 mm, saccular and slanting downwards
Stage IV	Diverticulum displaces and compresses the oesophagus

Source: data from Brombart M. Zenker's pharyngo-esophageal diverticulum; pathogenic considerations on radiological studies on 26 cases (23 cases in initial stage). *J Belge Radiol*. 1953;36:166–197.

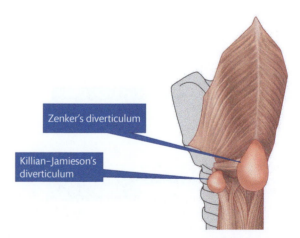

Figure 4.3 Topographic anatomy of Zenker's and Killian-Jamieson's diverticulum.

Pharyngo-oesophageal diverticulum

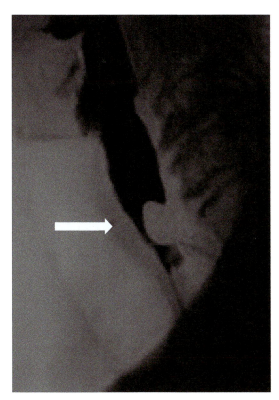

Figure 4.4 Contrast visualization of a cricopharyngeal bar (arrow).

of the upper oesophageal sphincter—may cause pouch formation. This theory was later confirmed by histological and complex manometric investigations.[20–22] Other theories emphasize anatomical or hereditary predispositions. Such theories are supported by reports of increased incidence in families[23] and certain geographical regions. An interesting observation in this regard is the higher prevalence in Northern Europe and North America,[24,25] probably owing to the above-average height of the resident population. Also, the presence and individual size of Killian's triangle seems to be a relevant pathogenetic factor.[24–26] Body size, length of the neck, and the extent of the descent of the larynx may give an explanation why men are more often affected than women. In an autopsy study, a Killian gap was present in 60% of men and 34% of women, and the area of this gap was significantly larger in males.[27]

Therapy and results

The first successful surgery for pharyngo-oesophageal diverticulum was performed by the Irish surgeon de Courcy Wheeler in 1886 by simple transcervical pharyngotomy with external drainage.[28] Most procedures that are still in use today were developed over the following decades, initially focusing solely on surgical elimination of the diverticular pouch. It was not until 1963 that the British surgeon Belsey recommended additional myotomy of the cricopharyngeal muscle and the upper oesophageal musculature to disrupt the pathogenic mechanism of pouch formation.[19] There are different recommendations regarding technique and extent of oesophageal myotomy,[28,29] and it is interesting that myotomy has no demonstrable influence on the functional outcome after the operation.[30] Nevertheless, myotomy is generally recommended by most experts today, because of increased recurrence rates after simple diverticulectomy.

The optimal therapeutic procedure is the subject of an ongoing discussion, which was further stimulated by the introduction of transoral endoscopic stapling techniques in 1993 by Collard[31] and Martin-Hirsch.[32] Rigid endoscopy was originally introduced by Mosher in 1917[33] and further improved by Dohlmann[34] in the 1960s. With the introduction of the carbon dioxide laser by van Overbeek[35] in the 1990s, the transoral access route increasingly won acceptance. Since the mid-1990s, flexible endoscopy has become popular, particularly among gastroenterologists.[36,37] The main benefit of the flexible approach is the possibility of performing the intervention without intubation anaesthesia and hyperextension of the neck.

A major problem for the scientific appraisal of the different therapeutic options is the limitation of available data: although large retrospective case series,[30,38] databases,[39] and meta-analyses[40–45] have been published, there are currently no randomized trials available. However, it may be concluded that both transcervical and transoral procedures have a success rate of 75–100%, and that recurrence rates after transoral techniques, particularly in small (<3 cm) diverticula, are higher.[30,38] Of note, the rate of persistent symptoms appears to be higher after transoral procedures; particularly when the full range of potential symptoms (dysphagia, regurgitation, and aspiration pneumonia) is taken into account. In addition, from our own experience we know that although patients usually report some improvement of symptoms after endoscopic therapy, complete freedom from symptoms is rarely achieved.[30] This phenomenon may be explained by the fact that the common wall between oesophageal and diverticular lumen is usually incompletely divided by transoral procedures, resulting in incomplete bolus clearance (Figure 4.5). In addition, particularly in small diverticula, cricopharyngeal and oesophageal myotomy is often inadequate and does not interrupt the underlying pathogenic mechanism. Another specific problem of the transoral therapy is

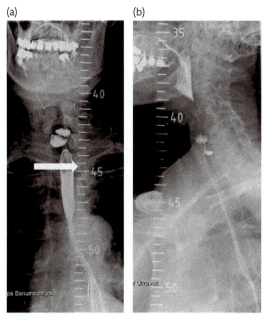

Figure 4.5 Contrast visualization of incomplete division of the common wall between oesophageal and diverticular lumen after flexible endoscopic access.

the fact that the immotile diverticular pouch remains in place, contributing to a poor bolus clearance in this area. This is particularly relevant for larger diverticula (>4 cm), and consequently some authors restrict indications for transoral therapy to medium-sized diverticula (3–4 cm), frail patients, and to cases after open cervicotomy because of the anticipated complex surgical preparation in this situation. The main techniques in open surgical treatment of Zenker's diverticulum established as standard practice are diverticular resection, cranial pexy, and invagination of the pouch. In all open techniques, it is recommended to perform a myotomy of the cricopharyngeal muscle including the top 2–3 cm of oesophageal muscles to avoid recurrences[30] and reduce the risk of leakage.[4] Simple myotomy is often sufficient, especially in small diverticula (<1 cm), since the mucosal level can compensate itself after this measure and the pouch disappears. Diverticulopexy and the invagination technique have the advantage of avoiding opening the oesophageal lumen. Oral feeding and even discharge from hospital may be possible early after surgery, with significant cost reduction.[30] In addition, the risk of oesophageal leakage can be minimized by these procedures. Therefore, in our service diverticulopexy with simultaneous myotomy represents the preferred technique in medium-sized diverticula (1–4 cm), and diverticular resection is reserved for large (>4 cm) diverticula.

Pulsion diverticula of the tubular oesophagus and epiphrenic diverticula

The majority of diverticula of the tubular oesophagus are due to oesophageal motility disorders.[46] Oesophageal pulsion diverticula are rare entities with a prevalence between 0.015% and 2% in radiological studies, and mainly occur in the sixth and seventh decades of life.[4,47] The most common entity is the epiphrenic diverticulum (Figure 4.6), which typically forms at the right side of the oesophagus.

Aetiology and pathophysiology

Manometric studies show a very high prevalence of specific and non-specific oesophageal dysmotility (75–100%),[48–54] and, therefore, simultaneous surgical treatment of the diverticulum and motility disorder (by myotomy) is generally recommended.[4,47] Patients with epiphrenic diverticula demonstrate variable symptoms such as dysphagia, regurgitation, weight loss, thoracic discomfort, and aspiration episodes.[55–59] Similar to pharyngo-oesophageal diverticula, patients with small pouches are often asymptomatic or show only minimal impairments which are usually well controlled by conservative measures. As mentioned by Belsey,[19] the spectrum of symptoms may also be caused by the underlying functional (motility) disorder of the oesophagus.

Therapy and results

For many years, transthoracic resection of the diverticulum was the treatment of choice. In 1959, Effler was the first to suggest a combination of diverticular resection and a long thoracic myotomy from the aortic arch to below the cardia,[60] taking into account the pathogenesis of the disease. However, this approach often resulted in impaired oesophageal clearance and severe reflux symptoms, ulceration, and stenosis. This experience led to today's standard of diverticulectomy,

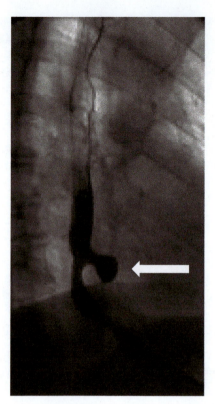

Figure 4.6 Contrast visualization of an epiphrenic diverticulum (arrow).

distal oesophageal myotomy, and an antireflux operation (fundoplication).[47] However, Dor's anterior hemi-fundoplication, which is typically used in this situation, does not provide adequate protection from reflux in all cases. Alternatively, Peracchia and colleagues from Milan suggested preoperative balloon dilation of the lower oesophageal sphincter to avoid myotomy-related reflux.[61] Pre- or intraoperative balloon dilation offers the advantage of preserving the oesophagogastric anatomy and is therefore believed to reduce the incidence of postinterventional reflux disease. However, the scientific evidence for this approach is weak. As an alternative to resection, diverticulopexy should also be mentioned here, which in selected situations makes it possible to eliminate the diverticulum without the risks of leaking from oesophageal sutures.[62,63]

With the advent of minimally invasive surgery in the 1990s, the transabdominal approach to an epiphrenic diverticulum has become increasingly popular. There are several hypothetical advantages of the laparoscopic approach, such as optimized patient comfort by reduced pain, shorter hospital stay, and faster return to normal activities.[61] Moreover, there are also technical arguments in favour of the transabdominal access route, such as an improved exposure of the oesophagogastric junction, potentially simplifying both the oesophageal myotomy and antireflux procedure compared with the transthoracic approach. On the other hand, full dissection of the diverticular neck, which is a prerequisite for accurate placement of the stapler and safe resection of the pouch, can be quite difficult in cases of large diverticula or a high exit point of the pouch. However, the limited data currently available do not permit a conclusive assessment.

Surgical treatment of oesophageal middle- and distal-third diverticula is associated with a perioperative morbidity of up to 50% and a mortality of 1–5%.[46] Suture leakage remains the most important complication with an incidence of up to one-third of patients. In a recent meta-analysis of a retrospective series, the leakage rates were significantly higher in cases without simultaneous myotomy.[54] The typical consequence of oesophageal leakage is the formation of purulent mediastinitis, mediastinal abscess, or pleural empyema, and delayed management is associated with a high risk of severe septicaemia and septic shock. Therefore, careful clinical surveillance and close monitoring of vital and laboratory parameters is paramount in the early postoperative phase. In the event of doubt, prompt and targeted radiological and endoscopic investigations are strongly recommended. In case of leakage, the therapeutic approach must be adapted to the individual postoperative situation and ranges from interventional measures (computed tomography-guided drainage, endoscopic stent placement, and/or endo-vacuum therapy) to surgical re-exploration.

The current published evidence does not allow clear recommendations as to whether a myotomy should be added in every case of an oesophageal pulsion diverticulum. However, this pathology carries a high risk of an underlying motility disorder and we may assume that a myotomy in principle makes sense in most cases. In the majority of patients, postoperative symptom control is 'good' to 'very good' with significant reduction of dysphagia.[54,57,64]

Summary

Oesophageal diverticula are rare entities that are often caused by motility disorders. Diverticular outpouchings may be observed over the entire length of the oesophagus, with a predilection (80% of cases) of the pharyngo-oesophageal region. The risk of malignancy is slightly increased compared with the standard population. Therapeutic management should be tailored to the location, size, symptomatology, and individual perioperative risk of the patient. Based on Herbella et al.,[1] one may summarize that asymptomatic diverticula need no therapy; small (<1 cm) diverticula usually need not be resected; and medium (1–3 cm) and large (>4 cm) diverticula should be treated by resection, diverticulopexy, invagination, or (in case of Zenker's diverticulum) by transoral diverticulo-oesophagostomy. In addition, a myotomy or (in the case of epiphrenic diverticula) alternatively a preoperative balloon dilatation of the sphincter region should be performed. Because of the rarity of oesophageal diverticula and due to the wide range of therapeutic options, expert experience is usually limited even in large hospitals. Therefore, we may conclude that management by an experienced multidisciplinary team using the complete spectrum of today's endoscopic and surgical options is a prerequisite for effective treatment of this rare disease.

REFERENCES

1. Herbella FAM, Patti MG. Modern pathophysiology and treatment of esophageal diverticula. *Langenbecks Arch Surg.* 2012;**397**:29–35.
2. Hoghooghi D, Coakley FV, Breiman RS, Qayyum A, Yeh BM. Frequency and etiology of midesophageal diverticula at barium esophagography. *Clin Imaging.* 2006;**30**:245–247.
3. Watanabe S, Matsuda K, Arima K. Detection of subclinical disorders of the hypopharynx and larynx by gastrointestinal endoscopy. *Endoscopy.* 1996;**28**:295–298.
4. Thomas ML, Anthony AA, Fosh BG, Finch JG, Maddern GJ. Oesophageal diverticula. *Br J Surg.* 2001;**88**:629–642.
5. Herter B, Dittler HJ, Wuttge-Hannig A, Siewert JR. Intramural pseudodiverticulosis of the esophagus: a case series. *Endoscopy.* 1997;**29**:109–113.
6. Lindholm EB, Hansbourgh F, Upp JR Jr, Cilloniz R, Lopoo J. Congenital esophageal diverticulum—a case report and review of literature. *J Pediatr Surg.* 2013;**48**:665–668.
7. Khan AS, Dwivedi RC, Sheikh Z, et al. Systematic review of carcinoma arising in pharyngeal diverticula: a 112-year analysis. *Head Neck.* 2014;**36**:1368–1375.
8. Hung JJ, Hsieh CC, Lin SC, Wang LS. Squamous cell carcinoma in a large epiphrenic esophageal diverticulum. *Dig Dis Sci.* 2009;**54**:1365–1368.
9. Khan AS, Dwivedi RC, Sheikh Z, et al. Systematic review of carcinoma arising in pharyngeal diverticula: a 112-year analysis. *Head Neck.* 2014;**36**:1368–1375.
10. Brombart M. Zenker's pharyngo-esophageal diverticulum; pathogenic considerations on radiological studies on 26 cases (23 cases in initial stage). *J Belge Radiol.* 1953;**36**:166–197.
11. D'Journo XB, Ferraro P, Martin J, Chen LQ, Duranceau A. Lower oesophageal sphincter dysfunction is part of the functional abnormality in epiphrenic diverticulum. *Br J Surg.* 2009;**96**:892–900.
12. Gockel I, Eckardt VF, Junginger T. Epiphrenisches Divertikel. Mögliche Ursachen und chirurgische Therapie. *Chirurg.* 2009;**76**:777–782.
13. Ludlow AA. A case of obstructed deglutition from a preternatural dilation of and bag formed in the pharynx. *Med Observ Inq.* 1769;**3**:85–101.
14. Zenker FZ. Dilatations of the esophagus. In: von Ziemssen H, ed. *Cyclopaedia of the Practice of Medicine, Vol. 3.* London: Low, Marston, Searle & Rivington; 1878:46–68.
15. Udare AS, Mondel PB, Badhe PV. Killian-Jamieson diverticulum. *Indian J Gastroenterol.* 2014;**33**:98.
16. Ferreira LEVVC, Simmons DT, Baron TH. Zenker's diverticula: pathophysiology, clinical presentation, and flexible endoscopic management. *Dis Esophagus.* 2008;**21**:1–8.
17. Cook I. Cricopharyngeal bar and Zenker diverticulum. *Gastroenterol Hepatol.* 2011;**7**:540.
18. Kühn D, Miller S, Ptok M. Cricopharyngeal bar and dysphagia. *Laryngo Rhino Otol.* 2013;**92**:230–233.
19. Belsey R. Functional disease of the oesophagus. *Postgrad Med J.* 1963;**39**:290–298.
20. Lerut T, Guelinckx P, Dom R, et al. Does the musculus cricopharyngeus play a role in the genesis of Zenker's diverticulum? Enzyme histochemical and contractility properties. In: Siewert JR, Hölscher AH, eds. *Diseases of the Esophagus.* Berlin: Springer Verlag; 1988:1018–1023.
21. Cook IJ, Blumbergs P, Cash K, et al. Structural abnormalities of the cricopharyngeus muscle in patients with pharyngeal (Zenker's) diverticulum. *J Gastroenterol Hepatol.* 1992;**7**:556–562.
22. Cook IJ, Gabb M, Panagopoulos V, et al. Pharyngeal (Zenker's) diverticulum is a disorder of upper esophageal sphincter opening. *Gastroenterology.* 1992;**103**:1229–1235.
23. Klockars T, Mäkitie A. Case report of Zenker's diverticulum in identical twins: further evidence for genetic predisposition. *J Laryngol Otol.* 2010;**124**:1129–1131.

24. van Overbeek JJ. Meditation on the pathogenesis of hypopharyngeal (Zenker's) diverticulum and a report of endoscopic treatment in 545 patients. *Ann Otol Rhinol Laryngol*. 1994;**103**:178–185.
25. van Overbeek JJ. Pathogenesis and methods of treatment of Zenker's diverticulum. *Ann Otol Rhinol Laryngol*. 2003;**112**:583–593.
26. Gutschow CA, Bauerfeind P. Pharyngoesophageal diverticulum. *Chirurg*. 2017;**88**:717–728.
27. Anagiotos A, Preuss SF, Koebke J. Morphometric and anthropometric analysis of Killian's triangle. *Laryngoscope*. 2010;**120**:1082–1088.
28. Wheeler W. Pharyngocoele and dilation of the pharynx, with existing diverticulum at lower portion of pharynx lying posterior to the oesophagus, cured by pharyngotomy, being the first of the kind recorded. *Dublin Journal of Medical Science*. 1886;**82**:349–356.
29. Yuan Y, Zhao YF, Hu Y, et al. Surgical treatment of Zenker's diverticulum. *Dig Surg*. 2013;**30**:207–218.
30. Gutschow CA, Hamoir M, Rombaux P, et al. Management of pharyngoesophageal (Zenker's) diverticulum: which technique? *Ann Thorac Surg*. 2002;**74**:1677–1682.
31. Collard JM, Otte JB, Kestens PJ. Endoscopic stapling technique of esophagodiverticulostomy for Zenker's diverticulum. *Ann Thorac Surg*. 1993;**56**:573–576.
32. Martin-Hirsch DP, Newbegin CJ. Autosuture GIA gun: a new application in the treatment of hypopharyngeal diverticula. *J Laryngol Otol*. 1993;**107**:723–725.
33. Jamieson GG, Duranceau AC, Payne WS. Pharyngo-oesophageal diverticulum. In: Jamieson GG, ed. *Surgery of the Oesophagus*. Edinburgh: Churchill Livingstone; 1988:435–443.
34. Dohlman G, Mattsson O. The endoscopic operation for hypopharyngeal diverticula: a roentgencinematographic study. *AMA Arch Otolaryngol*. 1960;**71**:744–752.
35. Wouters B, van Overbeek JJ. Pathogenesis and endoscopic treatment of the hypopharyngeal (Zenker's) diverticulum. *Acta Gastroenterol Belg*. 1990;**53**:323–329.
36. Mulder CJ, den Hartog G, Robijn RJ, Thies JE. Flexible endoscopic treatment of Zenker's diverticulum: a new approach. *Endoscopy*. 1995;**27**:438–442.
37. Ishioka S, Sakai P, Maluf-Filho F, Melo JM. Endoscopic incision of Zenker's diverticula. *Endoscopy*. 1995;**27**:433–437.
38. Bonavina L, Bona D, Abraham M, Saino G, Abate E. Long-term results of endosurgical and open surgical approach for Zenker diverticulum. *World J Gastroenterol*. 2007;**13**:2586–2589.
39. Onwugbufor MT, Obirieze AC, Ortega G, Allen D, Cornwell EE 3rd, Fullum TM. Surgical management of esophageal diverticulum: a review of the Nationwide Inpatient Sample database. *J Surg Res*. 2013;**184**:120–125.
40. Bizzotto A, Iacopini F, Landi R, Costamagna G. Zenker's diverticulum: exploring treatment options. *Acta Otorhinolaryngol Ital*. 2013;**33**:219–229.
41. Yuan Y, Zhao YF, Hu Y, Chen LQ. Surgical treatment of Zenker's diverticulum. *Dig Surg*. 2013;**30**:207–218.
42. Dzeletovic I, Ekbom DC, Baron TH. Flexible endoscopic and surgical management of Zenker's diverticulum. *Expert Rev Gastroenterol Hepatol*. 2012;**6**:449–465.
43. Leong SC, Wilkie MD, Webb CJ. Endoscopic stapling of Zenker's diverticulum: establishing national baselines for auditing clinical outcomes in the United Kingdom. *Eur Arch Otorhinolaryngol*. 2012;**269**:1877–1884.
44. Bonavina L, Rottoli M, Bona D, Siboni S, Russo IS, Bernardi D. Transoral stapling for Zenker diverticulum: effect of the traction suture-assisted technique on long-term outcomes. *Surg Endosc*. 2012;**26**:2856–2861.
45. Parker NP, Misono S. Carbon dioxide laser versus stapler-assisted endoscopic Zenker's diverticulotomy: a systematic review and meta-analysis. *Otolaryngol Head Neck Surg*. 2014;**150**:750–753.
46. Gutschow CA, Schmidt H. Esophageal diverticula (excluding cricopharyngeal diverticula). *Chirurg*. 2018;**89**:401–412.
47. Soares R, Herbella FA, Prachand VN, et al. Epiphrenic diverticulum of the esophagus. From pathophysiology to treatment. *J Gastrointest Surg*. 2010;**14**:2009–2015.
48. Yu L, Wu JX, Chen XH, et al. Laparoscopic diverticulectomy with the aid of intraoperative gastrointestinal endoscopy to treat epiphrenic diverticulum. *J Minim Access Surg*. 2016;**12**:366–369.
49. Fekete F, Vonns C. Surgical management of esophageal thoracic diverticula. *Hepatogastroenterology*. 1992;**39**:97–99.
50. Hudspeth DA, Thorne MT, Conroy R, et al. Management of epiphrenic esophageal diverticula. A fifteen-year experience. *Am Surg*. 1993;**59**:40–42.
51. Peracchia A, Fumagalli U, Rosati R. [Thoracoscopic techniques in treatment of esophageal diseases]. *Chirurg*. 1994;**65**:671–676.
52. Champion JK. Thoracoscopic Belsey fundoplication with 5-year outcomes. *Surg Endosc*. 2003;**17**:1212–1215.
53. Reznik SI, Rice TW, Murthy SC, et al. Assessment of a pathophysiology-directed treatment for symptomatic epiphrenic diverticulum. *Dis Esophagus*. 2007;**20**:320–327.
54. Chan DSY, Foliaki A, Lewis WG, et al. Systematic review and meta-analysis of surgical treatment of non-Zenker's oesophageal diverticula. *J Gastrointest Surg*. 2017;**21**:1067–1075.
55. Zaninotto G, Portale G, Costantini M, et al. Long-term outcome of operated and unoperated epiphrenic diverticula. *J Gastrointest Surg*. 2008;**12**:1485–1490.
56. Altorki NK, Sunagawa M, Skinner DB. Thoracic esophageal diverticula. Why is operation necessary? *J Thorac Cardiovasc Surg*. 1993;**105**:260–264.
57. Benacci JC, Deschamps C, Trastek VF, et al. Epiphrenic diverticulum: results of surgical treatment. *Ann Thorac Surg*. 1993;**55**:1109–1113.
58. Castrucci G, Porziella V, Granone PL, et al. Tailored surgery for esophageal body diverticula. *Eur J Cardiothorac Surg*. 1998;**14**:380–387.
59. Streitz JM Jr, Glick ME, Ellis FH Jr. Selective use of myotomy for treatment of epiphrenic diverticula. Manometric and clinical analysis. *Arch Surg*. 1992;**127**:585–587.
60. Effler DB, Barr D, Groves LK. Epiphrenic diverticulum of the esophagus—surgical treatment. *Arch Surg*. 1959;**79**:459–467.
61. Rosati R, Fumagalli U, Bona S, Bonavina L, Peracchia A. Diverticulectomy, myotomy, and fundoplication through laparoscopy: a new option to treat epiphrenic esophageal diverticula? *Ann Surg*. 1998;**227**:174–178.
62. Altorki NK, Sunagawa M, Skinner DB. Thoracic esophageal diverticula. Why is operation necessary? *J Thorac Cardiovasc Surg*. 1993;**105**:260–264.
63. Nehra D, Lord RV, DeMeester TR, et al. Physiologic basis for the treatment of epiphrenic diverticulum. *Ann Surg*. 2002;**235**:346–354.
64. Macke RA, Luketich JD, Pennathur A, et al. Thoracic esophageal diverticula: a 15-year experience of minimally invasive surgical management. *Ann Thorac Surg*. 2015;**100**:1795–1802.

5

Benign diseases of the stomach
Focus on dyspepsia

Kuniaki Aridome

Introduction

The term dyspepsia means impaired digestion; however, it is also used for a spectrum of symptoms localized by the patient in the epigastric region. The symptoms of dyspepsia may be acute or chronic, although they do not reliably distinguish between organic and functional forms of the disease (Figure 5.1).

Functional gastrointestinal disorders are common and characterized by persistent and recurrent gastrointestinal symptoms. The two most common functional gastrointestinal disorders are irritable bowel syndrome and functional dyspepsia (FD).[1,2] FD is the medical term for a condition that causes an upset stomach, or pain or discomfort in the upper abdomen, near the ribs. FD often recurs over time, and it is difficult for doctors to find a cause in most people. It is one of the most prevalent functional gastrointestinal disorders worldwide, with a prevalence of 11–30%, based on its different definitions (Rome criteria I, II, and III).[3,4]

Most benign diseases of the stomach are attributed to FD and acid-related disorders, such as gastro-oesophageal reflux disease and peptic ulcer disease (PUD). Dyspepsia is also the main manifestation of these acid-related conditions of the stomach. Proton pump inhibitors (PPIs) have dramatically improved the management options available for patients with acid-related disorders. The effectiveness of the currently available antisecretory therapies for these three acid-related diseases has recently gained attention worldwide. Meanwhile, the debate continues regarding the risk of adverse events related to long-term use of PPIs.

Functional dyspepsia

FD is a common gastrointestinal disorder and affects as many as 20% of the global population.[5] Both FD and organic conditions of the stomach or duodenum may provoke similar symptoms.[6] The diagnosis of FD remains one of exclusion, and oesophagogastroduodenoscopy is required to exclude peptic ulceration, oesophagitis, and malignancy (Figure 5.1).[7] In most

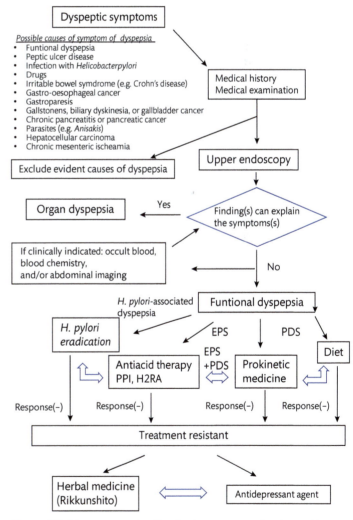

Figure 5.1 Management algorithm for the treatment of patients with functional dyspepsia. Dyspeptic symptoms include epigastric pain and burning, feeling bloated after a meal, early satiation, distension in the epigastric region, nausea, and vomiting. *H. pylori*, *Helicobacter pylori*; PPI, proton pump inhibitor; H2RA, histamine type-2 receptor antagonist.

cases, the cause of FD can be clarified by upper gastrointestinal endoscopy, which shows that less than 10% of patients with dyspepsia have peptic ulcer, less than 1% have gastro-oesophageal cancer, and more than 70% have FD.[8]

FD comprises three subtypes with presumed different pathophysiology and aetiology: postprandial distress syndrome (PDS), epigastric pain syndrome (EPS), and a subtype with overlapping PDS and EPS features. According to the recently revised Rome IV criteria,[9] FD is defined by persistent or recurring dyspepsia for more than 3 months within the past 6 months; no demonstration of a possible organic cause of the symptoms on endoscopy; and no sign that the dyspepsia is relieved by defecation alone or of an association with stool irregularities. The Rome IV criteria divide FD into two subgroups according to the cardinal symptoms: EPS (predominant epigastric pain or burning) and PDS (a feeling of fullness and early satiation).

One of the more prevalent theories currently being investigated is the possible relation between *Helicobacter pylori* infection and FD. Dyspepsia has been shown to occur after intentional *H. pylori* infection, suggesting a correlation with this symptom. However, the role of *H. pylori* in FD remains controversial.[10–13] The Kyoto consensus conference concluded that if patients with FD and *H. pylori* infection respond persistently to eradication therapy, the correct diagnosis is *H. pylori*-associated dyspepsia.[14] The majority who fail to obtain symptom relief despite successful eradication therapy are considered to have FD until proven otherwise. Nevertheless, recent studies have reported that long-term *H. pylori* eradication therapy improves the symptoms of FD.[15] According to the Kyoto consensus conference, FD symptoms are cured from 6 months to 1 year after *H. pylori* eradication therapy.[14] In FD patients with *H. pylori* infection, eradication therapy is recommended, if feasible, before preneoplastic changes develop, to minimize the risk of more serious complications of the infection.

The consensus guidelines recommend PPIs for the treatment of FD.[16] Empirical PPI treatment is expected to provide symptom relief to most patients with dyspepsia who present in clinical practice. The management of FD is often based on the predominant symptoms reported by patients. However, because of the significant overlap between symptoms of gastro-oesophageal reflux disease and FD, management of these conditions closely resembles that of gastro-oesophageal reflux disease, with the exception of surgical interventions. Patients with the EPS subtype can be treated with PPIs, whereas patients with the PDS subtype may be managed primarily with prokinetics, and patients with EPS and PDS can be co-administered PPIs and prokinetics. According to the Kyoto consensus conference, acotiamide–rabeprazole combination therapy, compared with rabeprazole monotherapy, significantly improves both PDS- and EPS-like symptoms.[14] These results suggest that combination therapy can stabilize both EPS and PDS symptoms.

Tricyclic antidepressants are particularly effective for some FD patients with chronic pain.[17,18] However, improvement of clinical symptoms of FD treated with antidepressants is reported to be limited.[19] The disease subtype might have a role in treatment efficacy. Epidemiological studies have shown that psychosocial factors (e.g. anxiety, depression, and stress) are more prevalent in patients with than without FD. A randomized controlled trial evaluated that standard medical therapy plus cognitive behaviour therapy improves short-term outcomes in patients with FD.[20]

Another emerging treatment option includes Rikkunshito, a herbal medicine that improves gastric emptying through 5-hydroxytryptamine-2B-mediated pharmacological action, and tricyclic antidepressants.[21] Rikkunshito improves symptoms of FD through elevation of deacylated ghrelin levels in *H. pylori*-negative patients, and the levels of deacylated ghrelin correlate with the efficacy of Rikkunshito.[22] Different drugs are needed to take account of the clinical symptoms and aetiology in individual patients[15,23] (Figure 5.1).

Peptic ulcer disease

PUD is characterized by a non-malignant lesion in the gastrointestinal mucosa that may be acute, subacute, or chronic. An ulcer in the stomach is called a gastric ulcer. The most common symptom of gastric ulcer is upper abdominal pain that may worsen with eating. The pain is often described as a burning or dull ache. Other symptoms have been described as discomfort characterized by fullness, bloating, distention, or nausea. Potential complications such as haemorrhage (15–20%), perforation (5%), and gastric outlet obstruction should be considered because they sometimes develop to a critical stage (2%).[24]

Two decades ago, almost all peptic ulcers were thought to be 'idiopathic' or caused by excess gastric acid, stress, or diet. The use of non-steroidal anti-inflammatory drugs (NSAIDs) and infection by *H. pylori* are both well-recognized contributors to the aetiology of PUD.[25] *H. pylori* infection has a high prevalence[26] and may be present in more than half of the world's population. It infects the stomach during childhood, and children in developing countries are more commonly infected. *H. pylori* may be passed from person to person through direct contact with saliva, vomit, or faecal matter.[25] *H. pylori* is an important major cause worldwide of PUD and gastric malignancies, such as mucosa-associated tissue lymphoma and gastric adenocarcinoma. Eradication of *H. pylori* improves gastric atrophy and intestinal metaplasia, and is therefore recommended in all patients with PUD.[26] First-line therapy should have an eradication rate of greater than 80%. With the decline in *H. pylori* infection rates and popularization of eradication treatment, the incidence of PUD is decreasing.[27]

Risk factors for gastrointestinal toxicity from NSAID use include older age; chronic use of high-dose NSAIDs; use of aspirin, anticoagulants, or corticosteroids; and a history of ulcers. When an active ulcer is suspected or confirmed, NSAID therapy should be stopped whenever possible; smoking should also be stopped to improve healing. PPIs are the preferred treatment because they provide rapid ulcer healing, especially with large, complicated ulcers.[28,29]

With the success of medical therapy, surgery now has a limited role in the management of PUD, and elective peptic ulcer surgery has been virtually abandoned. The indications for urgent surgery include failure to achieve haemostasis endoscopically, recurrent bleeding despite endoscopic attempts to achieve haemostasis (many surgeons advocate surgery after two failed endoscopic attempts), and perforation.

In the developing world, patients with PUD tend to be young male smokers, while in developed countries, affected patients tend to be adults of advanced age with multiple comorbidities and associated use of NSAIDs or steroids.[30,31] Surgical repair is the treatment of choice for perforated PUD and is a second- or third-line treatment for bleeding ulcers that cannot be managed by endoscopic and/or radiological means. Laparoscopic repair mirrors the techniques of open surgery, and sutureless techniques are more frequently used. This may be a result of training in intracorporeal knotting skills. A recent study compared the effectiveness of a sutureless onlay omental patch with a sutured omental patch.[32]

Disorders after long-term administration of proton pump inhibitors

PPIs are effective drugs that have revolutionized the treatment of peptic acid disorders over the last two decades.[33] Omeprazole was first introduced for clinical use in 1988.[34,35] There is no consensus about how to define chronic PPI use, although most health professionals consider chronic use to be longer than 12 continuous months.[33] PPI-induced inhibition of hydrochloric acid secretion causes iatrogenic hypochlorhydria and hypergastrinaemia. Therefore, long-term use of PPIs may cause various adverse events.

In the stomach, chronic use of PPIs has been associated with the growth of fundic gland polyps that may result in parietal cell hypertrophy.[36-39] The parietal cell changes are believed to be caused by hypergastrinaemia induced by long-term omeprazole intake, because gastrin has a trophic effect on parietal cells. Although the parietal cell abnormalities appear to be reversed after stopping therapy, questions remain regarding the long-term effects of PPIs on parietal cells and the natural history of fundic gland polyps induced by overuse and long-term therapy of PPIs. Several case reports have described PPI-induced neuroendocrine tumours that may result in enterochromaffin-like cell hyperplasia, exposing patients to rebound hydrochloric acid hypersecretion.[40] PPIs have been linked via retrospective studies to an increased risk of enteric infections, including *Clostridium difficile*-associated diarrhoea,[41] community-acquired pneumonia,[42] and chronic kidney disease.[43] The benefits of PPI therapy for appropriate indications need to be considered, along with the likelihood of the proposed risks. Reduction of inappropriate prescribing of PPIs in inpatient and outpatient settings can minimize the potential for adverse events.[44,45]

REFERENCES

1. Drossman DA. The functional gastrointestinal disorders and the Rome III process. *Gastroenterology*. 2006;**130**:1377–1390.
2. Talley NJ. Irritable bowel syndrome. *Intern Med J*. 2006;**36**:724–728.
3. Tack J, Talley NJ, Camilleri M, et al. Functional gastroduodenal disorders. *Gastroenterology*. 2006;**130**:1466–1479.
4. Enck P, Azpiroz F, Boeckxstaens G, et al. Functional dyspepsia. *Nat Rev Dis Primers*. 2017;**3**:17081.
5. Ford AC, Marwaha A, Sood R, et al. Global prevalence of, and risk factors for, uninvestigated dyspepsia: a meta-analysis. *Gut*. 2015;**64**:1049–1057.
6. Halder SL, Talley NJ. Functional dyspepsia: a new Rome III paradigm. *Curr Treat Options Gastroenterol*. 2007;**10**:259–272.
7. Moayyedi P, Talley NJ, Fennerty MB, et al. Can the clinical history distinguish between organic and functional dyspepsia? *JAMA*. 2006;**295**:1566–1576.
8. Ford AC, Marwaha A, Lim A, et al. What is the prevalence of clinically significant endoscopic findings in subjects with dyspepsia? Systematic review and meta-analysis. *Clin Gastroenterol Hepatol*. 2010;**8**:830–837.
9. Stanghellini V, Chan F, Hasler WL, et al. Gastroduodenal disorders. *Gastroenterology*. 2016;**150**:1380–1392.
10. McColl K, Murray L, El-Omar E, Dickson A, et al. Symptomatic benefit from eradicating Helicobacter pylori infection in patients with nonulcer dyspepsia. *N Engl J Med*. 1998;**339**:1869–1874.
11. Laine L, Schoenfeld P, Fennerty MB. Therapy for Helicobacter pylori in patients with nonulcer dyspepsia; a meta-analysis of randomized, controlled trials. *Ann Intern Med*. 2001;**134**:361–369.
12. Talley NJ, Janssens J, Lauritsen K, Rácz I, Bolling-Sternevald E. Eradication of Helicobacter pylori in functional dyspepsia: randomized, double blind placebo-controlled trial with 12 months' follow up. The Optimal Regimen Cures Helicobacter Induced Dyspepsia (ORCHID) Study Group. *BMJ*. 1999;**318**:833–837.
13. Blum AL, Talley NJ, O'Morain C, et al. Lack of effect of treating Helicobacter pylori infection inpatients with nonulcer dyspepsia. *N Engl J Med*. 1998;**339**:1875–1881.
14. Sugano K, Tack J, Kuipers EJ, et al. Kyoto global consensus report on Helicobacter pylori gastritis. *Gut*. 2015;**64**:1353–1367.
15. Du LJ, Chen BR, Kim JJ, et al. Helicobacter pylori eradication therapy for functional dyspepsia: systematic review and meta-analysis. *World J Gastroenterol*. 2016;**22**:3486–3495.
16. Talley NJ, Vakil N; Practice Parameters Committee of the American College of Gastroenterology. Guidelines for the management of dyspepsia. *Am J Gastroenterol*. 2005;**100**:2324–2337.
17. Saarto T, Wiffen PJ. Antidepressants for neuropathic pain. *Cochrane Database Syst Rev*. 2007;**4**:CD005454.
18. Talley NJ, Locke GR, Saito YA, et al. Effect of amitriptyline and escitalopram on functional dyspepsia; a multicenter, randomized controlled study. *Gastroenterology*. 2015;**149**:340–349.
19. Talley NJ, Herrick L, Locke GR. Antidepressants in functional dyspepsia. *Expert Rev Gastroenterology Hepatol*. 2010;**4**:5–8.
20. Orive M, Barrio I, Orive VM. A randomized controlled trial of a 10 week group psychotherapeutic treatment added to standard medical treatment in patients with functional dyspepsia. *J Psychosom Res*. 2015;**78**:563–568.
21. Tatsuta M, Iishi H. Effect of treatment with liu-jun-zi-tang (TJ-43) on gastric emptying and gastrointestinal symptoms in dyspeptic patients. *Aliment Pharmacol Ther*. 1993;**7**:459–462.
22. Togawa K, Matsuzaki J, Kobayakawa M, et al. Association of baseline plasma des-acyl ghrelin level with the response to rikkunshito in patients with functional dyspepsia. *J Gastroenterol Hepatol*. 2016;**31**:334–341.
23. Yamawaki H, Futagami S, Wakabayashi M, et al. Management of functional dyspepsia: state of the art and emerging therapies. *Ther Adv Chronic Dis*. 2018;**9**:23–32.
24. Silverstein F, Graham D, Senior J, et al. Misoprostol reduces gastrointestinal complications in patients with rheumatoid arthritis receiving nonsteroidal anti-inflammatory drugs. A randomized, double-blind, placebo-controlled trial. *Ann Intern Med*. 1995;**123**:241–249.
25. Shiotani A, Graham DY. Pathogenesis and therapy of gastric and duodenal ulcers disease. *J Med Clin N Am*. 2002;**86**:1447–1466.
26. Talley NJ, Vakil N; Practice Parameters Committee of the American College of Gastroenterology. Guidelines for the management of dyspepsia. *Am J Gastroenterol*. 2005;**100**:2324–2337.

27. Lanza FL, Chan FK, Quigley EM; Practice Parameters Committee of the American College of Gastroenterology. Guidelines for prevention of NSAID-related ulcer complications. *Am J Gastroenterol*. 2009;**104**:728–738.
28. Kuipers EJ, Thijs JC, Festen HP. The prevalence of Helicobacter pylori in peptic ulcer disease. *Aliment Pharmacol Ther*. 1995;**9**(Suppl 2):59–69.
29. Wolfe MM, Lichtenstein DR, Singh G. Gastrointestinal toxicity of nonsteroidal anti-inflammatory drugs. *N Engl J Med*. 1999;**340**:1888–1899.
30. Windsor JA, Hill AG. The management of perforated duodenal ulcer. *N Z Med J*. 1995;**108**:47–48.
31. Kang JY, Elders A, Majeed A. Recent trends in hospital admissions and mortality rates for peptic ulcer in Scotland 1982–2002. *Aliment Pharmacol Ther*. 2006;**24**:65–79.
32. Wang YC, Hsieh CH, Lo HC. Sutureless onlay omental patch for the laparoscopic repair of perforated peptic ulcers. *World J Surg*. 2014;**38**:1917–1921.
33. Raugnunath AS, O'Morain C, McLoughlin RC. Review article: the long-term use of proton-pump inhibitors. *Aliment Pharmacol Ther*. 2005;**22**(Suppl 1):S55–S63.
34. Dias MGM, Dani R, Lima EJM. Farmacoterapia, aparelho digestivo e o paciente geriatrico. In: Dani R, ed. *Gastroenterologia Essencial*. 4th ed. Rio de Janeiro: Guanabara Koogan; 2011:1168–1178.
35. Freeman HJ. Proton pump inhibitors and an emerging epidemic of gastric fundic gland polyposis. *World J Gastroenterol*. 2008;**7**:1318–1320.
36. el-Zimaity HM, Jackson FW, Graham DY. Fundic gland polyps developing during omeprazole therapy. *Am J Gastroenterol*. 1997;**92**:1858–1860.
37. Jalving M, Koornstra JJ, Wesseling J, Boezen HM, De Jong S, Kleibeuker JH. Increased risk of fundic gland polyps during long-term proton pump inhibitor therapy. *Aliment Pharmacol Ther*. 2006;**24**:1341–1348.
38. Hongo M, Fujimoto K; Gastric Polyps Study Group. Incidence and risk factor of fundic gland polyp and hyperplastic polyp in long-term proton pump inhibitor therapy: a prospective study in Japan. *J Gastroenterol*. 2010;**45**:618–624.
39. Graham JR. Gastric polyposis: onset during long-term therapy with omeprazole. *Med J Aust*. 1992;**157**:287–288.
40. Jianu CS, Fossmark R, Viset T, et al. Gastric carcinoids after long-term use of a proton pump inhibitor. *Aliment Pharmacol Ther*. 2012;**36**:644–649.
41. Roughead EE, Chan EW, Choi NK, et al. Proton pump inhibitors and risk of Clostridium difficile infection: a multi-country study using sequence symmetry analysis. *Expert Opin Drug Saf*. 2016;**15**:1589–1595.
42. Jena AB, Sun E, Goldman DP, et al. Confounding in the association of proton pump inhibitor use with risk of community-acquired pneumonia. *J Gen Intern Med*. 2013;**28**:223–230.
43. Lazarus B, Chen Y, Wilson FP. Proton pump inhibitor use and the risk of chronic kidney disease. *JAMA Intern Med*. 2016;**176**:238–246.
44. Vaezi MF, Yang YX, Howden CW. Complications of proton pump inhibitor therapy. *Gastroenterology*. 2017;**153**:35–48.
45. Heidelbaugh JJ, Kim AH, Chang R, et al. Overutilization of proton-pump inhibitors: what the clinician needs to know. *Therap Adv Gastroenterol*. 2012;**5**:219–232.

6

Gastro-oesophageal reflux disease

Björn-Ole Stüben, Anna Duprée, and Oliver Mann

Introduction to gastro-oesophageal reflux disease

Gastro-oesophageal reflux disease (GORD) is widely prevalent and occasional GORD-like symptoms occur in 20–40% of adults. Only about 60% of patients with GORD symptoms have reflux, and symptoms from cardiopulmonary disease, gallstone disease, or peptic ulcer disease can mimic those produced by GORD.

The typical symptom of GORD is postprandial, epigastric, and substernal burning pain. Up to 50% of patients also report an acidic taste in their mouths. Chronic microaspirations lead to atypical GORD symptoms. These include reactive airway symptoms, recurrent pneumonias, and even pulmonary fibrosis. Patients on antisecretory medication are more likely to report atypical symptoms and less heartburn.

Some degree of reflux is physiological, and these reflux episodes typically occur postprandially. They are usually short-lived and asymptomatic. Physiological reflux episodes do not typically occur at night. GORD is a condition which develops when the reflux of stomach contents leads to symptoms or complications.

GORD is frequent during pregnancy and may begin at any point, with its severity usually increasing during pregnancy. Predictors are gestational age, pre-existing heartburn, and parity. Symptoms usually resolve after delivery. Additional diagnostic testing is not necessary during pregnancy, and symptom-orientated therapy is indicated.

GORD is classified based on endoscopic findings of the oesophageal mucosa into:

- Erosive reflux disease: characterized by visible breaks in the distal oesophageal mucosa.
- Non-erosive reflux disease: characterized by the presence of GORD symptoms without visible injury to the oesophageal mucosa.

Epidemiology of gastro-oesophageal reflux disease

A systematic review showed that the prevalence of GORD is 18.1–27.8% in North America, 8.8–25.9% in Europe, 8.7–33.1% in the Middle East, 11.6% in Australia, and 23.0% in South America.[1] Asia, where GORD was previously uncommon, has seen an increase in the prevalence of GORD in recent years, and rates of 6–10% have been reported.[2] This increase has been linked to the rise in obesity rates as well as metabolic syndrome.

Traditionally, GORD has been a disease of the middle-aged and older population. However, a recent study showed that there has been a significant increase in the number of younger adults, especially 30–39-year-olds, suffering from GORD.[3]

GORD also has a large socioeconomic impact. Patients with disruptive GORD (daily or greater than weekly symptoms) showed an increase in time off work and decrease in work productivity. GORD also leads to a decrease in physical functioning as well as a lower quality of life.[4]

There is a definite relationship between GORD and obesity. Several meta-analyses suggest an association between body mass index, waist circumference, weight gain, and the presence of symptoms and complications of GORD including erosive reflux disease and Barrett's oesophagus (BO).[5] It is of concern that there has been a well-documented association between body mass index and carcinoma of the oesophagus and gastric cardia.

Clinical features and symptoms of gastro-oesophageal reflux disease

The classical symptoms of GORD are heartburn (pyrosis) and regurgitation:

- Heartburn:
  - Classically described as a retrosternal, burning sensation.
  - Commonly occurs after food intake.
  - Considered significant when:
    - Mild symptoms occur on 2 days or more per week.
    - Moderate or severe symptoms occur on more than 1 day a week.
- Regurgitation:
  - Perception of flow of refluxed gastric content into the mouth or hypopharynx.
  - Typically, patients regurgitate acid material mixed with undigested food (small amounts).

Other symptoms include:

- Dysphagia:
  - Usually present in patients with long-standing heartburn.
  - Can be an indicator of an oesophageal stricture.
  - Commonly seen in patients with erosive oesophagitis.
- GORD-related chest pain:
  - Can mimic angina pectoris, lasting for brief periods or up to hours.
  - Described by patients as burning or squeezing, usually post-prandial or nocturnally.
  - Commonly located substernally, radiating to the back, neck, jaw, or arms.
  - Resolves spontaneously or after the intake of antacids.
- Hypersalivation:
  - Uncommon symptom with patients producing up to 10 mL of saliva per minute in response to reflux.
- Globus sensation:
  - The almost constant sensation of having a lump in the throat.
  - The role of oesophageal reflux in globus symptoms is still uncertain.
- Nausea:
  - Infrequently reported.
  - GORD should be considered in patients with otherwise unexplained nausea.

Diagnosis of gastro-oesophageal reflux disease

The presumptive diagnosis of GORD can often be based on clinical symptoms alone in patients with classic symptoms. The diagnosis is usually made using a combination of typical symptom presentation, testing with endoscopy and ambulatory reflux monitoring, and response to lifestyle modification or therapy with antisecretory drugs.

Patients with mild GORD symptoms that respond to lifestyle modification and/or pharmacological treatment may simply be monitored without further diagnostic work-up. Patients with chest pain should have further diagnostic tests to exclude a cardiac cause before a gastrointestinal evaluation is commenced. Additional evaluation is required for patients with risk factors for BO or abnormal gastrointestinal imaging performed for the evaluation of their symptoms.

A response to proton pump inhibitor (PPI) therapy is not a diagnostic criterion for GORD, as a response to PPIs does not correlate well with objective measures of GORD, such as 24-hour pH monitoring.[6]

Other symptoms listed above may be seen in patients with GORD, but are not sufficient to clinically diagnose GORD, and other disorders need to be excluded before these symptoms can be attributed to GORD. Additional diagnostic tests should be carried out in selected patients with suspected GORD to:

- Rule out alternative diseases mimicking GORD-like symptoms.
- Confirm the diagnosis of GORD.
- Assess for complications of GORD (BO, oesophageal strictures).

Upper gastrointestinal endoscopy

Upper endoscopy is not required to diagnose GORD. However, it can detect oesophageal manifestations of GORD and can rule out malignancies of the upper gastrointestinal tract. Therefore, it is indicated in patients with 'alarm' symptoms and to screen patients who are at a high risk for complications. In the absence of BO, repeat endoscopies are not necessary unless new symptoms arise.

Upper gastrointestinal endoscopy may be normal in patients with GORD or may show varying degrees of oesophagitis. Among patients with untreated GORD, up to 30% show oesophagitis. The degree of oesophagitis does not correlate well with the duration or severity of symptoms.

The ulcerations in peptic oesophagitis are usually located in the distal oesophagus, are irregularly shaped or linear, and usually multiple lesions are present. These findings contrast with the appearance usually seen in patients with infectious or drug-induced oesophagitis. In patients with a long history of GORD, oesophageal strictures, Barrett's metaplasia, or even oesophageal neoplasms may be present.

There are several classifications used to grade the severity of oesophagitis. Of these, the Los Angeles classification is the most thoroughly evaluated and thus most widely applied (Table 6.1).[7] Examples of oesophagitis of increasing severity are shown in Figures 6.1–6.3.

Alternatively, the Savary–Miller classification is historically the most referenced grading of oesophagitis (Table 6.2).[8]

Histological findings

Routine biopsies are not recommended to diagnose GORD but should be performed if macroscopic findings are irregular. This is because histological findings show a low sensitivity, and there are currently no studies examining the efficacy of PPI therapy based on microscopic findings alone. Obtaining mucosal biopsies from normal-appearing gastro-oesophageal junctions (GOJs) has not been shown to be useful in patients with GORD.

Two-thirds of patients with no visible endoscopic findings have histological evidence of oesophageal injury due to GORD and respond to acid suppression. Histological findings are not specific for GORD and may also be seen in patients with eosinophilic oesophagitis, with the dilation of the intercellular spaces (visible on transmission electron microscopy) being the most common finding in

Table 6.1 Los Angeles classification of oesophagitis

Grade	Endoscopic findings
A	One or more mucosal breaks each ≤5 mm in length
B	One or more mucosal breaks >5 mm in length but not continuous between the tops of adjacent mucosal folds
C	One or more mucosal breaks that are continuous between the tops of adjacent mucosal folds
D	Mucosal breaks that involve ≥75% of the luminal circumference

Source: data from Lundell LR, Dent J, Bennett JR, et al. Endoscopic assessment of oesophagitis: clinical and functional correlates and further validation of the Los Angeles classification. *Gut.* 1999;45:172–180; and Armstrong D, Bennett JR, Blum AL, et al. The endoscopic assessment of esophagitis: a progress report on observer agreement. *Gastroenterology.* 1996;111(1):85–92.

Diagnosis of gastro-oesophageal reflux disease

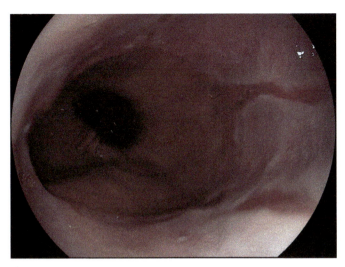

Figure 6.1 Oesophagitis grade B.

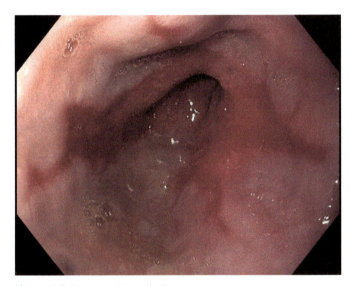

Figure 6.2 Oesophagitis grade C.

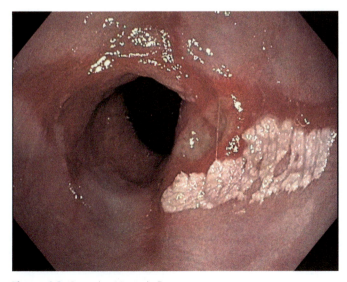

Figure 6.3 Oesophagitis grade D.

Table 6.2 Savary–Miller classification of oesophagitis

Grade	Endoscopic findings
I	One or more non-confluent red spots, with or without exudate
II	Erosive and exudative lesions that may be confluent but not circumferential
III	Circumferential lesions covered by haemorrhagic/pseudomembranous exudate
IV	Deep ulcerations, stenosis, scarring or Barrett's metaplasia

Source: data from Miller G, Savary M, Monnier P, eds. *Notwendige Diagnostik: Endoskopie.* Berlin: Springer.

patients with GORD. Cytokine-triggered inflammation causes other changes typically seen in patients with GORD, including the presence of neutrophils and eosinophils, dilated vascular channels in the papillae of the lamina propria, thickening of the basal cell layer with the presence of pale, squamous cells, and elongation of the papillae of the epithelium.

Radiographic findings

Double-contrast barium swallow is of limited utility and is no longer recommended. The reflux of barium during the study can be provoked in 25–71% of symptomatic patients and 20% of normal controls.[9] This makes it an inaccurate diagnostic method.

However, double-contrast barium swallow allows the identification of the GOJ in relation to the diaphragm and identifies hiatal hernias. This diagnostic method also evaluates for gastric outlet obstruction (in which case fundoplication would be contraindicated). Further, luminal imaging abnormalities can be a sign of upper gastric tract malignancy or achalasia and warrant further diagnostic tests including upper gastrointestinal endoscopy.

Oesophageal manometry

Oesophageal manometry has no role in the diagnosis of GORD. A decreased lower oesophageal sphincter pressure is not specific enough to diagnose GORD. To exclude oesophageal motility disorders, patients with suspected GORD and chest pain and/or dysphagia should have an oesophageal manometry preoperatively, and it is used to evaluate peristaltic function prior to antireflux surgery. Specifically, it is used to rule out achalasia or severe hypomotility, which would be a contraindication to a Nissen fundoplication.

Oesophageal pH monitoring

Ambulatory pH monitoring is used to confirm the diagnosis of GORD or to monitor the adequacy of treatment in those with continued symptoms. It is also indicated prior to surgical or endoscopic treatment in patients with non-erosive reflux disease. It is the only test that allows for correlation of reflux episodes and symptoms. Ambulatory reflux monitoring is not required in patients who present with short- or long-segment BO.

Ambulatory pH monitoring can be performed with a transnasally placed catheter (24 hours) or a wireless, capsule-shaped device (48 hours) that is affixed to the distal oesophageal mucosa. In both cases, the pH sensor is coupled with compact portable data recorders, and computerized data analyses performed. Impedance added to pH monitoring increases the sensitivity for reflux monitoring to close to 90%.

The patients are advised to consume an unrestricted diet during the test period. Studies with wireless devices are conducted over 2–4 days and increasing the monitoring period increases the yield of the study for detecting reflux episodes and correlating those events with symptoms.

The DeMeester score is measured following the testing period. This score, first reported by Johnson and DeMeester in 1974, is a composite score that measures acid exposure during pH monitoring. Acid reflux is defined when the pH of the oesophagus measured 5 cm above the lower oesophageal sphincter drops to 4 or lower. The calculation of the score is based on the standard deviation above the reference values obtained from healthy individuals for six parameters. These include:

- Total number of reflux episodes.
- Total time oesophageal pH is lower than 4.
- Percentage of upright time where oesophageal pH is lower than 4.
- Percentage of supine time where oesophageal pH is lower than 4.
- Number of reflux episodes lasting 5 minutes or longer.
- Longest reflux episode.

When the sum of all parameters leads to the threshold value (14.7) being exceeded, the diagnosis of pathological reflux is confirmed.

Differential diagnosis of gastro-oesophageal reflux disease

Infectious oesophagitis and eosinophilic oesophagitis are differential diagnosis of GORD. Other causes of dysphagia include impaired peristalsis due to an oesophagus motility disorder, and slowly progressive dysphagia for solids with obstruction is suggestive of either a stricture or an oesophageal cancer. Odynophagia may be due to infectious or medication-induced oesophagitis. GORD can be distinguished from these conditions by oesophageal manometry and upper endoscopy with biopsies and ambulatory pH monitoring.

Treatment of gastro-oesophageal reflux disease

Overall treatment strategies

Treatment approaches are based on the frequency and severity of the symptoms reported by patients, as well as the presence of erosive oesophagitis or BO.

A step-up approach is warranted for patients with mild and intermittent symptoms, where the potency of therapy is stepped up until symptom control is achieved.

In treatment naïve patients, lifestyle modifications combined with the use of low-dosage histamine-2 receptor antagonists (H2RAs) should be applied. If symptoms persist despite this treatment, an increase of the H2RAs to twice-daily intake (standard dose) is recommended. Any further increases in the dosage are unlikely to alleviate symptoms.

If symptoms of GORD persist, a switch to PPIs should be initiated at low doses and increased to standard dose if symptoms persist. If symptom control is achieved, treatment should be continued for at least 8 weeks.

For patients suffering from erosive oesophagitis, frequent symptoms (two or more episodes per week, and/or severe symptoms that impair quality of life), step-down approaches are implemented to achieve symptom control. Therapy begins with potent antisecretory agents and then involves decreases in the potency until symptom control is achieved. PPIs should be started in standard doses for 8 weeks once daily in addition to lifestyle modification. Acid suppression can be decreased to low-dose PPIs and subsequently to H2RAs if patients report only mild symptoms. Acid suppression can be discontinued if patients are asymptomatic except for patients with severe oesophagitis or BO.

The advantage of the step-up approach is that minimizes the use of PPIs and their side effects, whereas the step-down therapy provides faster symptom relief. Both therapeutic strategies can be used for patients suffering from GORD.

Lifestyle and dietary modifications

Of all lifestyle or dietary modifications applied in clinical practice, only weight loss and elevation of the head of the bed have been shown to significantly improve oesophageal pH-metry and/or GORD symptoms.[10-12]

The following lifestyle and dietary modifications are applied in clinical practice:

- Weight loss.
- Elevation of the head of the bed especially for patients with nocturnal or laryngeal symptoms (cough, hoarseness).
- Avoidance of meals 2–3 hours before bedtime.
- Selective elimination of dietary triggers, such as caffeine, spicy food, carbonated beverages, and foods with high fat content. For example, substitution of two servings per day of coffee, tea, or carbonated beverages with water led to a reduction in GORD symptoms.[13]
- Promotion of salivation by chewing gum or through lozenges.
- Avoidance of tobacco and alcohol.

Antacids

Antacids do not prevent GORD and their use is therefore limited to intermittent symptom relief. They usually contain a combination of magnesium trisilicate, aluminium hydroxide, or calcium carbonate. These neutralize the gastric pH, and thereby decrease the exposure of the oesophageal mucosa to gastric acid during reflux episodes.

Surface agents and alginates

Surface agents, such as sucralfate, adhere to the mucosal surface and protect from peptic injury. They also promote healing. Both mechanisms are not yet fully understood. The limited efficacy and short duration of symptom relief compared to PPIs limit the use of these agents to management of GORD during pregnancy.[14]

Sodium alginate forms a viscous gum which neutralizes postprandial acid in the stomach. Studies suggest this may be beneficial especially for mild postprandial reflux symptoms, and sodium alginate can also be used as an add-on therapy for patients with refractory GORD.[15,16]

Histamine-2 receptor antagonists

H2RAs decrease acid secretion by inhibiting the histamine-2 receptor on the gastric parietal cell. Tachyphylaxis within 2–6 weeks of initiation limit the use of H2RAs in the treatment of GORD.

Compared to antacids, H2RAs have a slower onset (2 hours) of action but significantly longer duration (4–10 hours) and are also more effective in decreasing the severity and frequency of heartburn symptoms when compared to antacids. While H2RAs show 10–24 times higher healing rates in mild erosive oesophagitis, they are ineffective in patients with severe oesophagitis.[17,18]

H2RA therapy can be used as a maintenance option if patients experience symptom relief and do not suffer from erosive reflux disease. Bedtime H2RA therapy can be used as an add-on to daytime PPI therapy if patients suffer from nocturnal GORD.

Proton pump inhibitors

PPIs are the most potent inhibitors of acid secretion in the stomach by irreversibly binding the hydrogen–potassium ATPase pump. They should be taken 30 minutes prior to food intake in the morning, as the amount of hydrogen–potassium ATPase present in the parietal cell is greatest following long fasting periods. They should be administered daily to provide continuous symptom control.

In patients who fail twice-daily H2RA therapy and patients with erosive oesophagitis, PPIs should be used. Therapy is initiated on standard-dose PPI once daily for 8 weeks. Patients with a partial response should be administered a tailored therapy with adjustment of dose timing or twice-daily application in patients with nocturnal symptoms. Alternatively, a switch to an alternative PPI may be warranted.

There are no major differences in the efficacy of different PPIs. Slow-release PPI should be taken 30 minutes prior to the first meal, while newer PPIs offer dosing flexibility. Most patients report symptom relief under standard-dose PPI therapy, and healing rates of erosive oesophagitis of up to 86% have been reported after this time.[19]

PPIs provide faster symptom relief and are more effective compared to H2RAs.[20] They are also more effective in healing erosive oesophagitis regardless of the severity and the dose and duration of therapy.[21]

Patients with erosive oesophagitis Los Angeles grade C or D should undergo follow-up endoscopy after a 2-month course of PPI therapy. This is performed to assess healing and rule out BO. In the absence of BO, repeat endoscopy after this is not warranted, unless complications such as bleeding, dysphagia, or a significant change in symptoms occurs while on therapy for GORD.

Non-responders following PPI therapy should be further evaluated.

Add-on therapies

In addition to PPIs, prokinetic therapy such as metoclopramide is another medical option. Patients receiving metoclopramide have shown a higher lower oesophagus sphincter pressure as well as enhanced oesophageal peristaltic and faster gastric emptying. However, clinical data confirming the therapeutic effect of metoclopramide in addition to PPI therapy are lacking. The same can be said for the combination with H2RAs. In the clinical setting, there is no role for metoclopramide in patients suffering from GORD unless gastroparesis is present.

The use of GABA antagonists such as baclofen has been demonstrated to be effective in patients suffering from GORD. Baclofen reduces transient relaxations of the lower oesophageal sphincter.[22] There is also evidence that it reduces postprandial reflux events[23] and nocturnal reflux activity.[24] Based on this evidence, a trial of baclofen therapy can be attempted in patients with objective documentation of symptomatic reflux despite PPI therapy. This therapy is off-label and is limited by the side effects of baclofen, including obstipation, dizziness, and somnolence.

Duration of therapy

Patients without BO or severe oesophagitis should receive PPIs in the lowest dose for the shortest appropriate duration. Acid suppression should be discontinued in all asymptomatic patients. Patients with non-complicated GORD can be managed with on-demand or intermittent PPI therapy.

Patients with severe oesophagitis or BO usually require ongoing acid suppression with a PPI at a standard dose, as discontinuing or decreasing acid suppression often leads to recurrence of symptoms and/or complications. Patients found to have Los Angeles grade B–C oesophagitis relapse in nearly 100% of cases within 6 months of pausing PPI therapy.[25] Additionally, patients with BO have been shown to have a decreased risk of dysplasia when continuing PPI therapy.[26]

Risks of PPI therapy

Adverse events associated with PPI therapy include headache, diarrhoea, and dyspepsia. In these patients and patients who fail to respond to PPI therapy, the use of an alternative PPI may be considered. Vitamin or mineral deficiencies and association with community-acquired pneumonia as well as an increased risk for osteoporosis with an increase in hip fractures have also been described.

By increasing gastric pH levels, PPIs may encourage the growth of gut microflora and thereby increase the susceptibility to gastrointestinal infections caused by microorganisms such as *Campylobacter jejuni*, *Escherichia coli*, *Salmonella*, *Clostridium difficile*, and *Vibrio cholerae*. A review found that PPI users were more susceptible to *Salmonella*, *Campylobacter*, and *C. difficile* infections.[27] PPIs should be used with caution in patients at risk from these infections.

The correlation of community-acquired pneumonia and PPI therapy is not clearly documented. A recent meta-analysis showed that short-term PPI use was associated with an increased risk of pneumonia, while long term-use was not.[28] The current literature allows for the recommendation that PPI therapy should not be withheld from patients requiring therapy due to the risk of community-acquired pneumonia.

There are insufficient data to suggest that PPI therapy leads to a significant increase for osteoporosis. While physiological data have in the past suggested that PPIs may inhibit osteoclast-mediated bone resorption by inhibiting the release of ionized calcium from calcium salts and protein-bound calcium, bone analysis of patients with PPI use over 5 years did not demonstrate decreased mineral bone density at the hip or lumbar spine.[29] The increase in hip fractures among PPI users is most likely associated with other risk factors.

The concerns for adverse cardiovascular events due to concomitant use of PPIs and clopidogrel arise from the fact that clopidogrel requires the activation of the enzyme cytochrome P450 2C19. This is the same pathway required for the metabolism of most PPIs.

However, several meta-analyses demonstrated that PPI use did not in fact lead to an increase in adverse cardiovascular events in patients using clopidogrel.[30,31]

Recurrent symptoms

Approximately two-thirds of patients with non-erosive reflux disease report symptom recurrence following the discontinuation of acid suppression. These patients should be treated with acid-suppressive medication at the dose at which they reported symptom control before the therapy was discontinued. If necessary, a step-up approach is necessary for patients reporting inadequate symptom control, with more potent medication being needed.

For patients showing an incomplete response to PPI therapy, medical options are limited. H2RAs can be added as a bedtime medication for patients with symptoms refractory under PPI therapy. However, a study has shown tachyphylaxis towards H2RA after 1 month of therapy.[32] Therefore, H2RAs may be most beneficial when applied on-demand for patients with provocable night-time symptoms.

Refractory gastro-oesophageal reflux disease

Patients who do not respond to PPI therapy and show persistent symptoms associated with GORD can be classed as suffering from refractory GORD.

Any patient that presents with symptoms associated with GORD despite antisecretory medication requires further evaluation. The goal of this evaluation is to differentiate those patients who have reflux as the cause of ongoing symptoms from those who have non-GORD aetiologies.

Endoscopic treatment options

Endoscopic treatment techniques for GORD do not have proven long-term efficacy. These include lower oesophagus sphincter radiofrequency augmentation, the injection of silicone into the lower oesophagus sphincter, and endoscopic suturing. Of these, none showed long-term improvement in symptoms or objective tests such as oesophageal pH measurements and cannot be recommended as therapeutic approaches.

Surgical treatment options

Surgical techniques to treat GORD include laparoscopic fundoplication or bariatric surgery for obese patients. Recently, augmentation of the lower oesophagus sphincter using the LINX Reflux Management System has also gained popularity.

Obese patients who are eligible for surgical therapy for GORD should be considered for bariatric surgery rather than fundoplication. Studies assessing GORD symptoms following Roux-en-Y gastric bypass showed improved symptom control following surgery.[33] Gastric bypass was more effective in reducing reflux symptoms compared to gastric banding.

Fundoplication or LINX implantation is an option for patients with a desire to discontinue medical therapy or patients who suffer from side effects associated with this treatment. Therapy-refractory oesophagitis or persistent symptoms caused by refractory GORD are also referral reasons for surgical therapy.

Fundoplication offers a long-term therapeutic approach to GORD. The best results are seen in patients who demonstrate a good response to PPI therapy and with abnormal pH monitoring with clear symptom correlation.[34] In these patients, good remission results can be expected and are in some cases superior to medical therapy. Fundoplication has also been shown to reduce the use of antisecretory medication. A study with long-term follow-up of patients with GORD showed that 92% of patients in the medical arm were using medical therapy compared to 62% of patients who had undergone antireflux surgery.[35]

Sphincter augmentation using the LINX system constructed of titanium beads has shown a significant reduction in pathological acid oesophageal acid exposure following surgery.[36] This technique has been demonstrated to show consistent symptom relief and pH control with fewer side effects than fundoplication and should be considered in patients with GORD.

It is critical to evaluate for response to PPI prior to surgery. Patients who do not respond to PPI therapy will likely not benefit from surgical therapy, even with an abnormal pH study.[37] These patients suffer from so-called laryngopharyngeal reflux and should not be considered for surgical therapy.

Surgical outcomes are also less encouraging for patients suffering from extraoesophageal symptoms. No significant improvement in pulmonary function was demonstrated in GORD patients after 1 year following Nissen fundoplication.[38] A randomized controlled trial for non-allergic, GORD-related asthma symptoms demonstrated equivalent results for surgical and medical therapy compared with placebo.[39]

Nissen fundoplication

Dr Rudolf Nissen (1896–1981) first described this procedure in the 1950s for the treatment of patients suffering from severe reflux oesophagitis.[40] Initially, a 360° wrap of the stomach around the oesophagus by plication of the anterior and posterior walls of the gastric fundus around the lesser curvature was performed. The laparoscopic Nissen fundoplication is now considered the standard surgical approach for the treatment of GORD, with success rates of 80% being reported in a 20-year follow-up.[41] Despite general reflux alleviation, bloating and inability to belch are the main complications of the Nissen procedure.[42]

Numerous options exist for port placement during a laparoscopic Nissen fundoplication, with all ports being inserted either umbilically or subcostally. The umbilical port is used as the port for the 30° laparoscope.

An atraumatic liver retractor is inserted at the beginning of the operation through the epigastric port. This allows the left hemiliver to be retracted, exposing the hiatus. With the liver retractor inserted, the hiatus should now be visible. Typically, the left triangular ligament is left *in situ* and is only divided if further mobilization is required. A laparoscopic atraumatic instrument is inserted which grasps the stomach or epiphrenic fat in order to retract it caudally.

The lesser omentum is opened above and below the hepatic branch of the anterior vagus nerve, which should be preserved during the procedure.

Dissection continues toward the diaphragm exposing the right crus. The right crus is then dissected bluntly from the oesophagus. The posterior vagus nerve is identified and preserved. The dissection can be continued over the anterior surface of the oesophagus down to the left crus. This should be done carefully in order to avoid a possible accessory left gastric artery running with the hepatic branch of the anterior vagus nerve.

The phreno-oesophageal ligament is divided. The anterior vagus nerve should be identified and preserved. It may be necessary to dissect an mobilize up to 6 cm of the intrathoracic oesophagus in order to gain adequate length. The branches of the vagus nerves should be identified and preserved accordingly. Blunt dissection of the posterior branches from the distal oesophagus is then performed.

Once the oesophagus has been freed, a nylon tape, Penrose drain, or instrument can be used to circumferentially hold the oesophagus. The oesophagus is then retracted anteriorly to expose the posterior hiatus.

The hiatus should be dissected to identify and delineate the diaphragmatic crus. Six centimetres of the distal posterior oesophagus must be fully mobilized. Care should be taken to preserve the inferior phrenic artery; in some cases, the left inferior phrenic artery arises from the left gastric artery and runs along the edge of the right hiatal pillar, and in some cases must be ligated.

In some centres the hiatus is repaired routinely, while others propagate a repair only when necessary. If hiatal repair is performed, sutures should be placed from posterior to anterior and with the hiatus having a diameter of approximately 2.5 cm following repair.

The fundus of the stomach is now grabbed by a blunt instrument and brought behind the oesophagus.

The traditional Nissen procedure involves uniting the posterior and anterior walls of the stomach anteriorly around the gastric fundus to provide a complete 360° 4–5 cm wrap around the lower oesophagus, with or two stitches including the wall of the oesophagus sufficing to prevent slippage of the cardia.

The Nissen–Rossetti modification includes the anterior wall of the fundus alone being used to construct a 360° wrap around the distal oesophagus as illustrated in Figure 6.4. Dividing the short gastric vessels is not recommended in the initial Nissen–Rossetti modification. However, this may be required if tension is present during the wrap.

Toupet fundoplication

Toupet described his technique of fundoplication in 1963.[43] While originally performed through a midline incision, the technique has since been modified and is now mainly performed via laparoscopic techniques.

Comparing the Toupet and Nissen procedures at 6 and 12 months, similar efficacy on GORD symptoms have been observed, with less dysphagia and gas bloat with the former (3% and 23%, respectively) than with the latter (7% and 36%, respectively).[44,45]

For the operation, five trocars are usually inserted, with the 30° laparoscope being inserted umbilically and the other incisions placed in the upper abdomen.

The initial operative steps are performed like the Nissen procedure. After complete mobilization, a posterior hiatoplasty is performed, usually by z-formed sutures with thick polyfilament sutures in order to put adequate tension on a large region. A part of the fundus is pulled behind the oesophagus to the right side. The right part of the fundus is fixed to the right crus with a running suture. Another suture fixes this part of the wrap to the right side of the oesophagus. The corresponding left part of the fundus is chosen and fixed to the left side of the oesophagus as seen in Figure 6.5. A single suture fixes the left fundus to the diaphragm. Vagal nerves should stay out of the sutures.

LINX surgery

The LINX Reflux Management System for the treatment of GORD was first described in 2012 by Bonavina et al.[46] The LINX device is composed of a string of ten or more beads containing a sealed core of magnetic neodymium iron boride. These magnets augment the closure of the lower oesophageal sphincter as illustrated in Figure 6.6. The beads are interconnected by small mobile wires that permit the device to expand, allowing for the passage of food as well as physiological functions such as belching or vomiting.

Various approaches to placement of the LINX device have been described, but the principal steps of the procedure are consistent. The procedure is performed laparoscopically with port placement like fundoplication. Exposure of the GOJ is then necessary. In order

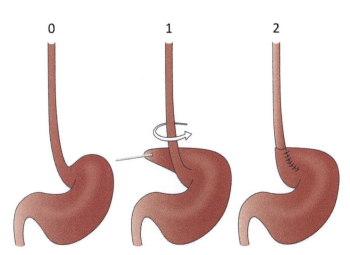

Figure 6.4 Nissen fundoplication.

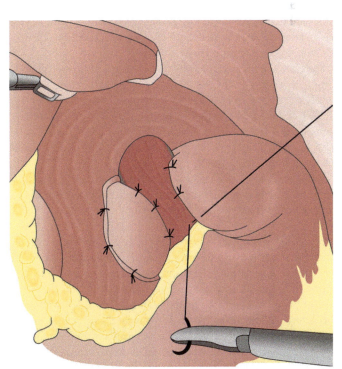

Figure 6.5 Toupet fundoplication.

6 Gastro-oesophageal reflux disease

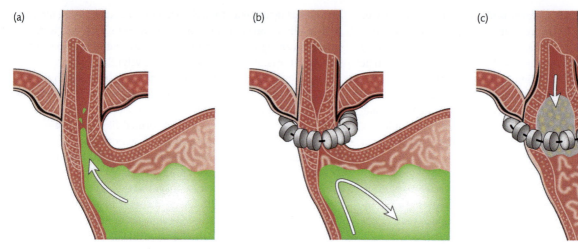

Figure 6.6 LINX antireflux system.

to do this, traction is applied to the stomach, and the peritoneal reflection is divided along the anterior surface of the GOJ. The lateral surface of the left crus is dissected from the fundus, avoiding injury to the short gastric vessels. The gastrohepatic ligament is opened above and below the hepatic branch of the vagus nerve. The posterior vagus nerve is identified and a small opening created between the nerve and the oesophagus. Tissue overlying the oesophageal musculature is dissected. A custom sizing instrument with a numerical indicator corresponding to the size range of the LINX device is used for device selection. The device should fit snugly around the oesophagus without causing an indentation of the tissue. Following selection of an appropriately sized device, the LINX is passed in a right to left direction through the tunnel. Both ends of the LINX device come together on the anterior surface of the oesophagus. The device should be placed at the bottom of the lower oesophageal sphincter just above the peritoneal reflection. Higher placement may cause persistent damage to the distal oesophagus. The ends of the device have a latch mechanism that, once properly aligned, allows the implant to be permanently secured in place.

Posterior crural repair may also be performed during the procedure depending on the size of the observed hiatal defect.

LINX therapy has been shown to be an effective treatment for GORD, and according to the current literature can be carefully recommended.[47] In case of recurrence symptoms, radiographs can be used to verify the correct subdiaphragmic positioning of the LINX system as shown in Figure 6.7.

Bonavina et al. showed that the device decreased oesophageal acid exposure, improved reflux symptoms and quality of life, and allowed cessation of PPIs in the majority of patients.[48]

Surgical risks

Patients undergoing surgery for GORD face some specific procedure-related risks, with the most common adverse event following antireflux surgery being the gas-bloat syndrome which occurs in 15–20% of patients undergoing fundoplication. The risk of developing this, along with the inability to belch, was significantly lower in patients who had undergone partial fundoplication compared to total fundoplication.[49] Small numbers of patients also report persistent postoperative dysphagia following surgery. It must be said that overall rates of postoperative complications are low in the existing studies.

Hiatal hernia

Introduction

Hiatal hernia is a common disorder, characterized by a protrusion of any abdominal structure other than the oesophagus into the thoracic cavity through a widening of the hiatus of the diaphragm.

Migration of the GOJ may result from weakening of the phreno-oesophageal ligament, leading to a proximal displacement of the GOJ. Most cases of hiatal hernia are acquired, though familial clustering has been reported.

Classification

The current anatomical classification has evolved to include a categorization of hiatal hernias into types I–IV. Types II–IV are all referred to as paraoesophageal hernias.

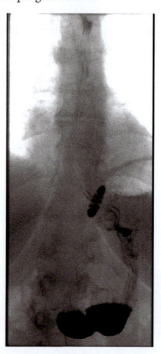

Figure 6.7 LINX system X-ray.

- Type I: sliding hiatal hernias, where the GOJ migrates above the diaphragm with the fundus remaining below the GOJ.
- Type II: pure paraoesophageal hernias; the GOJ remains in its normal anatomical position but a portion of the fundus herniates through the diaphragmatic hiatus adjacent to the oesophagus.
- Type III: combination of types I and II, with both the GOJ and the fundus herniating through the hiatus. The fundus lies above the GOJ.
- Type IV: defined as the presence of an intra-abdominal structure other than stomach within the hernia sac (bowel, omentum, etc.).

Diagnosis

Chest radiographs: a plain chest X-ray may identify soft tissue opacity with or without an air–fluid level within the chest. A retrocardiac air–fluid level is pathognomonic for paraoesophageal hernia. In case of intestinal herniation, visceral gas may also be visible.

Contrast studies: these studies are helpful to evaluate the size and reducibility of the hiatal hernia and to localize precisely the GOJ in relation to the oesophageal hiatus.

Barium is the contrast agent most frequently used for this purpose. Given the increased aspiration risk of patients with paraoesophageal hernias presenting with acute gastric outlet obstruction, ionic water-soluble contrast should be generally avoided.

Computed tomography: this may be carried out to visualize suspected complications from a volvulized paraoesophageal hernia. If intestinal obstruction and strangulation occur, dilated intestinal segments will be visualized with air–fluid levels within the chest cavity and abdomen. The migration of the GOJ above the oesophageal hiatus can be clearly seen.

Oesophagogastroduodenoscopy: this allows for visual assessment of the mucosa of the oesophagus, stomach, and duodenum. Possible reflux oesophagitis or BO can be detected during the exam. Additionally, the size and type of hernia can be determined. In case of an incarcerated volvulized paraoesophageal hernia, evaluation of gastric viability is important among patients undergoing emergency surgery.

Oesophageal manometry: manometry can demonstrate the level of the diaphragmatic crura as well as the location of the lower oesophageal sphincter. The size of the sliding component of a hiatal hernia can then be calculated. Placement of the manometry catheter distal to the lower oesophageal sphincter or below the diaphragm can be difficult in patients with a paraoesophageal hiatal hernia.[50] In patients with a paraoesophageal hiatal hernia, contrast swallow therefore replaces manometry. However, in patients with sliding hiatal hernia, an oesophageal motility study is critical to enable a pH probe to be properly positioned above the lower oesophageal sphincter.

pH testing: this is of limited relevance in the diagnosis of a hiatal hernia but is critical to identify patients who may benefit from antireflux surgery in the presence of increased oesophageal acid exposure.

Nuclear medicine studies, transoesophageal echocardiogram, and endoscopic ultrasound: these can also be used to demonstrate hiatal hernias but are not routinely used for diagnosis.

In summary, upper endoscopy and barium swallow examination are the most used diagnostic tools when assessing for hiatal hernia. Contrast studies are reported to be more sensitive than endoscopy in detecting sliding hiatal hernia, at least in the bariatric population.[51] Incidentally detected hiatal hernias, or those hernias which are minimally symptomatic, may be assessed by endoscopy and contrast radiology. If needed, computed tomography scans can be used to provide additional information to aid with clinical decision-making. Patients with known hiatal hernia and acute abdominal pain should be assessed for gastric volvulus with plain radiographs and endoscopy.[52] Excessive investigation in emergency presentation may lead to delay in treatment with suboptimal outcomes.[53]

Indications for surgery

The major clinical significance of a type I hernia is its association with reflux disease. The indication for repair of a sliding (type I) hiatal hernia is GORD, not the hernia itself. However, the hernia must be repaired during the procedure. A fundoplication to address the reflux disease is mandatory.[54] While there are studies reporting severe symptoms and complications related to sliding hernias, such as dysphagia or gastric ulceration, these are rare.[55,56] Therefore, if gastro-oesophageal reflux is not present, type I sliding hiatal hernias have been thought to be almost inconsequential and not warranting surgical repair.[57]

Many patients with a hiatal hernia are symptomatic.[58] However, these symptoms are usually mild and the condition is detected incidentally on a chest radiograph performed for another reason.[59] Symptoms associated with gastro-oesophageal reflux are usually the reason why patients with sliding hernias are symptomatic. Patients with paraoesophageal hernias often report postprandial chest fullness or shortness of breath, due to increasing portions of the stomach moving up into the thorax, causing respiratory symptoms secondary to pulmonary compression and reduction in forced vital capacity.[58] Reflux symptoms in these patients are uncommon.

In the latter stages, with vascular compromise from volvulus, gastric mucosal ischaemia may cause ulceration, bleeding, and anaemia, and iron deficiency anaemia can be seen in up to 50% of patients with a paraoesophageal hiatal hernia.[60]

When obstruction occurs, symptoms from mild nausea, bloating, or postprandial fullness to acute distress with dysphagia and retching are possible. Patients often describe a full or heavy feeling in the upper abdomen or severe postprandial pain which is often relieved by vomiting. Dysphagia and postprandial fullness can be explained by the compression of the adjacent oesophagus by a progressively expanding herniated stomach and by angulation of the GOJ that occurs as the stomach becomes progressively displaced in the chest.

The natural course of untreated hiatal hernias is unclear as very little data have been published regarding this topic. Only hernias where the gastric fundus has migrated above the diaphragm (paraoesophageal hernias) are at risk of obstruction. The risk of progression from asymptomatic to symptomatic paraoesophageal hernia is approximately 14% per year.[61] Reports of near-universal mortality due to complications, particularly from gastric necrosis, has meant that in the past elective repair of all paraoesophageal hernias in suitable surgical candidates was seen as the standard of care.[62] Patient with symptomatic hernias are thought to be at greater risk of developing complications, and elective repair in these patients is particularly important.[63] Recent reports have shown that mortality rates for emergency paraoesophageal hernias operations are much lower than previously reported,[64] with mortality rates as low as 0–5.4%,[65] though average mortality rates for emergency hiatal hernia surgery are high at around 17%.[66] The risk of developing acute symptoms requiring emergency surgery is thought to be less than 2% per year.[66,67]

The recent data suggest that, contrary to past dictum, routine elective repair of completely asymptomatic paraoesophageal hernias may not be indicated.[66] Based on recent studies, repair should be reserved for patients with symptoms of gastric outlet obstruction, severe gastro-oesophageal reflux, or anaemia, and those with possible gastric strangulation.[67,68]

Strangulation of the stomach can result from acute gastric volvulus with ischaemia, necrosis, and perforation of the stomach. Treatment includes laparoscopic or open reduction of the stomach and limited gastric resection in cases of gastric necrosis.

Technical approach

Large hiatal hernias can be repaired either transabdominally (open or laparoscopic) or via thoracotomy, usually through the left chest. There are no randomized trials comparing open transthoracic versus open transabdominal hiatal hernia repair. Laparoscopic approaches have shown decreased perioperative morbidity and mortality compared to open transthoracic repair.[69] The transthoracic approach allows for good visualization of the oesophagus as well as maximal mobilization, but the increased morbidity and prolonged recovery have rendered this technique almost obsolete except in rare circumstances. Therefore, the laparoscopic approach is the current standard of care. Transabdominal open repair may be most appropriate in an emergency where there is peritoneal contamination or gastric necrosis.[65]

Laparoscopic hiatal hernia repair results in less postoperative pain compared with the open approach. Postoperative respiratory complications are reduced, and studies have shown shorter hospital stay and less morbidity resulting from the minimally invasive approach.[70–72] Recurrence rates between laparoscopic and open repair are similar.

Sac dissection during paraoesophageal hernia repair is thought to release the tethering of the oesophagus, facilitating intraoperative reduction of the hernia and decreasing early recurrence, as well as protecting the oesophagus from iatrogenic damage.[73] Prior to addressing the sac on the right side of the oesophagus, the left gastric vessels should be reduced into the abdomen to prevent injury. Subsequent excision of the peritoneal hernia sac may be performed routinely.

Sac excision can be difficult in large hiatal hernias, and excision in these circumstances may predispose to vagal injury. When comparing complete with partial sac excision, partial sax excision has shown trends towards higher recurrence without showing a significant statistical difference.[74] When complete sac excision is not safely possible, partial sac excision should be performed to allow the fundoplication to be performed without excess bulk by a large residual sac.

Primary sutured crural repair has been the mainstay of practice for many years, but objective follow-up has suggested very high recurrence rates of 42% and higher after laparoscopic paraoesophageal hernia repair.[75] This has prompted many authors to advocate that the crural repair be reinforced. The ideal mesh and technique are unknown at this point. Most are applied in onlay technique following sutured crural repair.

Short-term results are supportive of reinforced hiatoplasty, but no long-term evidence is available to support this and is necessary to safely advocate the use of mesh reinforcement in patients with hiatal hernia.[76,77]

Similarities have been drawn to the Angelchik prosthesis, used in past decades as an antireflux barrier. These were shown to cause erosions into the oesophageal lumen.[78] Available data considering mesh complications are from studies with short-term follow-up. In these, complications are reported for both biological and synthetic meshes.[79,80] Of the possible complications, mesh erosion of the oesophagus is by far the most feared complication.[81] Other complications include oesophageal stenosis, pericardial tamponade, and effusion.

There have been reports on varying techniques for the fixation of meshes, including glues, tacks, and sutures.[82,83] Inadequate evidence exists for a recommendation to be made regarding optimal fixation techniques.

Many surgeons see fundoplication as a step of the repair for hiatal hernia. This is performed to aid in prevention of postoperative gastro-oesophageal reflux and to buttress the repair to prevent recurrence.[84] This is supported by findings that most patients with paraoesophageal hernias have an incompetent lower oesophageal sphincter.[85] There is, however, no high-level evidence to support this practice of routine fundoplication; case reports form most of the evidence base, with mixed conclusions. The current literature in respect to hernia recurrence following fundoplication is also inconclusive.

Extensive oesophageal mobilization is essential in preventing hiatal hernia recurrence, and bringing the GOJ 2–3 cm into the abdomen without tension is recommended.[86,87] High mediastinal dissection may be necessary to facilitate this. Failure to bring the GOJ into the abdomen by mobilization necessitates an oesophageal lengthening procedure.[88] A Collis gastroplasty is suggested in cases where a short oesophagus is encountered during hiatal hernia repair.[89] However, dysphagia has been shown to be a problem following Collis gastroplasty, as the neo-oesophagus does not display normal peristaltic activity.[90]

Gastropexy

Patients with large hiatal hernias undergoing laparoscopic repair and additionally receiving anterior gastropexy show significantly reduced hernia recurrence rates.[91] There have been other reports showing patients having laparoscopic paraoesophageal hernia repair with and without gastropexy, with no significant difference in recurrence rates.[92]

There have been studies on patients receiving hernia reduction and gastropexy alone without cruroplasty or sac excision, particularly in high-risk symptomatic patients. At radiological recurrence rates of 22% at 3 months postoperatively,[93,94] gastropexy alone should not be the aim of surgery but rather a fallback option.

Recurrent hiatal hernia

If symptoms match anatomical findings, recurrent hiatal hernia repair is indicated.[88] In experienced hands, revisional surgery is possible laparoscopically.[95] If fundoplication was primarily carried out, it should be taken down in its entirety, the right and left crura exposed, and the hernia sac excised, ensuring adequate intraabdominal oesophagus length.[95] Success rates of surgical interventions for laparoscopic revisional hiatal hernia approaches that of primary repair[76] but recurrence rates are higher. Although mesh can be used during these operations, the data to recommend their use are under-powered.

Barrett's disease

Introduction

BO is among the most common conditions encountered in clinical practice. This is a change of the normal squamous epithelium of the distal oesophagus to a columnar-lined intestinal metaplasia (IM).

Recent studies suggest that GORD is increasing in prevalence worldwide.[1] The diagnosis of GORD is associated with a 10–15% risk of BO, thus the increase of GORD will most likely be associated with a subsequent increase in the incidence of BO. There are various risk factors associated with the development of BO apart from GORD including male sex, obesity,[96] and age over 50 years.[97,98] The goal of a screening and surveillance programme for BO is to identify individuals at risk for progression to oesophageal adenocarcinoma, a malignancy which has been increasing for years.[99]

Definition

According to the British Society of Gastroenterology, BO is defined as the presence of 1 cm or more of metaplastic columnar epithelium replacing the stratified squamous epithelium which normally lines the distal oesophagus. The reasons why segments less than 1 cm have been classified as 'specialized IM of the oesophagogastric junction' and not BO are the high interobserver variability, as well as the low risk for oesophageal adenocarcinoma in these cases.[100]

In order to properly diagnose BO, it is essential to correctly identify the GOJ during endoscopy. This is possible by visualizing the distal end of the palisade vessels, which lie in the oesophageal mucosa but penetrate the submucosal layer at the GOJ, or by identifying the proximal end of the gastric folds. These two landmarks should coincide with the GOJ. The identification of these landmarks can be inconsistent due to peristalsis, the degree of insufflation during endoscopy, as well as anatomical vascular variants.

Studies have shown that using the gastric folds to identify the GOJ leads to a significant improvement in diagnostic compared to the palisading criteria.[101] Therefore, it is recommended that the proximal limit of the gastric folds be delineated under minimal insufflation to identify the GOJ during endoscopy.

From a histopathological perspective, the true GOJ is distal to the end of the tubular oesophagus and proximal to rugal folds as shown by the presence of submucosal oesophageal glands in this region. Hence, the distinction between columnar-lined oesophagus and intestinal metaplasia at the gastric cardia can only be made when columnar mucosa with or without IM is seen juxtaposed with native anatomical oesophageal structures such as submucosal glands and/or gland ducts. However, native structures are often lacking in biopsy samples, making the histopathological identification of the GOJ difficult. While the presence of IM in biopsy samples is highly corroborative for the diagnosis of BO, IM at the gastric cardia cannot be ruled out in samples lacking native structures.

Recent population studies suggest that of the types of metaplastic columnar epithelium in the oesophagus, intestinal is biologically most unstable and therefore presents the greatest risk of neoplastic progression to adenocarcinoma following dysplasia.[102] This has led to the American Gastroenterological Association making the presence of IM a requirement for the diagnosis of BO. The British Society of Gastroenterology, by contrast, does not see IM as a requirement, as sampling errors in biopsy samples may lead to underreporting of the disease.

Currently, the British Society of Gastroenterology recommends that IM is not a requirement for the diagnosis of BO, but should be considered when deciding on follow-up and surveillance of patients with IM.

Classification

The Prague classification was first described in 2006 and assesses the circumferential (C) and maximal extent (M) of the endoscopically visualized Barrett's segment as well as endoscopic landmarks such as diaphragmatic pinch and the proximal extent of the gastric folds. It is based on validated and consensus-driven criteria.[103]

Segments of BO measuring greater than 3 cm are classified as long-segment BO, with segments less than 3 cm classified as short-segment BO.[103] It is recommended that a uniform classification measuring length and shape of the columnar-lined segment be used to facilitate diagnosis to help determine the level of diagnostic confidence and aid communication between clinicians. These criteria are also important when evaluating for the risk of adenocarcinoma development, which can differ with segment length.

There are minimum endoscopic requirements when reporting the finding of BO apart from the Prague classification. These include describing the distance of the Barrett's islands from the incisors, documenting the number of lesions, as well as the visual description of the lesions according to the Paris classification,[104] where these lesions are classified as:

- Protruded pedunculated.
- Protruded sessile.
- Superficial elevated.
- Superficial depressed.
- Flat.
- Excavated.

Biopsies of these lesions should be taken according to the Seattle biopsy protocol, which requires four-quadrant biopsies every 2 cm as well as targeted biopsies on macroscopically visible lesions.[105]

Epidemiology

The majority of BO cases presumably go unrecognized.[106] Estimates of the prevalence in the general population vary widely, and rates of up to 20% have been described depending on the criteria used to establish the diagnosis and the population studied.[107–109] The mean age at diagnosis for patients with BO is approximately 55 years,[110] and male sex has been consistently identified as a risk factor for BO, with BO being twice as common in men than in women.[111] In the Western world, white individuals are more likely to have BO than Hispanic or Asian people, while the prevalence appears to be lowest in black individuals.[112,113] In Asia, BO has previously been considered a rare condition. However, a meta-analysis showed a remarkably high pooled prevalence (1.3%) of BO confirmed by histology.[114]

Risk factors

GORD

In patients with chronic GORD, 15% have been shown to suffer from BO.[115] Symptom duration has been shown to be a risk factor for the development of BO. The odds ratio for BO increased to 3.0 and 6.4 when symptoms were present for greater than 5 and greater than 10 years, respectively.[116]

Age

The risk for BO increases with age. In a retrospective study, the yield of BO in white men with GORD was 2% in the third decade of life but increased to 9% in the sixth decade.[97] Patients reporting GORD symptoms at least weekly before the age of 30 years have shown to have the highest risk for BO.[117]

Sex

Men have consistently shown higher BO rates than women, with a pooled male/female ratio of 2:1.[111]

Tobacco usage and alcohol consumption

A 2013 meta-analysis based on 39 studies demonstrated tobacco usage as a risk factor for the development of BO, possibly due to an increased risk of GORD.[118] In contrast to tobaccos use, no increase of BO has been demonstrated in patients consuming alcohol, with date suggesting that wine consumption may even have a protective effect.[119,120]

Obesity

Obesity is an independent risk factor for BO and oesophageal adenocarcinoma. Central obesity in particular is a risk factor for BO for both men and women compared to individuals with a normal body habitus.[96,121]

Family history

The presence of a family history for BO shows a strong association with BO.[122] Compared to controls, BO was more common in individuals with first- or second-degree relatives who also suffered from BO. Recently, single nucleotide polymorphisms on gene loci which may increase the susceptibility to BO development have been described.[123,124]

Screening

Survival rate for invasive oesophageal adenocarcinoma is very poor with less than 13% survival at 5 years.[125] The aim of endoscopic surveillance is to detect cancer at a stage when curative therapy is possible. Specifically, surveillance should detect cancer before invasion of the submucosa when the risk of lymph node metastases significantly increases.

Endoscopic screening is standard for patients with BO. This is based on the unproven assumption that the practice may reduce deaths from a progression into oesophageal adenocarcinoma, thereby prolonging or improving survival. Guidelines generally have recommended endoscopic surveillance for patients with BO at intervals that vary with grade of dysplasia found in the metaplastic epithelium as well as the segment length. Intervals of 3–5 years have been suggested for patients who have no dysplasia, 6–12 months for those found to have low-grade dysplasia, and every 3 months for patients with high-grade dysplasia who have not undergone endoscopic ablation therapy. The existing evidence, derived from retrospective or poorly controlled studies, suggests that endoscopic surveillance can reduce mortality from oesophageal adenocarcinoma when attention is paid to standard biopsy protocols like the Seattle biopsy protocol.

Chemoprevention

The use of pharmacological agents or surgical techniques to prevent the development of cancer is referred to as chemoprevention. Most patients with BO have reflux symptoms and are recommended to take medical therapy for symptomatic control. Of these drugs, PPIs show the best results in terms of symptomatic relief. While these drugs are recommended for symptom control, there is not yet sufficient evidence from the current data to advocate acid suppression as chemopreventive agents in BO.

Antireflux surgery, especially the Nissen fundoplication, has been suggested to promote the regression of BO and prevent progression to dysplasia.[126,127] However, this is based on small retrospective studies. Antireflux surgery has not been shown to be superior to pharmacological acid suppression for the prevention of neoplastic progression of BO.

Endoscopic treatment

The goal of endoscopic eradication therapy for patients with dysplasia in BO is to permanently eliminate all IM and achieve a complete reversion to squamous epithelium. Complete eradication appears to be more effective than therapy that removes only a localized area of dysplasia. The data to date show that reversion to squamous epithelium can persist for up to 5 years following endoscopic treatment.

In the absence of dysplasia, endoscopic eradication therapy is not suggested for the general population of patients with BO. However, radiofrequency ablation with or without endoscopic mucosal resection should be considered as a therapeutic option for select individuals with non-dysplastic BO who are at an increased risk for progression to high-grade dysplasia or cancer. Standardized criteria to identify this population have not been fully defined at this time. Endoscopic eradication therapy with radiofrequency ablation should also be a therapeutic option for treatment of patients with confirmed low-grade dysplasia in BO, as radiofrequency ablation therapy for patients with low-grade dysplasia leads to reversion to normal squamous epithelium in more than 90% of cases.

Radiofrequency ablation therapy for high-grade dysplasia reduces progression to oesophageal cancer. Several uncontrolled trials have shown a reduction in cancer development and sustained reversion to squamous mucosa in a large percentage of patients.

EMR is both a staging procedure and a potentially therapeutic procedure that should be performed in patients who have dysplasia associated with visible mucosal irregularities in BO.

Alternative therapeutic approaches such as endoscopic eradication therapy with cryotherapy for patients with confirmed low-grade or high-grade dysplasia within BO have not been studied long term, and further studies are needed to assess whether reversion to squamous epithelium can persist after cryotherapy.

Oesophagectomy

Although surgery is an effective treatment for Barrett's neoplasia, it is associated with significant morbidity and mortality compared with endoscopic therapy. The current literature suggests that endoscopic therapy for mucosal oesophageal adenocarcinoma has similar long-term disease-specific survival to surgery, but lower death rates.[128]

However, surgical treatment is considered the treatment of choice for early adenocarcinoma which has extended into the submucosa because of the risk of lymph node metastasis.

REFERENCES

1. El-Serag HB, Sweet S, Winchester CC, Dent J. Update on the epidemiology of gastro-oesophageal reflux disease: a systematic review. *Gut*. 2014;**63**:871–880.
2. Goh KL. Gastroesophageal reflux disease in Asia: a historical perspective and present challenges. *J Gastroenterol Hepatol*. 2011;**26**(Suppl 1):2–10.
3. Yamasaki T, Hemond C, Eisa M, Ganocy S, Fass R. The changing epidemiology of gastroesophageal reflux disease: are patients getting younger? *J Neurogastroenterol Motil*. 2018;**24**:559–569.
4. Becher A, El-Serag H. Systematic review: the association between symptomatic response to proton pump inhibitors and health-related quality of life in patients with gastro-oesophageal reflux disease. *Aliment Pharmacol Ther*. 2011;**34**:618–627.
5. Corley DA, Kubo A. Body mass index and gastroesophageal reflux disease: a systematic review and meta-analysis. *Am J Gastroenterol*. 2006;**101**:2619–2628.
6. Numans ME, Lau J, de Wit NJ, Bonis PA. Short-term treatment with proton-pump inhibitors as a test for gastroesophageal reflux disease: a meta-analysis of diagnostic test characteristics. *Ann Intern Med*. 2004;**140**:518–527.
7. Lundell LR, Dent J, Bennett JR, et al. Endoscopic assessment of oesophagitis: clinical and functional correlates and further validation of the Los Angeles classification. *Gut*. 1999;**45**:172–180.
8. Miller G, Savary M, Monnier P, eds. *Notwendige Diagnostik: Endoskopie*. Berlin: Springer; 1981.
9. Sellar RJ, De Caestecker JS, Heading RC. Barium radiology: a sensitive test for gastro-oesophageal reflux. *Clin Radiol*. 1987;**38**:303–307.
10. Kaltenbach T, Crockett S, Gerson LB. Are lifestyle measures effective in patients with gastroesophageal reflux disease? An evidence-based approach. *Arch Intern Med*. 2006;**166**:965–971.
11. Aslam M, Slaughter JC, Goutte M, Garrett CG, Hagaman D, Vaezi MF. Nonlinear relationship between body mass index and esophageal acid exposure in the extraesophageal manifestations of reflux. *Clin Gastroenterol Hepatol*. 2012;**10**:874–878.
12. Ness-Jensen E, Lindam A, Lagergren J, Hveem K. Weight loss and reduction in gastroesophageal reflux. A prospective population-based cohort study: the HUNT study. *Am J Gastroenterol*. 2013;**108**:376–382.
13. Mehta RS, Song M, Staller K, Chan AT. Association between beverage intake and incidence of gastroesophageal reflux symptoms. *Clin Gastroenterol Hepatol*. 2019;**18**:2226–2233.
14. Simon B, Ravelli GP, Goffin H. Sucralfate gel versus placebo in patients with non-erosive gastro-oesophageal reflux disease. *Aliment Pharmacol Ther*. 1996;**10**:441–446.
15. Poynard T, Vernisse B, Agostini H. Randomized, multicentre comparison of sodium alginate and cisapride in the symptomatic treatment of uncomplicated gastro-oesophageal reflux. *Aliment Pharmacol Ther*. 1998;**12**:159–165.
16. Chiu CT, Hsu CM, Wang CC, et al. Randomised clinical trial: sodium alginate oral suspension is non-inferior to omeprazole in the treatment of patients with non-erosive gastroesophageal disease. *Aliment Pharmacol Ther*. 2013;**38**:1054–1064.
17. Sabesin SM, Berlin RG, Humphries TJ, Bradstreet DC, Walton-Bowen KL, Zaidi S. Famotidine relieves symptoms of gastroesophageal reflux disease and heals erosions and ulcerations. Results of a multicenter, placebo-controlled, dose-ranging study. USA Merck Gastroesophageal Reflux Disease Study Group. *Arch Intern Med*. 1991;**151**:2394–2400.
18. Cloud ML, Offen WW, Robinson M. Nizatidine versus placebo in gastro-oesophageal reflux disease: a 12-week, multicentre, randomised, double-blind study. *Br J Clin Pract Suppl*. 1994;**76**:3–10.
19. Hunt R. Acid suppression for reflux disease: 'off-the-peg' or a tailored approach? *Clin Gastroenterol Hepatol*. 2012;**10**:210–213.
20. Chiba N, De Gara CJ, Wilkinson JM, Hunt RH. Speed of healing and symptom relief in grade II to IV gastroesophageal reflux disease: a meta-analysis. *Gastroenterology*. 1997;**112**:1798–1810.
21. Wang WH, Huang JQ, Zheng GF, et al. Head-to-head comparison of H2-receptor antagonists and proton pump inhibitors in the treatment of erosive esophagitis: a meta-analysis. *World J Gastroenterol*. 2005;**11**:4067–4077.
22. Grossi L, Spezzaferro M, Sacco LF, Marzio L. Effect of baclofen on oesophageal motility and transient lower oesophageal sphincter relaxations in GORD patients: a 48-h manometric study. *Neurogastroenterol Motil*. 2008;**20**:760–766.
23. Vela MF, Tutuian R, Katz PO, Castell DO. Baclofen decreases acid and non-acid post-prandial gastro-oesophageal reflux measured by combined multichannel intraluminal impedance and pH. *Aliment Pharmacol Ther*. 2003;**17**:243–251.
24. Orr WC, Goodrich S, Wright S, Shepherd K, Mellow M. The effect of baclofen on nocturnal gastroesophageal reflux and measures of sleep quality: a randomized, cross-over trial. *Neurogastroenterol Motil*. 2012;**24**:553–559.
25. Schindlbeck NE, Klauser AG, Berghammer G, Londong W, Muller-Lissner SA. Three year follow up of patients with gastrooesophageal reflux disease. *Gut*. 1992;**33**:1016–1019.
26. El-Serag HB, Aguirre TV, Davis S, Kuebeler M, Bhattacharyya A, Sampliner RE. Proton pump inhibitors are associated with reduced incidence of dysplasia in Barrett's esophagus. *Am J Gastroenterol*. 2004;**99**:1877–1883.
27. Bavishi C, Dupont HL. Systematic review: the use of proton pump inhibitors and increased susceptibility to enteric infection. *Aliment Pharmacol Ther*. 2011;**34**:1269–1281.
28. Johnstone J, Nerenberg K, Loeb M. Meta-analysis: proton pump inhibitor use and the risk of community-acquired pneumonia. *Aliment Pharmacol Ther*. 2010;**31**:1165–1177.
29. Targownik LE, Lix LM, Leung S, Leslie WD. Proton-pump inhibitor use is not associated with osteoporosis or accelerated bone mineral density loss. *Gastroenterology*. 2010;**138**:896–904.
30. Kwok CS, Jeevanantham V, Dawn B, Loke YK. No consistent evidence of differential cardiovascular risk amongst proton-pump inhibitors when used with clopidogrel: meta-analysis. *Int J Cardiol*. 2013;**167**:965–974.
31. Yacoub R. A meta-analysis of impact of proton pump inhibitors on antiplatelet effect of clopidogrel. *Cardiovasc Ther*. 2012;**30**:357.

32. Fackler WK, Ours TM, Vaezi MF, Richter JE. Long-term effect of H2RA therapy on nocturnal gastric acid breakthrough. *Gastroenterology*. 2002;**122**:625–632.
33. De Groot NL, Burgerhart JS, Van De Meeberg PC, de Vries DR, Smout AJ, Siersema PD. Systematic review: the effects of conservative and surgical treatment for obesity on gastro-oesophageal reflux disease. *Aliment Pharmacol Ther*. 2009;**30**:1091–1102.
34. Oelschlager BK, Quiroga E, Parra JD, Cahill M, Polissar N, Pellegrini CA. Long-term outcomes after laparoscopic antireflux surgery. *Am J Gastroenterol*. 2008;**103**:280–287.
35. Spechler SJ, Lee E, Ahnen D, et al. Long-term outcome of medical and surgical therapies for gastroesophageal reflux disease: follow-up of a randomized controlled trial. *JAMA*. 2001;**285**:2331–2338.
36. Lipham JC, DeMeester TR, Ganz RA, et al. The LINX(R) reflux management system: confirmed safety and efficacy now at 4 years. *Surgic Endosc*. 2012;**26**:2944–2949.
37. Swoger J, Ponsky J, Hicks DM, et al. Surgical fundoplication in laryngopharyngeal reflux unresponsive to aggressive acid suppression: a controlled study. *Clin Gastroenterol Hepatol*. 2006;**4**:433–441.
38. Spechler SJ, Gordon DW, Cohen J, Williford WO, Krol W. The effects of antireflux therapy on pulmonary function in patients with severe gastroesophageal reflux disease. Department of Veterans Affairs Gastroesophageal Reflux Disease Study Group. *Am J Gastroenterol*. 1995;**90**:915–918.
39. Larrain A, Carrasco E, Galleguillos F, Sepulveda R, Pope CE 2nd. Medical and surgical treatment of nonallergic asthma associated with gastroesophageal reflux. *Chest*. 1991;**99**:1330–1335.
40. Gutschow CA, Holscher AH. Surgical treatment of gastroesophageal reflux disease. *Langenbecks Arch Surg*. 2013;**398**:661–667.
41. Mardani J, Lundell L, Engström C. Total or posterior partial fundoplication in the treatment of GERD: results of a randomized trial after 2 decades of follow-up. *Ann Surg*. 2011;**253**:875–878.
42. Humphries LA, Hernandez JM, Clark W, Luberice K, Ross SB, Rosemurgy AS. Causes of dissatisfaction after laparoscopic fundoplication: the impact of new symptoms, recurrent symptoms, and the patient experience. *Surg Endosc*. 2013;**27**:1537–1545.
43. Wenck C, Zornig C. Laparoscopic Toupet fundoplication. *Langenbecks Arch Surg*. 2010;**395**:459–461.
44. Broeders JA, Bredenoord AJ, Hazebroek EJ, Broeders IA, Gooszen HG, Smout AJ. Reflux and belching after 270 degree versus 360 degree laparoscopic posterior fundoplication. *Ann Surg*. 2012;**255**:59–65.
45. Broeders JA, Mauritz FA, Ahmed Ali U, et al. Systematic review and meta-analysis of laparoscopic Nissen (posterior total) versus Toupet (posterior partial) fundoplication for gastro-oesophageal reflux disease. *Br J Surg*. 2010;**97**:1318–1330.
46. Bonavina L, DeMeester TR, Ganz RA. LINX(™) Reflux Management System: magnetic sphincter augmentation in the treatment of gastroesophageal reflux disease. *Expert Rev Gastroenterol Hepatol*. 2012;**6**:667–674.
47. Loh Y, McGlone ER, Reddy M, Khan OA. Is the LINX reflux management system an effective treatment for gastro-oesophageal reflux disease? *Int J Surg*. 2014;**12**:994–997.
48. Bonavina L, Saino G, Lipham JC, Demeester TR. LINX(®) Reflux Management System in chronic gastroesophageal reflux: a novel effective technology for restoring the natural barrier to reflux. *Ther Adv Gastroenterol*. 2013;**6**:261–268.
49. Ramos RF, Lustosa SA, Almeida CA, Silva CP, Matos D. Surgical treatment of gastroesophageal reflux disease: total or partial fundoplication? Systematic review and meta-analysis. *Arq Gastroenterol*. 2011;**48**:252–260.
50. Swanstrom LL, Jobe BA, Kinzie LR, Horvath KD. Esophageal motility and outcomes following laparoscopic paraesophageal hernia repair and fundoplication. *Am J Surg*. 1999;**177**:359–363.
51. Fornari F, Gurski RR, Navarini D, Thiesen V, Mestriner LH, Madalosso CA. Clinical utility of endoscopy and barium swallow X-ray in the diagnosis of sliding hiatal hernia in morbidly obese patients: a study before and after gastric bypass. *Obes Surg*. 2010;**20**:702–708.
52. Gourgiotis S, Vougas V, Germanos S, Baratsis S. Acute gastric volvulus: diagnosis and management over 10 years. *Dig Surg*. 2006;**23**:169–172.
53. Shafii AE, Agle SC, Zervos EE. Perforated gastric corpus in a strangulated paraesophageal hernia: a case report. *J Med Case Rep*. 2009;**3**:6507.
54. Stefanidis D, Hope WW, Kohn GP, Reardon PR, Richardson WS, Fanelli RD. Guidelines for surgical treatment of gastroesophageal reflux disease. *Surg Endosc*. 2010;**24**:2647–2669.
55. Al-Tashi M, Rejchrt S, Kopácová M, et al. Hiatal hernia and Barrett's oesophagus impact on symptoms occurrence and complications. *Casopis Lekaru Ceskych*. 2008;**147**:564–568.
56. Fujiwara Y, Nakao K, Inoue T, et al. Clinical significance of hiatal hernia in the development of gastroesophageal reflux after distal gastrectomy for cancer of the stomach. *J Gastroenterol Hepatol*. 2006;**21**:1103–1107.
57. Gordon C, Kang JY, Neild PJ, Maxwell JD. The role of the hiatus hernia in gastro-oesophageal reflux disease. *Aliment Pharmacol Ther*. 2004;**20**:719–732.
58. Awais O, Luketich JD. Management of giant paraesophageal hernia. *Minerva Chir*. 2009;**64**:159–168.
59. Hashemi M, Sillin LF, Peters JH. Current concepts in the management of paraesophageal hiatal hernia. *J Clin Gastroenterol*. 1999;**29**:8–13.
60. Low DE, Simchuk EJ. Effect of paraesophageal hernia repair on pulmonary function. *Ann Thorac Surg*. 2002;**74**:333–337.
61. Treacy PJ, Jamieson GG. An approach to the management of para-oesophageal hiatus hernias. *Aust N Z Surg*. 1987;**57**:813–817.
62. Hill LD. Incarcerated paraesophageal hernia. A surgical emergency. *Am J Surg*. 1973;**126**:286–291.
63. Harriss DR, Graham TR, Galea M, Salama FD. Paraoesophageal hiatal hernias: when to operate. *J R Coll Surg Edinb*. 1992;**37**:97–98.
64. Polomsky M, Jones CE, Sepesi B, et al. Should elective repair of intrathoracic stomach be encouraged? *J Gastrointest Surg*. 2010;**14**:203–210.
65. Bawahab M, Mitchell P, Church N, Debru E. Management of acute paraesophageal hernia. *Surg Endosc*. 2009;**23**:255–259.
66. Stylopoulos N, Gazelle GS, Rattner DW. Paraesophageal hernias: operation or observation? *Ann Surg*. 2002;**236**:492–500.
67. Allen MS, Trastek VF, Deschamps C, Pairolero PC. Intrathoracic stomach. Presentation and results of operation. *J Thorac Cardiovasc Surg*. 1993;**105**:253–258.
68. Hallissey MT, Ratliff DA, Temple JG. Paraoesophageal hiatus hernia: surgery for all ages. *Ann R Coll Surg Engl*. 1992;**74**:23–25.
69. Yano F, Stadlhuber RJ, Tsuboi K, Gerhardt J, Filipi CJ, Mittal SK. Outcomes of surgical treatment of intrathoracic stomach. *Dis Esophagus*. 2009;**22**:284–288.

70. Chrysos E, Tsiaoussis J, Athanasakis E, Zoras O, Vassilakis JS, Xynos E. Laparoscopic vs open approach for Nissen fundoplication. A comparative study. *Surg Endosc.* 2002;**16**:1679–1684.
71. Cuschieri A, Shimi S, Nathanson LK. Laparoscopic reduction, crural repair, and fundoplication of large hiatal hernia. *Am J Surg.* 1992;**163**:425–430.
72. Congreve DP. Laparoscopic paraesophageal hernia repair. *J Laparoendosc Surg.* 1992;**2**:45–48.
73. Edye MB, Canin-Endres J, Gattorno F, Salky BA. Durability of laparoscopic repair of paraesophageal hernia. *Ann Surg.* 1998;**228**:528–35.
74. Leeder PC, Smith G, Dehn TC. Laparoscopic management of large paraesophageal hiatal hernia. *Surg Endosc.* 2003;**17**:1372–1375.
75. Hashemi M, Peters JH, DeMeester TR, et al. Laparoscopic repair of large type III hiatal hernia: objective followup reveals high recurrence rate. *J Am Coll Surg.* 2000;**190**:553–560.
76. Frantzides CT, Madan AK, Carlson MA, Stavropoulos GP. A prospective, randomized trial of laparoscopic polytetrafluoroethylene (PTFE) patch repair vs simple cruroplasty for large hiatal hernia. *Arch Surg.* 2002;**137**:649–652.
77. Granderath FA, Schweiger UM, Kamolz T, Asche KU, Pointner R. Laparoscopic Nissen fundoplication with prosthetic hiatal closure reduces postoperative intrathoracic wrap herniation: preliminary results of a prospective randomized functional and clinical study. *Arch Surg.* 2005;**140**:40–48.
78. Angelchik JP, Cohen R. A new surgical procedure for the treatment of gastroesophageal reflux and hiatal hernia. *Surg Gynecol Obstet.* 1979;**148**:246–248.
79. Griffith PS, Valenti V, Qurashi K, Martinez-Isla A. Rejection of goretex mesh used in prosthetic cruroplasty: a case series. *Int J Surg.* 2008;**6**:106–109.
80. Stadlhuber RJ, Sherif AE, Mittal SK, et al. Mesh complications after prosthetic reinforcement of hiatal closure: a 28-case series. *Surg Endosc.* 2009;**23**:1219–1226.
81. Rumstadt B, Kähler G, Mickisch O, Schilling D. Gastric mesh erosion after hiatoplasty for recurrent paraesophageal hernia. *Endoscopy.* 2008;**40**(Suppl 2):E70.
82. Fortelny RH, Petter-Puchner AH, Glaser KS. Fibrin sealant (Tissucol) for the fixation of hiatal mesh in the repair of giant paraesophageal hernia: a case report. *Surg Laparosc Endosc Percutan Tech.* 2009;**19**:E91–E94.
83. Zehetner J, Lipham JC, Ayazi S, et al. A simplified technique for intrathoracic stomach repair: laparoscopic fundoplication with Vicryl mesh and BioGlue crural reinforcement. *Surg Endosc.* 2010;**24**:675–679.
84. Wu JS, Dunnegan DL, Soper NJ. Clinical and radiologic assessment of laparoscopic paraesophageal hernia repair. *Surg Endosc.* 1999;**13**:497–502.
85. Fuller CB, Hagen JA, DeMeester TR, Peters JH, Ritter M, Bremner CG. The role of fundoplication in the treatment of type II paraesophageal hernia. *J Thorac Cardiovasc Surg.* 1996;**111**:655–661.
86. Awad ZT, Filipi CJ, Mittal SK, et al. Left side thoracoscopically assisted gastroplasty: a new technique for managing the shortened esophagus. *Surg Endosc.* 2000;**14**:508–512.
87. Furnée EJ, Draaisma WA, Simmermacher RK, Stapper G, Broeders IA. Long-term symptomatic outcome and radiologic assessment of laparoscopic hiatal hernia repair. *Am J Surg.* 2010;**199**:695–701.
88. Hunter JG, Smith CD, Branum GD, et al. Laparoscopic fundoplication failures: patterns of failure and response to fundoplication revision. *Ann Surg.* 1999;**230**:595–604.
89. Rathore MA, Andrabi SI, Bhatti MI, Najfi SM, McMurray A. Metaanalysis of recurrence after laparoscopic repair of paraesophageal hernia. *JSLS.* 2007;**11**:456–460.
90. Légner A, Tsuboi K, Bathla L, Lee T, Morrow LE, Mittal SK. Reoperative antireflux surgery for dysphagia. *Surg Endosc.* 2011;**25**:1160–1167.
91. Poncet G, Robert M, Roman S, Boulez JC. Laparoscopic repair of large hiatal hernia without prosthetic reinforcement: late results and relevance of anterior gastropexy. *J Gastrointest Surg.* 2010;**14**:1910–1916.
92. Diaz S, Brunt LM, Klingensmith ME, Frisella PM, Soper NJ. Laparoscopic paraesophageal hernia repair, a challenging operation: medium-term outcome of 116 patients. *J Gastrointest Surg.* 2003;**7**:59–67.
93. Rosenberg J, Jacobsen B, Fischer A. Fast-track giant paraoesophageal hernia repair using a simplified laparoscopic technique. *Langenbecks Arch Surg.* 2006;**391**:38–42.
94. Agwunobi AO, Bancewicz J, Attwood SE. Simple laparoscopic gastropexy as the initial treatment of paraoesophageal hiatal hernia. *Br J Surg.* 1998;**85**:604–606.
95. Haider M, Iqbal A, Salinas V, Karu A, Mittal SK, Filipi CJ. Surgical repair of recurrent hiatal hernia. *Hernia.* 2006;**10**:13–19.
96. Singh S, Sharma AN, Murad MH, et al. Central adiposity is associated with increased risk of esophageal inflammation, metaplasia, and adenocarcinoma: a systematic review and meta-analysis. *Clin Gastroenterol Hepatol.* 2013;**11**:1399–1412.
97. Rubenstein JH, Mattek N, Eisen G. Age- and sex-specific yield of Barrett's esophagus by endoscopy indication. *Gastrointest Endosc.* 2010;**71**:21–27.
98. Rubenstein JH, Morgenstern H, Appelman H, et al. Prediction of Barrett's esophagus among men. *Am J Gastroenterol.* 2013;**108**:353–362.
99. Devesa SS, Blot WJ, Fraumeni JF, Jr. Changing patterns in the incidence of esophageal and gastric carcinoma in the United States. *Cancer.* 1998;**83**:2049–2053.
100. Jung KW, Talley NJ, Romero Y, et al. Epidemiology and natural history of intestinal metaplasia of the gastroesophageal junction and Barrett's esophagus: a population-based study. *Am J Gastroenterol.* 2011;**106**:1447–1455.
101. Amano Y, Ishimura N, Furuta K, et al. Which landmark results in a more consistent diagnosis of Barrett's esophagus, the gastric folds or the palisade vessels? *Gastrointest Endosc.* 2006;**64**:206–211.
102. Bhat S, Coleman HG, Yousef F, et al. Risk of malignant progression in Barrett's esophagus patients: results from a large population-based study. *J Natl Cancer Inst.* 2011;**103**:1049–1057.
103. Sharma P, Dent J, Armstrong D, et al. The development and validation of an endoscopic grading system for Barrett's esophagus: the Prague C & M criteria. *Gastroenterology.* 2006;**131**:1392–1399.
104. Endoscopic Classification Review Group. Update on the Paris classification of superficial neoplastic lesions in the digestive tract. *Endoscopy.* 2005;**37**:570–578.
105. Levine DS, Blount PL, Rudolph RE, Reid BJ. Safety of a systematic endoscopic biopsy protocol in patients with Barrett's esophagus. *Am J Gastroenterol.* 2000;**95**:1152–1157.
106. Hayeck TJ, Kong CY, Spechler SJ, Gazelle GS, Hur C. The prevalence of Barrett's esophagus in the US: estimates from

a simulation model confirmed by SEER data. *Dis Esophagus*. 2010;**23**:451–457.
107. Hirota WK, Loughney TM, Lazas DJ, Maydonovitch CL, Rholl V, Wong RK. Specialized intestinal metaplasia, dysplasia, and cancer of the esophagus and esophagogastric junction: prevalence and clinical data. *Gastroenterology*. 1999;**116**:277–285.
108. Cameron AJ, Zinsmeister AR, Ballard DJ, Carney JA. Prevalence of columnar-lined (Barrett's) esophagus. Comparison of population-based clinical and autopsy findings. *Gastroenterology*. 1990;**99**:918–922.
109. Ormsby AH, Kilgore SP, Goldblum JR, Richter JE, Rice TW, Gramlich TL. The location and frequency of intestinal metaplasia at the esophagogastric junction in 223 consecutive autopsies: implications for patient treatment and preventive strategies in Barrett's esophagus. *Mod Pathol*. 2000;**13**:614–620.
110. Spechler SJ. Barrett's esophagus. *Semin Gastrointest Dis*. 1996;**7**:51–60.
111. Cook MB, Wild CP, Forman D. A systematic review and meta-analysis of the sex ratio for Barrett's esophagus, erosive reflux disease, and nonerosive reflux disease. *Am J Epidemiol*. 2005;**162**:1050–1061.
112. Abrams JA, Fields S, Lightdale CJ, Neugut AI. Racial and ethnic disparities in the prevalence of Barrett's esophagus among patients who undergo upper endoscopy. *Clin Gastroenterol Hepatol*. 2008;**6**:30–34.
113. Corley DA, Kubo A, Levin TR, et al. Race, ethnicity, sex and temporal differences in Barrett's oesophagus diagnosis: a large community-based study, 1994-2006. *Gut*. 2009;**58**:182–188.
114. Shiota S, Singh S, Anshasi A, El-Serag HB. Prevalence of Barrett's esophagus in Asian countries: a systematic review and meta-analysis. *Clin Gastroenterol Hepatol*. 2015;**13**:1907–1918.
115. Johansson J, Håkansson HO, Mellblom L, et al. Prevalence of precancerous and other metaplasia in the distal oesophagus and gastro-oesophageal junction. *Scand J Gastroenterol*. 2005;**40**:893–902.
116. Lieberman DA, Oehlke M, Helfand M. Risk factors for Barrett's esophagus in community-based practice. GORGE consortium. Gastroenterology Outcomes Research Group in Endoscopy. *Am J Gastroenterol*. 1997;**92**:1293–1297.
117. Thrift AP, Kramer JR, Qureshi Z, Richardson PA, El-Serag HB. Age at onset of GERD symptoms predicts risk of Barrett's esophagus. *Am J Gastroenterol*. 2013;**108**:915–922.
118. Andrici J, Cox MR, Eslick GD. Cigarette smoking and the risk of Barrett's esophagus: a systematic review and meta-analysis. *J Gastroenterol Hepatol*. 2013;**28**:1258–1273.
119. Anderson LA, Cantwell MM, Watson RG, et al. The association between alcohol and reflux esophagitis, Barrett's esophagus, and esophageal adenocarcinoma. *Gastroenterology*. 2009;**136**:799–805.
120. Kubo A, Levin TR, Block G, et al. Alcohol types and sociodemographic characteristics as risk factors for Barrett's esophagus. *Gastroenterology*. 2009;**136**:806–815.
121. Kubo A, Cook MB, Shaheen NJ, et al. Sex-specific associations between body mass index, waist circumference and the risk of Barrett's oesophagus: a pooled analysis from the international BEACON consortium. *Gut*. 2013;**62**:1684–1691.
122. Chak A, Lee T, Kinnard MF, et al. Familial aggregation of Barrett's oesophagus, oesophageal adenocarcinoma, and oesophagogastric junctional adenocarcinoma in Caucasian adults. *Gut*. 2002;**51**:323–328.
123. Orloff M, Peterson C, He X, et al. Germline mutations in MSR1, ASCC1, and CTHRC1 in patients with Barrett esophagus and esophageal adenocarcinoma. *JAMA*. 2011;**306**:410–419.
124. Ek WE, Levine DM, D'Amato M, et al. Germline genetic contributions to risk for esophageal adenocarcinoma, Barrett's esophagus, and gastroesophageal reflux. *J Natl Cancer Inst*. 2013;**105**:1711–1718.
125. Eloubeidi MA, Mason AC, Desmond RA, El-Serag HB. Temporal trends (1973–1997) in survival of patients with esophageal adenocarcinoma in the United States: a glimmer of hope? *Am J Gastroenterol*. 2003;**98**:1627–1633.
126. O'Riordan JM, Byrne PJ, Ravi N, Keeling PW, Reynolds JV. Long-term clinical and pathologic response of Barrett's esophagus after antireflux surgery. *Am J Surg*. 2004;**188**:27–33.
127. Hofstetter WL, Peters JH, DeMeester TR, et al. Long-term outcome of antireflux surgery in patients with Barrett's esophagus. *Ann Surg*. 2001;**234**:532–538.
128. Pech O, Bollschweiler E, Manner H, Leers J, Ell C, Hölscher AH. Comparison between endoscopic and surgical resection of mucosal esophageal adenocarcinoma in Barrett's esophagus at two high-volume centers. *Ann Surg*. 2011;**254**:67–72.

7

Upper gastrointestinal bleeding
Non-surgical and surgical management

Zaheer Nabi and D. Nageshwar Reddy

Introduction

Upper gastrointestinal (GI) bleeding is one of the most common emergencies that require hospitalization. It has been traditionally defined as bleeding arising from a site proximal to the ligament of Treitz (i.e. oesophagus, stomach, and duodenum). The aetiologies of upper GI bleeding can be divided into variceal and non-variceal causes. This differentiation is important as management strategies and outcomes are different in variceal upper GI bleeding (VUGIB) and non-variceal upper GI bleeding (NVUGIB). Over the last two decades, the incidence of hospitalization and in-hospital mortality due to upper GI bleeding has reduced significantly.[1] This decreasing trend has been accompanied by a parallel rise in the rate of endoscopy and endoscopic therapy. Improved access to endoscopy, availability of potent acid-suppressive medications, and recognition of the role of *Helicobacter pylori* in peptic ulcer disease have contributed to the better outcomes in patients with upper GI bleeding. In contrast, bleeding from oesophageal varices appears to have increased as evident in a nationwide audit in the UK.[2]

In the following sections, we discuss the epidemiology and endoscopic and surgical management of upper GI bleeding.

Epidemiology

Common causes of upper GI bleeding include peptic ulcer disease, gastritis, oesophagitis, and gastro-oesophageal varices (GOVs).[2] Other less common causes include a Mallory–Weiss tear, angiodysplasia, Dieulafoy's lesions, and neoplasms (Table 7.1 and Figure 7.1) The incidence of NVUGIB decreased from 2006 to 2014 (from 112.3 to 94.4 per 100,000) before increasing to 116.2 per 100,000 by 2019.[3] The mortality rate has also decreased from 4.5% to 2.1% along with a parallel increase in the rates of endoscopy (70% to 85%) and endoscopic therapy (10% to 27%) over last two decades.[1] These trends reflect the widespread availability and utilization of proton pump inhibitors (PPIs), anti-*H. pylori* therapy, and endoscopy.

VUGIB is less common than NVUGIB and accounts for 4–20% of all cases of upper GI bleeding. VUGIB can be attributed to bleeding from oesophageal or gastric varices. Bleeding from oesophageal varices is far more common than gastric variceal bleeding which accounts for 10–20% of variceal bleeding cases. The in-hospital mortality due to VUGIB has reduced from 40–50% in older studies to 15% in recent studies.[4]

Management of upper gastrointestinal bleeding

Initial management and fluid resuscitation

In patients presenting with acute upper GI bleeding (variceal or non-variceal), the first aim is fluid resuscitation to achieve haemodynamic stability. Haemorrhagic shock is associated with multiorgan failure and death.[5] Therefore, fluid resuscitation should precede pharmacological and endoscopic management. Colloids (e.g. albumin, dextran, hydroxyethyl starch, and modified gelatin) are expensive and have no substantial advantage over crystalloids (Ringer's lactate or normal saline). Airway protection is equally important and

Table 7.1 Aetiological spectrum of upper gastrointestinal bleeding

Aetiology	Incidence (%) US	Incidence (%) UK
Peptic ulcer disease	47.1	36
Gastritis	18.1	7.2
Oesophagitis	15.2	8.9
Angiodysplasia	6.2	1.6
Mallory–Weiss tear	6.9	2.1
Neoplasm	3.7	3.7
Oesophageal varices	1.8	11
Dieulafoy lesion	1.5	–
No abnormality	–	17

Source: data from Hearnshaw SA, Logan RF, Lowe D, et al. Acute upper gastrointestinal bleeding in the UK: patient characteristics, diagnoses and outcomes in the 2007 UK audit. *Gut*. 2011;60:1327-1335; and Wuerth BA, Rockey DC. Changing epidemiology of upper gastrointestinal hemorrhage in the last decade: a nationwide analysis. *Dig Dis Sci*. 2018;63:1286-1293.

7 Upper gastrointestinal bleeding: management

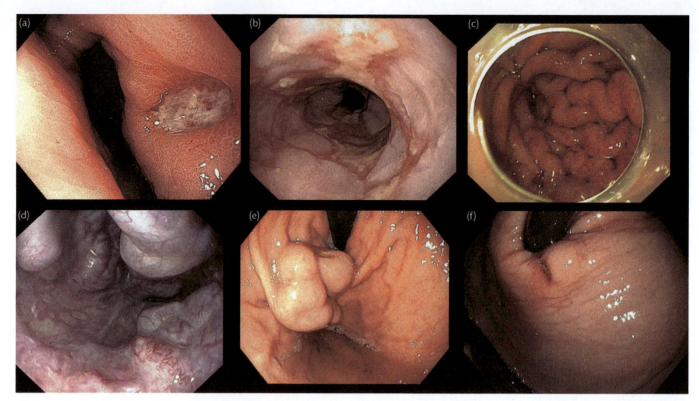

Figure 7.1 Common aetiologies of upper gastrointestinal bleeding. (a) Peptic ulcer disease. (b) Severe erosive oesophagitis. (c). Gastric erosions or gastritis. (d) Large oesophageal varices. (e) Gastric varices. (f) Mallory–Weiss tear.

consideration should be given to endotracheal intubation especially in patients with an altered sensorium.

Blood transfusion should be given to maintain a haemoglobin level between 7 and 8 g/dL. Over-transfusion should be avoided as it is associated with higher re-bleeding rates and increased mortality.[6,7] Exceptions to this strategy include those with coronary artery disease and haemodynamically unstable patients with severe ongoing bleeding. Blood transfusion appears to be more detrimental in variceal bleeders than in non-variceal bleeders.[7] Correction of international normalized ratio with fresh frozen plasma or factor VIIa concentrates is not beneficial and, therefore, not recommended routinely.[8] The UK guidelines recommend transfusion of fresh frozen plasma in selected cases with low fibrinogen levels (<1 g/L) and high prothrombin time or international normalized ratio (>1.5 times upper limit of normal).[4] Similarly, platelet transfusion may be given in cases with active bleeding and a platelet count less than 50×10^9/L.[4] It is important to note that the level of evidence supporting the transfusion of these blood products in patients with VUGIB is very low (level 5, grade D recommendation).[4]

Management of variceal bleeding

Non-surgical management
Pharmacological

Pharmacological management in patients with active variceal bleeding includes infusion of vasoactive peptides, intravenous (IV) antibiotics, and IV prokinetic agents.

Vasoactive drugs should be initiated without delay in patients with confirmed or suspected VUGIB. These include somatostatin, octreotide, and terlipressin. These agents act by reduction in portal blood flow by causing splanchnic vasoconstriction or inhibiting the release of vasodilatory peptide glucagon. All three drugs have similar efficacy in controlling variceal bleeding when combined with endoscopic therapy.[9] However, terlipressin is the only vasoactive agent that has been shown to reduce all-cause mortality in these patients. In countries where terlipressin is not available (such as the US and Japan), other agents can also be used effectively. The dosages and durations of different vasoactive agents are listed in Table 7.2. Patients with cirrhosis and variceal bleeding are at a higher risk of bacterial infections. Therefore, IV antibiotics (ceftriaxone 1 g/day) should be administered up to a maximum period of 7 days. Besides reduction in infection, re-bleeding rates and mortality are lower in those receiving IV antibiotics. IV prokinetic agents (e.g. erythromycin or metoclopramide) are administered within 30–60 minutes of planned endoscopy in cases with ongoing bleeding with a high likelihood of finding clots and blood in the stomach.

Endoscopic treatment

Endoscopy should be performed within 12 hours of presentation in a case with acute variceal bleeding after haemodynamic resuscitation. Endoscopic treatment options for VUGIB include endoscopic band ligation (EBL), sclerotherapy (sodium morrhuate or ethanolamine), and injection of tissue adhesives (e.g. *n*-butyl cyanoacrylate).

Oesophageal varices

EBL and endoscopic sclerotherapy are effective in 80–90% of cases. EBL is preferred over endoscopic sclerotherapy for acute bleeding

Table 7.2 Management options for variceal upper gastrointestinal bleeding

Therapy	Specific modality	Comments
Pharmacological[a]	Somatostatin Octreotide Terlipressin[b]	250 mcg IV bolus → 250 mcg/hour infusion 50 mcg IV bolus followed by 50 mcg/hour infusion 2 mg IV 4-hourly, 1 mg IV 4-hourly after haemostasis
Mechanical tamponade	Balloon tamponade (Sengstaken–Blakemore, Linton–Nachlas, Minnesota)	High adverse event and re-bleeding rates, used as temporary measure (≤24 hours)
	Covered self-expandable metal stent	See text
Endoscopic	Band ligation, sclerotherapy	Band ligation preferred over sclerotherapy
	Glue injection, glue + coil injection	TIPSS is an alternative if glue not available
Interventional radiology	TIPSS	Refractory bleeding, primary therapy in high risk
	BRTO	Gastric varices with splenorenal shunt and patent portal vein
Surgical	Shunt surgeries: non-selective, selective, partial, Rex shunt	In cases with preserved liver function, non-selective shunts avoided in future transplant candidates, Rex shunt utilized in extrahepatic portal vein obstruction
	Non-shunt surgeries: Sugiura surgery, Hassab's operation	In cases with contraindication to TIPSS and shunt surgeries not feasible

[a] Vasoactive peptides should be given up to a period of 5 days. [b] Monitor serum sodium while using terlipressin.

from oesophageal varices. The major advantages of EBL over sclerotherapy include requirement of fewer sessions, lower incidence of recurrent bleeding, and fewer complications.[10] Sclerotherapy is useful in selected cases with fibrosed varices and a bloody field where band ligation may be difficult. Commonly used sclerosants include ethanolamine oleate (5%) and polidocanol (1–2%).

In cases with early re-bleeding within 5 days, a second session of endotherapy can be attempted. Whereas in cases with persistent or refractory bleeding (10–20%) after vasoactive peptides and endoscopic therapy, transjugular intrahepatic portosystemic shunt (TIPSS) should be considered (see later). Balloon tamponade and placement of a covered metal stent can be considered as bridging options in these cases. Balloon tamponade is achieved by any of the three types of available balloons: Sengstaken–Blakemore tube (oesophageal and gastric balloon), Minnesota tube, and Linton–Nachlas tube (only gastric balloon). Although effective, balloon tamponade is associated with a high failure rate (35.5%), and excess adverse events (20%). Therefore, it is used as a temporary measure pending more definitive therapies such as band ligation. On the other hand, specially designed covered oesophageal stents (SX-Ella Danis stent, ELLA-CS, Hradec Kralove, Czech Republic) are superior in terms of safety profile and short-term control of bleeding.[11] In recent studies, the pooled rates of immediate bleeding control and re-bleeding with metal stents were 84.5% and 19.4%, respectively.[12] The other advantage of metal stents is that they can be kept *in situ* for a longer duration (up to 2 weeks) in contrast to balloons which must be removed within 24–48 hours.

Gastric varices

Gastric varices are found in 20% of patients with portal hypertension and bleeding from gastric varices accounts for 10–20% of all cases with variceal bleeding. Gastric varices are classified as GOV types 1 or 2 (GOV1 or GOV2) and isolated gastric varices types 1 or 2 (IGV1 or IGV2).[13] This classification has implications for management and prognosis of bleeding from gastric varices. Gastric variceal bleeding is more severe than bleeding from oesophageal varices and patients with bleeding from IGVs fare worse than those bleeding from GOVs.

Initial management of gastric variceal bleeding is similar to that for bleeding from oesophageal varices (i.e. haemodynamic resuscitation, airway protection, administration of IV antibiotics, and vasoactive drugs). In cases with massive ongoing bleeding, balloon tamponade can be used as a temporary measure until definitive therapies can be administered. The endoscopic management options for bleeding from gastric varices include EBL (GOV1), injection of tissue adhesives (*n*-butyl cyanoacrylate), endoscopic ultrasound-guided injection of glue and coil, and endoscopic injection of thrombin (Figure 7.2). Cyanoacrylate glue injection is more effective than EBL especially in GOV2 and IGVs. Primary haemostasis is achieved in 86–100%, with re-bleeding rates of 7–28%.[4] Major complications with glue injection especially pulmonary and cerebral emboli are uncommon but can be potentially fatal. Endoscopic ultrasound-guided injection of glue and coil has emerged as an effective and safe alternative to endoscopic glue injection.[14] In a systematic review, the pooled treatment efficacy and gastric varices obliteration after endoscopic ultrasound-guided therapy was 93.7% (95% confidence interval (CI) 89.5–96.3%; I^2 = 53.7) and 84.4% (95% CI 74.8–90.9%; I^2 = 77), respectively. The recurrence of gastric varices, early re-bleeding, and late re-bleeding were 9.1%, 7.0%, and 11.6%, respectively.[15] Combined glue injection with coil embolization is superior to coil embolization alone with fewer re-bleeding episodes (3.3% vs 20%; p = 0.04).[14] In cases refractory to endoscopic management, TIPSS should be considered.

Prevention of re-bleeding

In oesophageal varices, the combination of EBL and non-selective beta blockers (NSBB: propranolol, nadolol, and carvedilol) is the best strategy to prevent re-bleeding. In cases with contraindication or intolerance to NSBB, EBL alone can be used as secondary prophylaxis.

Repeated sessions (usually three or four) of EBL at 1–2-week intervals are required for complete variceal obliteration (Figure 7.3). Consideration should be given to stop or reduce the dose of NSBB in selected situations such as refractory ascites with hypotension (systolic blood pressure <90 mmHg), acute kidney injury, and hyponatraemia (<130 mEq/L).[16]

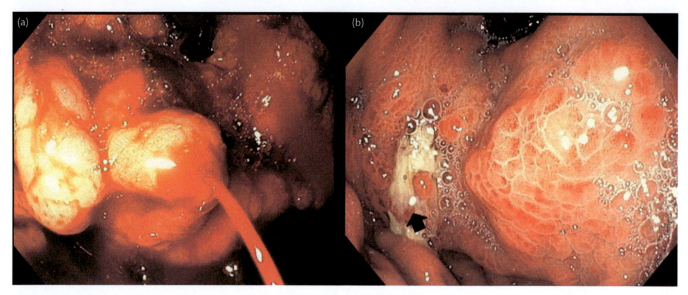

Figure 7.2 Gastric variceal bleeding. (a) Active spurting from large fundal varices. (b) Haemostasis after cyanoacrylate glue injection.

In order to prevent bleeding from gastric varices, glue injection can be repeated after 2–4 weeks. The role of NSBBs is less clear in the secondary prophylaxis of gastric variceal bleed. TIPSS or balloon-occluded retrograde transvenous obliteration (BRTO) should be considered in cases with recurrent bleeding after glue injection.

Transjugular intrahepatic portosystemic shunt

The indications for TIPSS include persistent bleeding, re-bleeding after two sessions of endotherapy, failure of secondary prophylaxis, and selected high-risk cases with high hepatic venous pressure gradient greater than 20 mmHg, Model for End-Stage Liver Disease (MELD) score of at least 19 and Child's C (score 10–13) cirrhosis.[17] As a salvage therapy, TIPSS is effective in controlling bleeding in 90% of the patients. However, re-bleeding at 1 month (15%) and high mortality (40%) remain a concern after TIPSS.[18] More recently, early TIPSS (i.e. within 72 hours of presentation) has been shown to be effective and better as compared to standard management (endotherapy plus NSBB) in preventing re-bleeding and in improving transplant-free survival rates in high-risk patients with hepatic venous pressure gradient greater than 20 mmHg or Child's C cirrhosis.[19,20] The use of polytetrafluoroethylene-covered stents has further improved the outcomes of TIPSS with less frequent stent dysfunction as compared to the use of bare stents in initial studies[21] (**Figure 7.4a,b**).

Common complications associated with TIPSS include hepatic encephalopathy (20–40%) and shunt dysfunction (15–20%). Other complications are uncommon and include puncture of the liver capsule, cholangitis and haemobilia due to biliary puncture, liver decompensation, and stent infection or 'tipsitis'. It is important to check the patency of the shunt at regular intervals (e.g. 1–4 weeks followed by every 3–6-monthly) using Doppler ultrasonography which has a high sensitivity and specificity (>90%) for detecting shunt dysfunction. Although effective, TIPSS is not feasible in all the patients with refractory VUGIB. Contraindications to TIPSS include congestive heart failure, severe tricuspid regurgitation, uncontrolled sepsis, severe pulmonary hypertension, obstructed biliary system, and multiple hepatic cysts.[18] Poor prognostic factors associated with high post-TIPSS mortality include decompensated cirrhosis (Child C score >13), bilirubin concentration greater than 3 mg/dL, encephalopathy, and elevated alanine transaminase levels (>100 IU/L).[18]

In gastric variceal bleeding, TIPSS is an effective option either as a primary therapy or in cases with failure of medical and endoscopic

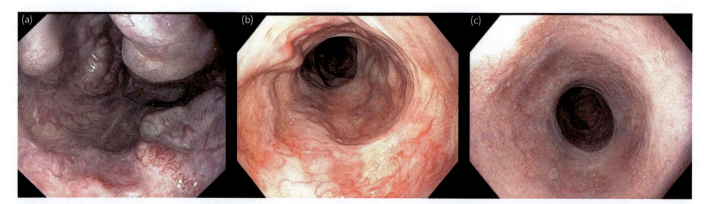

Figure 7.3 Outcome of endoscopic variceal ligation for large oesophageal varices. (a) Large oesophageal varices. (b) Endoscopic view after two sessions of endoscopic band ligation. (c) Endoscopic view after complete variceal obliteration.

Management of variceal bleeding | 69

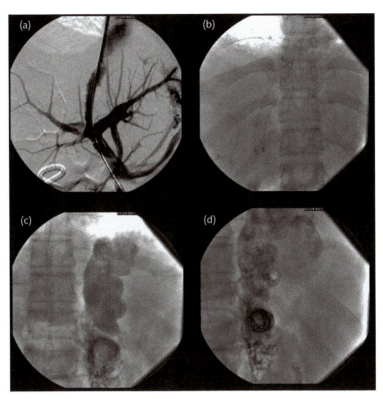

Figure 7.4 Interventional radiology in variceal bleeding (TIPSS and BRTO). (a) Contrast opacification after catheterization of portal vein. (b) Placement of covered metal stent connecting portal vein and inferior vena cava. (c) Cannulation of left renal vein and contrast opacification of large collaterals after inflation of balloon (note that these collaterals represent gastrorenal shunt). (d) Occlusion of the shunt with coil embolization.

therapies. TIPSS is also indicated when cyanoacrylate glue is not available or not approved for use in gastric variceal bleeding and where expertise is inadequate for glue injection. Practice guidelines from the American Association for the Study of Liver Diseases recommend TIPSS as the primary therapy in the control of bleeding from cardiofundal varices (GOV2 or IGV1).[8]

Balloon-occluded retrograde transvenous obliteration

BRTO is an option in cases where TIPSS is contraindicated or not advisable due to the various factors described above. The technique of BRTO is as follows: the left renal vein and gastrorenal shunt are accessed via the internal jugular or right femoral vein. Subsequently, the balloon is inflated and a venogram obtained to define the anatomy of the collaterals. Finally, a sclerosing agent (ethanolamine oleate iopamidol or sodium tetradecyl sulphate) is injected to completely opacify the varix.[22] (Figure 7.4c,d). Various other agents can be used in place of sclerosants and include Gelfoam, cyanoacrylate, coils, and vascular plugs.

BRTO and TIPSS have similar technical success rates (91.4% vs 89.7%) and immediate bleeding control rates (97.7% vs 95.9%). Re-bleeding rates (10.6% vs 18.7%) and hepatic encephalopathy (0% vs 23.1%) have been shown to be lower with BRTO as compared to TIPSS.[23] BRTO may be more effective than cyanoacrylate injection in preventing re-bleeding from gastric varices.[24]

However, portal pressure gradients may increase after BRTO which in turn may increase the likelihood of bleeding from oesophageal varices and aggravation of ascites (22.4% vs 4.3%).[23] An absolute contraindication to the BRTO procedure is complete portal vein thrombosis. Relative contraindications include an absence of a gastrorenal shunt, uncontrolled bleeding from oesophageal varices, splenic vein thrombosis, and severe uncorrected coagulopathy.[22]

The choice between BRTO and TIPSS is largely dictated by the patient's clinical status, contraindications to the procedure, and the available expertise.

Surgical management

Surgery is not commonly performed in patients with VUGIB due to the high risk of liver decompensation, encephalopathy, and mortality (20–50%) when performed in emergency settings. TIPSS is a safer and equally effective alternative to shunt surgery in refractory cases.[25] In the current era, surgery is utilized in non-cirrhotic patients (e.g. pre-hepatic portal hypertension), those with preserved liver function (Child A, low MELD score), and where TIPSS is not available or contraindicated. Surgical options for patients with VUGIB include shunt surgeries and non-shunt or devascularization surgeries.

Portosystemic shunts

Shunt surgeries include selective (distal splenorenal shunt), non-selective (portocaval shunt), and partial shunt surgeries. Shunt surgeries are highly effective in achieving control of active bleeding and preventing recurrent bleeding.[26]

Portocaval shunt (synonym: total or non-selective shunt)

An end-to-side or side-to-side portocaval shunt (>12 mm) effectively decompresses the entire portal venous system and controls variceal bleeding effectively. The procedure is technically easier and quicker than a distal splenorenal shunt which is difficult in unstable, actively bleeding patients. However, due to diversion of the entire portal blood flow away from the liver, the incidence of hepatic encephalopathy is high (30–40%). In addition, portocaval shunt surgery involves dissection at the porta hepatis which may pose problems during future liver transplantation. Other non-selective shunts include a mesocaval shunt and proximal or central splenorenal shunt. Since these latter shunts do not involve dissection at the porta hepatis, future liver transplantation is not complicated. Currently, portocaval shunts are not commonly utilized in cases with refractory VUGIB.

Distal splenorenal shunt (DSRS; synonym: selective shunt or Warren shunt)

DSRSs are now widely performed. As the name suggests, these shunts selectively decompress the spleen and gastro-oesophageal collaterals. Therefore, the incidence of hepatic encephalopathy and liver decompensation is lower as compared to total shunts. In a randomized trial, DSRS was similarly efficacious to TIPSS in controlling refractory variceal bleeding and preventing re-bleeding (5.5% vs 10.5%).[25] The main drawback of DSRSs is their loss of selectivity over a period of time. DSRS cannot be performed in those with splenic vein thrombosis and a history of splenectomy. In addition, ascites may get aggravated after DSRS due to persistently elevated hepatic sinusoidal pressures. Therefore, this shunt is contraindicated in patients with moderate to severe ascites.

Partial portocaval shunt

This type of shunt is performed with the aim to preserve some blood flow to the liver by using a smaller (8 or 10 mm) interposition graft between the portal vein and inferior vena cava. Encephalopathy is less common with partial shunts compared to total portocaval shunts.

Mesentericoportal venous bypass (Rex shunt)

This is performed in patients, especially children, with extrahepatic portal vein obstruction. Prerequisites include a patent left portal vein and superior mesenteric vein or any other suitable collateral. The shunt between intrahepatic portal vein and superior mesenteric vein improves liver perfusion, minimizing the risk of encephalopathy after shunt surgery.

Non-shunt surgeries

Various type of non-shunt procedures include splenectomy for left-sided portal hypertension and oesophagogastric devascularization including the Sugiura procedure (classical and modified) and Hassab's operation (described later).

The basic difference between shunt and non-shunt surgeries is that the portal blood flow is not diverted in the latter. Consequently, the blood flow to the liver is preserved and the incidence of hepatic encephalopathy is lower.

- Splenectomy: in cases with chronic splenic vein thrombosis or left-sided portal hypertension complicated by VUGIB, splenectomy is a safe and effective option. Splenectomy reduces the blood flow in the collateral circulation thereby decompressing the GOVs and preventing future re-bleeding episodes. Since, liver function is usually preserved in cases with left-sided portal hypertension major postoperative complications related to liver decompensation are rare.
- Sugiura procedure: this procedure involves transection of the lower oesophagus with devascularization of the oesophagogastric junction and splenectomy. The Sugiura procedure is performed in two stages: thoracic and abdominal. The thoracic stage involves extensive interruption or devascularization of the oesophagus and oesophageal transection. While in the abdominal stage, devascularization of the abdominal oesophagus along with cardia, splenectomy, selective vagotomy, and pyloroplasty are performed.
- Hassab's operation is similar to the Sugiura procedure except that it is a single-stage operation as oesophageal transection is not performed. Recurrence of oesophageal varices is higher after Hassab's surgery. Therefore, this surgery is preferred in those with only gastric varices.

Management of non-variceal upper gastrointestinal bleeding

Non-surgical management

Pre-endoscopy risk stratification

Hospitalization and inpatient management are not required in all the patients who present with upper GI bleeding. Several pre-endoscopic risk assessment scores are available for directing patients to an outpatient management including the Glasgow Blatchford score, pre-endoscopic Rockall score, and AIMS65 score. Of these, a Glasgow Blatchford score of 1 or less is considered optimal to identify patients who are at a very low risk for re-bleeding or mortality and thus may not require hospitalization or inpatient endoscopy.[5,27,28]

Pre-endoscopy pharmacotherapy

IV PPIs are not recommended in stable patients with suspected NVUGIB prior to endoscopy.[29] PPIs reduce the high-risk stigmata (PPIs vs control: 37.2% vs 46.5%) and the requirement of subsequent endoscopic treatment (8.6% vs 11.7%). However, this benefit does not translate into prevention of re-bleeding (PPI vs no PPI: 13.9% vs 16.6%), requirement for surgery (9.9% vs 10.2%), and reduction in mortality (6.1% vs 5.5%).[30] The exception to this rule is inability to perform an endoscopy within 24 hours due to unavailability or other reasons. In these cases, IV PPIs should be given as an 80 mg bolus, followed by 8 mg/hour continuous infusion (Table 7.3).

The use of antithrombotics is associated with increased the risk of GI bleeding. Preliminary data suggest that the risk of NVUGIB may be higher with warfarin (vs direct oral anticoagulants) and rivaroxaban (vs dabigatran and apixaban).[31,32] The decision to stop antithrombotic agents after an episode of upper GI bleeding should be individualized according to the coagulation risk of patients. In cases with severe bleeding and high risk of thrombosis, early resumption of antithrombotic agents is recommended once endoscopic haemostasis has been achieved[33] (Table 7.4).

Endoscopic management

Endoscopy should be performed within 24 hours (early endoscopy) of admission after haemodynamic resuscitation. Very early (≤12 hours) or urgent endoscopy (≤6 hours) do not appear to be superior to early endoscopy.[34] In a well-conducted randomized trial

Table 7.3 Management options in cases with non-variceal upper gastrointestinal bleeding

Management options	Subcategories	Comments
Pharmacological	PPIs	As an adjunct to endoscopic haemostasis in high-risk cases
	Erythromycin	250 mg IV, half hour before endoscopy
Endoscopic		
(a) Injection	Epinephrine, sclerosants	High recurrent bleeding (20–30%), used in combination with thermal/mechanical modalities
(b) Thermal	Heater probe, bipolar probes, haemostatic forceps, APC	Thermal and mechanical modalities equally effective, risk of perforation with thermal haemostasis
(c) Mechanical	TTSC, OTSC, banding device, covered metal stents	Endoclips application challenging in posterior duodenal ulcer and high lesser curvature
(d) Haemostatic powder	Hemospray (TC-325)	High re-bleeding rates (10–40%), used as a temporary or salvage modality
Angiographic embolization	Coil, Gelfoam	Indicated in refractory bleeding and poor surgical risk, high re-bleeding rates
Surgery		
Minimal surgery	Underrunning/suture plication, wedge excision (gastric ulcer)	Preferred over definitive surgery, re-bleeding risk higher than definitive surgeries
Definitive surgery	Underrunning+ truncal vagotomy + drainage or gastric resection	Lower re-bleeding risk, higher morbidity, less commonly performed

(516 patients), urgent endoscopy (≤6 hours) had no advantage over early endoscopy (6–24 hours) in reducing mortality or requirement for surgery and angioembolization.[35] Importantly, patients with persistent haemodynamic instability despite resuscitation were excluded from this trial. Therefore, in a selected group of patients with high-risk clinical features like persistent haemodynamic instability despite resuscitation and a bloody nasogastric aspirate, very early (≤12 hours) endoscopy may be indicated.[28]

During endoscopy the peptic ulcers should be classified according to Forrest's classification which has therapeutic and prognostic importance (Figure 7.5). The Forrest classification classifies ulcers into high-risk (Ia: spurting; Ib: oozing; IIa: non-bleeding visible vessel) and low-risk (IIc: flat pigmented spot; III: clean ulcer base) types according to the risk of persistent bleeding and re-bleeding. In cases with an adherent clot (IIb), the ulcer can be re-classified into high- or low-risk types after removing the clot. Endoscopic therapy is beneficial in ulcers with high-risk stigmata including Forrest Ia, Ib, and IIa.[36] The decision for endotherapy in Forrest IIb (adherent clot) should be individualized as the literature shows conflicting evidence with regard to the benefits of endoscopic haemostasis in this group.

The low-risk group (Forrest IIc and III) do not require endotherapy and oral PPIs are sufficient in these patients.

After endoscopic therapy, all the high-risk patients should receive IV PPIs (80 mg bolus followed by 8 mg/hour infusion). The use of high-dose PPI infusion substantially reduces the incidence of recurrent bleeding after initial endoscopic haemostasis (PPI infusion vs placebo: 22.5% vs 6.7%).[37]

The predictors of mortality in bleeding peptic ulcers after endoscopic haemostasis include advanced age, multiple comorbidities, hypovolaemic shock, in-hospital bleeding, re-bleeding, and need for surgery.[38]

Endoscopic haemostasis procedures

Endoscopic haemostasis is superior to PPI therapy in ulcers with high-risk stigmata (i.e. Forrest Ia and Ib). Endoscopic haemostasis is achieved via injection (epinephrine (adrenaline) or sclerosant), contact thermal, and mechanical modalities. Epinephrine injection is not used alone due to high re-bleeding rates. Whereas endoclips or thermal coagulation are effective modalities when used with or without epinephrine injection and achieve haemostasis in greater than 80% of cases.[39]

Table 7.4 Recommendations for stopping antithrombotic agents in patients with non-variceal upper gastrointestinal bleeding

Patient category	Strategy to stop antithrombotic agents	Time of resuming antiplatelets or anticoagulants
Single antiplatelet agent	• Withhold aspirin in severe bleeding	Within 3–5 days of endoscopic haemostasis
Dual antiplatelet agents	• Continue both in those with coronary stents • Withhold clopidogrel, continue aspirin	Within 5 days especially in those with drug-eluting coronary stents
Warfarin	• Withhold until haemostasis; prothrombin complex concentrate and low-dose vitamin K (<5 mg) if international normalized ratio >2.5 • Bridging anticoagulation if high thromboembolic risk	Resume after haemostasis
Direct oral anticoagulants (DOACs)	• Withhold until haemostasis • Activated charcoal if DOAC consumed within 3 hours • Consider idarucizumab in cases on dabigatran	Resume after haemostasis

Source: data from Chan FKL, Goh KL, Reddy N, et al. Management of patients on antithrombotic agents undergoing emergency and elective endoscopy: joint Asian Pacific Association of Gastroenterology (APAGE) and Asian Pacific Society for Digestive Endoscopy (APSDE) practice guidelines. *Gut*. 2018;67:405–417.

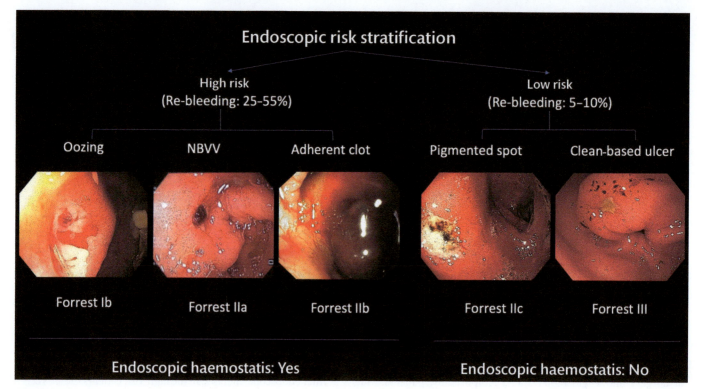

Figure 7.5 Endoscopic risk stratification in cases with peptic ulcer bleeding.

Injection therapy

Injection therapy with diluted epinephrine (1:10,000 to 1:20,000) is among the most commonly utilized haemostatic methods. Epinephrine injection is given as 1 mL aliquots in four quadrants of the bleeding ulcer using a sclerotherapy needle. Large-volume injections (>13 mL) are more effective in reducing recurrent bleeding.[40] The advantages of injection therapy are low cost, universal availability, and technical ease. In addition, it facilitates the use of a second haemostatic modality by improving the visualization of the bleeding site. The downside of epinephrine injection is that the injected solution dissipates over time resulting in a high re-bleeding rate (30–40%) when used alone. The combination of epinephrine with another haemostatic modality like a thermal or mechanical procedure is superior to epinephrine injection alone in preventing re-bleeding and the requirement for surgery in high-risk cases.[41] Other sclerosants (alcohol, polidocanol) are effective but result in severe tissue damage and are therefore not commonly utilized in clinical practice.

Thermal haemostatic modalities

Thermal methods of haemostasis include contact and non-contact haemostatic devices. Contact thermal devices include the multipolar electrocoagulation probe (also called the bipolar probe), heater probe, and haemostatic forceps. The non-contact thermal modalities include argon plasma coagulation (APC) and laser.

Contact probes achieve haemostasis by mechanical tamponade and coaptive coagulation or sealing of the blood vessels. Thermal coagulation modalities are effective in achieving haemostasis in cases with NVUGIB either alone or in combination with epinephrine injection. However, the combination appears superior to thermal coagulation alone in achieving primary haemostasis.[42] Haemostatic forceps are commonly utilized to control intraprocedural bleeding during procedures like endoscopic mucosal resection and endoscopic submucosal dissection. Limited data show their efficacy in peptic ulcer bleeding as well. In a randomized trial, haemostatic forceps was non-inferior to APC in bleeding peptic ulcers.[43] In another randomized trial, haemostatic forceps was superior to haemoclips in achieving primary haemostasis (98.2% vs 80.4%; $p = 0.004$). The re-bleeding rate was lower in the haemostatic forceps group (3.6% vs 17.7%; $p = 0.04$).[44] More data are required to support the routine use of haemostatic forceps for this indication. Caution is advised while using thermal devices as injudicious use may lead to deep tissue injury and perforation.

APC is a non-contact method of coagulation and is especially useful in cases with diffuse blood oozing like gastric antral vascular ectasia and tumour bleeds (Figure 7.6).

Mechanical haemostatic modalities

Mechanical devices for haemostasis include through-the-scope clips (TTSCs), over-the-scope clips (OTSCs), and banding devices. TTSC or haemoclips are effective haemostatic devices and achieve haemostasis in 85–90% of patients.[39] There is probably no benefit of combining injection therapy with haemoclips. In a systematic review and meta-analysis of randomized trials (28 trials, 2988 patients), the combination of injection therapy and haemoclips was not superior to haemoclips alone.[42] The advantages of haemoclips are high efficiency and avoidance of thermal injury. The notable disadvantages include technical difficulty of haemoclip application in large fibrotic ulcers and certain locations like higher along the lesser curvature and posterior wall of the duodenal bulb. In these cases, thermal coagulation modalities are reasonable alternatives.

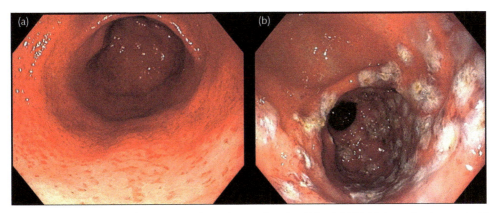

Figure 7.6 Endoscopic haemostasis in a case with gastric antral vascular ectasia-related bleed. (a) Multiple small red spots studding the antrum. (b) Endoscopic appearance after endoscopic haemostasis using argon plasma coagulation.

EBL provides mechanical compression at the bleeding site and has been successfully utilized in bleeding due to certain aetiologies like a Dieulafoy lesion and gastric antral vascular ectasia. In a randomized trial, there was no difference in efficacy or safety between the band ligation and endoscopic haemoclip groups in cases with bleeding Dieulafoy lesions.[45] In another retrospective study, primary haemostasis was achieved equally after EBL and haemoclips. Re-bleeding rates (3.1% vs 14.7%) and procedure duration (11.5 vs 19.1 minutes) were shorter in the EBL group.[46] The data on the role of EBL in gastric antral vascular ectasia-related bleeding are more limited. Few retrospective studies indicate that EBL may be superior to APC with less frequent re-bleeding rates and reduced need of blood transfusions.[46] Large, prospective trials are required to define the role of EBL in the management of upper GI bleeding related to Dieulafoy lesions and gastric antral vascular ectasia.

Recurrent bleeding: prediction, prevention, and treatment

Predictors of recurrent bleeding

Recurrent bleeding occurs in 8–15% of patients after initial endoscopic haemostasis and is associated with a high mortality. Major predictors for re-bleeding include haemodynamic instability, active bleeding at endoscopy, large ulcer size (>2 cm), ulcer location (posterior duodenum or high lesser curvature), a very low haemoglobin concentration, and the need for transfusion.[47,48]

Prevention of re-bleeding

With increasing use of PPIs as potent acid suppressants, the incidence of recurrent bleeding has reduced. Patients with bleeding ulcers and high-risk stigmata should receive high-dose PPI infusion, that is, IV loading dose (80 mg) followed by continuous infusion (8 mg/hour) for 72 hours after endoscopy.[5] In a well-conducted randomized trial, high-dose IV esomeprazole infusion reduced re-bleeding (5.9% vs 10.3%), requirement of endoscopic re-treatment (6.4% vs 11.6%), surgery (2.7% vs 5.4%), and all-cause mortality (0.8% vs 2.1%) compared to placebo.[49] Other regimens including intermittent IV bolus and double-dose oral PPIs have also been shown to be effective in preventing re-bleeding.[50–52] After 72 hours, twice-daily PPIs should be used for 2 weeks followed by once-daily PPIs in high-risk patients.[5] In addition, H. pylori should be checked in peptic ulcer-related bleeding and appropriate therapy initiated if detected. Since the sensitivity of H. pylori testing is lower in acute settings, it is recommended to re-check for H. pylori if the initial result is negative.[28]

The role of second-look endoscopy to prevent re-bleeding has been a subject of debate for several decades. In the absence of a strong benefit, routine endoscopy is not recommended for the prevention of re-bleeding. Moreover, high-dose IV PPI therapy is effective in preventing re-bleeding obviating the need for re-look endoscopy.[53] On the other hand, repeat endoscopy may be useful in selected cases where initial endoscopic haemostasis was considered suboptimal, there is a history of use of non-steroidal anti-inflammatory drugs, and large amounts of blood have been transfused.[53]

Management of re-bleeding

Re-bleeding can be managed with endoscopy in the majority of cases. In a randomized trial, re bleeding could be controlled with endoscopy in 35 out of 48 patients (73%). Hypotension and an ulcer size of at least 2 cm were independent factors predictive of the failure of endoscopic retreatment.[54] The use of OTSCs is an alternative in cases who fail with conventional endoscopic haemostatic modalities.[55]

Novel endoscopic haemostatic modalities

In this section, we shall briefly discuss upcoming techniques and devices for the management of NVUGIB. These include the use of a Doppler endoscopic probe (DEP), haemostatic spray, and OTSCs.

The DEP allows the assessment of arterial blood flow in ulcers with high-risk stigmata. Therefore, it potentially improves the risk stratification of high-risk ulcers over endoscopic visual impression alone and guides further management.[56,57] In a randomized trial (148 patients), re-bleeding rates were compared between visual-guided endoscopic haemostasis and DEP-guided haemostasis in patients who presented with severe NVUGIB.[56] The rates of re-bleeding within 30 days were significantly lower in the Doppler probe-guided group (11.1% vs 26.3%; $p = 0.021$). In a systematic review and meta-analysis, DEP-guided management yielded decreased overall re-bleeding, bleeding-related mortality, and need for surgery.[58] At present the data are limited and the use of a DEP may be affected by availability and expertise.[5] The current guidelines (Asia-Pacific Working Group (2018) and International Consensus Group (2019)) do not recommend the use of DEP-guided endotherapy.[5,29]

Nevertheless, the DEP appears to be a promising technique and should be evaluated further.

Haemostatic spray (Hemospray, TC-325) is an inorganic inert powder that forms a mechanical barrier and enhances clot formation when it comes into contact with blood. The notable advantages of haemostatic spray are that it is easy to use and achieves high intraprocedural haemostasis (80–95%) in GI bleeding due to various causes.[29] In a recent multicentre, randomized trial, TC-325 was non-inferior to standard endoscopic treatment in the control of NVUGIB.[59] However, most of the Hemospray powder gets washed away within 24–48 hours explaining the high re-bleeding rate (10–40%) which is a major drawback.[60,61] The risk factors for re-bleeding after Hemospray include spurting type of bleed and hypotension at presentation. The guidelines from the International Consensus Group recommend against using TC-325 as a single therapeutic strategy.[5] Hemospray can be useful in cases with GI bleeding due to malignant causes and as a temporary haemostatic method pending more definitive approaches. Preliminary data show that Hemospray use may improve outcomes in patients with acute variceal bleeding as well.[62]

The OTSC is a novel clip that is larger and has a greater compressing force than conventional endoclips. The complete set consists of an applicator cap with a mounted OTSC clip, thread, thread retriever, and a hand wheel for clip release. The applicator cap is mounted over the tip of the endoscope and the clip is released by rotating the handwheel akin to endoscopic variceal ligation. In a multicentre randomized trial, the OTSC was compared with standard endoscopic treatment (endoclips and thermocoagulation) in 66 patients with recurrent peptic ulcer bleeding. Further re-bleeding was significantly less frequent in the OTSC group (15.2% 57.6%; $p = 0.001$).[55] However, there was no difference in the requirement for surgery or mortality between the two groups. As a primary modality, OTSC is superior to standard haemostatic modalities especially in cases with major stigmata for recent haemorrhage (active spurting bleeding, visible vessel, or clot).[63] A recent systematic review including 21 studies and 851 patients analysed the efficacy and safety of the OTSC in GI bleeding. The primary clinical success rate was 96.6% (95% CI 95.1–98.2%) and re-bleeding rate 10.3% (95% CI 6.5–14.1%). The failure rate of OTSCs was 9% and 26% when used as primary modality and rescue modality, respectively.[64] In another very recent systematic review and meta-analysis, haemostasis with OTSC was associated with a higher clinical success rates and lower 7-day and 30-day re-bleeding rate in cases with high-risk NVUGIB.[65] The Asia-Pacific Working Group consensus recommends the use of OTSCs in treating bleeding refractory to conventional endoscopic therapy.[29]

Transcatheter arterial embolization

Transcatheter arterial embolization (TAE) is an effective option in refractory peptic ulcer bleeding and in cases where the site of bleeding cannot be localized on endoscopy. Prophylactic TAE (after endoscopic therapy) may be considered in selected high-risk peptic ulcer bleeds.[66,67] In addition, it can also be used in poor surgical risk cases as a bridge for patient optimization before definitive surgery. Although TAE does not completely eliminate the need for surgery, it is increasingly being preferred over surgery especially because many patients with refractory NVUGIB are elderly with multiple comorbidities. In a large study (282 patients), 97 patients underwent TAE for uncontrolled peptic ulcer bleeding. The overall hazard of death was decreased by 34% in the TAE group (adjusted hazard ratio 0.66, 95% CI 0.46–0.96). In addition, the complications were fewer as compared to surgery (8.3% vs 32.2%). However, the risk of re-bleeding was higher after TAE compared with surgery (hazard ratio 2.48, 95% CI 1.33–4.62).[68] In patients with angiographically negative acute upper GI bleeding, empiric TAE has been shown to be an effective option with a clinical success and re-bleeding rates of 75% and 36%, respectively.[69] The main drawback with TAE is re-bleeding which occurs in up to one-third of the patients.[68,70] In the absence of high-quality data, the choice between TAE and surgery should be individualized based on availability and candidacy for surgery. TAE is preferable in patients who are poor candidates for surgery.

Surgical management

Over the last few decades, the use of endoscopic haemostasis and potent acid-suppressive medications has increased with a parallel decline in the rate of salvage surgeries especially definitive surgeries like vagotomy, gastric resection, or pyloroplasty.[71]

In the current era, surgery is indicated in the following scenarios: refractory bleeding after two endoscopic sessions and non-availability or failure of TAE (Figure 7.7). Hypotension and ulcer size of 2 cm or greater are predictive factors for failure of endoscopic treatment and may predict the possible requirement for surgery in NVUGIB.[54]

The major concern with emergency surgery is high mortality (10–30%) mainly due to patient-related factors such as comorbid illnesses.[72,73] In a nationwide cohort study, the mortality after emergency surgery for bleeding peptic ulcers was 17.8%.[73] Similar mortality rates have been reported in the 2007 UK audit and nationwide in hospital data from the US.[2,71]

There are two main types of surgeries that are performed in patients with refractory NVUGIB. These include definitive surgeries which intend to achieve haemostasis as well as prevent recurrent bleeding in future. Definitive surgery includes underrunning or excision of the ulcer for achieving haemostasis in combination with vagotomy (truncal or selective) and gastrectomy or drainage procedure. Vagotomy and gastrectomy result in reduced acid secretion in the postoperative period and are performed with an intention to prevent future recurrences. Definitive surgeries are usually avoided in patients with severe comorbidities and haemodynamic instability.

The minimal surgical approach aims at rapid control of bleeding by ligating the culprit vessel. Different methods of suture plication include two-quadrant (6 and 12 o'clock), four-quadrant plication, and 'U'-shaped plication.[74] Regardless of the technique used, the aim is to control bleeding from major branches of the gastroduodenal artery and the transverse pancreatic artery. Ulcer excision is used especially in cases with gastric ulcer with high suspicion of malignancy. The minimal approach is especially useful in poor surgical risk patients with multiple comorbidities. However, the risk of recurrent bleeding is higher as compared to the definitive approach, such as vagotomy/drainage or antrectomy.[75]

Choice of surgery: definitive versus minimal approach

The optimal surgical approach in cases with refractory NVUGIB is not clear in the light of current evidence. The differences in re-bleeding and mortality rates in the published studies are probably due to differences in study population and comorbidities. In a large

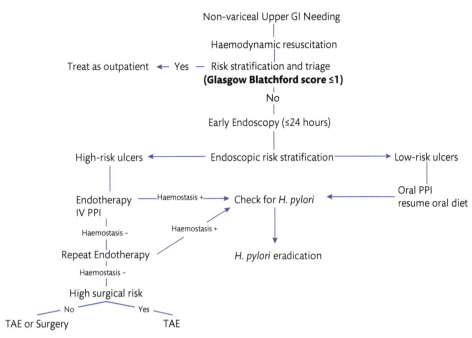

Figure 7.7 Management algorithm in cases with non-variceal upper gastrointestinal bleeding.

retrospective study, vagotomy/drainage was found to be superior to local oversewing in patients who required emergency surgery for bleeding peptic ulcers. Vagotomy/drainage was associated with a significantly lower postoperative mortality rate (9.1% vs 21.3%).[76] There was no demonstrable advantage of vagotomy/gastric resection procedure with respect to early postoperative outcomes in the same study. In addition, a longer hospital stay is a disadvantage of vagotomy/gastric resection in these patients.[76,77] In contrast, re-bleeding rates were lower (3% vs 17%) and mortality rates were similar (23% vs 22%) in the gastric resection group as compared to oversewing with vagotomy in an earlier study.[78] In another study, there was no significant difference in mortality between vagotomy/pyloroplasty (10%), gastric resection (12%), and vagotomy/antrectomy (6%).[79]

In conclusion, the requirement of salvage surgery has declined with the availability of PPIs and advancements in endoscopic haemostatic techniques. The choice of surgery in refractory bleeding ulcers is guided by the available expertise and patient comorbidities. A minimal surgical approach is a reasonable alternative in high surgical risk patients. The other argument in favour of a minimal approach is that the majority of the studies depicting poor outcomes with this approach were conducted before the PPI era. With the availability of potent acid-suppressive medications and *H. pylori* eradication regimens, the requirement of definitive surgeries is likely to decline.[80] In otherwise fit patients, a definitive approach such as vagotomy/drainage is an option due to lower re-bleeding rates (0–10%). Gastric resection with Billroth I or II anastomosis may be required in some cases with large distal gastric ulcers (>2 cm) along the lesser curvature.

Upper gastrointestinal bleeding (other than varices and peptic ulcer related)

Other causes of upper GI bleeding can be broadly divided into acid related (e.g. gastritis, oesophagitis) and non-acid related (angiodysplasia and Mallory–Weiss tear). Bleeding related to gastritis and oesophagitis is usually not severe, often does not require endotherapy, and can usually be managed with acid-suppressing medications. The requirement and type of endotherapy for other lesions is dictated by the type of lesions and the severity of bleeding. The options for endoscopic haemostasis are similar to those available for peptic ulcer-related bleeding. The notable exception to the conventional management protocol for upper GI bleeding is aortoenteric fistula which is a rare but fatal cause of upper GI bleeding. Aortoenteric fistula should be suspected in cases with a history of graft repair for aortic aneurysm. Endoscopic haemostasis is not effective in these cases. Urgent computed tomography angiography and surgery can be life-saving.

Summary

The incidence of emergency hospitalization for upper GI bleeding has reduced over the last few decades. This reflects improved availability of upper GI endoscopy, increasing use of PPIs and *H. pylori* eradication therapies, and routine screening of patients with portal hypertension. The primary aim in patients presenting with upper GI bleeding is haemodynamic stabilization, irrespective of the underlying cause. Endoscopic haemostasis is effective in the majority of patients with variceal and non-variceal bleeding. In the current era, surgery is rarely required for refractory variceal or non-variceal GI bleeding.

REFERENCES

1. Abougergi MS, Travis AC, Saltzman JR. The in-hospital mortality rate for upper GI hemorrhage has decreased over 2 decades in the United States: a nationwide analysis. *Gastrointest Endosc.* 2015;**81**:882–888.

2. Hearnshaw SA, Logan RF, Lowe D, Travis SP, Murphy MF, Palmer KR. Acute upper gastrointestinal bleeding in the UK: patient characteristics, diagnoses and outcomes in the 2007 UK audit. *Gut*. 2011;**60**:1327–1335.
3. Zheng NS, Tsay C, Laine L, Shung DL. Trends in characteristics, management, and outcomes of patients presenting with gastrointestinal bleeding to emergency departments in the United States from 2006 to 2019. *Aliment Pharmacol Ther*. 2022;**56**:1543–1555.
4. Tripathi D, Stanley AJ, Hayes PC, et al. U.K. guidelines on the management of variceal haemorrhage in cirrhotic patients. *Gut*. 2015;**64**:1680–1704.
5. Barkun AN, Almadi M, Kuipers EJ, et al. Management of nonvariceal upper gastrointestinal bleeding: guideline recommendations from the International Consensus Group. *Ann Intern Med*. 2019;**171**:805–822.
6. Villanueva C, Colomo A, Bosch A, et al. Transfusion strategies for acute upper gastrointestinal bleeding. *N Engl J Med*. 2013;**368**:11–21.
7. Radadiya D, Devani K, Rockey DC. The impact of red blood cell transfusion practices on inpatient mortality in variceal and non-variceal gastrointestinal bleeding patients: a 20-year US nationwide retrospective analysis. *Aliment Pharmacol Ther*. 2022;**56**:41–55.
8. Garcia-Tsao G, Abraldes JG, Berzigotti A, Bosch J. Portal hypertensive bleeding in cirrhosis: risk stratification, diagnosis, and management: 2016 practice guidance by the American Association for the Study of Liver Diseases. *Hepatology*. 2017;**65**:310–335.
9. Seo YS, Park SY, Kim MY, et al. Lack of difference among terlipressin, somatostatin, and octreotide in the control of acute gastroesophageal variceal hemorrhage. *Hepatology*. 2014;**60**:954–963.
10. Laine L, Cook D. Endoscopic ligation compared with sclerotherapy for treatment of esophageal variceal bleeding. A meta-analysis. *Ann Intern Med*. 1995;**123**:280–287.
11. Rodrigues SG, Cardenas A, Escorsell A, Bosch J. Balloon tamponade and esophageal stenting for esophageal variceal bleeding in cirrhosis: a systematic review and meta-analysis. *Semin Liver Dis*. 2019;**39**:178–194.
12. Mohan BP, Chandan S, Khan SR, et al. Self-expanding metal stents versus TIPS in treatment of refractory bleeding esophageal varices: a systematic review and meta-analysis. *Endosc Int Open*. 2020;**8**:E291–E300.
13. Sarin SK, Lahoti D, Saxena SP, Murthy NS, Makwana UK. Prevalence, classification and natural history of gastric varices: a long-term follow-up study in 568 portal hypertension patients. *Hepatology*. 1992;**16**:1343–1349.
14. Robles-Medranda C, Oleas R, Valero M, et al. Endoscopic ultrasonography-guided deployment of embolization coils and cyanoacrylate injection in gastric varices versus coiling alone: a randomized trial. *Endoscopy*. 2020;**52**:268–275.
15. Mohan BP, Chandan S, Khan SR, et al. Efficacy and safety of endoscopic ultrasound-guided therapy versus direct endoscopic glue injection therapy for gastric varices: systematic review and meta-analysis. *Endoscopy*. 2020;**52**:259–267.
16. Sheibani S, Khemichian S, Kim JJ, et al. Randomized trial of 1-week versus 2-week intervals for endoscopic ligation in the treatment of patients with esophageal variceal bleeding. *Hepatology*. 2016;**64**:549–555.
17. Tripathi D, Stanley AJ, Hayes PC, et al. Transjugular intrahepatic portosystemic stent-shunt in the management of portal hypertension. *Gut*. 2020;**69**:1173–1192.
18. Hung ML, Lee EW. Role of transjugular intrahepatic portosystemic shunt in the management of portal hypertension: review and update of the literature. *Clin Liver Dis*. 2019;**23**:737–754.
19. Hernandez-Gea V, Procopet B, Giraldez A, et al. Preemptive-TIPS improves outcome in high-risk variceal bleeding: an observational study. *Hepatology*. 2019;**69**:282–293.
20. Lv Y, Yang Z, Liu L, et al. Early TIPS with covered stents versus standard treatment for acute variceal bleeding in patients with advanced cirrhosis: a randomised controlled trial. *Lancet Gastroenterol Hepatol*. 2019;**4**:587–598.
21. Bureau C, Garcia-Pagan JC, Otal P, et al. Improved clinical outcome using polytetrafluoroethylene-coated stents for TIPS: results of a randomized study. *Gastroenterology*. 2004;**126**:469–475.
22. Lee EW, Shahrouki P, Alanis L, Ding P, Kee ST. Management options for gastric variceal hemorrhage. *JAMA Surg*. 2019;**154**:540–548.
23. Yu Q, Liu C, Raissi D. Balloon-occluded retrograde transvenous obliteration versus transjugular intrahepatic portosystemic shunt for gastric varices: a meta-analysis. *J Clin Gastroenterol*. 2021;**55**:147–158.
24. Luo X, Xiang T, Wu J, et al. Endoscopic cyanoacrylate injection versus balloon-occluded retrograde transvenous obliteration for prevention of gastric variceal bleeding: a randomized controlled trial. *Hepatology*. 2021;**74**:2074–2084.
25. Henderson JM, Boyer TD, Kutner MH, et al. Distal splenorenal shunt versus transjugular intrahepatic portal systematic shunt for variceal bleeding: a randomized trial. *Gastroenterology*. 2006;**130**:1643–1651.
26. Orloff MJ. Fifty-three years' experience with randomized clinical trials of emergency portacaval shunt for bleeding esophageal varices in cirrhosis: 1958–2011. *JAMA Surg*. 2014;**149**:155–169.
27. Stanley AJ, Laine L, Dalton HR, et al. Comparison of risk scoring systems for patients presenting with upper gastrointestinal bleeding: international multicentre prospective study. *BMJ*. 2017;**356**:i6432.
28. Gralnek IM, Dumonceau JM, Kuipers EJ, et al. Diagnosis and management of nonvariceal upper gastrointestinal hemorrhage: European Society of Gastrointestinal Endoscopy (ESGE) Guideline. *Endoscopy*. 2015;**47**:a1–a46.
29. Sung JJ, Chiu PW, Chan FKL, et al. Asia-Pacific working group consensus on non-variceal upper gastrointestinal bleeding: an update 2018. *Gut*. 2018;**67**:1757–1768.
30. Sreedharan A, Martin J, Leontiadis GI, et al. Proton pump inhibitor treatment initiated prior to endoscopic diagnosis in upper gastrointestinal bleeding. *Cochrane Database Syst Rev*. 2010;**10**:CD005415.
31. Ingason AB, Hreinsson JP, Agustsson AS, et al. Rivaroxaban is associated with higher rates of gastrointestinal bleeding than other direct oral anticoagulants: a nationwide propensity score-weighted study. *Ann Intern Med*. 2021;**174**:1493–1502.
32. Ingason AB, Hreinsson JP, Agustsson AS, et al. Warfarin is associated with higher rates of upper but not lower gastrointestinal bleeding compared to direct oral anticoagulants: a population-based propensity-weighted cohort study. *Clin Gastroenterol Hepatol*. 2022. 14 Aug. doi: 10.1016/j.cgh.2022.06.033. Epub ahead of print.

33. Chan FKL, Goh KL, Reddy N, et al. Management of patients on antithrombotic agents undergoing emergency and elective endoscopy: joint Asian Pacific Association of Gastroenterology (APAGE) and Asian Pacific Society for Digestive Endoscopy (APSDE) practice guidelines. *Gut*. 2018;**67**:405–417.
34. Guo CLT, Wong SH, Lau LHS, et al. Timing of endoscopy for acute upper gastrointestinal bleeding: a territory-wide cohort study. *Gut*. 2022;**71**:1544–1550.
35. Lau JYW, Yu Y, Tang RSY, et al. Timing of endoscopy for acute upper gastrointestinal bleeding. *New England Journal of Medicine*. 2020;**382**:1299–1308.
36. Laine L, McQuaid KR. Endoscopic therapy for bleeding ulcers: an evidence-based approach based on meta-analyses of randomized controlled trials. *Clin Gastroenterol Hepatol*. 2009;**7**:33–47.
37. Lau JY, Sung JJ, Lee KK, et al. Effect of intravenous omeprazole on recurrent bleeding after endoscopic treatment of bleeding peptic ulcers. *N Engl J Med*. 2000;**343**:310–316.
38. Chiu PW, Ng EK, Cheung FK, et al. Predicting mortality in patients with bleeding peptic ulcers after therapeutic endoscopy. *Clin Gastroenterol Hepatol*. 2009;**7**:311–316.
39. Sung JJ, Tsoi KK, Lai LH, Wu JC, Lau JY. Endoscopic clipping versus injection and thermo-coagulation in the treatment of non-variceal upper gastrointestinal bleeding: a meta-analysis. *Gut*. 2007;**56**:1364–1373.
40. Lin HJ, Hsieh YH, Tseng GY, Perng CL, Chang FY, Lee SD. A prospective, randomized trial of large- versus small-volume endoscopic injection of epinephrine for peptic ulcer bleeding. *Gastrointest Endosc*. 2002;**55**:615–619.
41. Vergara M, Bennett C, Calvet X, Gisbert JP. Epinephrine injection versus epinephrine injection and a second endoscopic method in high-risk bleeding ulcers. *Cochrane Database Syst Rev*. 2014;**10**:CD005584.
42. Baracat F, Moura E, Bernardo W, et al. Endoscopic hemostasis for peptic ulcer bleeding: systematic review and meta-analyses of randomized controlled trials. *Surg Endosc*. 2016;**30**:2155–2168.
43. Kim JW, Jang JY, Lee CK, Shim JJ, Chang YW. Comparison of hemostatic forceps with soft coagulation versus argon plasma coagulation for bleeding peptic ulcer—a randomized trial. *Endoscopy*. 2015;**47**:680–687.
44. Toka B, Eminler AT, Karacaer C, Uslan MI, Koksal AS, Parlak E. Comparison of monopolar hemostatic forceps with soft coagulation versus hemoclip for peptic ulcer bleeding: a randomized trial (with video). *Gastrointest Endosc*. 2019;**89**:792–802.
45. Park CH, Joo YE, Kim HS, Choi SK, Rew JS, Kim SJ. A prospective, randomized trial of endoscopic band ligation versus endoscopic hemoclip placement for bleeding gastric Dieulafoy's lesions. *Endoscopy*. 2004;**36**:677–681.
46. Ahn DW, Lee SH, Park YS, et al. Hemostatic efficacy and clinical outcome of endoscopic treatment of Dieulafoy's lesions: comparison of endoscopic hemoclip placement and endoscopic band ligation. *Gastrointest Endosc*. 2012;**75**:32–38.
47. Elmunzer BJ, Young SD, Inadomi JM, Schoenfeld P, Laine L. Systematic review of the predictors of recurrent hemorrhage after endoscopic hemostatic therapy for bleeding peptic ulcers. *Am J Gastroenterol*. 2008;**103**:2625–2632.
48. Garcia-Iglesias P, Villoria A, Suarez D, et al. Meta-analysis: predictors of rebleeding after endoscopic treatment for bleeding peptic ulcer. *Aliment Pharmacol Ther*. 2011;**34**:888–900.
49. Sung JJ, Barkun A, Kuipers EJ, et al. Intravenous esomeprazole for prevention of recurrent peptic ulcer bleeding: a randomized trial. *Ann Intern Med*. 2009;**150**:455–464.
50. Sung JJ, Suen BY, Wu JC, et al. Effects of intravenous and oral esomeprazole in the prevention of recurrent bleeding from peptic ulcers after endoscopic therapy. *Am J Gastroenterol*. 2014;**109**:1005–1010.
51. Sachar H, Vaidya K, Laine L. Intermittent vs continuous proton pump inhibitor therapy for high-risk bleeding ulcers: a systematic review and meta-analysis. *JAMA Intern Med*. 2014;**174**:1755–1762.
52. Laine L, Shah A, Bemanian S. Intragastric pH with oral vs intravenous bolus plus infusion proton-pump inhibitor therapy in patients with bleeding ulcers. *Gastroenterology*. 2008;**134**:1836–1841.
53. Park SJ, Park H, Lee YC, et al. Effect of scheduled second-look endoscopy on peptic ulcer bleeding: a prospective randomized multicenter trial. *Gastrointest Endosc*. 2018;**87**:457–465.
54. Lau JY, Sung JJ, Lam YH, et al. Endoscopic retreatment compared with surgery in patients with recurrent bleeding after initial endoscopic control of bleeding ulcers. *N Engl J Med*. 1999;**340**:751–776.
55. Schmidt A, Golder S, Goetz M, et al. Over-the-scope clips are more effective than standard endoscopic therapy for patients with recurrent bleeding of peptic ulcers. *Gastroenterology*. 2018;**155**:674–686.
56. Jensen DM, Kovacs TOG, Ohning GV, et al. Doppler endoscopic probe monitoring of blood flow improves risk stratification and outcomes of patients with severe nonvariceal upper gastrointestinal hemorrhage. *Gastroenterology*. 2017;**152**:1310–1318.
57. Barkun AN, Adam V, Wong RCK. Use of Doppler probe in nonvariceal upper-gastrointestinal bleeding is less costly and more effective than standard of care. *Clin Gastroenterol Hepatol*. 2019;**17**:2463–2470.
58. Chapelle N, Martel M, Bardou M, Almadi M, Barkun AN. Role of the endoscopic Doppler probe in nonvariceal upper gastrointestinal bleeding: systematic review and meta-analysis. *Dig Endosc*. 2022. 22 May. doi: 10.1111/den.14356. Epub ahead of print.
59. Lau JYW, Pittayanon R, Kwek A, et al. Comparison of a hemostatic powder and standard treatment in the control of active bleeding from upper nonvariceal lesions: a multicenter, noninferiority, randomized trial. *Ann Intern Med*. 2022;**175**:171–178.
60. Rodriguez de Santiago E, Burgos-Santamaria D, Perez-Carazo L, et al. Hemostatic spray powder TC-325 for GI bleeding in a nationwide study: survival and predictors of failure via competing risks analysis. *Gastrointest Endosc*. 2019;**90**:581–590.
61. Chahal D, Lee JGH, Ali-Mohamad N, Donnellan F. High rate of re-bleeding after application of Hemospray for upper and lower gastrointestinal bleeds. *Dig Liver Dis*. 2020;**52**:768–772.
62. Ibrahim M, El-Mikkawy A, Abdel Hamid M, et al. Early application of haemostatic powder added to standard management for oesophagogastric variceal bleeding: a randomised trial. *Gut*. 2019;**68**:844–853.
63. Jensen DM, Kovacs T, Ghassemi KA, Kaneshiro M, Gornbein J. Randomized controlled trial of over-the-scope clip as initial treatment of severe nonvariceal upper gastrointestinal bleeding. *Clin Gastroenterol Hepatol*. 2021;**19**:2315–2323.

64. Chandrasekar VT, Desai M, Aziz M, et al. Efficacy and safety of over-the-scope clips for gastrointestinal bleeding: a systematic review and meta-analysis. *Endoscopy*. 2019;**51**:941–949.
65. Bapaye J, Chandan S, Naing LY, et al. A systematic review and meta-analysis of safety and efficacy of over the scope clips versus standard therapy for high-risk non-variceal upper gastrointestinal bleeding. *Gastrointest Endosc*. 2022;**96**:712–720.
66. Boros E, Sipos Z, Hegyi P, et al. Prophylactic transcatheter arterial embolization reduces rebleeding in non-variceal upper gastrointestinal bleeding: a meta-analysis. *World J Gastroenterol*. 2021;**27**:6985–6999.
67. Chang JHE, Lye TJY, Zhu HZ, et al. Systematic review and meta-analysis of prophylactic transarterial embolization for high-risk bleeding peptic ulcer disease. *J Vasc Interv Radiol*. 2021;**32**:576–584.
68. Sverden E, Mattsson F, Lindstrom D, Sonden A, Lu Y, Lagergren J. Transcatheter arterial embolization compared with surgery for uncontrolled peptic ulcer bleeding: a population-based cohort study. *Ann Surg*. 2019;**269**:304–309.
69. Yu Q, Funaki B, Navuluri R, et al. Empiric transcatheter embolization for acute arterial upper gastrointestinal bleeding: a meta-analysis. *AJR Am J Roentgenol*. 2021;**216**:880–893.
70. Wong TC, Wong KT, Chiu PW, et al. A comparison of angiographic embolization with surgery after failed endoscopic hemostasis to bleeding peptic ulcers. *Gastrointest Endosc*. 2011;**73**:900–908.
71. Wang YR, Richter JE, Dempsey DT. Trends and outcomes of hospitalizations for peptic ulcer disease in the United States, 1993 to 2006. *Ann Surg*. 2010;**251**:51–58.
72. Jairath V, Kahan BC, Logan RF, et al. National audit of the use of surgery and radiological embolization after failed endoscopic haemostasis for non-variceal upper gastrointestinal bleeding. *Br J Surg*. 2012;**99**:1672–1680.
73. Byrne BE, Bassett M, Rogers CA, et al. Short-term outcomes after emergency surgery for complicated peptic ulcer disease from the UK National Emergency Laparotomy Audit: a cohort study. *BMJ Open*. 2018;**8**:e023721.
74. Chiu PW, Ng EK, Wong SK, et al. Surgical salvage of bleeding peptic ulcers after failed therapeutic endoscopy. *Dig Surg*. 2009;**26**:243–248.
75. Poxon VA, Keighley MR, Dykes PW, Heppinstall K, Jaderberg M. Comparison of minimal and conventional surgery in patients with bleeding peptic ulcer: a multicentre trial. *Br J Surg*. 1991;**78**:1344–1345.
76. Schroder VT, Pappas TN, Vaslef SN, De La Fuente SG, Scarborough JE. Vagotomy/drainage is superior to local oversew in patients who require emergency surgery for bleeding peptic ulcers. *Ann Surg*. 2014;**259**:1111–1118.
77. de la Fuente SG, Khuri SF, Schifftner T, Henderson WG, Mantyh CR, Pappas TN. Comparative analysis of vagotomy and drainage versus vagotomy and resection procedures for bleeding peptic ulcer disease: results of 907 patients from the Department of Veterans Affairs National Surgical Quality Improvement Program database. *J Am Coll Surg*. 2006;**202**:78–86.
78. Millat B, Hay JM, Valleur P, Fingerhut A, Fagniez PL. Emergency surgical treatment for bleeding duodenal ulcer: oversewing plus vagotomy versus gastric resection, a controlled randomized trial. French Associations for Surgical Research. *World J Surg*. 1993;**17**:568–573.
79. Hunt PS, McIntyre RL. Choice of emergency operative procedure for bleeding duodenal ulcer. *Br J Surg*. 1990;**77**:1004–1006.
80. Abe N, Takeuchi H, Yanagida O, Sugiyama M, Atomi Y. Surgical indications and procedures for bleeding peptic ulcer. *Dig Endosc*. 2010;**22**(Suppl 1):S35–S37.

8

Upper gastrointestinal perforation
Non-surgical and surgical management

Alexander Hendricks, Mark Ellrichmann, and Clemens Schafmayer

Introduction

Perforations of the upper intestinal tract and specifically those of the oesophagus are serious conditions. There are multiple reasons for perforations but the most frequent causes are iatrogenic injuries.[1] Localization of perforations are thoracic in 70%, cervical in 15%, and abdominal in 12% of cases.[2] The clinical symptoms are diverse and this often leads to delayed diagnosis and initiation of adequate treatment.[3-5] Due to a number of severe comorbidities, for instance, mediastinitis with subsequent sepsis, the general mortality rate of oesophageal perforations can be between 15% and 50%.[6-8] The chance of mortality depends on the location of the oesophageal perforation—for instance, perforations of the cervical and also the lower thoracic and abdominal oesophagus have mortality rates of 6–20%[6,9,10] and 3–22%,[3,6,11,12] respectively. Patients suffering from perforation of the middle oesophageal segment experience significantly higher mortality rates of 5.4–36%[6,10,13] (Figure 8.1). In addition to location, multiple studies have demonstrated that the time span between time of diagnosis and initiation of treatment is significantly related to mortality.[14,15] If adequate intervention is started earlier than 24 hours after the time of diagnosis, there is a substantial decrease in mortality, hospital stay, and treatment duration.[16-18] In these cases, mortality may be as low as 0–18%. If the time interval exceeds 24 hours, mortality rates of 7–37.5% have been observed, essentially due to progressive local sepsis.[3,19]

Causes of oesophageal perforation

Iatrogenic oesophageal perforation is the most common cause with frequencies around 59–63% because of advances in medical innovation and the increasing frequency of minimally invasive endoscopic treatment and diagnostic approaches and options. These include procedures in patients with spontaneous reflux oesophagitis tumours, after radio-chemotherapy (16%), foreign body ingestion (12%), and trauma-associated (9%) perforation.[6,9,20,21] A special variant of the oesophageal perforation is the Boerhaave syndrome, which is caused by excessive vomiting.[22]

Diagnosis of oesophageal perforation

Due to the varied and non-specific symptoms, the diagnosis of oesophageal rupture is challenging and often delayed.[23] In general, patients report non-specific chest pain, and later, with progression of the illness, fever and shivering; subsequently, with no intervention taking place, there is severe septicaemia. Clinical signs of mediastinitis often manifest in arrhythmia and anomalies in blood pressure. In terms of instrumental diagnosis, radiological as well as endoscopic techniques are often utilized. Computed tomography (CT) scanning is undoubtedly superior to fluoroscopy.

The gold standard in adequately and precisely diagnosing oesophageal rupture is indeed the endoscopy. This allows an accurate analysis and diagnosis of the perforation, its location, and its extent. Furthermore, endoscopy as the initial diagnostic approach allows immediate therapeutic intervention. A CT scan should also be performed to allow the diagnosis of comorbidities, such as mediastinitis, pneumothorax, pleural effusion or empyema, and pneumonia.

Therapeutic options in oesophageal ruptures

In general, there are three possible regimens for the treatment of oesophageal perforations: (1) conservative/watch-and-wait, (2) endoscopy, and (3) surgery. When deciding on the most suitable therapeutic management strategy, several key parameters must be considered: the clinical state of the patient, inflammatory status, extent and localization of the perforation, potential pathogenic mechanism,[9,16] time interval from diagnosis to initiation of therapy, and lastly the individual's experience of interventional endoscopy.[24,25]

Conservative approach

In rare cases, conservative management is adequate for the treatment of oesophageal ruptures. This may be indicated for perforations of a small size, located in the upper third of the oesophagus, but must be accompanied by gastric tube feeding (or

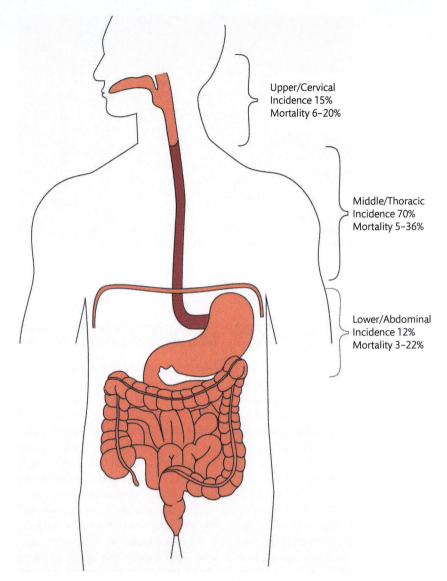

Figure 8.1 Depiction of the gastrointestinal tract showing apportionment of the oesophagus with the rates of incidence for perforation and concordant mortality rates.

even parenteral feeding) and by broad-spectrum antibiotics.[26] It has been reported that the mortality of conservative management is 17% and the need for surgical intervention during the course of illness is 20%.[9,13,27] A major weakness of non-intervention is the lack of the possibility of wound lavage. Hence, this choice must be restricted to those in whom the contamination is moderate and there is little inflammation.

Endoscopy

In general, endoscopic treatment is the gold standard for closing and adequately treating most oesophageal perforations. Before deciding on the most suitable therapeutic strategy, non-operative management criteria have to be considered.[28] Novel endoscopic techniques including clips, stents, and vacuum therapy have emerged over the last decades and have been shown to be excellent and effective treatment regimens.[29] In patients who present early and have contained oesophageal disruption and minimal contamination, non-operative management is indicated.[28]

Application of fibrin adhesives and plugs

The application of fibrin adhesives and plugs has been described in a few experimental studies.[30,31] After initial insertion of the fibrin adhesive, a plug is administered. However, in several cases, the non-invasive intervention was followed by an add-on surgical intervention or stent application. Undoubtedly, this concept is only suitable for minor perforations with confined surrounding inflammatory reaction. The treatment of gastrointestinal fistulae would be an appropriate indication. Valid analyses and assumptions cannot be drawn due to the small sample sizes and few existing studies and case reports. Ultimately, the practitioner/clinician must opt for this method on an individual non-empiric basis.

Clip application

Application of clips by endoscopy has been performed for decades. In general, this is a very thoroughly investigated and studied method of sealing perforations. Continuous developmental approaches have led to a safe and enhanced technique of endoscopic intervention. In

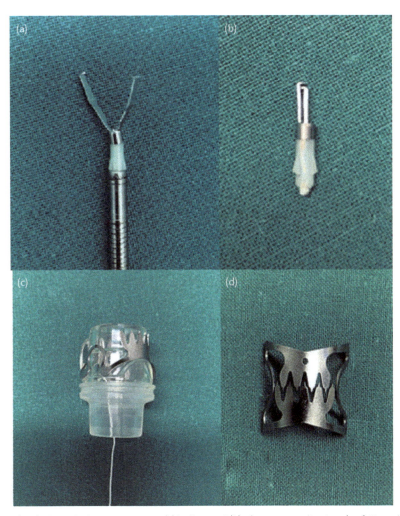

Figure 8.2 Endoscopic stenting. (a, b) Through-the-scope stents, (a) before and (b) after stent application. (c, d) Over-the-scope stents, (c) before and (d) after stent application.

principle, two key types of clips and their application can be specified: through-the-scope clips (TTSCs) (Figure 8.2a,b) and over-the-scope clips (OTSCs) (Figure 8.2c,d).

TTSCs are applied through the working channel of the endoscope. They are designed to seal small mucosal defects and lessen intense haemorrhage. Fully opened and ready for application they span 11 mm and are hence indicated for defects of <10 mm. TTSCs only grasp the tissue. As a consequence, multiple TTSCs may be necessary for sufficient treatment of a defect or bleeding. With larger defects (10–20 mm), OTSCs may be useful.[32] This clip device consists of an over-the-scope applicator cap with a mounted Nitinol clip. The clip itself is fitted with anchors which compress the tissue safely and appropriately. To start with, the tissue or perforation is fully loaded into the cap at the distal end of the endoscope either by suction or with the help of a grasper device. Then by manual force the clip is released.[33] Overall the rate of complications is stated to be 1%, making this method a safe approach in the entire gastrointestinal tract.[32,34,35] According to the guidelines of the European Society of Gastrointestinal Endoscopy, in patients with oesophageal perforations, clips should only be applied in clinically stable patients with perforations smaller than 2 cm and no signs of general inflammation.[36] However, these recommendations are based on small sample studies and are empiric. Large, robust studies comparing the use and effectiveness of TTSCs and OTSCs are lacking. Lázár et al. summarized the current data and case reports.[32] If TTSC was applied in patients with an oesophageal perforation, an effective closure was reported in 88.8% (24/27). In patients treated with an OTSC, successful healing was achieved in 92.8% (26/28) with no statistically significant difference ($p = 0.12$).[32] An example of effective application of TTSCs is in patients after peroral endoscopic myotomy for treating achalasia and other oesophageal motility disorders. In 100% of the patients a complete closure was observed after clip application.[37] The long-term outcome after clip application is rarely monitored. A large retrospective study in which 188 patients were followed up after OTSC application revealed the following information on outcome: median follow-up of 146 days, complete sealing of perforations in 90% and of leakages in 73.3%. If OTSCs are employed in the initial therapeutic intervention, the long-term outcome is significantly superior.[15] Chronic transmural defects (e.g. in fistulae or anastomotic leaks) pose a difficult challenge for successful clip application. Due to the thickening and scarring of connective tissue, the technique is demanding. OTSCs and TTSCs have been studied in this setting in small trials and case reports. In 57.7% (15/26) of patients with fistulae and 77.7% (12/18) of patients with leaks, the application and the outcome were successful. Deploying TTSCs, in 100% (4/4) of patients with chronic fistulae a positive outcome was obtained and 54.4% (6/11) of patients with a leak were treated effectively.[38,39]

Combination techniques

This method uses a combination of two techniques for sealing larger perforations in the gastrointestinal tract, which cannot be sufficiently handled by stand-alone clip application due to the diameter restrictions of the clips. In general, TTSCs are applied around the circumference of the intestinal wall defect, are then enclosed by an endoloop and lastly pulled together—analogous to a pouch suture. In the beginning this technique was described and applied after large endoscopic mucosal resections, but later also for the treatment of the Mallory–Weiss syndrome.[40,41] To date, only a few case studies have reported on this technique, hence there is no reference for general application and its use should be indicated on an individual basis.

Endoscopic suturing

Endoscopically driven suturing is an innovative approach of sealing. For over a decade various many approaches have been evaluated, but few have been used on a large scale.[42] Using an experimental animal model, a metal anchor in the shape of a T (T-tags; Ethicon Endo-Surgery, Cincinnati, OH, USA) was developed for sealing oesophageal leaks. At the tip of each T-tag a polypropylene thread is mounted. By using a hollow needle, the T-tag and thread are put into place by puncturing the tissue a few millimetres away from the perforation. Then the contralateral gastrointestinal wall is punctured, and another T-tag is ejected. Afterwards, the threads are tied together with a locking cinch. In the earlier mentioned animal model study, this approach achieved an equivalent outcome to established thoracoscopically based sutures.[43–45] This technique has an advantage over the other procedures, as it limits the manoeuvring of the endoscope and hence allows for more precise movement. However, the depth of penetration of the needle and T-tag application is not predictable, and may cause extraluminal bleeding or perforation of neighbouring structures. Moreover, in another study the authors questioned whether the sealing of the perforation was sufficient because their data and experience suggested there was leakage of air after application of the T-tags.[41] T-tags have not yet received approval for clinical use. Various other methods of endoscopic suturing have been developed, but their clinical application in treating oesophageal perforations in particular is limited. Up-to-date valid data can only be found regarding the OverStitch Endoscopic Suturing System (Apollo Endosurgery, Austin, TX, USA). Referring to this, case reports have been published in which encouraging outcomes were described. The system's needle driver attaches to the distal end of an endoscope, whereas the OverStitch handle that triggers the needle driver is placed at the proximal end of the endoscope, allowing for endoluminal suturing. Both absorbable and non-absorbable threads can be used, and suturing can be performed either by a single stitch or continuously.[46] Halvax et al. published data in which they demonstrated adequate and sufficient closure of transmural defects of up to 3 cm in an animal model at a rate of 100%.[47] Deploying the OverStitch system to incidents in the oesophagus, only case reports have been published. The scope of allocation includes transmural perforations, postoperative anastomotic leakages, and the fixation of self-expanding metal stents in order to overcome their migration.[48–51] The OverStitch method undoubtedly offers a technique of sealing transmural defects of the gastrointestinal tract in centres with experience in interventional endoscopy.

Endoscopic stenting

Stent application is widely accepted and deployed in the treatment of oesophageal perforation and anastomotic leakages. Over the last decades it has become the standard treatment mode. Historically, this practice is not really innovative. In 1878, Symonds applied a prothesis as an oesophageal stent made of iron and silver[52] and in 1914, the palliative treatment of stenotic oesophageal lesions by oesophageal tubes was first described. Placement happened once the oesophageal lumen could be viewed directly. After this, stents or rigid tubes were regularly used in patients with stenosis in the oesophagus when there was no option for surgical resection. A major disadvantage of these inflexible stents was their proneness to migration, and due to the stent stiffness their initial placement as well as replacement was challenging. In the 1990s, a significant advance was made by the use of self-expanding stents composed of either Elgiloy (cobalt, nickel, chrome) or Nitinol (nickel, titanium) (Figure 8.3). Placement of these novel stents can be done by flexible endoscopy with much less risk and higher comfort for the patient. Additionally, the radial pressure in the oesophageal tube is lower, leading to less dilation of the oesophagus and consequently less frequent stent migration.

A medical breakthrough was the development of coated flexible stents. These self-expanding and flexible stents were covered with polymers like silicon, polyurethane, or other biomaterials. After this there was a steady utilization of endoscopic stenting in oesophageal perforations or anastomotic leakages with the first case series published around the turn of the millennium. The outcomes in terms of associated morbidity and mortality and treatment success were variable. Following the initial case series, larger cohorts of patient data were pooled and analysed and a standard procedure regimen was developed. The overall successful outcome on endoscopic stenting was reported to be 81–86% and it was generally recommended that the stent should be removed after 6–8 weeks of therapy[53–59]—in some animal experiments complete healing was observed only 4 weeks after initial stent application.[53,56] Furthermore, continuous advancements in the evolution of endoscopic stenting led to a decrease of

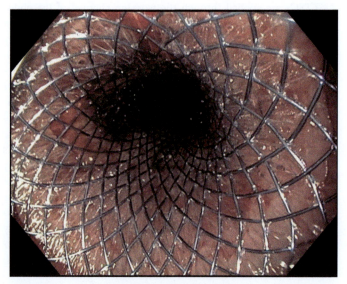

Figure 8.3 Oesophageal stent after submission. A covered Nitinol stent was applied to seal an oesophageal perforation.

linked mortality and complications to 10–13% and 13–34%, respectively.[53,54,56,58] Freeman et al. proposed oesophageal stenting potentially to be just as effective as surgery for oesophageal perforations.[60] Only in 13% of cases is surgical intervention needed, mainly to deal with stent-related complications or incomplete healing of the initial injury.[54,58] In general, a positive outcome is affected not only by the time interval between initial diagnosis and induction of stenting, but also by the subsequent degree of inflammation, localization, and the extent of perforation. Extensive perforations, those across the gastro-oesophageal junction, or perforations of the very proximal oesophagus have a worse outcome. Some patients do not tolerate the stent easily and greater rates of failure of therapy are observed in them.[58] Data on the threshold of the extent of the rupture at which treatment failure occurs are inconsistent and vague. In their study, Ong and Freeman stated the maximum diameter of ruptures in which successful treatment was achieved was 6 cm. Perforations larger than this treated by endoscopic stenting have a worse outcome.[58] Van Halsema et al. described an increased risk of therapy failure in septic patients with a defect larger than 1.5 cm that had persisted for several weeks.[57] In general, there is a consensus that for a beneficial outcome after applying endoscopic stenting in oesophageal perforations, there must be certain conditions present: (1) early insertion of large lumen thoracic drains, (2) immediate initiation of antibiotics, and (3) enteral feeding either via a triluminal tube or via a percutaneous endoscopic gastrostomy.[58,61] In addition to this, soon after initial endoscopic treatment, a CT scan should be performed to assess whether drainage of an abscess or other inflammatory formation now covered by the stent is necessary. Furthermore, complications such as mediastinitis, pneumonia, pleural effusion, or pleural empyema should be detected by the CT scan, allowing for rapid intervention and hence improving the outcome. Technically sound oesophageal stent implantation is reported to have a success rate of 91–100% in the literature. Adverse events following stenting are dislocation in 2–3% and migration in 18–31%, where endoscopic or surgical intervention is indicated in 21% of these cases.[53–57,61] In order to minimize stent dislocation or migration and hence achieve a stable closure of the perforation, there have been many options described—the stent can be attached by endoscopic clipping or fixed by suturing or heat sealing to the mucosa by an argon plasma beam. In summary, covered stents are an established option for adequately treating oesophageal perforations. The outcome monitored and reported by multiple studies is sound, though to some degree not appropriately consistent. Various studies are non-controlled, sample sizes limited, and patients heterogeneous. As a consequence, it is crucial to constantly monitor the patient's state and to evaluate interim goals achieved by stenting. The clinician should consider alternative endoscopic options as well as surgical intervention, particularly in case of deterioration of the patient's condition. All decision-making should be performed by a multidisciplinary team.

Endoluminal vacuum therapy

The first case of successful endoluminal vacuum therapy was reported in 2007.[62] In the following years, multiple studies of its use in postoperative anastomotic leaks and perforations in the upper gastrointestinal tract were reported in Germany,[14,63–68] although the commencement of endoluminal vacuum therapy was seen in the treatment of anastomotic leaks after operations on the lower gastrointestinal tract.[62,69,70] As a consequence of successful outcomes

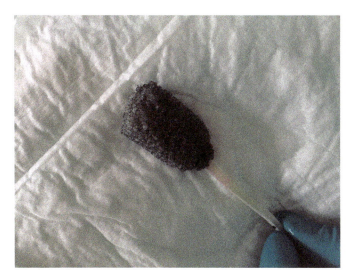

Figure 8.4 Endoscopic vacuum therapy. A polyurethan sponge as depicted here is introduced into the cavity and replaced on a regular basis.

and in some areas even superior ways of handling leaks and perforations compared to the conventional treatment options, in 2014 the Eso-Sponge (B. Bruan, Aesculap AG, Germany) was introduced (Figure 8.4).

This device presents a standardized and for the first time CE-certified product that permits the universal application of an adequate treatment regimen. At a set procedure, a size-adjusted polyurethane sponge is endoscopically inserted into the cavernous defect lining the entire perforation. Via a flexible tube, which is placed transnasally, a constant negative pressure of approximately 75–125 mmHg is applied by a vacuum pump.[71] The vacuum administered by the sponge leads to a build-up and conditioning of granulation tissue resulting in faster cleaning and complete healing of the wound[72,73] (Figures 8.5 and 8.6). Every 2–3 days the sponge has to be exchanged endoscopically.

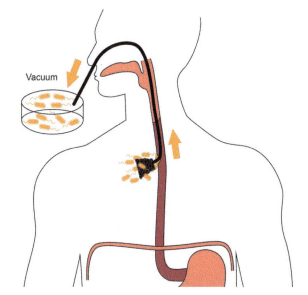

Figure 8.5 Schematic depiction of the fundamentals of endoscopic vacuum therapy. The polyurethan sponge is inserted into the cavity and transnasally discharged. A continuous negative pressure is applied to the sponge for wound healing.

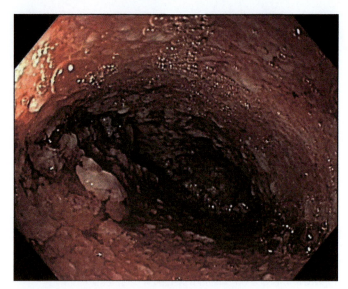

Figure 8.6 Wound cavity after endoscopic vacuum therapy. The wound closure at the base is sufficient and a significant granulation is implemented.

Experience showed that an extension of the intervals led to a more frequent ingrowth of the sponge leading to a technically more challenging endoscopic intervention, hence putting the patient at more risk with less benefit at the same time.[74] Distinct advantages of the replicate endoscopic endoluminal vacuum therapies include being on-site, allowing repeated lavage, inspection over a period of time, and a direct closure of the septic defect with simultaneous drainage.

The primary end point of this treatment scheme is the state of the fully sealed wound bed. Several studies performed over recent years have clearly demonstrated a positive outcome for patients with septicaemia and mediastinitis due to oesophageal perforations that were treated by endoluminal vacuum therapy[72,73] and in comparison to endoscopic stenting, superior results in terms of patient survival (80–96%)[67,68,75–77] and complete healing of the wound cavity (84–100%)[14,63,64,66,78–80] have been reported. The secondary effects of the endoluminal vacuum therapy are excessive stenosis as a result of scaring, which is mostly reversible by endoscopic dilatation.[65,67,68,77,81] The on-site sponge can presumably lead to a disproportionate degree of granulation, hence resulting in stenosis. Despite the exceptional short- and long-term outcomes of endoluminal vacuum therapy, after initial endoscopic intervention and sponge placement, a CT scan of the thorax should be performed to detect the extent of mediastinitis and other local consequences. In addition, it is important to perform a multidisciplinary evaluation of the patient's present state, the continuous therapeutic success, and treatment approach including endoscopists, intensive care physicians, and surgeons. Nevertheless, on the basis of recent literature, endoluminal vacuum therapy is clearly the most effective method of dealing with perforations of the upper gastrointestinal tract. In the event of failure or clinical deterioration of the patient, a surgical option should be considered.

Surgery

Surgical intervention still plays an important part in the treatment of major oesophageal perforations and ensures suitable prompt handling of the condition.[6] It should be performed in all patients who do not meet the non-operative management criteria.[28] The mortality of the surgical intervention largely depends on the timespan between point of diagnosis and start of surgery—it is crucial to try for early intervention. Patients being admitted to the operative room within 24 hours after time of diagnosis show a significantly reduced mortality of under 10%, compared to 30% in those operated later.[6,20,82,83]

In general, the advantages and indications for surgical oesophageal perforation management include clear exposure of the defect, possibility of debridement of non-viable tissue, chance of closure of the perforation and adequate wound drainage, haemodynamic instability, intra-abdominal perforation, and presence of an underlying malignancy.[28]

Various reports and studies have been published to date regarding the surgical approach to dealing with oesophageal perforations, indicating that there is an ongoing debate on the appropriate procedures. Surgical strategy depends on the location of the oesophageal perforation—cervical, thoracic, or abdominal.

Summary

An oesophageal perforation results in an acute clinical problem which is often associated with significant mortality and morbidity. Adequate handling of this involves immediate and diagnostic and therapeutic interventions using an interdisciplinary approach. The role of surgical intervention is rare nowadays and reserved for severe injuries. Endoscopy plays a key role in diagnosis and treating the vast majority. Some variables should be considered in the evaluation of the appropriate endoscopic treatment: (1) time to point of diagnosis, (2) time span between diagnosis and start of possible treatment, (3) size of the perforation, (4) secondary infectious focus, and (5) local expertise of the treating physician. Based on our experience, we have established the following workflow for handling perforations of the upper gastrointestinal tract: for small lesions (<1 cm), which have been diagnosed early (within 24 hours) and do not show inflammation, we usually apply an endoclip, and for slightly larger lesions (1–2 cm) we apply an OTSC. In case of an oesophageal perforation larger than 2 cm, but without any inflammation, we stent the defect, and in rare cases also overstitch it. If the patient deteriorates with this approach, and therapy monitoring shows unsatisfactory results, the treatment is changed to endoscopic vacuum therapy. In cases of a late primary diagnosis (>24 hours) or inflammation of the wound, endoscopic vacuum therapy is our primary approach. Small perforations (<1 cm) are dealt with by endoluminal sponge placement. In case of larger defects (>1 cm), the sponge is initially placed inside the cavity. If necessary, more than one sponge is used. If despite the vacuum therapy there is deterioration of the patient, or the cavity is not granulating and healing sufficiently, the therapeutic regimen can be changed to a surgical intervention. In sum, to guarantee the most optimal outcome for the patient, it is crucial to pursue an interdisciplinary approach involving specialists from endoscopy, intensive care medicine, and surgery.

REFERENCES

1. Baron TH, Wong Kee Song LM, Zielinski MD, Emura F, Fotoohi M, Kozarek RA. A comprehensive approach to the management of acute endoscopic perforations (with videos). *Gastrointest Endosc.* 2012;**76**:838–859.

2. Sdralis EIK, Petousis S, Rashid F, Lorenzi B, Charalabopoulos A. Epidemiology, diagnosis, and management of esophageal perforations: systematic review. *Dis Esophagus*. 2017;**30**:1–6.
3. Griffiths EA, Yap N, Poulter J, Hendrickse MT, Khurshid M. Thirty-four cases of esophageal perforation: the experience of a district general hospital in the UK. *Dis Esophagus*. 2009;**22**:616–625.
4. Wang N, Razzouk AJ, Safavi A, et al. Delayed primary repair of intrathoracic esophageal perforation: is it safe? *J Thorac Cardiovasc Surg*. 1996;**111**:114–122.
5. Søreide JA, Konradsson A, Sandvik OM, Øvrebø K, Viste A. Esophageal perforation: clinical patterns and outcomes from a patient cohort of Western Norway. *Dig Surg*. 2012;**29**:494–502.
6. Abbas G, Schuchert MJ, Pettiford BL, et al. Contemporaneous management of esophageal perforation. *Surgery*. 2009;**146**:749–756.
7. Hermansson M, Johansson J, Gudbjartsson T, et al. Esophageal perforation in South of Sweden: results of surgical treatment in 125 consecutive patients. *BMC Surgery*. **10**:31.
8. Markar SR, Mackenzie H, Wiggins T, et al. Management and outcomes of esophageal perforation: a national study of 2,564 patients in England: *Am J Gastroenterol*. 2015;**110**:1559–1566.
9. Brinster CJ, Singhal S, Lee L, Marshall MB, Kaiser LR, Kucharczuk JC. Evolving options in the management of esophageal perforation. *Ann Thorac Surg*. 2004;**77**:1475–1483.
10. Gupta NM, Kaman L. Personal management of 57 consecutive patients with esophageal perforation. *Am J Surg*. 2004;**187**:58–63.
11. Braghetto MI, Rodríguez NA, Csendes JA, Korn BO. Perforación esofágica: Experiencia clínica y actualización del tema. *Rev Méd Chile*. 2019;**133**:1233–1241.
12. Eroglu A, Turkyilmaz A, Aydin Y, Yekeler E, Karaoglanoglu N. Current management of esophageal perforation: 20 years experience. *Dis Esophagus*. 2009;**22**:374–380.
13. Vogel SB, Rout WR, Martin TD, Abbitt PL. Esophageal perforation in adults: aggressive, conservative treatment lowers morbidity and mortality. *Ann Surg*. 2005;**241**:1016–1023.
14. Weidenhagen R, Hartl WH, Gruetzner KU, Eichhorn ME, Spelsberg F, Jauch KW. Anastomotic leakage after esophageal resection: new treatment options by endoluminal vacuum therapy. *Ann Thorac Surg*. 2010;**90**:1674–1681.
15. Biancari F, D'Andrea V, Paone R, et al. Current treatment and outcome of esophageal perforations in adults: systematic review and meta-analysis of 75 studies. *World J Surg*. 2013;**37**:1051–1059.
16. Schmidt SC, Strauch S, Rösch T, et al. Management of esophageal perforations. *Surg Endosc*. 2010;**24**:2809–2813.
17. Heits N, Bernsmeier A, Reichert B, et al. Long-term quality of life after endovac-therapy in anastomotic leakages after esophagectomy. *J Thorac Dis*. 2018;**10**:228–240.
18. Hauge T, Kleven OC, Johnson E, Hofstad B, Johannessen HO. Outcome after iatrogenic esophageal perforation. *Scand J Gastroenterol*. 2019;**54**:140–144.
19. Wang Y, Zhang R, Zhou Y, et al. Our experience on management of Boerhaave's syndrome with late presentation. *Dis Esophagus*. 2009;**22**:62–67.
20. Chirica M, Champault A, Dray X, et al. Esophageal perforations. *J Visc Surg*. 2010;**147**:e117–e128.
21. Nirula R. Esophageal perforation. *Surg Clin North Am*. 2014;**94**:35–41.
22. de Schipper JP, Pull ter Gunne AF, Oostvogel HJM, van Laarhoven CJHM. Spontaneous rupture of the oesophagus: Boerhaave's syndrome in 2008. Literature review and treatment algorithm. *Dig Surg*. 2009;**26**:1–6.
23. Lin Y, Jiang G, Liu L, et al. Management of thoracic esophageal perforation. *World J Surg*. 2014 May;**38**:1093–1099.
24. Carrott PW, Low DE. Advances in the management of esophageal perforation. *Thorac Surg Clin*. 2011;**21**:541–555.
25. Kuppusamy MK, Hubka M, Felisky CD, et al. Evolving management strategies in esophageal perforation: surgeons using nonoperative techniques to improve outcomes. *J Am Coll Surg*. 2011;**213**:164–171.
26. Amir AI, van Dullemen H, Plukker JTM. Selective approach in the treatment of esophageal perforations. *Scand J Gastroenterol*. 2004;**39**:418–422.
27. Altorjay A, Kiss J, Vörös A, Bohák A. Nonoperative management of esophageal perforations. Is it justified? *Ann Surg*. 1997;**225**:415–421.
28. Chirica M, Kelly MD, Siboni S, et al. Esophageal emergencies: WSES guidelines. *World J Emerg Surg*. 2019;**14**:26.
29. Watkins JR, Farivar AS. Endoluminal therapies for esophageal perforations and leaks. *Thorac Surg Clin*. 2018;**28**:541–554.
30. Harries K, Masoud A, Brown TH, Richards DG. Endoscopic placement of fibrin sealant as a treatment for a long-standing Boerhaave's fistula. *Dis Esophagus*. 2004;**17**:348–350.
31. Rábago LR, Castro JL, Joya D, et al. [Esophageal perforation and postoperative fistulae of the upper digestive tract treated endoscopically with the application of Tissucol]. *Gastroenterol Hepatol*. 2000;**23**:82–86.
32. Lázár G, Paszt A, Mán E. Role of endoscopic clipping in the treatment of oesophageal perforations. *World J Gastrointest Endosc*. 2016;**8**:13–22.
33. Kirschniak A, Kratt T, Stüker D, Braun A, Schurr M-O, Königsrainer A. A new endoscopic over-the-scope clip system for treatment of lesions and bleeding in the GI tract: first clinical experiences. *Gastrointest Endosc*. 2007;**66**:162–167.
34. Baron TH, Song LMWK, Ross A, Tokar JL, Irani S, Kozarek RA. Use of an over-the-scope clipping device: multicenter retrospective results of the first U.S. experience (with videos). *Gastrointest Endosc*. 2012;**76**:202–208.
35. Voermans RP, Le Moine O, von Renteln D, et al. Efficacy of endoscopic closure of acute perforations of the gastrointestinal tract. *Clin Gastroenterol Hepatol*. 2012;**10**:603–608.
36. Paspatis GA, Dumonceau JM, Barthet M, et al. Diagnosis and management of iatrogenic endoscopic perforations: European Society of Gastrointestinal Endoscopy (ESGE) position statement. *Endoscopy*. 2014;**46**:693–711.
37. Inoue H, Minami H, Kobayashi Y, et al. Peroral endoscopic myotomy (POEM) for esophageal achalasia. *Endoscopy*. 2010;**42**:265–271.
38. Mönkemüller K, Peter S, Toshniwal J, et al. Multipurpose use of the 'bear claw' (over-the-scope-clip system) to treat endoluminal gastrointestinal disorders. *Dig Endosc*. 2014;**26**:350–357.
39. Hagel AF, Naegel A, Lindner AS, et al. Over-the-scope clip application yields a high rate of closure in gastrointestinal perforations and may reduce emergency surgery. *J Gastrointest Surg*. 2012;**16**:2132–2138.
40. Ivekovic H, Rustemovic N, Brkic T, et al. The esophagus as a working channel: successful closure of a large Mallory-Weiss tear with clips and an endoloop. *Endoscopy*. 2011;**43**(Suppl 2):E170.
41. Luigiano C, Ferrara F, Polifemo AM, et al. Endoscopic closure of esophageal fistula using a novel 'clips and loop' method. *Endoscopy*. 2009;**41**(Suppl 2):E249–E250.
42. Stavropoulos SN, Modayil R, Friedel D. Current applications of endoscopic suturing. *World J Gastrointest Endosc*. 2015;**7**:777–789.

43. Austin RCT, Mosse CA, Swain P. A novel use of T-tag sutures for the safe creation and closure of the NOTES gastrotomy using a hybrid technique. *Surg Endosc.* 2009;**23**:2827–2830.
44. Fritscher-Ravens A, Hampe J, Grange P, et al. Clip closure versus endoscopic suturing versus thoracoscopic repair of an iatrogenic esophageal perforation: a randomized, comparative, long-term survival study in a porcine model (with videos). *Gastrointest Endosc.* 2010;**72**:1020–1026.
45. Mori H, Kobara H, Fujihara S, et al. Feasibility of pure EFTR using an innovative new endoscopic suturing device: the double-arm-bar suturing system (with video). *Surg Endosc.* 2014;**28**:683–690.
46. ASGE Technology Committee, Banerjee S, Barth BA, et al. Endoscopic closure devices. *Gastrointest Endosc.* 2012;**76**:244–251.
47. Halvax P, Diana M, Lègner A, et al. Endoluminal full-thickness suture repair of gastrotomy: a survival study. *Surg Endosc.* 2015;**29**:3404–3408.
48. Henderson JB, Sorser SA, Atia AN, Catalano MF. Repair of esophageal perforations using a novel endoscopic suturing system. *Gastrointest Endosc.* 2014;**80**:535–537.
49. Gaur P, Lyons C, Malik TM, Kim MP, Blackmon SH. Endoluminal suturing of an anastomotic leak. *Ann Thorac Surg.* 2015;**99**:1430–1432.
50. Lim BS, Eskandari A. Weaving through the twists and turns of the fish bone case: demonstration of 2 different indications for endoscopic suturing in a single case of esophageal leak. *Gastrointest Endosc.* 2016;**83**:826–827.
51. Maselli R, Viale E, Fanti L, Testoni P. Successful endoscopic suturing of esophageal perforation after surgical suturing failure. *Endoscopy.* 2017;**49**:E202–E203.
52. Symonds CJ. The treatment of malignant stricture of the oesophagus by tubage or permanent catheterism. *Br Med J.* 1887;**1**:870–873.
53. van Boeckel PGA, Sijbring A, Vleggaar FP, Siersema PD. Systematic review: temporary stent placement for benign rupture or anastomotic leak of the oesophagus. *Aliment Pharmacol Ther.* 2011;**33**:1292–1301.
54. Law R, Prabhu A, Fujii-Lau L, Shannon C, Singh S. Stent migration following endoscopic suture fixation of esophageal self-expandable metal stents: a systematic review and meta-analysis. *Surg Endosc.* 2018;**32**:675–681.
55. Vermeulen BD, Siersema PD. Esophageal stenting in clinical practice: an overview. *Curr Treat Options Gastroenterol.* 2018;**16**:260–273.
56. Dasari BVM, Neely D, Kennedy A, et al. The role of esophageal stents in the management of esophageal anastomotic leaks and benign esophageal perforations. *Ann Surg.* 2014;**259**:852–860.
57. van Halsema EE, Rauws EAJ, Fockens P, van Hooft JE. Self-expandable metal stents for malignant gastric outlet obstruction: a pooled analysis of prospective literature. *World J Gastroenterol.* 2015;**21**:12468–12481.
58. Ong GKB, Freeman RK. Endoscopic management of esophageal leaks. *J Thorac Dis.* 2017;**9**(Suppl 2):S135–S145.
59. Shah ED, Hosmer AE, Patel A, Morales S, Law R. Valuing innovative endoscopic techniques: endoscopic suturing to prevent stent migration for benign esophageal disease. *Gastrointest Endosc.* 2020;**91**:278–285.
60. Freeman RK, Herrera A, Ascioti AJ, Dake M, Mahidhara RS. A propensity-matched comparison of cost and outcomes after esophageal stent placement or primary surgical repair for iatrogenic esophageal perforation. *J Thorac Cardiovasc Surg.* 2015;**149**:1550–1555.
61. Licht E, Markowitz AJ, Bains MS, et al. Endoscopic management of esophageal anastomotic leaks after surgery for malignant disease. *Ann Thorac Surg.* 2016;**101**:301–304.
62. Weidenhagen R, Gruetzner KU, Wiecken T, Spelsberg F, Jauch KW. Endoscopic vacuum-assisted closure of anastomotic leakage following anterior resection of the rectum: a new method. *Surg Endosc.* 2008;**22**:1818–1825.
63. Heits N, Stapel L, Reichert B, et al. Endoscopic endoluminal vacuum therapy in esophageal perforation. *Ann Thorac Surg.* 2014;**97**:1029–1035.
64. Kuehn F, Schiffmann L, Rau BM, Klar E. Surgical endoscopic vacuum therapy for anastomotic leakage and perforation of the upper gastrointestinal tract. *J Gastrointest Surg.* 2012;**16**:2145–2150.
65. Schorsch T, Müller C, Loske G. Endoscopic vacuum therapy of anastomotic leakage and iatrogenic perforation in the esophagus. *Surg Endosc.* 2013;**27**:2040–2045.
66. Smallwood NR, Fleshman JW, Leeds SG, Burdick JS. The use of endoluminal vacuum (E-Vac) therapy in the management of upper gastrointestinal leaks and perforations. *Surg Endosc.* 2016;**30**:2473–2480.
67. Laukoetter MG, Mennigen R, Neumann PA, et al. Successful closure of defects in the upper gastrointestinal tract by endoscopic vacuum therapy (EVT): a prospective cohort study. *Surg Endosc.* 2017;**31**:2687–2696.
68. Möschler O, Nies C, Mueller MK. Endoscopic vacuum therapy for esophageal perforations and leakages. *Endosc Int Open.* 2015;**3**:E554–E558.
69. Nagell CF, Holte K. Treatment of anastomotic leakage after rectal resection with transrectal vacuum-assisted drainage (VAC). A method for rapid control of pelvic sepsis and healing. *Int J Colorectal Dis.* 2006;**21**:657–660.
70. Yousaf M, Witherow A, Gardiner KR, Gilliland R. Use of vacuum-assisted closure for healing of a persistent perineal sinus following panproctocolectomy: report of a case. *Dis Colon Rectum.* 2004;**47**:1403–1407.
71. Ahrens M, Schulte T, Egberts J, et al. Drainage of esophageal leakage using endoscopic vacuum therapy: a prospective pilot study. *Endoscopy.* 2010;**42**:693–698.
72. Nguyen NT, Rudersdorf PD, Smith BR, Reavis K, Nguyen X-MT, Stamos MJ. Management of gastrointestinal leaks after minimally invasive esophagectomy: conventional treatments vs. endoscopic stenting. *J Gastrointest Surg.* 2011;**15**:1952–1960.
73. Pennathur A, Luketich JD. Resection for esophageal cancer: strategies for optimal management. *Ann Thorac Surg.* 2008;**85**:S751–S756.
74. Schniewind B, Schafmayer C, Both M, Arlt A, Fritscher-Ravens A, Hampe J. Ingrowth and device disintegration in an intralobar abscess cavity during endosponge therapy for esophageal anastomotic leakage. *Endoscopy.* 2011;**43**(Suppl 2):E64–E65.
75. Feith M, Gillen S, Schuster T, Theisen J, Friess H, Gertler R. Healing occurs in most patients that receive endoscopic stents for anastomotic leakage; dislocation remains a problem. *Clin Gastroenterol Hepatol.* 2011;**9**:202–210.
76. Schweigert M, Dubecz A, Stadlhuber RJ, Muschweck H, Stein HJ. Treatment of intrathoracic esophageal anastomotic leaks by means of endoscopic stent implantation. *Interact Cardiovasc Thorac Surg.* 2011;**12**:147–151.

77. Bludau M, Hölscher AH, Herbold T, et al. Management of upper intestinal leaks using an endoscopic vacuum-assisted closure system (E-VAC). *Surg Endosc.* 2014;**28**:896–901.
78. Schniewind B, Schafmayer C, Voehrs G, et al. Endoscopic endoluminal vacuum therapy is superior to other regimens in managing anastomotic leakage after esophagectomy: a comparative retrospective study. *Surg Endosc.* 2013;**27**:3883–3890.
79. Wedemeyer J, Brangewitz M, Kubicka S, et al. Management of major postsurgical gastroesophageal intrathoracic leaks with an endoscopic vacuum-assisted closure system. *Gastrointest Endosc.* 2010;**71**:382–386.
80. Loske G, Schorsch T, Müller C. Endoscopic vacuum sponge therapy for esophageal defects. *Surg Endosc.* 2010;**24**:2531–2535.
81. Brangewitz M, Voigtländer T, Helfritz FA, et al. Endoscopic closure of esophageal intrathoracic leaks: stent versus endoscopic vacuum-assisted closure, a retrospective analysis. *Endoscopy.* 2013;**45**:433–438.
82. Biancari F, Saarnio J, Mennander A, et al. Outcome of patients with esophageal perforations: a multicenter study. *World J Surg.* 2014;**38**:902–909.
83. Ivatury RR, Moore FA, Biffl W, et al. Oesophageal injuries: position paper, WSES, 2013. *World J Emerg Surg.* 2014;**9**:9.

9

Obesity
Non-surgical treatment and bariatric surgery

Rishabh Shah, Lisandro Montorfano, Emanuele Lo Menzo, Samuel Szomstein, and Raul J. Rosenthal

Introduction

Obesity is a growing international health epidemic. In fact, as human society across the globe has become more sedentary and food sources more manufactured and processed, the rates of obesity have increased exponentially. The World Health Organization's data show a threefold increase in obesity since 1975, with nearly 2 billion adults being overweight or obese in 2016.[1] According to the Centers for Disease Control and Prevention, in the United States nearly 42% of adults were obese in 2017–2018.[2]

Besides the social implications of obesity, the burden of weight-related medical disorders has become one of the major concerns in modern medicine, as obesity affects nearly every organ system in the body (Table 9.1). Worldwide, more people die every year from obesity-related diseases than from complications of underweight. Consequently, the World Health Organization has prioritized halting the rise in obesity and diabetes as one of their nine targets in preventing and controlling non-communicable diseases.

Despite the recognition of obesity as a disease, it remains mistakenly viewed as a failure of character of the obese person. However, more and more evidence is available on the aspects of the genetic imprint and the environmental influences as key factors in the development of obesity.[3–5]

To date, surgical management of obesity has proven to be the most effective and long-lasting method of weight loss in the morbidly obese. However, despite the availability of a large body of literature on its effectiveness and safety, surgical treatment is still considered by many to be a secondary option. Every surgeon should understand the basic anatomy and pitfalls of bariatric operations as they may be called to treat patients who have a history of these procedures. Among the several historical and novel operations described in the literature, only the most common weight loss operations will be reviewed here. These include the Roux-en-Y gastric bypass (RNYGB), the sleeve gastrectomy (SG), the one-anastomosis gastric bypass (OAGB), the biliopancreatic diversion with duodenal switch (BPDDS), and the single-anastomosis duodeno-ileal bypass (SADI). The growing field of endoscopic obesity interventions will also be discussed. This chapter will also describe the most common non-operative interventions utilized against obesity.

Non-operative methods of weight loss

Diet and exercise

Diet has long been the most touted method to attain weight loss. Among a myriad of dietary interventions, caloric restriction, and the increase in roughage consumption, in the form of fruit and vegetables, have shown the best results in the short term. By contrast, the increase in calorie consumption with exercise has also been recommended, not only for the purpose of weight loss, but also to improve cardiovascular health. However, both dietary and exercise interventions have failed to result in robust and sustainable weight loss by themselves, mainly due to the difficult sustainability of such interventions over time.[6–9] In fact, even in well-conducted and strictly regulated clinical trials, such as the Surgical Treatment And Medications Potentially Eradicate Diabetes Efficiently (STAMPEDE), in which patients were prospectively randomized between bariatric surgery (RNYGB and SG) and intensive lifestyle therapy alone, the surgical

Table 9.1 Medical conditions related to obesity

Cardiac	Coronary artery disease, hypertension, hyperlipidaemia, pulmonary hypertension
Endocrine	Diabetes, infertility
Gastrointestinal	Gastro-oesophageal reflux disease, gallstone disease, steatosis, and cirrhosis
Integumentary	Intertriginous cellulitis, hidradenitis suppurativa
Musculoskeletal	Osteoarthritis, gout, risk of fracture
Neurological	Stroke, pseudotumor cerebri, depression
Oncological	Endometrial, breast, ovarian, prostate, liver, gallbladder, kidney, and colon cancers
Pulmonary	Obstructive sleep apnoea
Renal	Chronic and end-stage renal disease

arm results were more effective than the medical arm for weight loss and diabetes treatment for up to 5 years.[10] Also, the addition of weight loss surgery increases the results of the non-surgical interventions exponentially, as demonstrated in the Diabetes Surgery Study (DSS), another observational study examining RNYGB added to intensive lifestyle therapy and medical management of type 2 diabetes. This randomized observational study showed significant benefit of adding RNYGB to intensive lifestyle and medical management to the triple end point at 5 years (systolic blood pressure of <130 mmHg, haemoglobin A1C level of <7%, and low-density lipoprotein cholesterol concentration of <100 mg/dL).[11]

Drugs

Several medications with different mechanisms of action are currently approved by the US Food and Drug Administration for weight loss.[12] In addition to the modest results, some of these drugs can have significant side effects.

Among the drugs that limit intestinal absorption, orlistat, an inhibitor of pancreatic lipase, remains one of the most popular. This inhibition of lipase leads to an excretion in the faeces of up to 30% of the fat calories ingested. Studies on the use of orlistat have shown a 10% excess body weight loss, versus around 5% for placebo.[13] However, because of the indiscriminate reduction of fat absorption and the consequent excretion of fat in the stool, gastrointestinal side effects, such as abdominal boating, cramps, and flatulence, are common. In addition, fat-soluble vitamin deficiency can also occur.[13]

The more centrally acting noradrenergic sympathomimetics, such as phentermine, diethylpropion, benzphetamine, and phendimetrazine, cause early satiety by either increasing the release, or by blocking the uptake of norepinephrine (noradrenaline) at the nerve terminals. In the US, they are only approved for use up to 12 weeks, as they can increase heart rate and blood pressure. They also have a risk for potential abuse. Sibutramine, another potent inhibition of norepinephrine, serotonin (5-hydroxytryptamine), and to a lesser extent, dopamine reuptake at the neuronal synapse, was removed from the market in the US after being found to lead to an increased risk of myocardial infarction. Despite their serious potential side effects and based on their short time of utilization, this class of medications has been shown to lead to a modest 7.5 kg average weight loss.[14]

Glucagon-like peptide 1 (GLP-1) receptor agonists, such as liraglutide, stimulate insulin secretion, and inhibit glucagon release. In addition to their positive effects on diabetes, this class of drugs has resulted in weight loss. The use of this class of medications in obese patients with type 2 diabetes has the double benefit of improved glycaemic control and weight loss. Even for these medications, however, the weight loss remains only 2–4 kg greater than placebo. In addition, several gastrointestinal side effects, such as nausea and vomiting, are common.[15]

Serotonin antagonists, like lorcaserin, activate the central serotonin 2-C receptor, which reduces food intake. The reported weight loss for this class of drugs was found to be around 4 kg greater than placebo. Additional benefits also included reduction in the onset of obesity, improved blood pressure and cholesterol levels, and stabilization of chronic kidney disease, though the overall effects were modest. Side effects are mild and include upper respiratory infection and headache.[16]

Mechanism of surgical weight loss

While there is no doubt about the efficacy of bariatric surgery in terms of rapid and durable weight loss, less is known regarding the physiological changes that lead to that weight loss.

The most readily apparent mechanism of action of the metabolic procedures is the reduction in intake of calories. This seems to be the common element of all the metabolic procedures herein described. Normally the stretch receptors in the wall of the stomach mediate a gastro-hypothalamic feedback loop via the vagus nerve. A sensation of satiety ensues 10–20 minutes after gastric distension. Hence, patients after bariatric surgery learn a negative feedback loop if they overeat, and, consequently, experience emesis.[17]

The next common mechanism of action of the metabolic surgical procedures is the hypoabsorption of nutrients. In the BPDDS, RNYGB, and OAGB procedures, variable lengths of intestine are bypassed, where the nutrients are not absorbed or properly digested because of lack of pancreatic enzymes, bile, and gastrointestinal enterohormones. Consequently, the length of the remaining common channel, where chyme and pancreatic enzymes and bile mix, leads to variable amounts of nutrient absorption. However, restriction and malabsorption cannot by themselves explain the sometimes immediate onset of metabolic improvements, such as improved insulin sensitivity.[18–20]

Hormonal changes are the key in explaining the metabolic and satiety effects of bariatric surgery. The unusual presence of nutrients in the distal ileum due to the bypass of intestine and subsequent malabsorption lead to increased levels of certain enterohormones (GLP-1, peptide YY, etc.) that increase sensitivity and increase insulin release. By contrast, other substances, like the gastric-produced appetite-stimulating hormone ghrelin, are reduced in production.[21,22]

With the effectiveness of weight loss, regardless of mechanism, the resolution of the comorbidities follows. In fact, as previously mentioned, bariatric surgery has proven to be more effective than optimal medical therapy at treating (and sometimes curing) diabetes. Weight loss also positively affects other medical conditions proper of the metabolic syndrome, such as diabetes and coronary artery disease, and others closely related to it, such as obstructive sleep apnoea. Recent retrospective and prospective studies have shown improvement or halting in the progression of chronic kidney disease, improvement in left ventricular ejection fraction, and a decrease in cardiovascular risk.[10,11,23–28]

Bariatric surgery

Roux-en-Y gastric bypass

Long considered the gold standard in weight loss surgery, the RNYGB (Figure 9.1) for weight loss has decades of proven safety and efficacy. By creating both restriction (through the small gastric pouch) and malabsorption (as anywhere from 150 to 200 cm of small intestine is bypassed before pancreatic enzymes and bile mix with chyme), it creates significant weight loss. Although its popularity in recent years is lower compared to the SG, it remains the operation of choice for severe metabolic syndrome, severe gastro-oesophageal reflux disease, or the extremes of obesity. It also has the benefit of

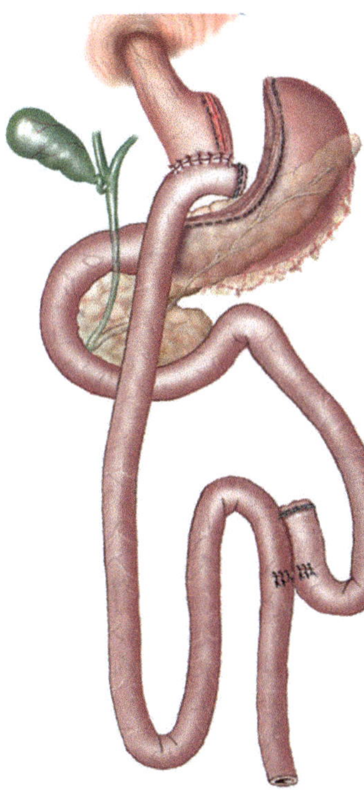

Figure 9.1 Roux-en-Y gastric bypass.
Reproduced with permission from Nuzzo A, Czernichow S, Hertig A, et al. Prevention and treatment of nutritional complications after bariatric surgery. *Lancet Gastroenterol Hepatol.* 2021;6(3):238–251.

reversibility, and it is the most common revisional procedure from other bariatric operations.

From a technical standpoint, the gastric bypass can be broken down into three major components: the creation of a gastric pouch, the creation of a gastrojejunostomy, and the creation of a jejunojejunostomy. The gastric pouch is based on the less stretchable lesser curvature of the stomach and it is created with several firings of a linear stapler with a full exclusion of the gastric fundus. When properly constructed, it should have a volume of approximately 30–60 mL. The alimentary (or Roux) limb is then constructed by dividing the jejunum at a variable distance of 50–100 cm distal to the ligament of Treitz. The distal portion of the divided jejunum is used to create a gastrojejunostomy. This has been historically described as being performed either through a created defect in the transverse mesocolon with the limb brought behind the remnant stomach (retrocolic retrogastric) or antecolic antegastric. Nowadays the antecolic antegastric route is preferred as it is technically easier, it creates one less mesenteric defect, and allows for easier revisional surgery. The gastrojejunostomy is performed either with a linear or circular stapler, or is completely handsewn. The diameter of the anastomosis is purposely kept small to enhance restriction. An air leak test is commonly performed to ensure integrity of the gastrojejunostomy.

Finally, the jejunojejunostomy is created by anastomosing the alimentary limb to the biliopancreatic limb at a variable length, but typically around 15–200 cm distal to the gastrojejunostomy.

Gastric bypass has been shown to result in 75% excess body weight loss. The not fully understood hormonal effects of bypassing the duodenum have also shown to result in a dramatic improvement in diabetes mellitus, especially type 2.[10,11] However, long-term complications can result in reoperation in 3–20% of patients after gastric bypass.[29]

Sleeve gastrectomy

Nowadays, the laparoscopic SG has become the most commonly performed operation worldwide. Initially designed as the first step of the biliopancreatic diversion, it was long ago recognized to be a free-standing procedure. The exponential popularity of the SG derives from its relative technical simplicity, its safety profile, and the excellent results, in terms of weight loss and comorbidity resolution. The SG now constitutes 70–80% of all bariatric operations performed. Due to its preservation of the gastrointestinal physiology, patients adapt more easily to the postoperative changes determined by the SG.

An SG (Figure 9.2) is a tubularization of the body of the stomach over a sizer (36–40 Fr bougie) resulting in the removal of the majority of the body and fundus of the organ. The division of the stomach is based on the less distensible lesser curvature. This accomplishes multiple goals. The first is to reduce the volume of the stomach. Second, the lesser curvature has less ability to distend and has a faster transit time than the greater curvature. The third is to drastically reduce the production of ghrelin, which in turn decreases the hunger drive in the body. Less clear is the mechanism that leads to the changes of the other enterohormones, such as GLP-1, seen early after such procedures.

The first step is the devascularization of the greater curvature of the stomach starting about 3–5 cm from the pylorus. The lesser sac is entered and the greater curve mesogastrium is divided along the greater curve up to the left crus of the diaphragm. In the presence of a hiatal hernia, this should be repaired posterior to the gastro-oesophageal junction. Attachments between the stomach and the retroperitoneum should also be divided without compromising the left gastric artery.

At this point, a bougie is passed to the level of the antrum and serial gastrointestinal stapler firings are used to create the gastric sleeve. The first and last firings are the most critical. The first should

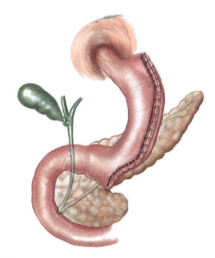

Figure 9.2 Sleeve gastrectomy.
Reproduced with permission from Nuzzo A, Czernichow S, Hertig A, et al. Prevention and treatment of nutritional complications after bariatric surgery. *Lancet Gastroenterol Hepatol.* 2021;6(3):238–251.

not narrow the stomach at the level of the incisura, as this can lead to gastric outlet obstruction. The last should stay lateral to the fat pad at the angle of His (Murphy's fat pad). The most dreaded complication of SG, in fact, is a leak at the proximal staple line. This complication derives from both distal obstruction and close stapling to the angle of His, determining ischaemia.

Multiple techniques are used to reinforce the staple line. If reinforcement seems to decrease the chance of bleeding, its benefit on decreasing leakage rates remains controversial.

The SG on average induces a weight loss of 60% excess body weight, with excellent metabolic results as well. The overall long-term complication rate is less than 5%, with severe gastro-oesophageal reflux disease being the most concerning.[30,31]

One-anastomosis gastric bypass

The OAGB has been more recently popularized as being a technically easier version of the traditional gastric bypass (Figure 9.3). Initially it was known as the 'mini-bypass' because it used to be performed through a small upper midline laparotomy. A gastric pouch is fashioned in a similar manner as to that previously described for the RNYGB, except intentionally left longer in order to minimize bile reflux to the oesophagus. A loop of jejunum is then identified to create the single-anastomosis loop gastrojejunostomy, similar to a Billroth II configuration. The length chosen for this limb has even more variability than that for the RNYGB. Some surgeons measure from the ligament of Treitz and use a 200 cm afferent limb. Others advocate for measuring a set length of common channel (400–500 cm) to maximize malabsorption without causing malnutrition. The jejunal loop is then advanced to the pouch in an antegastric fashion and an end-to-side gastrojejunostomy is constructed either via gastrointestinal anastomosis stapler or handsewn. The advantages of this technique include its relative simplicity, the presence of only one anastomosis, and the virtual absence of internal hernias.[32,33] By contrast, the long-term nutritional side effects are more pronounced because of the higher degree of hypoabsorption.

Biliopancreatic diversion with duodenal switch

Although considered the most metabolically effective bariatric operation, the BPDDS (Figure 9.4) is also the most technically challenging one. Based on this dichotomy, the BPDDS is usually reserved for patients with higher body mass index or severe metabolic comorbidities such as brittle diabetes mellitus.

After a higher volume SG is performed similar to the earlier description, the next step is the division of the duodenum at the first portion using a linear stapler. Care must be taken to avoid injury to the right gastric artery, the right gastroepiploic artery, and the gastroduodenal artery. The duodenal cuff should be as long as possible to aid in creating the duodeno-ileostomy.

Next, the small bowel is divided 250 cm proximal to the ileocaecal valve, and the distal ileum is anastomosed to the proximal duodenum to create a Roux limb, by using a gastrointestinal anastomosis stapler, end-to-end anastomosis stapler, or handsewn technique.

Then a segment of distal ileum is selected 100 cm proximal to the ileocaecal valve. A side-to-side ileoileostomy similar to the jejunojejunostomy in the RNYGB is created. The mesenteric defect is then closed.

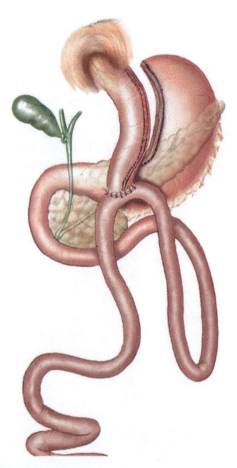

Figure 9.3 One-anastomosis gastric bypass.
Reproduced with permission from Nuzzo A, Czernichow S, Hertig A, et al. Prevention and treatment of nutritional complications after bariatric surgery. *Lancet Gastroenterol Hepatol.* 2021;6(3):238–251.

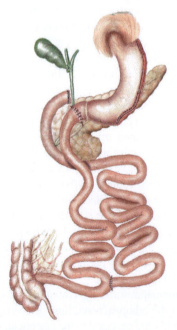

Figure 9.4 Biliopancreatic diversion with duodenal switch.
Reproduced with permission from Nuzzo A, Czernichow S, Hertig A, et al. Prevention and treatment of nutritional complications after bariatric surgery. *Lancet Gastroenterol Hepatol.* 2021;6(3):238–251.

BPDDS has a higher total weight loss compared to the RNYGB. More impressively (likely due to the enterohormonal mechanisms described above), up to 98% of diabetics are cured of their disease.[34,35] However, similarly to the OAGB, the long-term metabolic derangements are more pronounced, and closer follow-up is necessary.

Single-anastomosis duodeno-ileal bypass

The SADI combines an SG with a loop duodeno-ileostomy about 200–300 cm proximal to the ileocaecal valve (Figure 9.5). This allows for a competent pylorus and a single anastomosis. This approach obviates the concern for bile reflux as well as potentially giving the metabolic effects of BPDDS without the surgical complexity.[36–38] More reports are becoming available regarding its efficacy; however, the metabolic consequences remain more severe than in other, less hypoabsorptive operations.

Bariatric complications

The most important topic of discussion for the general surgeon who will not be performing bariatric surgery is the care of complications secondary to bariatric surgery.

Gastrointestinal leaks can occur at any staple line or anastomosis that is created during bariatric surgery. Probably the most feared is the proximal gastric leak after SG. The high-pressure system determined by the narrow gastric lumen, and the relative distal obstruction determined by the intact pylorus, makes spontaneous closure of the leak unlikely. As a consequence, therapeutic options for these chronic leaks require morbid procedures, such as the proximal gastrectomy and oesophagojejunostomy. Fistulae to the bronchus, pleura, and colon have also been described. Other anastomotic leaks in haemodynamically stable patients and in the absence of distal obstruction, while a worrisome complication, many times can be treated with wide drainage, *nil per os*, and total parenteral nutrition. However, any anastomotic leak if unrecognized and not properly treated can lead to significant morbidity and mortality.[39–41]

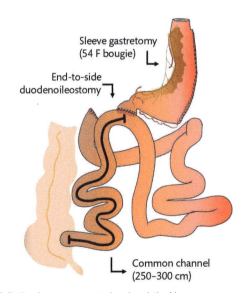

Figure 9.5 Single anastomosis duodenal-ileal bypass.
Reproduced with permission from Ruano-Campos A, Lasses B, Ser bariatric surg, et al. SADI (single-anastomosis duodeno-ileal bypass): current evidence. *Curr Surg Rep.* 2020;8:20.

Marginal ulcers occur at any anastomosis between the small intestine and stomach (RNYGB, OAGB). The presence of the pylorus usually prevents this complication. The ulcer is on the intestinal side of the anastomosis. The aetiology is typically multifactorial. Tension on the gastrojejunostomy or use of tobacco products can lead to ischaemia and reduction in mucosal protective factors. Frequent use of non-steroidal anti-inflammatory drugs or *Helicobacter pylori* infection also decreases mucosal protective factors. Also, the presence of a foreign object, such as an anastomotic ring, or permanent sutures can create chronic inflammation. The ulcer can cause pain, usually in the epigastrium, as well as dysphagia from an associated stricture, and haematemesis. The treatment is usually non-operative and includes discontinuation of the precipitating factors, the use of proton pump inhibitors, and cytoprotective medication such as sucralfate. In the acute setting, a full-thickness penetration of the marginal ulcer can lead to a free intraperitoneal perforation, often necessitating emergent operation. Also, the chronic scarring of healed ulcers can lead to narrowing of the anastomosis non-responsive to endoscopic dilatation. In these cases, a surgical gastrojejunostomy revision may also be necessary.[42–44]

Although adhesions after laparoscopic surgery are significantly rarer than open operations, small bowel obstruction can still occur from internal herniation. The potential spaces are the jejunojejunal mesenteric defect, the retrocolic mesocolon defect, and Petersen's space (between the Roux limb and the transverse colon in antecolic reconstructions). Most internal hernias occur at the small bowel intestinal defect. As for other complications, the early diagnosis is paramount to reduce the morbidity. Obese patients often present more subtle signs and symptoms, delaying the diagnosis. Tachycardia is a worrisome finding in these patients as it could be the first sign of compromised bowel and internal hernia should be ruled out.[45–48]

Strictures at any of the above-described anastomoses or in the gastric body in an SG can lead to persistent vomiting, dysphagia, and dehydration. Gastrojejunostomy strictures can be dilated endoscopically with good results. Jejunojejunostomy strictures are rare, but when symptomatic require surgical correction. Endoscopic dilatation and stenting has been reported as successful in certain types of strictures after SG; however, revision to a RNYGB is often necessary.[49,50]

Gastro-oesophageal reflux disease and oesophagitis can occur in 5–10% of SG patients. In some cases, the symptoms are not controlled by medication and the sleeve needs to be converted to a RNYGB. In fact, the high intraluminal pressure system created by the SG, the presence of an intact pylorus, and often incompetent lower oesophageal sphincter, can increase reflux of acid into the oesophagus. The long-term fears of Barrett's oesophagus and cancer mandate treatment. Bile reflux is a potentially worrisome complication exclusive of the OAGB. Bile is known to be much more caustic than acid in causing oesophagitis.[51–54]

Deep vein thrombosis is of major concern in obese patients undergoing surgery, and pulmonary embolus is the number one cause of mortality in post-bariatric patients. While there is no consensus regarding deep vein thrombosis prophylaxis, the current recommendations include chemical and mechanical thromboprophylaxis. Some surgeons will prescribe an outpatient extended prophylactic course for the super morbidly obese (body mass index >55–60 kg/m^2).[55–58]

Protein, vitamin, and mineral malnutrition are inversely related to the length of the common channel. Thus, true malnutrition is unlikely in the gastric sleeve, whereas micronutrient deficiencies are present in up to 70% of patients undergoing BPDDS. Consistent vitamin and minerals supplementation, frequent serum level checks, and strict professional follow-up are key to avoid serious deficiencies.[59–62]

Finally, the development of cholelithiasis is a potential occurrence not only for bariatric surgery patients, but also in any individual undergoing rapid weight loss. The pathogenesis of cholelithiasis is thought to be related to the alteration in fat metabolism and increased stasis of bile in the gallbladder. About 30% of patients who develop cholelithiasis will develop biliary symptoms. For this reason, it is recommended to perform concomitant cholecystectomy during the index bariatric operation for any patient with a known history of symptomatic cholelithiasis. This is particularly important during those operations that bypass the second portion of the duodenum (RNYGB, BPDDS, OAGB, and SADI). In fact, the altered postoperative anatomy makes the treatment of choledocholithiasis more difficult as oral endoscopic techniques cannot be used.[63–66]

Conclusion

Obesity is a growing international health epidemic. It has genetic, behavioural, and environmental causes. It is a well-studied risk factor for major chronic illnesses, including heart disease, renal disease, diabetes, and many cancers. Approximately 21% of US healthcare expenditures are attributable to obesity.[67] Due to its complexity, this epidemic requires multilevel integrated solutions. Both dietary and exercise interventions by themselves have failed to result in robust and sustainable weight loss. Numerous medications with different mechanisms of action are currently approved for weight loss, yet modest results and significant side effects have been reported. Surgical weight loss continues to provide the most effective and most durable results. With the effectiveness of weight loss, regardless of mechanism, the resolution of the comorbidities follows. Nowadays, the laparoscopic SG has become the most commonly performed operation worldwide, due to its relative technical simplicity, its safety profile, and the excellent results. Yet, other bariatric surgery options are available and are as effective. A basic understanding of surgical anatomy and potential complications is essential. Surgeons and gastroenterologists should be familiar with these procedures and complication management strategies.

REFERENCES

1. World Health Organization. Fact sheet: obesity and overweight. 2018. https://www.who.int/news-room/fact-sheets/detail/obesity-and-overweight
2. Centers for Disease Control and Prevention. Prevalence of obesity and severe obesity among adults: United States, 2017–2018. 2020. https://www.cdc.gov/nchs/products/databriefs/db360.htm
3. Bray MS, Loos RJ, McCaffery JM, et al. NIH working group report—using genomic information to guide weight management: from universal to precision treatment. *Obesity (Silver Spring)*. 2016;**24**:14–22.
4. Lee A, Cardel M, Donahoo WT. Social and Environmental Factors Influencing Obesity. In: Endotext. MDText.com, Inc., South Dartmouth (MA); 2000. PMID: 25905211.
5. Look AHEAD Research Group. Eight-year weight losses with an intensive lifestyle intervention: the look AHEAD study. *Obesity (Silver Spring)*. 2014;**22**:5–13.
6. Henry RR, Wiest-Kent TA, Scheaffer L, et al. Metabolic consequences of very-low-calorie diet therapy in obese non-insulin-dependent diabetic and nondiabetic subjects. *Diabetes*. 1986;**35**:155–164.
7. Jackness C, Karmally W, Febres G, et al. Very low-calorie diet mimics the early beneficial effect of Roux-en-Y gastric bypass on insulin sensitivity and β-cell function in type 2 diabetic patients. *Diabetes*. 2013;**62**:3027–3032.
8. Jakobsen GS, Småstuen MC, Sandbu R, et al. Association of bariatric surgery vs medical obesity treatment with long-term medical complications and obesity-related comorbidities. *JAMA*. 2018;**319**:291–301.
9. Caudwell P, Hopkins M, King NA, et al. Exercise alone is not enough: weight loss also needs a healthy (Mediterranean) diet? *Public Health Nutr*. 2009;**12**:1663–1666.
10. Schauer PR, Bhatt DL, Kirwan JP, et al. Bariatric surgery versus intensive medical therapy for diabetes—5-year outcomes. *N Engl J Med*. 2017;**376**:641–651.
11. Ikramuddin S, Korner J, Lee W, et al. Lifestyle intervention and medical management with vs without Roux-en-Y gastric bypass and control of hemoglobin A1c, LDL cholesterol, and systolic blood pressure at 5 years in the Diabetes Surgery Study. *JAMA*. 2018;**319**:266–278.
12. Saunders KH, Umashanker D, Igel LI, Kumar RB, Aronne LJ. Obesity pharmacotherapy. *Med Clin North Am*. 2018;**102**:135–148.
13. Heck AM, Yanovski JA, Calis KA. Orlistat, a new lipase inhibitor for the management of obesity. *Pharmacotherapy*. 2000;**20**:270–279.
14. Joo JK, Lee KS. Pharmacotherapy for obesity. *J Menopausal Med*. 2014;**20**:90–96.
15. Tran KL, Park YI, Pandya S, et al. Overview of glucagon-like peptide-1 receptor agonists for the treatment of patients with type 2 diabetes. *Am Health Drug Benefits*. 2017;**10**:178–188.
16. Gustafson A, King C, Rey JA. Lorcaserin (Belviq): a selective serotonin 5-HT2C agonist in the treatment of obesity. *P T*. 2013;**38**:525–534.
17. Lips MA, de Groot GH, van Klinken JB, et al. Calorie restriction is a major determinant of the short-term metabolic effects of gastric bypass surgery in obese type 2 diabetic patients. *Clin Endocrinol (Oxf)*. 2014;**80**:834–842.
18. Billeter AT, Fischer L, Wekerle AL, Senft J, Müller-Stich B. Malabsorption as a therapeutic approach in bariatric surgery. *Viszeralmedizin*. 2014;**30**:198–204.
19. Van Hee RH. Biliopancreatic diversion in the surgical treatment of morbid obesity. *World J Surg*. 2004;**28**:435–444.
20. Marceau P, Biron S, Bourque RA, Potvin M, Hould FS, Simard S. Biliopancreatic diversion with a new type of gastrectomy. *Obes Surg*. 1993;**3**:29–35.
21. Ionut V, Burch M, Youdim A, Bergman RN. Gastrointestinal hormones and bariatric surgery-induced weight loss. *Obesity (Silver Spring)*. 2013;**21**:1093–1103.
22. Valverde I, Puente J, Martín-Duce A, et al. Changes in glucagon-like peptide-1 (GLP-1) secretion after biliopancreatic diversion or vertical banded gastroplasty in obese subjects. *Obes Surg*. 2005;**15**:387–397.
23. Ortiz-Gomez C, Romero-Funes D, Gutierrez-Blanco D, et al. Impact of rapid weight loss after bariatric surgery on the prevalence of arterial hypertension in severely obese patients with chronic kidney disease. *Surg Endosc*. 2019;**34**:3197–3203.

24. Gutierrez Blanco D, Romero Funes D, Giambartolomei G, Lo Menzo E, Szomstein S, Rosenthal RJ. Impact of rapid weight loss on risk reduction of developing arterial hypertension in severely obese patients undergoing bariatric surgery. A single-institution experience using the Framingham Hypertension Risk Score. *Surg Obes Relat Dis*. 2019;15:920–925.
25. Gutierrez-Blanco D, Romero Funes D, Castillo M, Lo Menzo E, Szomstein S, Rosenthal RJ. Bariatric surgery reduces the risk of developing type 2 diabetes in severe obese subjects undergoing sleeve gastrectomy. *Surg Obes Relat Dis*. 2019;15:168–172.
26. Gutierrez-Blanco D, Funes-Romero D, Madiraju S, et al. Reduction of Framingham BMI score after rapid weight loss in severely obese subjects undergoing sleeve gastrectomy: a single institution experience. *Surg Endosc*. 2018;32:1248–1254.
27. Funes DR, Blanco DG, Gómez CO, et al. Metabolic surgery reduces the risk of progression from chronic kidney disease to kidney failure. *Ann Surg*. 2019;270:511–518.
28. de Raaff CAL, de Vries N, van Wagensveld BA. Obstructive sleep apnea and bariatric surgical guidelines: summary and update. *Curr Opin Anaesthesiol*. 2018;31:104–109.
29. Daellenbach L, Suter M. Jejunojejunal intussusception after Roux-en-Y gastric bypass: a review. *Obes Surg*. 2011;21:253–263.
30. Rosenthal RJ; International Sleeve Gastrectomy Expert Panel, Diaz AA, et al. International Sleeve Gastrectomy Expert Panel Consensus Statement: best practice guidelines based on experience of >12,000 cases. *Surg Obes Relat Dis*. 2012;8:8–19.
31. Alvarenga ES, Lo Menzo E, Szomstein S, Rosenthal RJ. Safety and efficacy of 1020 consecutive laparoscopic sleeve gastrectomies performed as a primary treatment modality for morbid obesity. A single-center experience from the metabolic and bariatric surgical accreditation quality and improvement program. *Surg Endosc*. 2016;30:2673–2678.
32. De Luca M, Tie T, Ooi G, et al. Mini gastric bypass-one anastomosis gastric bypass (MGB-OAGB)—IFSO position statement. *Obes Surg*. 2018;28:1188–1206.
33. Carbajo MA, Luque-de-León E, Jiménez JM, et al. Laparoscopic one-anastomosis gastric bypass: technique, results, and long-term follow-up in 1200 patients. *Obes Surg*. 2017;27:1153–1167.
34. Risstad H, Søvik TT, Engström M, et al. Five-year outcomes after laparoscopic gastric bypass and laparoscopic duodenal switch in patients with body mass index of 50 to 60: a randomized clinical trial. *JAMA Surg*. 2015;150:352–361.
35. Hedberg J, Sundström J, Sundbom M. Duodenal switch versus Roux-en-Y gastric bypass for morbid obesity: systematic review and meta-analysis of weight results, diabetes resolution and early complications in single-centre comparisons. *Obes Rev*. 2014;15:555–563.
36. Cylke R, Skrzypek P, Ziemiański P, Domieniek-Karlowicz J, Kosieradzki M, Lisik W. Single-anastomosis duodeno-ileal—new revision procedure in a patient with insufficient weight loss after sleeve gastrectomy. *Wideochir Inne Tech Maloinwazyjne*. 2018;13:407–411.
37. Shoar S, Poliakin L, Rubenstein R, Saber A. Single anastomosis duodeno-ileal switch (SADIS): a systematic review of efficacy and safety. *Obes Surg*. 2018;28:104–113.
38. Sánchez-Pernaute A, Rubio MÁ, Cabrerizo L, Ramos-Levi A, Pérez-Aguirre E, Torres A. Single-anastomosis duodenoileal bypass with sleeve gastrectomy (SADI-S) for obese diabetic patients. *Surg Obes Relat Dis*. 2015;11:1092–1098.
39. Court I, Wilson A, Benotti P, Szomstein S, Rosenthal RJ. T-tube gastrostomy as a novel approach for distal staple line disruption after sleeve gastrectomy for morbid obesity: case report and review of the literature. *Obes Surg*. 2010;20:519–522.
40. Sasson M, Ahmad H, Dip F, Menzo EL, Szomstein S, Rosenthal RJ. Comparison between major and minor surgical procedures for the treatment of chronic staple line disruption after laparoscopic sleeve gastrectomy. *Surg Obes Relat Dis*. 2016;12:969–975.
41. Thompson CE 3rd, Ahmad H, Lo Menzo E, Szomstein S, Rosenthal RJ. Outcomes of laparoscopic proximal gastrectomy with esophagojejunal reconstruction for chronic staple line disruption after laparoscopic sleeve gastrectomy. *Surg Obes Relat Dis*. 2014;10:455–459.
42. Clapp B, Hahn J, Dodoo C, Guerra A, de la Rosa E, Tyroch A. Evaluation of the rate of marginal ulcer formation after bariatric surgery using the MBSAQIP database. *Surg Endosc*. 2019;33:1890–1897.
43. Qiu J, Lundberg PW, Javier Birriel T, Claros L, Stoltzfus J, El Chaar M. Revisional bariatric surgery for weight regain and refractory complications in a single MBSAQIP accredited center: what are we dealing with? *Obes Surg*. 2018;28:2789–2795.
44. Ribeiro-Parenti L, Arapis K, Chosidow D, Marmuse JP. Comparison of marginal ulcer rates between antecolic and retrocolic laparoscopic Roux-en-Y gastric bypass. *Obes Surg*. 2015;25:215–221.
45. Cho M, Pinto D, Carrodeguas L, et al. Frequency and management of internal hernias after laparoscopic antecolic antegastric Roux-en-Y gastric bypass without division of the small bowel mesentery or closure of mesenteric defects: review of 1400 consecutive cases. *Surg Obes Relat Dis*. 2006;2:87–91.
46. Szomstein S, Lo Menzo E, Simpfendorfer C, Zundel N, Rosenthal RJ. Laparoscopic lysis of adhesions. *World J Surg*. 2006;30:535–540.
47. Nimeri AA, Maasher A, Al Shaban T, Salim E, Gamaleldin MM. Internal hernia following laparoscopic Roux-en-Y gastric bypass: prevention and tips for intra-operative management. *Obes Surg*. 2016;26:2255–2256.
48. Lopera CA, Vergnaud JP, Cabrera LF, et al. Preventative laparoscopic repair of Petersen's space following gastric bypass surgery reduces the incidence of Petersen's hernia: a comparative study. *Hernia*. 2018;22:1077–1081.
49. Buchwald H, Avidor Y, Braunwald E, et al. Bariatric surgery: a systematic review and meta-analysis. *JAMA*. 2004;292:1724–1737.
50. Nelson DW, Blair KS, Martin MJ. Analysis of obesity-related outcomes and bariatric failure rates with the duodenal switch vs gastric bypass for morbid obesity. *Arch Surg*. 2012;147:847–854.
51. El-Hadi M, Birch DW, Gill RS, Karmali S. The effect of bariatric surgery on gastroesophageal reflux disease. *Can J Surg*. 2014;57:139–144.
52. Rebecchi F, Allaix ME, Patti MG, Schlottmann F, Morino M. Gastroesophageal reflux disease and morbid obesity: to sleeve or not to sleeve? *World J Gastroenterol*. 2017;23:2269–2275.
53. Laffin M, Chau J, Gill RS, Birch DW, Karmali S. Sleeve gastrectomy and gastroesophageal reflux disease. *J Obes*. 2013;2013:741097.
54. Khan A, Kim A, Sanossian C, Francois F. Impact of obesity treatment on gastroesophageal reflux disease. *World J Gastroenterol*. 2016;22:1627–1638.
55. Escalante-Tattersfield T, Tucker O, Fajnwaks P, Szomstein S, Rosenthal RJ. Incidence of deep vein thrombosis in morbidly obese patients undergoing laparoscopic Roux-en-Y gastric bypass. *Surg Obes Relat Dis*. 2008;4:126–130.

56. Safdie FM, Dip F, Ardila-Gatas J, et al. Incidence and clinical implications of upper extremity deep vein thrombosis after laparoscopic bariatric procedures. *Obes Surg*. 2015;**25**:1098–1101.
57. Moon RC, Ghanem M, Teixeira AF, et al. Assessing risk factors, presentation, and management of portomesenteric vein thrombosis after sleeve gastrectomy: a multicenter case-control study. *Surg Obes Relat Dis*. 2018;**14**:478–483.
58. Jamal MH, Corcelles R, Shimizu H, et al. Thromboembolic events in bariatric surgery: a large multi-institutional referral center experience. *Surg Endosc*. 2015;**29**:376–380.
59. Kwon Y, Kim HJ, Lo Menzo E, Park S, Szomstein S, Rosenthal RJ. Anemia, iron and vitamin B12 deficiencies after sleeve gastrectomy compared to Roux-en-Y gastric bypass: a meta-analysis. *Surg Obes Relat Dis*. 2014;**10**:589–597.
60. Kaidar-Person O, Rosenthal RJ. Malnutrition in morbidly obese patients: fact or fiction? *Minerva Chir*. 2009;**64**:297–302.
61. Kaidar-Person O, Person B, Szomstein S, Rosenthal RJ. Nutritional deficiencies in morbidly obese patients: a new form of malnutrition? Part A: vitamins. *Obes Surg*. 2008;**18**:870–876.
62. Kaidar-Person O, Person B, Szomstein S, Rosenthal RJ. Nutritional deficiencies in morbidly obese patients: a new form of malnutrition? Part B: minerals. *Obes Surg*. 2008;**18**:1028–1034.
63. Tucker ON, Fajnwaks P, Szomstein S, Rosenthal RJ. Is concomitant cholecystectomy necessary in obese patients undergoing laparoscopic gastric bypass surgery? *Surg Endosc*. 2008;**22**:2450–2454.
64. Li VK, Pulido N, Martinez-Suartez P, et al. Symptomatic gallstones after sleeve gastrectomy. *Surg Endosc*. 2009;**23**:2488–2492.
65. Lalor PF, Tucker ON, Szomstein S, Rosenthal RJ. Complications after laparoscopic sleeve gastrectomy. *Surg Obes Relat Dis*. 2008;**4**:33–38.
66. Aiolfi A, Asti E, Rausa E, Bernardi D, Bonitta G, Bonavina L. Trans-gastric ERCP after Roux-en-Y gastric bypass: systematic review and meta-analysis. *Obes Surg*. 2018;**28**:2836–2843.
67. Cawley J, Meyerhoefer C. The medical care costs of obesity: an instrumental variables approach. *J Health Econ*. 2012;**31**:219–230.

PART 2
Oesophageal cancer

10. Oesophageal cancer: epidemiology, symptoms, diagnostics, and staging 99
    Andrew Tang, Thomas Rice, and Usman Ahmad

11. Oesophageal cancer: multimodal treatment 105
    Ben M. Eyck, Berend J. van der Wilk, Maurice J.C. van der Sangen, Ate van der Gaast, and J. Jan B. van Lanschot

12. Oesophageal cancer: endoscopic treatment 129
    Thomas Rösch

13. Oesophageal cancer: surgery 137
    Björn-Ole Stüben, Karl-Frederick Karstens, Michael Nentwich, Jakob R. Izbicki, and Matthias Reeh

14. Oesophageal cancer: minimally invasive surgery and robotic surgery 155
    Gijsbert van Boxel, Pieter C. van der Sluis, Peter P. Grimminger, and Richard van Hillegersberg

15. Oesophageal cancer: future aspects of treatment 169
    Thorsten Oliver Goetze and Salah-Eddin Al-Batran

10

Oesophageal cancer
Epidemiology, symptoms, diagnostics, and staging

Andrew Tang, Thomas Rice, and Usman Ahmad

Epidemiology

The incidence of oesophageal cancer varies geographically, reflecting the influence of genetics and environmental risk factors on the pathogenesis of these cancers. While other types of cancers can arise from the various cells within the oesophagus, epithelial malignancies are by far the most common. The World Health Organization estimates over 600,000 new cases of oesophageal cancer worldwide during 2020.[1]

Oesophageal cancers occur most frequently in Eastern Asia, as these populations appear to be at higher risk of developing these upper gastrointestinal cancers (Figure 10.1). Additionally, males are twice as likely to develop oesophageal cancer compared to their female counterparts (Figure 10.1). After Eastern Asia, the

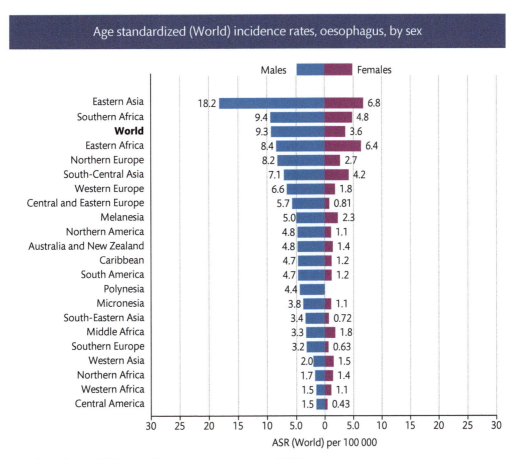

Figure 10.1 Global incidence (per 100,000 people) of oesophageal cancer in 2020 by sex.
Reproduced with permission from International Agency for Research on Cancer. Oesophagus (C15) fact sheet: Globocan 2020. World Health Organization. 2020. https://gco.iarc.fr/today/data/factsheets/cancers/6-Oesophagus-fact-sheet.pdf

age-standardized incidence of oesophageal cancer was highest in Southern Africa and Eastern Africa.[1]

Within the oesophagus, the two most common forms of cancer are squamous cell carcinoma (~85%) and adenocarcinoma (~15%).[2] Unlike lung cancer where both histologies share similar risk factors, in the oesophagus, the risk factors and clinical phenotypes are quite unique among the histological subtypes. Alcohol, tobacco, and hot beverage consumption are the strongest risk factors for squamous cell carcinoma, which is the predominant form of oesophageal cancer in East Asia. Globally, countries with lower sociodemographic indices tend to have higher age-adjusted incidence rates of squamous cell oesophageal carcinoma.[2] This is thought to be secondary to extrinsic factors in the environment, lifestyle, and diet. Over the past several decades as social and environmental factors have changed, the age-standardized incidence rates of oesophageal squamous cell carcinoma have been decreasing. However, there is an increasing incidence of adenocarcinoma, which happens to be the predominant form of oesophageal cancer in North America and Europe. This typically develops in the setting of central obesity, smoking, and gastro-oesophageal reflux disease.[2] Uncontrolled gastro-oesophageal reflux disease can lead to columnar intestinal metaplasia of the distal oesophagus, or Barrett's oesophagus. Persistent damage from acid reflux can cause low-grade dysplasia that can ultimately progress to high-grade dysplasia and adenocarcinoma. The American Society for Gastrointestinal Endoscopy recommends screening for Barrett's oesophagus for patients with gastro-oesophageal reflux disease and high-risk individual factors, including male sex, central adiposity, smoking history, or a family history of oesophageal cancer/Barrett's oesophagus.[3] A population-based study from Denmark suggests that the absolute annual risk of developing oesophageal adenocarcinoma in the setting of Barrett's oesophagus is 0.12% annually.[4] Patients with Barrett's oesophagus are 11 times more likely to develop adenocarcinoma compared to patients without Barrett's oesophagus.[4] Additionally, the relative risk of developing adenocarcinoma is significantly greater in patients with dysplasia in the setting of Barrett's oesophagus.[4] The authors concluded that routine surveillance for adenocarcinoma in the setting of Barrett's oesophagus without dysplasia was not justified given the low absolute annual risk of cancer transformation. However, this study was performed in a relatively homogeneous patient population and findings should be carefully extrapolated to individual patients with additional risk factors for cancer development. The American College of Gastroenterologists recommends surveillance intervals of 3–5 years for non-dysplastic Barrett's oesophagus and endoscopic ablation for high-grade dysplasia.[5] Patients with low-grade dysplasia may undergo either endoscopic surveillance or ablation.[5]

Symptoms

For the upper gastrointestinal tract, symptoms are related to the degree of intraluminal obstruction. Oesophageal cancer symptoms may include dysphagia, odynophagia, chest pain, and worsening reflux. Dysphagia symptoms typically progress as the tumour grows, which leads to weight loss over time. Worsening reflux can lead to hoarseness and coughing. Occasionally, these tumours may be found on work-up for anaemia, upper gastrointestinal bleeding, or melaena.

Diagnostics

The gold standard of diagnosing upper gastrointestinal cancers involves oesophagogastroduodenoscopy. Oesophagogastroduodenoscopy allows for direct visualization and biopsy of oesophageal lesions. It is also a safe method of surveillance for patients with Barrett's oesophagus. To accurately track this disease, it is important to utilize a uniform method of reporting. In 2006, an international group of researchers developed the Prague criteria to report endoscopic findings in a simple manner.[6] Patients with Barrett's oesophagus on endoscopy may have a circumferential (C) and maximum (M) extent of metaplasia (Figure 10.2). Endoscopic ultrasound (EUS) is an adjunct to oesophagogastroduodenoscopy and allows for assessment of the depth of tissue invasion (Figure 10.3). Skilled endoscopists can also use EUS to assess regional lymph node involvement as well; however, the accuracy of this is user dependent.[7,8] There is some concern that EUS may not be accurate in early-stage oesophageal cancer ($\leq$cT2N0M0) compared to relatively larger tumours.[7] This inaccuracy has major implications in terms of treatment options, as a patient with a cT1a tumours may opt for endoscopic mucosal resection, only to realize that they actually had a tumour with deeper invasion and pathologically positive lymph nodes.[9] One study found that 26% of patients with cT1b tumours, who ultimately underwent oesophagectomy after endoscopic mucosal resection, actually had lymph node metastases in their surgical specimen.[9] Computed tomography of the chest and abdomen and positron emission tomography are adjuncts used to assess for regional lymph node involvement in the chest and abdomen for oesophageal cancer. Reliable tumour markers for the diagnosis of oesophageal cancer have not yet been identified.[10]

From a clinical perspective, patients with distal oesophageal tumours on endoscopy, who have dysphagia or are obstructed, are considered to have at least stage III disease. In this setting, an EUS

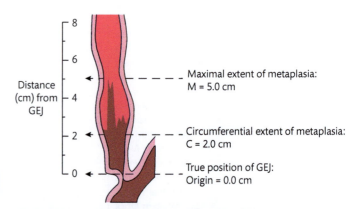

Figure 10.2 Schematic depicting the Prague criteria that reports the circumferential extent of metaplasia (C) and the maximal extent of metaplasia (M). GEJ, gastro-oesophageal junction.

Reproduced with permission from Sharma P, Dent J, Armstrong D, et al. The development and validation of an endoscopic grading system for Barrett anesophagus: the Prague C & M criteria. *Gastroenterology.* 2006;131(5):1392–1399. doi:10.1053/j.gastro.2006.08.032

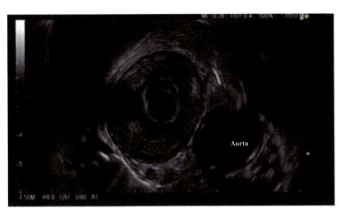

Figure 10.3 Endosonographic image showing the five layers of the oesophageal wall: mucosa (1), muscularis mucosa (2), submucosa (3), muscularis propria (4), and adventitia (5). This lesion was staged as T2N0.
Reproduced with permission from Sooklal S, Chahal P. Endoscopic ultrasound. *Surg Clin North Am.* 2020;100(6):1133–1150. doi:10.1016/j.suc.2020.07.003

can be avoided and the patient can proceed directly to the intended stage-based therapy.

Staging

Cancer staging should serve to provide patients and providers with the anatomical extent of disease which in turn guides the choice of therapy. The prognostic role of staging is becoming more popular and hence a patient may be assigned multiple clinical stages at various steps of treatment (c stage, u stage, p stage, yp stage). Early iterations of oesophageal cancer staging were crudely based on tumour size and length for T1 (<5 cm and non-circumferential) and T2 (>5 cm and circumferential) cancers, and did not account for tumour depth until T3 (extra-oesophageal invasion).[11] Lymph node metastasis was simply categorized as N0 or N1 regardless of the number of positive lymph nodes or location of positive lymph node stations.[11] Eventually, the staging system was refined to account for the depth of tumour invasion, number of positive lymph nodes, and location of positive lymph nodes (e.g. cervical lymph node metastases in upper thoracic oesophagus cancers count as M1a).

Because carcinomas are the most common forms of cancer in the oesophagus, we will refer to the American Joint Commission on Cancer (AJCC) *AJCC Cancer Staging Manual* for these cancers.[12-16] While for the most part oesophagus and stomach cancers behave differently and therefore are staged separately, the gastro-oesophageal junction (GOJ) can overlap with the two.[17] How a GOJ tumour is defined has changed between staging editions, with Siewert type III GOJ tumours belonging to the oesophagus in the seventh edition and belonging to the stomach in the eighth edition. The exact tumour location is measured based on the epicentre of the tumour measuring the endoscopic distance from the incisors. Tumours with their epicentre within the proximal 2 cm of the gastric cardia (Siewert types I and II) are staged as oesophageal cancers (Figure 10.4).[18] Tumours with their epicentre more than 2 cm distal from the GOJ, even if the GOJ is involved, are staged as gastric cancers.[18] Controversies in how to stage and treat GOJ tumours will not be specifically addressed in this chapter as it is not within its scope. The general principles of oesophageal cancer staging follow gastrointestinal cancer staging principles: the tumour

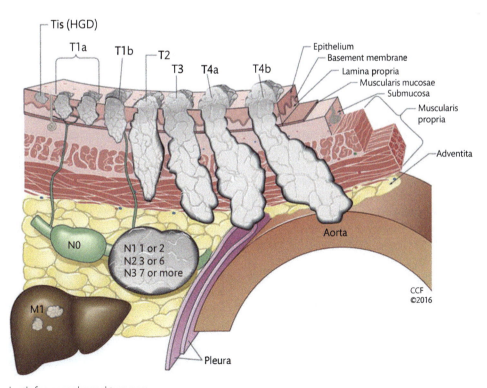

Figure 10.4 Tumour depth for oesophageal tumours.
Reproduced with permission from Rice TW, Ishwaran H, Ferguson MK, Blackstone EH, Goldstraw P. Cancer of the esophagus and esophagogastric junction: an eighth edition staging primer. *J Thorac Oncol.* 2016;12(1):36–42. doi:10.1016/j.jtho.2016.10.016

depth of invasion from the mucosa to the outer layers of the organ, number of regional lymph nodes involved, and distant metastases (Figure 10.4).

The seventh and eighth editions of the staging manual were designed to reflect patient-specific risks and prognosis, and to stratify staging based on homogeneous probability of survival rather than arbitrary anatomical definitions.[14,19] With this in mind, the staging group for the seventh and eighth editions of oesophageal cancer staging used machine learning analysis of the Worldwide Esophageal Cancer Collaborative (WECC; comprised of 33 institutions across six continents) data to generate uniform groups of subpopulations for staging based on anatomy, histology, and tumour grade (Figures 10.5–10.7). The eighth edition was designed to further provide prognosis across different time points: clinical, pathological, and pathological after neoadjuvant therapy (Figures 10.6 and 10.7). In the eighth edition of the staging manual, the prognosis of a clinical stage IA (cStageIA) adenocarcinoma is different from that of a pathological stage IA (pStageIA) adenocarcinoma, which is different from that of a post-neoadjuvant pathological stage IA (ypStageIA) adenocarcinoma.[20–22]

As previously mentioned, there are two predominant forms of oesophageal carcinoma, squamous cell carcinoma and adenocarcinoma, which rely on the same tumour, node, and metastasis (TNM) descriptors, but each have separate stage categorizations. Between the seventh and eighth edition staging systems, there have been a few changes.[11] Tumour location is now based on the tumour epicentre rather than its most proximal border. Additionally, tumour grading ranges from G1 through G3 in the eighth edition. Previous G4 (undifferentiated) tumours must now have additional pathological analysis to determine a histological subtype.

Clinical stage

Clinical staging is based on endoscopic and radiographic staging of biopsy-proven oesophageal cancers and does not factor in tumour grade, as it is difficult to determine this from the limited tissue obtained on biopsy (Figures 10.6a and 10.7a).[20] Patients with early-stage (cTis and cT0) adenocarcinoma have superior survival in comparison to their squamous cell carcinoma counterparts.[20] Generally, compared to previous staging iterations, patients with early clinical stage cancers had worse than expected survival compared to equivalent pathological categories from previous WECC data.[20] Additionally, patients with advanced clinical stage cancers had better than expected survival compared to equivalent pathological categories from previous WECC data.[20] This suggests that there are inherent limitations in clinical staging accuracy. For example, within the cT2N0M0 adenocarcinoma subgroup, the clinical staging accuracy was only 14% among all participating centres of the WECC database.[23] Although some of this is related to the inability to accurately clinically stage nodal disease, the degree of accuracy for tumour staging was only 24%.[23] After multivariable logistic regression, it was determined that longer tumour length was likely to be predictive for pathological nodal positivity (>3.5 cm).[23]

Pathological stage

Building upon the data from the WECC that was used for the seventh edition of the *AJCC Cancer Staging Manual*, the eighth edition was able to provide an even more homogeneous and uniform pathological staging groups for squamous cell carcinoma and

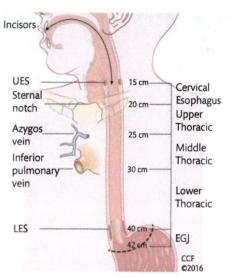

Figure 10.5 Location of oesophageal cancer primary site, including typical endoscopic measurements of each region measured from the incisors. Cancers involving the oesophagogastric junction (EGJ) that have their epicentre within the proximal 2 cm of the cardia (Siewert types I/II) are staged as oesophageal cancers. Cancers whose epicentre is more than 2 cm distal from the oesophagogastric junction, even if the oesophagogastric junction is involved, are staged using the gastric cancer staging scheme. LES, lower oesophageal sphincter; UES, upper oesophageal sphincter.
Reproduced with permission from Rice TW, Ishwaran H, Ferguson MK, Blackstone EH, Goldstraw P. Cancer of the esophagus and esophagogastric junction: an eighth edition staging primer. *J Thorac Oncol*. 2016;12(1):36–42. doi:10.1016/j.jtho.2016.10.016

adenocarcinoma groups (Figures 10.6b and 10.7b). Tumour grade plays a more prominent role in pathological staging, as even within the same pT and pN categories patients have different prognoses depending on tumour grade.[21,24] Additionally, in squamous cell carcinoma, tumour location changes the pathological stage in pN0 patients (Figure 10.7b).[21]

Post-neoadjuvant treatment

Previous staging iterations did not make the survival distinction between patients who underwent neoadjuvant therapy versus those who underwent resection alone. The eighth edition makes this distinction as there is a dramatic difference between pathological and post-neoadjuvant staging groups (Figures 10.6c and 10.7c). This is an important distinction, especially with the advent of neoadjuvant regimens that have shown improved survival compared to upfront resection (e.g. CROSS).[25] Interestingly, survival was much less distinctive for ypT, grade, and location than in pathologically staged cancers.[21] Survival was substantially worse for ypN+ patients versus those with ypN0.[21] Similarly, survival was substantially worse for ypM+ patients versus those with ypM0.[21] The survival benefit of lower histological grade is less evident in patients with ypTNM cancers than in those with similarly staged pTNM cancers, and therefore is not included in the post-neoadjuvant staging algorithm (Figures 10.6c and 10.7c).

Summary

The latest iteration of oesophageal cancer staging was designed to reflect the changes in tumour characteristics and behaviour over the course of time and treatments. As perioperative care continues to

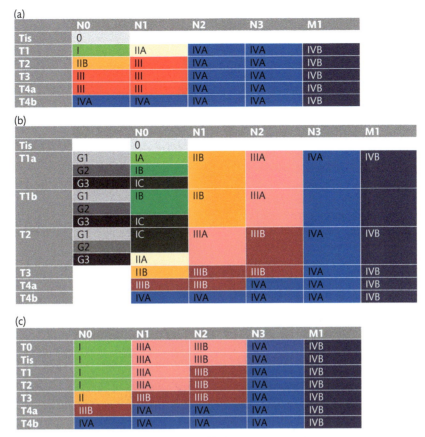

Figure 10.6 Adenocarcinoma staging: (a) clinical, (b) pathological, and (c) after neoadjuvant therapy.

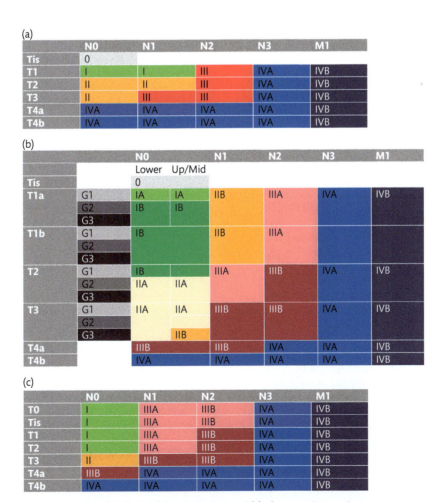

Figure 10.7 Squamous cell carcinoma staging: (a) clinical, (b) pathological, and (c) after neoadjuvant therapy.

improve and treatment options continue to expand, this will allow for finer tuning of staging. Future iterations of cancer staging are likely to incorporate tumour-specific biomarkers that will help provide patient-specific prognoses.

Conclusion

Internationally, squamous cell carcinoma of the upper third of the oesophagus, secondary to smoking and alcohol, is the most prevalent form of oesophageal cancer. However, in Western countries where gastro-oesophageal reflux and Barrett's oesophagus are more prevalent, adenocarcinoma is the more common form of oesophageal cancer. Dysphagia is the most common presenting symptom and is typically related to the degree of tumour growth. Oesophageal cancers are diagnosed with oesophagogastroduodenoscopy and staged with EUS and computed tomography. More recent staging iterations are able to provide homogeneous groupings based on survival at various timepoints in treatment. Future iterations of staging will require cooperation among head and neck surgeons for upper oesophageal cancers, and oncologists/radiation oncologists for patients who undergo definitive chemoradiation for unresectable cancers. Additionally, as we discover more biomarkers and targets for immunotherapy, these will naturally be factored into cancer survival and prognoses in the future.

REFERENCES

1. International Agency for Research on Cancer. Oesophagus cancer: Globocan 2020. World Health Organization. 2020. https://gco.iarc.fr/today/data/factsheets/cancers/6-Oesophagus-fact-sheet.pdf
2. Kamangar F, Nasrollahzadeh D, Safiri S, et al. The global, regional, and national burden of oesophageal cancer and its attributable risk factors in 195 countries and territories, 1990–2017: a systematic analysis for the Global Burden of Disease Study 2017. *Lancet Gastroenterol Hepatol.* 2020;**5**:582–597. doi:10.1016/s2468-1253(20)30007-8
3. Qumseya B, Sultan S, Bain P, et al. ASGE guideline on screening and surveillance of Barrett's esophagus. *Gastrointest Endosc.* 2019;**90**:335–359. doi:10.1016/j.gie.2019.05.012
4. Hvid-Jensen F, Pederson L, Drewes AM, Sorensen HT, Funch-Jensen P. Incidence of adenocarcinoma among patients with Barrett's esophagus. *N Engl J Med.* 2011;**365**:1375–1383. doi:10.1056/NEJMoa1103042.
5. Shaheen NJ, Falk GW, Iyer PG, Gerson LB. ACG clinical guideline: diagnosis and management of Barrett's esophagus. *Am J Gastroenterol.* 2016;**111**:30–50. doi:10.1038/ajg.2015.322
6. Sharma P, Dent J, Armstrong D, et al. The development and validation of an endoscopic grading system for Barrett's esophagus: the Prague C & M criteria. *Gastroenterology.* 2006;**131**:1392–1399. doi:10.1053/j.gastro.2006.08.032
7. Sooklal S, Chahal P. Endoscopic ultrasound. *Surg Clin North Am.* 2020;**100**:1133–1150. doi:10.1016/j.suc.2020.07.003
8. Rice TW, Boyce GA, Sivak MV, Adelstein DJ, Kirby TJ. Esophageal carcinoma: esophageal ultrasound assessment of preoperative chemotherapy. *Ann Thorac Surg.* 1992;**53**:972–977. doi:10.1016/0003-4975(92)90369-F
9. Molena D, DeMeester SR. When less is just less: endoscopic therapy for submucosal T1b esophageal cancer. *Gastrointest Endosc.* 2020;**92**:40–43. doi:10.1016/j.gie.2020.03.011
10. Shimada H, Noie T, Ohashi M, Oba K, Takahashi Y. Clinical significance of serum tumor markers for gastric cancer: a systematic review of literature by the Task Force of the Japanese Gastric Cancer Association. *Gastric Cancer.* 2014;**17**:26–33. doi:10.1007/s10120-013-0259-5
11. Rice TW, Blackstone EH. Esophageal cancer staging. past, present, and future. *Thorac Surg Clin.* 2013;**23**:461–469. doi:10.1016/j.thorsurg.2013.07.004
12. Amin MB, Edge SB, Greene FL, et al., eds. AJCC Cancer Staging Manual. 7th ed. New York: Springer; 2017.
13. Ahmad U, Tang A, Rice TW. Esophageal cancer staging. In: Sugarbaker DJ, Bueno R, Burt BM, et al., eds. *Sugarbaker's Adult Chest Surgery.* 3rd ed. New York: McGraw-Hill Education; 2020. http://accesssurgery.mhmedical.com/content.aspx?aid=1170405992
14. Amin MB, Greene FL, Edge SB, et al. The Eighth Edition AJCC Cancer Staging Manual: continuing to build a bridge from a population-based to a more 'personalized' approach to cancer staging. *CA Cancer J Clin.* 2017;**67**:93–99. doi:10.3322/caac.21388
15. Washington K. 7th edition of the AJCC cancer staging manual: stomach. *Ann Surg Oncol.* 2010;**17**:3077–3079. doi:10.1245/s10434-010-1362-z
16. Rice TW, Ishwaran H, Ferguson MK, Blackstone EH, Goldstraw P. Cancer of the esophagus and esophagogastric junction: an eighth edition staging primer. *J Thorac Oncol.* 2016;**12**:36–42. doi:10.1016/j.jtho.2016.10.016
17. Tang A, Sohal D, McNamara M, Murthy SC, Raja S. Siewert III adenocarcinoma: still searching for the right treatment combination. *Surg Oncol Clin N Am.* 2020;**29**:647–653. doi:10.1016/j.soc.2020.07.002
18. Rice TW, Gress DM, Patil DT, Hofstetter WL, Kelsen DP, Blackstone EH. Cancer of the esophagus and esophagogastric junction—major changes in the American Joint Committee on Cancer eighth edition cancer staging manual. *CA Cancer J Clin.* 2017;**67**:304–317. doi:10.3322/caac.21399
19. Rice TW, Lu M, Ishwaran H, Blackstone EH. Precision surgical therapy for adenocarcinoma of the esophagus and esophagogastric junction. *J Thorac Oncol.* 2019;**14**:2164–2175. doi:10.1016/j.jtho.2019.08.004
20. Rice TW, Apperson-Hansen C, DiPaola LM, et al. Worldwide Esophageal Cancer Collaboration: clinical staging data. *Dis Esophagus.* 2016;**29**:707–714. doi:10.1111/dote.12493
21. Rice TW, Lerut TEMR, Orringer MB, et al. Worldwide Esophageal Cancer Collaboration: neoadjuvant pathologic staging data. *Dis Esophagus.* 2017;**29**:715–723. doi:10.1111/dote.12513.Worldwide
22. Rice TW, Chen LQ, Hofstetter WL, et al. Worldwide Esophageal Cancer Collaboration: pathologic staging data. *Dis Esophagus.* 2017;**29**(7):724–733. doi:10.1111/dote.12520.Worldwide
23. Atay SM, Correa A, Hofstetter WL, et al. Predictors of staging accuracy, pathologic nodal involvement, and overall survival for cT2N0 carcinoma of the esophagus. *J Thorac Cardiovasc Surg.* 2019;**157**:1264–1272. doi:10.1016/j.jtcvs.2018.10.057
24. Nicholson AG, Tsao MS, Travis WD, et al. Eighth edition staging of thoracic malignancies: implications for the reporting pathologist. *Arch Pathol Lab Med.* 2018;**142**:645–661. doi:10.5858/arpa.2017-0245-RA
25. Shapiro J, van Lanschot JJB, Hulshof MCCM, et al. Neoadjuvant chemoradiotherapy plus surgery versus surgery alone for oesophageal or junctional cancer (CROSS): long-term results of a randomised controlled trial. *Lancet Oncol.* 2015;**16**:1090–1098. doi:10.1016/S1470-2045(15)00040-6

11

Oesophageal cancer
Multimodal treatment

Ben M. Eyck, Berend J. van der Wilk, Maurice J.C. van der Sangen, Ate van der Gaast, and J. Jan B. van Lanschot

Introduction

Improving the survival of patients with locally advanced oesophageal cancer without distant metastases is mostly achieved by resection of the oesophagus. Although improved staging, more radical surgical techniques, improved perioperative care, and better patient selection have resulted in survival improvement from approximately 12% to 39% between 1950 and 2000, microscopically tumour-positive resection margins were still present in 25–30% of patients, strongly worsening the prognosis of these patients.[1–3] Another striking observation after primary surgery for oesophageal cancer was the high rate of both distant metastases and locoregional recurrences. After primary surgery, nearly half of the patients developed distant metastases and nearly 40% developed locoregional recurrences, resulting in poor long-term survival.[4] Furthermore, the operation has a permanent negative impact on the health-related quality of life in these patients.[5–7] In order to improve the distant and locoregional disease control, therapies additional to surgery (multimodal treatments) have been extensively tested. Examples of such multimodal treatments additional to surgery are radiotherapy, chemotherapy, chemoradiotherapy, and, more recently, targeted therapy. Considerable variability exists in the nature and timing of these multimodal therapies among countries. While large parts of Europe and North America have adopted neoadjuvant chemoradiotherapy as the standard of care for patients with locally advanced oesophageal cancer, some Western and Asian countries advocate the use of pre- or perioperative chemotherapy. This chapter will provide the rationale for the usage of modern multimodal treatments in patients with locally advanced oesophageal cancer.

Radiotherapy

Mechanism of action

Radiotherapy is used to target tumour tissue using ionizing radiation mostly via X-rays or gamma rays while preserving the normal surrounding tissue. Currently, nearly half of the patients who have a malignancy undergo radiotherapy, either for cure or palliation—the latter for treating symptoms, for instance, pain due to metastatic disease.[8] Radiation therapy mostly uses low and high linear energy transfer which is a measurement used to approximate the number of ionizations it causes due to traversing tissue. The efficacy of the ionizing therapy depends on several biological mechanisms. The direct effects consist mostly of directly damaging of DNA in tumour cells, causing single- and double-strand breaks in the DNA and their subsequent lysis. The indirect effects are caused by free radicals that appear after ionization of the water within a cell (cells consist of about 80% water). These free radicals are subsequently able to damage the DNA within a cell (Figure 11.1).[9]

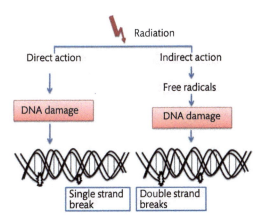

Figure 11.1 Direct and indirect effects of radiotherapy. The direct effects act by directly damaging DNA in tumour cells resulting in single- and double-strand breaks in the DNA and lysis of the tumour cell. Indirect effects result from damaging DNA by free radicals that are formed from ionization of water due to the radiotherapy.

Reproduced from Baskar R, Dai J, Wenlong N, Yeo R, Yeoh KW. Biological response of cancer cells to radiation treatment. *Front Mol Biosci*. 2014;1:24. Reproduced under a Creative Commons Attribution 4.0 International (CC BY 4.0) (https://creativecommons.org/licenses/by/4.0/)

The dose of radiation is expressed in grays (Gy) administered. In treatment of oesophageal cancer with curative intent, a total dose of 40–60 Gy is usually given, among other things depending on the setting of treatment (neoadjuvant or definitive, both of which will be discussed later). Fractionation of the radiotherapy total dose in smaller dose parts allows healthy tissue to recover, while tumour cells are generally less efficient in the intracellular repair mechanisms. As such, late side effects are partly prevented by using such a fractionated regimen. Furthermore, elimination of tumour cells can be improved by such a fractionated dose due to progression of the tumour cell from a radioresistant phase to a radiosensitive phase after one dose of radiotherapy (e.g. due to reoxygenation of a tumour cell).[10]

Applying radiotherapy to the primary tumour and its immediately adjacent lymph nodes results in increased locoregional control of radiosensitive tumours. As such, microscopically positive resection margins and the presence of positive locoregional lymph nodes in the resection specimen could be decreased.

Radiotherapy

The earliest research concerning radiotherapy for oesophageal cancer mostly consists of historical cohorts. In these reports, a complete response rate as assessed in the resection specimen was detected in 10% of cases when using 40–50 Gy. The pathological complete response rate increased up to 50% when using a dose of 50–60 Gy.[11–13] However, one of these high-dose studies reported an increased mortality rate of 21% in the irradiated group versus 13% in the control group.[11] A complete response is considered to have a better prognostic value compared to a non-complete response. However, several studies showed contradictory results concerning the overall survival in patients undergoing radiotherapy followed by surgery versus surgery alone. Comparative analysis of these historical cohort studies is difficult since insufficient information is available concerning the delay between radiation and surgery, the morbidity of the radiation, and the numbers of patients at risk during long-term follow-up. Therefore, several trials have been performed randomizing patients between 20 and 40 Gy radiotherapy prior to surgery versus surgery alone, as summarized in Table 11.1.[14–18]

None of these trials clearly showed a long-term survival advantage for patients undergoing higher-dose radiotherapy. All survival advantages observed were modest and not statistically significant. Also, the radical resectability rate did not significantly differ between the two groups. In 2005, a meta-analysis was performed combining the results of these randomized trials and confirmed these disappointing results.[19] After combining individual patient data from 1147 patients in these trials, the authors reported that there was a modest 5-year overall survival advantage of 3% (from 15% to 18%; $p = 0.062$, hazard ratio (HR) 0.89, with 95% confidence interval (CI) 0.78–1.01) after the addition of preoperative radiotherapy (Figure 11.2). However, due to the increased morbidity, costs, and duration of treatment, routinely performed preoperative radiotherapy was not recommended by the authors.

Postoperative radiotherapy in doses ranging from 45 to 60 Gy was tested in four trials randomizing between surgery followed by radiotherapy versus surgery alone as summarized in Table 11.1.[20–23] None of the studies reported a clear advantage in overall survival for patients undergoing postoperative radiotherapy. A meta-analysis combined the results of these small randomized trials and confirmed this conclusion.[24] Since no clear advantages have been reported for the addition of neoadjuvant or adjuvant radiotherapy to surgery in the treatment of oesophageal cancer, this specific combined therapy has no place in the guidelines for treatment of locally advanced oesophageal cancer.[25,26]

Neoadjuvant or perioperative chemotherapy

Mechanisms of action

Over the last decades, it has been shown that survival significantly improves when systemic chemotherapy is given in addition to surgery for the treatment of patients with locally advanced oesophageal cancer.[27] Chemotherapy can be given in the neoadjuvant, perioperative, or adjuvant setting. In the neoadjuvant setting, chemotherapy is given preoperatively to downstage the primary tumour and improve the chance of a radical resection. Additionally, chemotherapy

Table 11.1 Randomized controlled trials comparing preoperative radiotherapy followed by surgery versus surgery alone or postoperative radiotherapy following surgery versus surgery alone

	Author	Year	Period	Patients	Tumour histology	Dose radiotherapy	Survival[a]; HR (95% CI)	3-yOS[a]	5-yOS[a]
Preoperative radiotherapy	Launois et al.[16]	1981	1973–1976	124	SCC	40 Gy (8 × 5 Gy)	1.01 (0.67–1.53)	NR	10% vs 11%
	Gignoux et al.[15]	1988	1976–1982	229	SCC	33 Gy (10 × 3.3 Gy)	1.02 (0.78–1.33)	20% vs 14%	8% vs 9%
	Wang et al.[18]	1989	1977–1985	206	SCC	40 Gy (8 × 5 Gy)	0.81 (0.65–1.01)	47% vs 42%	37% vs 33%
	Arnott et al.[14]	1992	1979–1983	176	SCC (56)/AC (114)/other (7)	20 Gy (10 × 2 Gy)	1.19 (0.87–1.62)	13% vs 21%	10% vs 17%
	Nygaard et al.[17]	1992	1983–1988	108	SCC	35 Gy (20 × 1.75 Gy)	0.60 (1.40–0.91)	21% vs 9%	NR
Postoperative radiotherapy	Teniere et al.[21]	1991	1979–1985	221	SCC	45–55 Gy (fractions NR)	NR	27% vs 29%	21% vs 19%
	Fok et al.[20]	1993	1968–1981	81	SCC	45–53 Gy (fractions NR)	NR	17% vs 24%	10% vs 16%
	Zieren et al.[23]	1995	1988–1991	68	SCC	55.8 Gy (31 × 1.8 Gy)	NR	29% vs 31%	NR
	Xiao et al.[22]	2003	1986–1997	495	SCC	50–60 Gy (25–30 × 2 Gy)	NR	51% vs 44%	41% vs 37%

[a] Radiotherapy followed by surgery versus surgery alone.
AC, adenocarcinoma; CI, confidence interval; HR, hazard ratio; NR, not reported; SCC, squamous cell carcinoma; yOS, year overall survival.

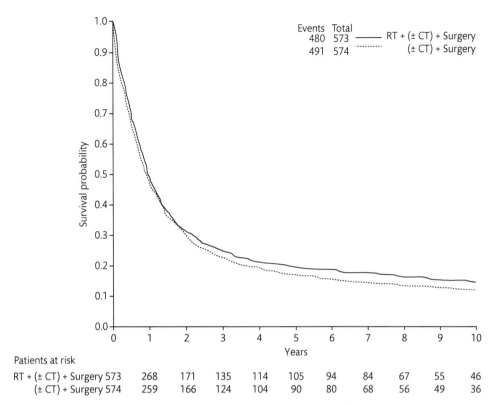

Figure 11.2 Survival curves from the meta-analysis of Arnott et al. representing individual data of 1147 patients either undergoing preoperative radiotherapy (with or without chemotherapy) followed by surgery or surgery alone.[19] Overall HR was 0.89 (95% CI 0.78–1.01; $p = 0.06$). RT, radiotherapy; CT, chemotherapy.
Reproduced with permission from Arnott SJ, Duncan W, Gignoux M, et al. Preoperative radiotherapy for esophageal carcinoma. *Cochrane Database Syst Rev.* 2005;4:CD001799.

can act systemically by eliminating subclinical metastases. In the adjuvant setting, chemotherapy is given postoperatively not only to eliminate micrometastatic disease but also to kill residual locoregional tumour cells that were not surgically removed. In the perioperative setting, chemotherapy is given both before and after surgery to combine the mechanisms of action of neoadjuvant and adjuvant chemotherapy.

Commonly used classes of chemotherapy for oesophageal cancer are platinum-based agents, taxanes, pyrimidine analogues, anthracyclines, bleomycins, etoposide, and/or vinca alkaloids. The antineoplastic mechanism of platinum-based agents (e.g. cisplatin, carboplatin, and oxaliplatin) is based on their ability to cause inter- and intra-strand DNA crosslinks. In this way, the agents interfere with DNA repair mechanisms and induce apoptosis in cancer cells. Because of the number of serious side effects of cisplatin, other platinum-based agents that have less side effects (i.e. carboplatin and oxaliplatin) are being increasingly used for cancer treatment nowadays.[28] The antineoplastic mechanism of taxanes (e.g. docetaxel, paclitaxel) is based on their ability to stabilize the microtubules and prevent depolymerization. Hence, taxanes cause cell-cycle arrest and prevent cell division. Since microtubules are also essential components of axonal structures, neurotoxic side effects are common for treatment with taxanes. Taxanes were first isolated from needles and bark of the yew tree (genus *Taxus*) but are now being synthesized artificially. For treatment of oesophageal cancer, paclitaxel and docetaxel have both been widely studied and used.[29] The antineoplastic mechanism of pyrimidine analogues (e.g. fluorouracil, capecitabine) is based on the incorporation of fluoronucleotides into RNA and DNA. In this way, the agents' metabolites compete with naturally occurring nucleotides. Moreover, pyrimidine analogues inhibit the nucleotide synthetic enzyme thymidylate synthase.[30] Through both mechanisms, DNA and RNA synthesis is inhibited and cell death is initiated. Folinic acid (leucovorin) can be given in combination with fluorouracil to enhance its inhibiting effect on thymidylate synthase. Anthracyclines (epirubicin, doxorubicin) and bleomycins (bleomycin) are part of a group of cytotoxic antibiotics and both have several antineoplastic mechanisms. The main mechanism of action of anthracyclines is their ability to intercalate into DNA, which inhibits DNA replication and transcription.[31] Moreover, they inhibit topoisomerase II. This enzyme normally creates transient double-strand DNA breaks which are necessary to change the winding of the DNA helix. Anthracyclines impede resealing of these DNA breaks and hence cause growth arrest and programmed cell death. Moreover, anthracyclines can bind to DNA and can generate free radicals that cause damage to cell membranes and DNA, all initiating cell death. Bleomycins act by binding metals and oxygen and causing single-strand and double-strand DNA breaks. In this way, they inhibit RNA and protein synthesis.[32] Similar to anthracyclines, the semisynthetic derivative of podophyllotoxin, etoposide, also acts through inhibition of topoisomerase II.[33] Vinca alkaloids (e.g. vindesine, vinblastine, and vinorelbine) have an antineoplastic effect through the inhibition of tubulin polymerization into microtubules.[34] Therefore, this class of drugs interferes with the formation of microtubules and thus with cell division. Although some can be semi-synthetically produced, most vinca alkaloids are isolated from the Madagascar or pink periwinkle (genus *Catharanthus*, which is related to the genus *Vinca*).

Neoadjuvant chemotherapy

From the early 1980s until the late 1990s, several trials were conducted that investigated chemotherapy in addition to surgery with regimens consisting of cisplatin in combination with fluorouracil, bleomycin, or bleomycin and vindesine/vinblastine (Table 11.2).[17,35–39] Although these early and mostly underpowered trials failed to show a survival benefit for patients treated with neoadjuvant or perioperative chemotherapy, patients who responded well to chemotherapy had significantly prolonged overall survival compared to non-responders and patients who did not receive chemotherapy.[35,36,38,39] Thereafter, several major trials have demonstrated the benefit of chemotherapy in addition to surgical treatment for locally advanced oesophageal cancer (Table 11.2).

Between 1992 and 1998, the OE02 trial randomized 802 patients with squamous cell carcinoma or adenocarcinoma between preoperative cisplatin and fluorouracil followed by surgery versus surgery alone. This was the first and largest trial that showed a significant survival benefit from neoadjuvant chemotherapy (HR 0.79, 95% CI 0.67–0.93; $p = 0.004$).[40,41] Surprisingly, using a regimen similar to the OE02 trial in a comparable group of 440 patients, the Radiation Therapy Oncology Group (RTOG) 8911 trial did not show a survival benefit from neoadjuvant chemotherapy (HR 1.07, 95% CI 0.87–1.32; $p = 0.49$).[42,43] Differences in outcome between the OEO2 and RTOG 8911 trials cannot be fully explained. However, in the preoperative chemotherapy group of the RTOG 8911 trial, 29% of patients had grade 3–4 neutropenia and 20% of patients did not undergo surgery. In the OE02 trial, graded adverse events were not reported but 8% of patients underwent dose reduction due to neutropenia and only 10% did not undergo surgery. These differences in toxicity profiles and number of patients proceeding to surgery could be a possible explanation. In the same period, Boonstra et al. showed that patients with squamous cell carcinoma can also benefit from neoadjuvant chemotherapy consisting of cisplatin and etoposide.[44] Overall survival was significantly better in the neoadjuvant chemotherapy group (HR 0.71, 95% CI 0.51–0.98; $p = 0.03$). Grade 3–4 haematological toxicity was reported in 27% of patients and 11% of patients did not undergo surgery. Interestingly, patients treated with preoperative chemotherapy in these trials did not have significantly fewer distant metastases than patients treated with surgery alone, suggesting that preoperative chemotherapy has its major effect through improving locoregional tumour control and to a lesser extent has a systemic effect.

After these major trials have shown that doublet neoadjuvant chemotherapy resulted in better overall survival, more aggressive regimens have been investigated (Table 11.2). Between 2005 and 2011, the OE05 trial randomized 897 patients with oesophageal adenocarcinoma between preoperative epirubicin, cisplatin, and capecitabine followed by surgery (ECX arm) versus preoperative cisplatin and fluorouracil followed by surgery (CF arm).[45] While the ECX regimen was more toxic than the CF regimen, with grade 3–4 toxicity occurring in 49% of patients compared to 31% in the CF arm ($p <0.0001$), overall survival did not differ significantly between both arms (HR 0.90, 95% CI 0.77–1.05; $p = 0.19$). Moreover, locoregional and distant disease progression was comparable between both arms. Between 2011 and 2013, the OGSG1003 trial randomized 162 patients with oesophageal squamous cell carcinoma between preoperative doxorubicin (anthracycline derivative), cisplatin, and fluorouracil followed by surgery (ACF arm) versus preoperative docetaxel, cisplatin, and fluorouracil followed by surgery (DCF arm).[46] Toxicity was high in both groups, with grade 3–4 neutropenia occurring in 69% of patients in the ACF arm and in 90% in the DCF arm ($p <0.01$).[47] Recurrence-free survival was better in the DCF arm than in the ACF arm (HR 0.53, 95% CI 0.33–0.83; $p = 0.0057$). Two-year overall survival did not significantly differ (78.6% vs 65.4%; $p = 0.08$). However, this phase II study was not powered on overall survival and it was not the primary outcome measure. Although the OE05 and OGSG1003 trials included patients with different histology, both trials showed that patients with resectable oesophageal cancer do not benefit from additional anthracyclines in the neoadjuvant regimen. However, the OGSG1003 trial showed a trend towards more effective treatment by addition of a taxane. A recent meta-analysis summarized the results of studies that investigated the addition of a taxane to platinum/fluoropyrimidine-based neoadjuvant chemotherapy in patients with adenocarcinoma or squamous cell carcinoma.[48] This meta-analysis showed that the addition of a taxane was associated with more grade 3–4 neutropenia (pooled odds ratio 13.28, 95% CI 1.37–129.01; $p = 0.03$), but also with better overall survival (pooled HR 0.50, 95% CI 0.37–0.68; $p < 0.0001$). Similar results were observed in the subgroup analysis for squamous cell carcinoma only. It should be noted, however, that this meta-analysis included mostly cohort studies and only a few randomized controlled trials.

Perioperative chemotherapy

Trials that investigated perioperative chemotherapy are summarized in Table 11.3. The first trial that showed a significant survival benefit from perioperative chemotherapy was the MAGIC trial.[49] Between 1994 and 2002, 503 patients with resectable adenocarcinoma of the distal oesophagus, oesophagogastric junction, or stomach were randomized between perioperative epirubicin, cisplatin, and fluorouracil (ECF) plus surgery versus surgery alone. At the start, the study was designed to include only gastric cancer. Later, the study was amended to include distal adenocarcinoma as well. Some 86% of patients in the perioperative chemotherapy group completed all three preoperative cycles and 91.6% proceeded to surgery. However, only 54.8% started postoperative chemotherapy, which was mainly due to disease progression or early death. Of the patients who started postoperative chemotherapy, 75.9% completed the three postoperative cycles. Postoperative mortality was 5.6% in the perioperative chemoradiotherapy group and 5.9% in the surgery alone group. Overall survival was better in the perioperative chemotherapy group than in the surgery alone group (HR 0.75, 95% CI 0.60–0.93; $p = 0.009$) with 5-year overall survival rates of 36.3% and 23.0%, respectively. No clear difference in effectivity could be observed between patients with gastric cancer and patients with distal oesophageal cancer. Between 1995 and 2003, the ACCORD07 trial included 224 patients with resectable adenocarcinoma of the distal oesophagus, oesophagogastric junction, or stomach.[50] Patients were randomized between perioperative cisplatin and fluorouracil plus surgery versus surgery

Table 11.2 Randomized controlled trials investigating neoadjuvant chemotherapy followed by surgery

Author	Year	Period	Patients	Tumour histology	Arm A	Arm B	Survival[a], HR (95% CI)	2-yOS[a]	3-yOS[a]	5-yOS[a]
Nygaard et al.[17]	1992	1983	91	SCC	Two 2-week cycles of cisplatin (20 mg/m²) on days 1–5 and bleomycin (5 mg/m²) on days 1–5	Surgery alone	1.22 (0.82–1.81)[b]	NR	NR	NR
Schlag et al.[39]	1992	NA	46	SCC	Three 3-week cycles of cisplatin (20 mg/m²) on days 1–5 and fluorouracil (1000 mg/m²) on days 1–5	Surgery alone	0.97 (0.60–1.57)[b]	NR	NR	NR
Maipang et al.[37]	1994	1988–1990	46	SCC	Two 4-week cycles of cisplatin (100 mg/m²) on day 1, bleomycin (10 mg/m²) on days 3–8, and vinblastine (3 mg/m² days) 1, 8, 15, and 22	Surgery alone	1.61 (0.79–3.27)[b]	NR	31% vs 36%	NR
Law et al.[36]	1997	1989–1995	147	SCC	Two 3-week cycles cisplatin (100 mg/m²) on day 1 and fluorouracil (1000 mg/m²) on days 1–5	Surgery alone	0.73 (0.53–1.00)[b]	44% vs 31%	NR	NR
Kelsen et al.[42,43] (RTOG 8911)	1998, 2007	1990–1995	440	SC + AC	Three 4-week cycles of cisplatin (100 mg/m²) on day 1 and continuous infusion of fluorouracil (1000 mg/m²) from day 1 to day 5 plus surgery	Surgery alone	1.07 (0.87–1.32)	35% vs 37%	23% vs 26%	NR
Ancona et al.[35]	2001	1992–1997	94	SCC	Two 3-week cycles of cisplatin (100 mg/m²) on day 1 and fluorouracil (1000 mg/m²) on days 1–5	Surgery alone	0.85 (0.50–1.44)[b]	NR	44% vs 41%	34% vs 22%
MRCOC Working Group[40,41] (OE02)	2002, 2009	1992–1998	802	SCC + AC	Two 3-week cycles of cisplatin (80 mg/m²) on day 1 and continuous infusion of fluorouracil (1000 mg/m²) from day 1 to day 4 plus surgery	Surgery alone	0.79 (0.67–0.93)	43% vs 34%	NR	23% vs 17%
Schuhmacher et al.[137] (EORTC 40954)	2010	1999–2004	144	AC	Two 48-day cycles of cisplatin (50 mg/m²) on days 1, 15, and 29 and d-L-folinic acid (500 mg/m²) followed by continuous 24-hour infusion of fluorouracil (2000 mg/m²) on days 1, 8, 15, 22, 29, and 36 plus surgery	Surgery alone	0.84 (0.52–1.35)	73% vs 70%	NR	NR
Boonstra et al.[44]	2011	1989–1996	169	SCC	Two 3-week cycles of cisplatin (80 mg/m²) on day 1 and etoposide (200 mg/m²) on days 3 and 5 plus surgery	Surgery alone	0.71 (0.51–0.98)	42% vs 30%	NR	26% vs 17%
Alderson et al.[45] (OEO5)	2017	2005–2011	897	AC	Two 3-week cycles of cisplatin (80 mg/m²) on day 1 and continuous infusion of fluorouracil (1000 mg/m²) from day 1 to day 4 plus surgery	Four 3-week cycles of epirubicin (50 mg/m²) and cisplatin (60 mg/m²) on day 1 and daily oral capecitabine (1250 mg/m²) throughout the four cycles plus surgery	0.90 (0.77–1.05)	NR	39% vs 42%	NR
Yamasaki et al.[46] (OGSG1003)	2017	2011–2013	162	SCC	Two 4-week cycles of Adriamycin (35 mg/m²) and cisplatin (70 mg/m²) on day 1 and continuous infusion of fluorouracil (700 mg/m²) from day 1 to day 7 plus surgery	Two 3-week cycles of docetaxel (70 mg/m²) and cisplatin (70 mg/m²) on day 1 and continuous infusion of fluorouracil (700 mg/m²) from day 1 to day 5 plus surgery	NR, NS	79% vs 65%	NR	NR

[a] Arm A vs arm B; [b] from Sjoquist et al.[27]

AC, adenocarcinoma; CI, confidence interval; HR, hazard ratio; NA, not available; NR, not reported; NS, not significant; SCC, squamous cell carcinoma; yOS, year overall survival.

Table 11.3 Randomized controlled trials investigating perioperative chemotherapy plus surgery

Author	Year	Period	Patients	Tumour histology	Arm A	Arm B	Survival[a]: HR (95% CI)	2-yOS[a]	3-yOS[a]	5-yOS[a]
Roth et al.[38]	1988	NA	39	SCC	Two cycles of cisplatin (120 mg/m²) on day 1, vindesine (3 mg/m²) on days 1, 8, and bleomycin (10 U/m²) on days 3–6	Surgery alone	0.71 (0.36–1.43)[b]	NA	NA	NA
Cunningham et al.[49] (MAGIC)	2006	1994–2002	503	AC	Three preoperative and three postoperative 3-week cycles of epirubicin (50 mg/m²) and cisplatin (60 mg/m²) on day 1 and continuous infusion of fluorouracil (200 mg/m²) from day 1 to day 21 plus surgery	Surgery alone	0.75 (0.60–0.93)	NR	NR	36% vs 23%
Ychou et al.[50] (ACCORD07-FFCD 9703)	2011	1995–2003	224	AC	Two or three preoperative and three or four postoperative 4-week cycles of cisplatin (100 mg/m²) on day 1 and continuous infusion of fluorouracil (800 mg/m²) from day 1 to day 5 followed by surgery	Surgery alone	0.69 (0.50–0.95)	NR	NR	38% vs 24%
Al-Batran et al.[51] (FLOT4)	2019	2010–2015	716	AC	Four preoperative and four postoperative 2-weekly cycles of docetaxel (50 mg/m²), oxaliplatin (85 mg/m²), leucovorin (200 mg/m²), and 24-hour continuous infusion of fluorouracil (2600 mg/m²) on day 1 plus surgery	Three preoperative and three postoperative 3-week cycles of epirubicin (60 mg/m²) and cisplatin (60 mg/m²) on day 1 plus either continuous infusion of fluorouracil (200 mg/m²) or oral capecitabine (1250 mg/m²) from day 1 to day 21 plus surgery	0.77 (0.63–0.94)	68% vs 59%	57% vs 48%	45% vs 36%
Zhao et al.[138]	2015	2005–2007	346	SCC	Two preoperative and two postoperative 3-week cycles of paclitaxel (100 mg/m²) on day 1, cisplatin (60 mg/m²) on day 1, and continuous infusion of fluorouracil (700 mg/m²) from day 1 to day 5	Two preoperative 3-week cycles of paclitaxel (100 mg/m²) on day 1, cisplatin (60 mg/m²) on day 1, and continuous infusion of fluorouracil (700 mg/m²) from day 1 to day 5	0.79 (0.59–0.95)	NR	NR	38% vs 22%

[a] Arm A versus arm B; [b] from Sjoquist et al.[27]
AC, adenocarcinoma; CI, confidence interval; HR, hazard ratio; NA, not available; NR, not reported; SCC, squamous cell carcinoma; yOS, year overall survival.

alone. Postoperative chemotherapy was given to 47.8% of patients. Overall survival was better in the perioperative chemotherapy group than in the surgery alone group (HR 0.69, 95% CI 0.50–0.95; $p = 0.02$). Five-year overall survival rates were 38% and 24%, respectively. From 2010 to 2015, the FLOT4 trial randomized 716 patients with locally advanced, resectable adenocarcinoma of the oesophagogastric junction or stomach between perioperative ECF or ECX versus perioperative fluorouracil, leucovorin, oxaliplatin, and docetaxel (FLOT).[51] In the ECF/ECX group, 91% of patients completed all three preoperative cycles and postoperative chemotherapy was given to 52% of patients. In the FLOT group, 90% of patients completed all four preoperative cycles and 60% started postoperative chemotherapy. Grade 3–4 neutropenia occurred more often (51%) in the FLOT group than in the ECF/ECX group (39%).[52] An overall survival benefit was observed for patients receiving FLOT (HR 0.77, 95% CI 0.63–0.94; $p = 0.012$), corresponding to estimated 5-year overall survival rates of 45% in the FLOT group and 36% in the ECF/ECX group.

After these trials, many countries adopted perioperative chemotherapy according to the MAGIC (ECF/ECX) trial and later according to the FLOT trial as standard treatment for adenocarcinoma of the oesophagogastric junction or stomach. Perioperative chemotherapy according to the ACCORD07 trial was widely adopted for adenocarcinoma of the distal oesophagus. Some countries also adopted the MAGIC and FLOT regimens for adenocarcinoma of the distal oesophagus. However, opinions differ on whether the MAGIC and FLOT regimens should be used to treat patients with adenocarcinoma of the distal oesophagus instead of neoadjuvant chemoradiotherapy or should only be used to treat gastric adenocarcinomas. In the MAGIC trial, the majority of patients had gastric adenocarcinoma (74%) and only 26% had oesophageal or junctional adenocarcinoma. Comparable to the MAGIC trial, most patients in the FLOT trial had junctional tumours of Siewert type II or III (33%) or gastric tumours (44%). Only 23% of patients included in the FLOT trial had adenocarcinoma of the distal oesophagus (Siewert type I). In contrast, most patients in the ACCORD07 trial had adenocarcinoma of the distal oesophagus or oesophagogastric junction (75%).

Adjuvant chemotherapy

Adjuvant chemotherapy, without any preoperative chemotherapy, has mostly been investigated by the Japan Clinical Oncology Group (JCOG) in patients with squamous cell carcinoma (Table 11.4). The JOCG showed that administration of cisplatin and vindesine after surgery did not significantly improve overall survival, compared to surgery alone; nor did a regimen of adjuvant cisplatin and fluorouracil.[53,54] Since neoadjuvant chemotherapy had already become the standard of care in several Western countries, from 2000 to 2006 the JCOG9907 trial compared adjuvant chemotherapy with neoadjuvant chemotherapy, both consisting of cisplatin and fluorouracil.[55] In the adjuvant group, patients only received chemotherapy if malignant lymph nodes were identified pathologically (pN+). In the neoadjuvant group, 97% of patients received chemotherapy. In the adjuvant group, 57% received chemotherapy. During interim analysis, it became clear that overall survival was significantly different, in favour of neoadjuvant chemotherapy (HR 0.64, 95% CI 0.45–0.91; $p = 0.01$). Final results showed that 5-year overall survival was 55% in the neoadjuvant group versus 43% in the adjuvant group. Based on these results, it was widely agreed that adjuvant chemotherapy without any preoperative

Table 11.4 Randomized controlled trials investigating adjuvant chemotherapy plus surgery

Author	Year	Period	Patients	Tumour histology	Arm A	Arm B	Survival[a]; HR (95% CI)	2-yOS[a]	3-yOS[a]	5-yOS[a]
Ando et al.[53]	1997	1988-1991	205	SCC	Surgery followed by two 3-week cycles of cisplatin (70 mg/m²) and vindesine (3 mg/m²) on day 1	Surgery alone	Relative risk = 0.89 (0.61–1.31)	NR	NR	48% vs 45%
Ando et al.[54] (JCOG9204)	2003	1992-1997	242	SCC	Surgery followed by two 3-week cycles of cisplatin (80 mg/m²) and continuous infusion of fluorouracil (800 mg/m²) from day 1 to day 5	Surgery alone	NR/NS	NR	NR	61% vs 52%
Ando et al.[55] (JCOG9907)	2012	2000-2006	330	SCC	Two preoperative 3-week cycles of cisplatin (80 mg/m²) on day 1 and continuous infusion of fluorouracil (800 mg/m²) from day 1 to day 5	Two postoperative 3-week cycles of cisplatin (80 mg/m²) on day 1 and continuous infusion of fluorouracil (800 mg/m²) from day 1 to day 5	0.64 (0.45–0.91)	NR	NR	55% vs 43%

[a] Arm A versus arm B; [b] from Sjoquist et al.[27]
AC, adenocarcinoma; CI, confidence interval; HR, hazard ratio; NA, not available; NR, not reported; SCC, squamous cell carcinoma; yOS, year overall survival.

chemotherapy should not be preferred over neoadjuvant or perioperative chemotherapy.

Neoadjuvant chemoradiotherapy

Mechanisms of action

Similar to chemotherapy, survival outcomes for patients with locally advanced oesophageal cancer are improved when chemoradiotherapy is given prior to surgery.[27] Neoadjuvant chemoradiotherapy can be given sequentially or concurrently. When given sequentially, chemotherapy and radiotherapy mostly work alone, having their own mechanisms of action. In this way, both therapies could cooperate spatially, where radiotherapy provides local control and chemotherapy mainly provides distant control (Figure 11.3). However, a meta-analysis showed that sequential neoadjuvant chemoradiotherapy did not provide a survival benefit for patients with squamous cell carcinoma or adenocarcinoma.[56] This is probably due to the fact that radiotherapy alone is not sufficiently effective in providing locoregional control prior to surgery. When given concurrently, however, both therapies can cooperate in-field, where chemotherapy has a radiosensitizing effect on tumour cells (Figure 11.3). Agents that are commonly given concurrently with radiotherapy for oesophageal cancers are cisplatin, carboplatin, oxaliplatin, fluorouracil, and paclitaxel. Multiple mechanisms are known for the synergistic effect of these chemotherapeutic agents. Several agents can increase radiation damage by incorporation of the agent into DNA (e.g. cisplatin, fluorouracil) or into RNA (cisplatin). Moreover, chemotherapy can cause cell-cycle arrests in radiosensitive phases (e.g. paclitaxel) and can eliminate radioresistant cells in their replication (S) phase (e.g. fluorouracil) (Figure 11.4). After radiotherapy, DNA repair processes can be inhibited (e.g. cisplatin, fluorouracil) and proliferation and repopulation can be prevented (e.g. fluorouracil). Also, it is known that hypoxic cells are more radioresistant. Chemotherapy can reoxygenate these cells by decreasing the tumour size which causes reperfusion of hypoxic areas (e.g. paclitaxel). Finally, chemotherapy can have a systemic effect even at low radiosensitizing doses.[57]

Neoadjuvant chemoradiotherapy

Similar to neoadjuvant chemotherapy, the first trials that investigated neoadjuvant chemoradiotherapy were started in the early 1980s.[17,58-61] Although these trials showed promising results with pathological complete response rates up to 28%, they failed to demonstrate a survival benefit. This could be explained by the fact that these early trials gave chemotherapy and radiotherapy sequentially instead of concurrently or were underpowered for detecting small differences in overall survival. Trials investigating neoadjuvant chemoradiotherapy are summarized in Table 11.5.

Between 1990 and 1995, Walsh et al. randomized 113 patients with oesophageal adenocarcinoma between two cycles of preoperative cisplatin and fluorouracil with concurrent 40 Gy radiotherapy followed by surgery versus surgery alone.[62] This was the first trial that demonstrated a survival benefit from neoadjuvant chemoradiotherapy (median overall survival: 16 vs 11 months; $p = 0.01$). However, survival in the surgery alone arm was poor. From 1994 to 2000, Burmeister et al. randomized 256 patients with squamous cell carcinoma or adenocarcinoma between one cycle of preoperative cisplatin and fluorouracil with concurrent 35 Gy radiotherapy followed

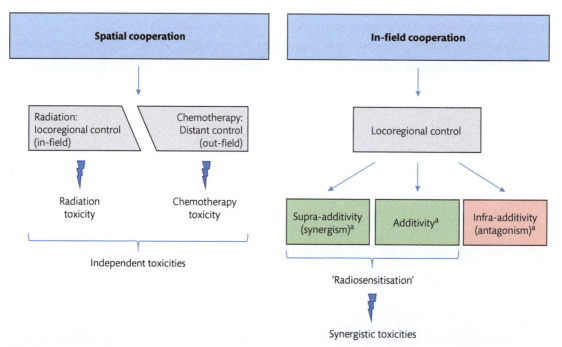

Figure 11.3 Rationale for concurrent chemoradiotherapy. Spatial cooperation and in-field cooperation are the hypothetical types of cooperation between chemotherapy and radiotherapy. Both mechanisms can contribute synergistically to clinical benefit.

[a] In-field interaction between radiotherapy and chemotherapy can result in cell death, either to a higher degree (supra-additive), the same degree (additivity), or to a lower degree (infra-additivity) than using both modalities sequentially. The latter is not desirable as this could protect the tumour.

Reproduced with permission from Seiwert TY, Salama JK, Vokes EE. The concurrent chemoradiation paradigm) than using both m. *Nat Clin Pract Oncol.* 2007;4:86.

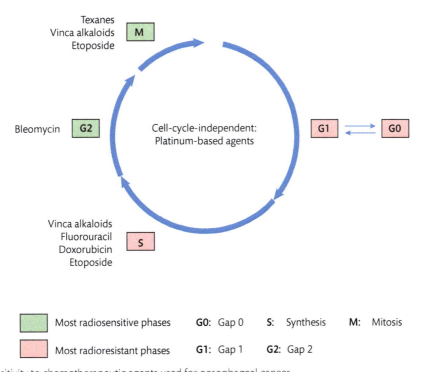

Figure 11.4 Cell-cycle sensitivity to chemotherapeutic agents used for oesophageal cancer.
Reproduced with permission from Seiwert TY, Salama JK, Vokes EE. The concurrent chemoradiation paradigmtic agents used for. *Nat Clin Pract Oncol.* 2007;4:86.

by surgery versus surgery alone.[63] In this trial, a significant difference in overall survival could not be observed (22.2 vs 19.3 months; $p = 0.570$). This could be explained by the rather low radiation dose and by the fact that only one cycle of chemotherapy was given. Although it should be noted that the trial was not powered to show survival differences in subgroups, Burmeister et al. were one of the first groups to show that neoadjuvant chemoradiotherapy seemed to have a more pronounced effect in patients with squamous cell carcinoma (HR 0.69, 95% CI 0.42–1.15; $p = 0.16$) than in patients with adenocarcinoma (HR 1.04, 95% CI 0.74–1.48; $p = 0.81$).

Table 11.5 Randomized controlled trials comparing concurrent neoadjuvant chemoradiotherapy plus surgery with surgery alone

Study	Year	Study period	Patients	Tumour histology	Radiotherapy	Chemotherapy	pCR rate	Survival[a]; HR (95% CI)	3-yOS[a]
Apinop et al.[58]	1994	1986–1992	69	SCC	40 Gy in 20 fractions	Cisplatin and fluorouracil	27%	0.80 (0.48–1.34)	26% vs 20%
Urba et al.[61]	2001	1989–1994	100	SCC + AC	45 Gy in 30 fractions	Cisplatin, fluorouracil, and vinblastine	28%	0.74 (0.48–1.12)	30% vs 16%
Walsh et al.[62]	1996	1990–1995	113	AC	40 Gy in 15 fractions	Cisplatin and fluorouracil	25%	0.58 (0.38–0.88)	32% vs 6%
Burmeister et al.[63]	2005	1994–2000	256	SCC + AC	35 Gy in 15 fractions	Cisplatin and fluorouracil	16%	0.94 (0.70–1.26)	36% vs 32%[b]
Tepper et al.[65] (CALGB 9781)	2008	1997–2000	56	SCC + AC	50.4 Gy in 28 fractions	Cisplatin and fluorouracil	40%	0.40 (0.18–0.87)	66% vs 20%[b]
Lv et al.[64]	2010	1997–2004	160	SCC	40 Gy in 20 fractions	Cisplatin and paclitaxel	NA	0.55 (0.36–0.84)	61% vs 49%
Lee et al.[66]	2004	1999–2002	101	SCC	45.6 Gy in 38 fractions	Cisplatin and fluorouracil	43%	0.88 (0.48–1.62)	48% vs 41%[b]
Van Hagen et al.[4,68] (CROSS)	2012, 2015	2004–2008	366	SCC + AC	41.4 Gy in 23 fractions	Carboplatin and paclitaxel	29%	0.66 (0.50–0.87)	58% vs 44%
Mariette et al.[67] (FFCD 9901)	2014	2000–2009	195	SCC + AC	45 Gy in 25 fractions	Cisplatin and fluorouracil	35.8%	0.92 (0.63–1.34)	48% vs 53%
Yang et al.[69] (NEOCRTEC5010)	2018	2007–2014	451	SCC	40.0 Gy in 20 fractions	Cisplatin and vinorelbine	43.2%	0.71 (0.53–0.96)	69% vs 59%

[a] Neoadjuvant chemoradiotherapy plus surgery versus surgery alone; [b] approximates extracted from Kaplan-Meier curves.
AC, adenocarcinoma; CI, confidence interval; HR, hazard ratio; NA, not available; pCR, pathological complete response; SCC, squamous cell carcinoma; yOS, year overall survival.

In 1997, two trials were initiated to further improve survival by investigating different regimens. A three-arm trial by Lv et al. replaced the classic agent fluorouracil for a taxane and assigned 238 patients with squamous cell carcinoma to neoadjuvant chemoradiotherapy consisting of paclitaxel and cisplatin with concurrent 40 Gy radiotherapy, or to adjuvant chemoradiotherapy consisting of the same regimen, or to surgery alone.[64] Five-year survival in the neoadjuvant, adjuvant, and surgery alone groups was 43.5%, 42.3% and 33.8%, respectively. While survival in both the neoadjuvant and adjuvant group was better than survival in the surgery alone group ($p = 0.0051$ and $p = 0.0209$, respectively), the survival of the neoadjuvant and adjuvant groups was comparable ($p = 0.4978$). The CALGB 9781 trial did not change the chemotherapeutic agents but increased the total dose of radiation to 50.4 Gy.[65] Unfortunately, after 56 patients had been enrolled, the trial had to be terminated prematurely due to poor accrual. Despite this small number, survival of patients treated with neoadjuvant chemoradiotherapy was significantly better than those treated with surgery alone ($p = 0.002$), with 5-year overall survival rates of 39% and 16%, respectively. A subsequent trial by Lee et al. intended to compare neoadjuvant cisplatin and fluorouracil with concurrent 45.6 Gy radiotherapy plus surgery versus surgery alone.[66] In the neoadjuvant chemoradiotherapy group only 69% of patients underwent surgery, compared to 96% in the surgery alone group. As a result, more locoregional failures occurred in the neoadjuvant chemoradiotherapy group which also led to premature termination of the trial.

Between 2000 and 2009, the French FFCD 9901 trial intended to randomize 380 patients with stage I or II oesophageal squamous cell carcinoma or adenocarcinoma between preoperative cisplatin and fluorouracil with concurrent 45 Gy radiotherapy followed by surgery versus surgery alone.[67] At interim analysis, however, a difference between both groups at completion of the trial was no longer expected. Therefore, the study was terminated prematurely after 195 patients had been enrolled because of futility. Overall survival did not differ between both groups (HR 0.99, 95% CI 0.69–1.40; $p = 0.94$). The comparable survival outcomes are rather surprising given the pathological complete response rate of 35.8% and the fact that 70% of patients had squamous cell carcinoma, which generally tends to be more radiosensitive than adenocarcinoma. A partial explanation for this finding could be the difference in postoperative mortality between the neoadjuvant chemoradiotherapy group and the surgery alone group (11.1% vs 3.4%; $p = 0.049$), which is big compared to other more recent trials. This high mortality rate could be explained by the low volume per centre (less than two included patients per centre per year). However, mortality in the surgery alone arm was according to modern standards.

Thus far, completed trials that investigated concurrent neoadjuvant chemoradiotherapy mostly used one or two cycles of cisplatin and fluorouracil with at least 3 weeks in between the cycles. Many trials had small sample sizes and were not adequately powered to show a survival benefit from neoadjuvant chemoradiotherapy. Moreover, the applied agents can induce severe toxicity. Only Lv et al. used a taxane instead of fluorouracil and first demonstrated the potential of this regimen for patients with squamous cell carcinoma. Unfortunately, limited toxicity data were reported.[64]

The promising antitumour effect of paclitaxel with concurrent radiotherapy as well as the lower toxicity of carboplatin compared to cisplatin led to the initiation of the CROSS trial in 2004.[4,68] In this trial, 366 patients with locally advanced squamous cell carcinoma or adenocarcinoma of the oesophagus or oesophagogastric junction were randomized between five cycles of carboplatin and paclitaxel with concurrent 41.4 Gy radiotherapy plus surgery versus surgery alone. Grade 3–4 neutropenia was observed in only 2% of patients. Overall survival was significantly better for patients in the neoadjuvant chemoradiotherapy group compared to the surgery alone group (HR 0.68, 95% CI 0.53–0.88; $p = 0.003$) with 5-year overall survival rates of 47% and 33%, respectively.[4] While only 23% of patients in the CROSS trial had squamous cell carcinoma, neoadjuvant chemoradiotherapy had a more pronounced effect on survival in patients with squamous cell carcinoma (HR 0.48, 95% CI 0.28–0.83; $p = 0.008$) than in patients with adenocarcinoma (HR 0.73, 95% CI 0.55–0.98; $p = 0.038$). Therefore, interpreting the results of these subgroups should be done with caution. After the CROSS trial was published, many countries adopted this regimen as standard of care for patients with oesophageal squamous cell carcinoma and adenocarcinoma.

More recently, the NEOCRTEC5010 trial investigated another neoadjuvant chemoradiotherapy regimen for patients with squamous cell carcinoma.[69] From 2007 to 2014, eight Chinese centres randomized 451 patients between preoperative cisplatin and vinorelbine with concurrent 40 Gy radiotherapy followed by surgery versus surgery alone. However, high toxicity was observed for this regimen, with grade 3–4 neutropenia occurring in 45.7% of patients. Although complications from these high toxicity rates were not reported, 82.6% of patients could complete the full chemoradiotherapy regimen. Patients in the neoadjuvant chemoradiotherapy group had better overall survival than patients in the surgery alone group (HR 0.71, 95% CI 0.53–0.96; $p = 0.025$).[4] Corresponding 5-year overall survival rates were 61% and 51%, respectively. The 5-year overall survival rate for patients receiving neoadjuvant chemoradiotherapy is comparable to the squamous cell carcinoma subgroup in the CROSS trial (approximately 62%, extracted from the Kaplan–Meier curve). However, toxicity reported in the CROSS trial from carboplatin/paclitaxel was substantially lower than the cisplatin/vinorelbine regimen.

Neoadjuvant chemotherapy versus chemoradiotherapy

Several randomized controlled trials that investigated neoadjuvant (or perioperative) chemotherapy and chemoradiotherapy were not sufficiently powered to show smaller differences in overall survival. Therefore, a meta-analysis of these studies was performed by Gebski et al.[56] and later updated by Sjoquist et al.[27] to clarify the benefits of neoadjuvant treatment. The latter showed that the pooled hazard ratio for all-cause mortality was 0.87 (95% CI 0.79–0.96; $p = 0.005$) for neoadjuvant chemotherapy and 0.78 (95% CI 0.70–0.88; $p <0.0001$) for neoadjuvant chemoradiotherapy. This can be translated into a 2-year overall survival benefit of 5.1% and 8.7%, respectively. Moreover, neoadjuvant chemotherapy and neoadjuvant chemoradiotherapy were compared indirectly, which resulted in a pooled hazard ratio for all-cause mortality of 0.88 (0.76–1.01; $p = 0.07$) (Figure 11.5). Thus, although this meta-analysis suggested a benefit of neoadjuvant chemoradiotherapy over chemotherapy, the survival advantage was

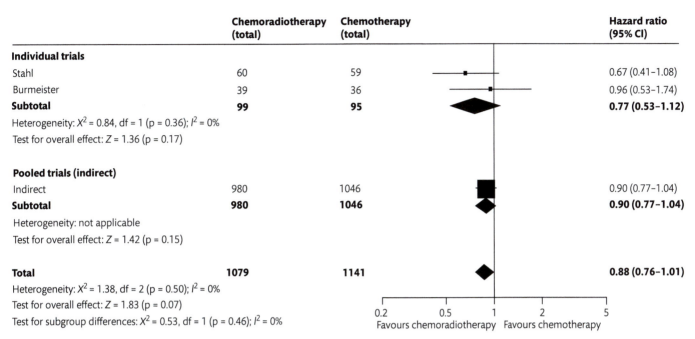

Figure 11.5 Indirect comparison of all-cause mortality for chemoradiotherapy and chemotherapy from the meta-analysis of Sjoquist et al.
Reproduced with permission from Sjoquist KM, Burmeister BH, Smithers BM, et al. Survival after neoadjuvant chemotherapy or chemoradiotherapy for resectable oesophageal carcinoma: an updated meta-analysis. *Lancet Oncol.* 2011;12(7):681–692.

not statistically significant and between-study heterogeneity was high. Also, chemotherapy regimens that are frequently used for oesophageal or junctional adenocarcinoma (MAGIC and FLOT) were not included since most patients in the MAGIC trial had gastric cancer and the FLOT trial was not yet finished at that time. Therefore, the Irish Neo-AEGIS and German ESOPEC trials are currently comparing perioperative chemotherapy according to the MAGIC and FLOT regimens versus neoadjuvant chemoradiotherapy according to the CROSS regimen for locally advanced oesophageal cancer.[70,71] Moreover, in the Japanese NExT trial, neoadjuvant chemotherapy consisting of cisplatin and fluorouracil with and without docetaxel is being compared with neoadjuvant chemotherapy consisting of cisplatin and fluorouracil with concurrent 41.4 Gy radiotherapy in patients with oesophageal squamous cell carcinoma.[72] Hopefully, results of these ongoing studies can provide evidence for the optimal neoadjuvant regimen.

Definitive chemoradiotherapy

Since oesophagectomy is a highly complicated surgical procedure possibly resulting in severe complications, substantial morbidity, and even mortality, patients should be in good condition before considering such potentially curative surgery. Patients for whom surgery is contraindicated still have another potentially curative option: definitive chemoradiotherapy. Definitive chemoradiotherapy aims to achieve a complete response and, as such, to prevent surgery. Definitive regimens rely on higher doses of radiotherapy (mostly >50 Gy) concurrently given with chemotherapy. This organ-preserving treatment with curative intent is an option especially for patients with contraindications to surgery, patients with tumours located at unfavourable locations (e.g. the cervical oesophagus), patients refusing surgery, or patients with cT4b tumours.

Current evidence on definitive chemoradiotherapy

Earlier studies concerning treatment with radiotherapy alone in patients with oesophageal cancer have reported disappointing results with very low 5-year overall survival rates.[73] Since subsequent studies suggested that chemotherapy combined with radiation therapy may result in improved survival, a large multicentre study was performed randomizing patients between definitive chemoradiotherapy, consisting of four cycles of fluorouracil and cisplatin with 50 Gy radiotherapy versus definitive radiotherapy alone, consisting of 64 Gy.[74,75] Some 121 patients with oesophageal cancer were enrolled in this study. The combined treatment seemed more toxic than the radiotherapy treatment alone since 20 of 60 patients (33%) in the combined therapy group had severe or life-threatening side effects versus 11 of 61 patients (18%) in the group undergoing radiotherapy alone. However, 44% of patients undergoing chemoradiotherapy showed recurrence of the tumour after 12 months versus 62% of patients undergoing radiotherapy alone. After a median follow-up of 17.9 months, patients undergoing chemoradiotherapy had a median overall survival of 12.5 months versus 8.9 months in the radiotherapy alone group. The trial was stopped after the interim analysis reported this statistically significant difference in favour of definitive chemoradiotherapy over definitive radiotherapy alone. A Cochrane review combining the results of 19 studies randomizing between chemoradiotherapy versus radiotherapy confirmed these results.[76]

Subsequent studies started to focus on the possibility to preserve the oesophagus by treating oesophageal cancer by high-dose chemoradiotherapy only, not performing surgery afterwards. This strategy originated after one study suggested that high-dose chemoradiotherapy alone could provide similar survival in patients with adenocarcinoma of the oesophagus compared to chemoradiotherapy followed by surgery.[77] This study included only 35 patients over a time span of 11 years (between 1981 and

Table 11.6 Randomized controlled trials comparing definitive chemoradiotherapy versus preoperative chemoradiotherapy followed by surgery

Author	Year	Period	Patients	Tumour histology	Definitive chemoradiotherapy	Preoperative chemoradiotherapy	Survival[a]; HR (95% CI)	3-yOS	5-yOS[a]
Stahl et al.[78]	2005	1994–2002	172	SCC	**Induction CT:** three cycles of fluorouracil (500 mg/m^2), leucovorin (300 mg/m^2), etoposide (80 mg/m^2)	**Induction CT:** three cycles of fluorouracil (500 mg/m^2), leucovorin (300 mg/m^2), etoposide (80 mg/m^2)	1.2 (0.81–1.84)	24% vs 31%	13% vs 29%
					CRT: cisplatin (50 mg/m^2) and etoposide (80 mg/m^2) with 65 Gy radiotherapy	**CRT:** cisplatin (50 mg/m^2) and etoposide (80 mg/m^2) with 40 Gy radiotherapy			
Bedenne et al.[79]	2007	1993–2000	444	SCC	**Induction CRT:** two cycles fluorouracil (800 mg/m^2) with cisplatin (15 mg/m^2) with either S.C. Rtx 30 Gy (10 × 3 Gy) or C. Rtx 46 Gy (23 × 2 Gy)	**Induction CRT:** two cycles fluorouracil (800 mg/m^2) with cisplatin (15 mg/m^2) with either S.C. Rtx 30 Gy (10 × 3 Gy) or C. Rtx 46 Gy (23 × 2 Gy)	0.90 ($p = 0.49^b$)	32% vs 29%	NR
					CRT: three cycles fluorouracil (800 mg/m^2) with cisplatin (15 mg/m^2) with either S.C. Rtx 15 Gy (5 × 3 Gy) or C. Rtx 20 Gy (10 × 2 Gy)				

[a] Definitive chemoradiotherapy versus preoperative chemoradiotherapy followed by surgery; [b] 95% CI not reported.
CI, confidence interval; CRT, chemoradiotherapy; C. Rtx, conventional radiotherapy; CT, chemotherapy; HR, hazard ratio; NR, not reported; SCC, squamous cell carcinoma; S.C. Rtx, split-course radiotherapy; yOS, year overall survival.

1992). Eleven patients were treated between 1981 and 1987 with high-dose chemoradiotherapy (two cycles of 5-fluorouracil and mytomycin-C with 60 Gy radiotherapy) and 24 patients were subsequently treated between 1987 and 1992 with the same regimen, followed by surgery. Randomized clinical trials were subsequently performed to assess the possibility for organ-sparing definitive chemoradiotherapy in patients with locally advanced oesophageal cancer (Table 11.6).

In 2005, Stahl et al. published the results of a clinical trial randomizing patients with oesophageal squamous cell cancer between induction chemotherapy (5-fluorouracil, leucovorin, etoposide, and cisplatin) followed by chemoradiotherapy (cisplatin, etoposide, and 40 Gy radiotherapy) and oesophagectomy versus the same induction chemotherapy followed by chemoradiotherapy alone (cisplatin, etoposide and at least 65 Gy radiotherapy).[78] A total of 172 eligible patients were included. Although treatment-related mortality was significantly higher in the chemoradiotherapy followed by surgery group (12.8% vs 3.5%), overall survival was reported to be comparable. After a median follow-up of 6 years, 2-year overall survival was 40% for patients undergoing chemoradiotherapy followed by surgery versus 35% for patients undergoing chemoradiotherapy alone (Figure 11.6). Although the authors also report an equivalence in 3-year overall survival (31% vs 24%, respectively), 5-year overall survival seems different with an overall survival of approximately 29% for patients undergoing chemoradiotherapy followed by surgery versus 13% for patients undergoing chemoradiotherapy alone. However, these results were not explicitly mentioned in the article. The authors did report a significantly improved locoregional progression-free survival for patients undergoing chemoradiotherapy followed by surgery versus chemoradiotherapy alone (2-year progression-free survival 64% vs 41%, respectively). Following the results of this trial, Bedenne et al.[79] published the results of a randomized trial in patients with oesophageal squamous cell cancer undergoing chemoradiotherapy with cisplatin and 5-fluorouracil concurrently with either 30 Gy or 45 Gy. Only patients with a clinically complete or partial response to induction chemoradiotherapy were considered for randomization. A complete response was objectified as the absence of dysphagia and the absence of a visible tumour on oesophagography only and

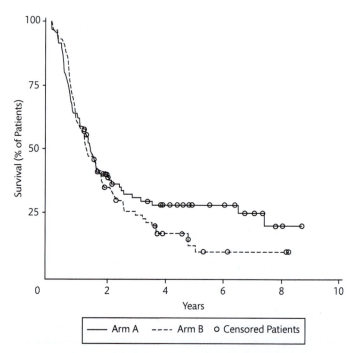

Figure 11.6 Survival curves from the randomized controlled trial by Stahl et al. of patients undergoing chemoradiotherapy followed by surgery (arm A) versus definitive chemoradiotherapy (arm B).
Reproduced with permission from Stahl M, Stuschke M, Lehmann N, et al. Chemoradiation with and without surgery in patients with locally advanced squamous cell carcinoma of the esophagus. *J Clin Oncol.* 2005;23(10):2310–2317.

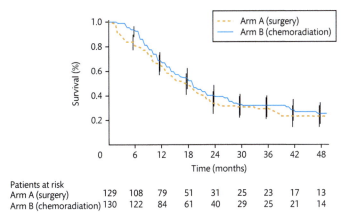

Figure 11.7 Bedenne et al. published these survival curves representing patients undergoing chemoradiation (using 30–45 Gy radiotherapy) followed by surgery (arm A) versus patients undergoing definitive chemoradiotherapy (up to 66 Gy radiotherapy).

Reproduced with permission from Bedenne L, Michel P, Bouche O, et al. Chemoradiation followed by surgery compared with chemoradiation alone in squamous cancer of the esophagus: FFCD 9102. *J Clin Oncol.* 2007;25(10):1160–1168.

a partial response was defined as a decrease of more than 30% of the tumour length on oesophagography and improvement of dysphagia. Patients were subsequently randomized between additional chemoradiotherapy (5-fluorouracil, cisplatin, and additional radiotherapy up to 45–66 Gy) versus immediate surgery. Some 444 patients were included of whom 259 patients were randomly assigned. The 3-month mortality rate was higher in the surgery group (9% vs 0.8%). However, after a median follow-up of 47 months the median overall survival of patients undergoing chemoradiotherapy followed by surgery versus chemoradiotherapy alone was 18 months versus 19 months, respectively (Figure 11.7). Even though the non-responders to chemoradiotherapy were excluded from further analysis in this trial, the 2-year overall survival was only 34% which seems relatively low. Furthermore, the authors later published overall survival rates of the patients who were non-responders to chemoradiotherapy and were therefore excluded from the trial.[80] This study reported that overall survival was not different between the responders and the non-responders in the trial, which is hard to explain.

Two randomized clinical trials have attempted to improve locoregional control and survival by increasing the total dose of radiotherapy in definitive chemoradiotherapy regimens. In 2002, the RTOG INT 0123 trial reported that cisplatin and 5-fluorouracil in combination with a total dose of 64.8 Gy radiotherapy compared to a total dose of 50.4 Gy did not significantly improve 2-year locoregional failure (56% vs 52%, respectively) nor 2-year overall survival (31% vs 40%).[81] In 2021, the ARTDECO study was published.[82] In this study, again dose escalation up to a total dose of 61.6 Gy was compared with a dose of 50.4 Gy. This time, however, carboplatin and paclitaxel were given concurrently instead of cisplatin and 5-fluorouracil. Also, more modern radiation techniques (intensity-modulated techniques and volumetric-modulated arc therapy) were used instead of conventional multiple field radiation. Furthermore, the fraction dose of the simultaneously integrated boost to the primary tumour was increased to 2.2 Gy to reach to the high total dose of 61.6 Gy in the same overall treatment time, instead of increasingly the number of fractions (and thus the length of the treatment regimen). Despite these adjustments, the ARTDECO study also reported comparable 3-year locoregional progression-free survival (73% vs 70%) and 3-year overall survival (39% vs 42%).[82] It was concluded that dose escalation over 50.4 Gy does not improve local control nor survival.

Salvage surgery

As previously mentioned, a substantial number of patients undergoing definitive chemoradiotherapy have persistence or recurrence of the tumour after 12 months.[75] Some patients become eligible for oesophagectomy during follow-up after definitive chemoradiotherapy. In this case, surgery could be considered after proven persistence or recurrence of the tumour; so-called salvage surgery. A non-randomized phase II study reported on the outcomes of salvage surgery after definitive chemoradiotherapy.[83] A total of 41 patients were included in the study and underwent induction chemotherapy (5-fluorouracil, cisplatin, and paclitaxel) followed by concurrent chemoradiotherapy (5-fluorouracil, cisplatin, with 50.4 Gy radiotherapy). Non-haematological toxicity was reported in 28 of 37 patients who completed induction chemotherapy followed by chemoradiotherapy. Four patients died due to treatment-related causes. Some 21 patients underwent salvage surgery due to recurrence or persistence (20 patients) or the patient's wish (one patient). After a median follow-up of 22 months, the 1-year survival of all 41 evaluable patients was 71%. At time of publication, 13 patients were still alive and disease free, of whom eight patients underwent salvage surgery. The initial plan of the authors of the study was to proceed with this salvage treatment strategy in a phase III randomized trial. However, since the hypothesized 77.5% 1-year survival was not reached, this trial was never initiated.

Several other studies reported that postoperative mortality and morbidity after salvage surgery following definitive chemoradiotherapy was increased when compared to mortality and morbidity in patients undergoing either neoadjuvant chemoradiotherapy followed by surgery or surgery alone.[84,85] The study by Miyata et al.[84] reported that postoperative mortality rate was 12% in patients undergoing definitive chemoradiotherapy versus 3.6% in patients undergoing neoadjuvant chemoradiotherapy ($p = 0.059$). Furthermore, a significant increase was reported in postoperative complications such as anastomotic leakage (39% vs 22%; $p = 0.049$) and bleeding (15% vs 1.7%; $p = 0.002$). The increased mortality and morbidity is perhaps acceptable considering that salvage surgery is the only potentially curative option for patients with persistent or recurrent disease after definitive chemoradiotherapy. However, the risks of salvage surgery should be discussed thoroughly with the patients and the indication should be considered cautiously and only for a highly selected group of patients in selected centres.

Targeted therapy

Monoclonal antibodies and their targets

Researchers have been extensively testing targeted therapy in the treatment of oesophageal cancer. An example of such therapy is the administration of monoclonal antibodies. These monoclonal antibodies are known for their potential to bind to target cell surface receptors and cause subsequent tumour response. By contrast, monoclonal antibodies can have severe side effects like autoimmune reactions (e.g. colitis, immune-induced hepatitis) due to the binding of antibodies to healthy tissue.[86] However, the specific binding of agents potentially results in the selective inhibition of molecular pathways or in the activation of a host's immune response in order to eliminate tumour cells. Examples of ligands to which monoclonal antibodies bind include vascular endothelial growth factor (VEGF), epithelial growth factor receptor (EGFR), human epidermal growth factor receptor 2 (HER2), programmed cell death protein 1 (PD-1), and PD-1 ligand (PD-L1). These receptors are present on the normal cell surface of healthy individuals. Normally, their functions include control and induction of cell proliferation, cell survival, cell-cycle progression, and apoptosis of a cell. However, these receptors have oncogenic potential when overexpressed on the cell surface, for example, resulting in excessive proliferation of the cell. In oesophageal cancer, varying percentages concerning overexpression of the receptors are mentioned, ranging from 9–60% for HER2 and VEGFR to greater than 70% for EGFR.[87,88] As such, binding to (and blocking) these overexpressed receptors could be a potentially valuable target in the treatment of oesophageal cancer.

VEGF

Inhibitors of VEGF have several mechanisms of action. VEGF inhibitors can act by binding VEGF directly, thus preventing VEGF from binding to VEGF receptors on the cell surface (e.g. bevacizumab).[89] Other agents can bind directly to the VEGF receptor (e.g. ramucirumab) or to the tyrosine kinase domain of the intracellular region of the receptor (i.e. tyrosine kinase inhibitors). Since overexpression of VEGF receptors can result in tumour growth due to increased angiogenesis in the tumour microenvironment, inhibition of angiogenesis potentially results in decreasing tumour growth. One of the key trials using bevacizumab is the STO3-trial. In this trial, 1063 patients with oesophagogastric or gastric cancer underwent either perioperative chemotherapy combined with bevacizumab or perioperative chemotherapy alone.[90] The addition of bevacizumab did not result in improvement of overall survival or improvement of any of the secondary outcomes. The REGARD trial, however, did report a survival benefit for patients with advanced gastric or oesophagogastric adenocarcinoma progressing after first-line chemotherapy compared to placebo.[91] The VEGF receptor inhibitor ramucirumab proved to be efficient in patients with advanced gastric or oesophagogastric junctional cancer.[91,92] Consequently, this agent has been approved by the US Food and Drug Administration (FDA) for second-line systemic treatment in these patients. However, there is as yet no place for VEGF inhibition in the treatment of resectable oesophageal cancer outside clinical trials.

EGFR

Two EGFR inhibitors that have been extensively tested in the treatment of metastatic or locally advanced oesophageal cancer are cetuximab and panitumumab. Both agents block EGFR, thus preventing its oncogenic functions when overexpressed on tumour cells.[93] Cetuximab was tested in patients with resectable oesophageal adeno- or squamous cell cancer in the SAKK 75/08 trial.[94] Some 300 patients were randomized between chemotherapy (docetaxel and cisplatin) followed by chemoradiation (docetaxel, cisplatin, and 45 Gy radiotherapy) plus surgery with versus without cetuximab. Although addition of cetuximab led to significantly improved

Table 11.7 Randomized controlled trials comparing neoadjuvant therapy with versus without cetuximab

Author	Year	Period	Patients	Tumour histology	Neoadjuvant + cetuximab	Neoadjuvant	pCR	Survival[a]; HR (95% CI)	3-yOS[a]	5-yOS[a]
Suntharalingam et al.[95]	2017	2008–2013	328	AC (62%)/ SCC (38%)	Six cycles of cisplatin (25 mg/m²), paclitaxel (50 mg/m²), and cetuximab (first week 400 mg/m² followed by a weekly dose of 250 mg/m²) with 50.4 Gy radiotherapy (28 × 1.8 Gy radiotherapy)	Six cycles of cisplatin (25 mg/m²), paclitaxel (50 mg/m²), with 50.4 Gy radiotherapy (28 × 1.8 Gy radiotherapy)	NR	0.90 (0.70–1.16)	34% vs 28%	NR
Ruhstaller et al.[94]	2018	2010–2013	300	AC (63%)/ SCC (37%)	**Induction CT:** two cycles of cisplatin (75 mg/2) and docetaxel (75 mg/m²) with six cycles of cetuximab (first week 400 mg/m² followed by a weekly dose of 250 mg/m²) **CRT:** five cycles of cisplatin (25 mg/m²) and docetaxel (20 mg/m²) and five cycles of cetuximab (first week 400 mg/m² followed by a weekly dose of 250 mg/m²) with 45 Gy radiotherapy (25 × 1.8 Gy) **Adjuvant:** weekly cetuximab (500 mg/m²) for 3 months	**Induction CT:** two cycles of cisplatin (75 mg/m²) and docetaxel (75 mg/m²) **CRT:** five cycles of cisplatin (25 mg/m²) and docetaxel (20 mg/m²) with 45 Gy radiotherapy (25 × 1.8 Gy)	37% vs 33%	0.73 (0.52–1.01)	62% vs 51%	53% vs 41%

[a] Neoadjuvant therapy with cetuximab versus neoadjuvant therapy alone.
AC, adenocarcinoma; CI, confidence interval; CRT, chemoradiotherapy; CT, chemotherapy; HR, hazard ratio; NR, not reported; pCR, pathological complete response; SCC, squamous cell carcinoma; yOS, year overall survival.

locoregional control of the disease, both progression-free survival and overall survival were not significantly prolonged. Concurrent addition of cetuximab to chemoradiotherapy in patients with locally advanced oesophageal cancer also failed to improve overall survival in the NRG Oncology RTOG 0436 randomized clinical trial.[95] The results of both randomized trials are summarized in Table 11.7. Panitumumab was also not able to improve overall survival or pathological complete response rates in patients with resectable oesophageal cancer during phase II trials.[96,97] Moreover, one randomized trial comparing chemotherapy (epirubicin, oxaliplatin, and capecitabine) with versus without panitumumab in patients with advanced oesophagogastric cancer reported a statistically significantly increased mortality for patients using panitumumab.[98] Since no improvements in outcomes were seen in several randomized or phase II trials using cetuximab or panitumumab, and some studies even reported increased mortality in subgroups of patients, EGFR blockage has mostly been abandoned in the treatment of oesophageal cancer.

HER2

The most widely investigated HER2 inhibitor is trastuzumab, which binds to and consequently inhibits the HER2 receptor and the downstream signalling pathway, of which overexpression results in increased and constant proliferative signalling.[99] After the introduction of trastuzumab for the treatment of metastatic breast cancer it became of interest for other malignancies.[100] Trastuzumab was proven to be effective in metastatic gastric and oesophagogastric junction cancer in the ToGa trial.[101] However, no trials have proved efficacy of trastuzumab in locally advanced oesophageal cancer. Most recently, the NRG Oncology/RTOG-1010 trial was published.[102] This randomized phase III trial investigated the addition of trastuzumab to neoadjuvant chemoradiotherapy according to the CROSS regimen in patients with HER2 overexpression. Median disease-free survival (the primary end point) was comparable with or without the addition of trastuzumab (19.6 months vs 14.2 months, respectively; $p = 0.97$). The group who received trastuzumab had less treatment-related adverse events at grade 3 or greater (69% vs 79%). Given the addition of trastuzumab did not lead to increased toxicity, the authors concluded that research into HER2 blockage should still be continued, but with other or multiple agents. The TRAP study was a phase II trial that added both trastuzumab and pertuzumab (dual-agent HER2 blockade) to neoadjuvant chemoradiotherapy for treatment of patients with oesophageal adenocarcinoma that showed overexpression of HER2.[103] A pathological complete response rate of 34% was seen (compared to 23% after conventional neoadjuvant chemoradiotherapy). Toxicity was similar to the CROSS regimen with the exception of increased incidences of rash and grade 3 diarrhoea. The authors concluded that the addition of trastuzumab and pertuzumab to neoadjuvant chemoradiotherapy is feasible and demonstrates potentially promising activity compared with historical controls. The subsequent phase III trial (TRAP-2 study) investigating this same dual-agent regimen is currently recruiting (NCT05188313).

PD-1 and PD-L1

Nivolumab and pembrolizumab are both immune checkpoint inhibitors that block PD-1 and which have been investigated in clinical trials for advanced non-resectable and locally advanced resectable oesophageal cancer. PD-1 is normally expressed on immune cells and has an immunoregulatory role in the immune system response. PD-1 on the immune cell binds to the PD-1 ligand (PD-L1) on the host's own cells preventing autoimmune reactions.[104] However, tumour cells often overexpress PD-L1 preventing immune cells from eliminating those tumour cells.[105] Targeting PD-1 on the immune cells could prevent the immunosuppressive binding from PD-L1 of the tumour cells to PD-1 on the immune cells, thus breaking the protective shield and enhancing the immune response against the tumour cells, possibly increasing tumour control.

In patients with non-resectable oesophageal cancer, nivolumab was tested in the randomized phase III ATTRACTION-3 trial including 419 patients with treatment-refractory advanced squamous cell carcinoma.[106] Median overall survival was significantly improved in patients undergoing nivolumab compared to chemotherapy. Also for patients with oesophageal and/or gastric adenocarcinoma, nivolumab has been investigated. The CheckMate 649 study showed that nivolumab plus chemotherapy has yielded better overall survival as first-line treatment than chemotherapy alone in those patients with high PD-L1 expression (PD-L1 combined positive score of ≥5).[107] The CheckMate 648 study has shown that nivolumab as well as nivolumab plus ipilimumab in addition to chemotherapy as first-line treatment leads to better overall survival than chemotherapy alone in patients with advanced oesophageal squamous cell carcinoma.[108] Based on these studies, nivolumab has been FDA approved for advanced squamous cell carcinoma and adenocarcinoma. An ongoing four-arm trial is currently randomizing patients with locally advanced oesophageal adenocarcinoma between neoadjuvant chemoradiotherapy with versus without nivolumab with adjuvant nivolumab with versus without ipilimumab (NCT03604991).

The phase III KEYNOTE-181 trial randomized 628 patients with treatment-refractory advanced squamous cell carcinoma and adenocarcinoma of the oesophagus between pembrolizumab or investigator's choice of chemotherapy. The median overall survival for patients with high PD-L1-expressing tumours (combined positive score ≥10) who received pembrolizumab was 9.3 months compared to 6.7 months in patients who received chemotherapy alone ($p = 0.007$). Median overall survival of patients with squamous cell carcinoma was 8.2 versus 7.1 months, respectively ($p = 0.009$).[109] In 2021, the phase III, placebo-controlled KEYNOTE-590 trial was published.[110] In this study, first-line treatment with pembrolizumab in addition to chemotherapy was studied in patients with locally unresectable or metastatic adenocarcinoma or squamous cell carcinoma. Median overall survival of patients who received pembrolizumab was 12.4 months compared to 9.8 months in patients receiving chemotherapy alone ($p <0.001$). Based on the results of the KEYNOTE-181 and KEYNOTE-590 trials, the FDA has approved pembrolizumab for the treatment of patients with metastatic or locally advanced oesophageal or oesophagogastric cancer in combination with platinum- and fluoropyrimidine-based chemotherapy, or as a single agent after one or more prior lines of systemic therapy for patients with tumours of squamous cell histology that express PD-L1 (combined positive score ≥10). For treatment of patients with locally advanced resectable oesophageal cancer, these immune checkpoint inhibitors have also been studied. The CheckMate 577 trial investigated adjuvant nivolumab in patients who received neoadjuvant chemoradiotherapy and radical resection, but who had residual disease in the resection specimen.[111] Administration of nivolumab for 1 year after surgery led to a median disease-free survival (primary end point) of 22.4 months, compared to 11.0 months in patients who received a placebo (p <0.001). Longer-term follow-up will be required to demonstrate an improvement in overall survival. Either below or 1% or greater PD-L1 expression in tumour cells yielded comparable survival. Grade 3 or 4 adverse events occurred in 34% of patients receiving nivolumab, and in 32% of patients receiving the placebo. Grade 3 or 4 adverse events that were related to nivolumab or the placebo by the investigators occurred in 13% of patients receiving nivolumab, and in 6% of patients receiving the placebo. Based on this trial, nivolumab has been approved by the FDA and the European Medicines Agency as adjuvant treatment for patients with incomplete pathological response after neoadjuvant chemoradiotherapy and radical surgery for oesophageal cancer.

Studies are also ongoing using pembrolizumab concurrently with chemoradiotherapy in patients with locally advanced oesophageal cancer.[112] A phase II study treated 28 patients with locally advanced oesophageal squamous cell carcinoma with pembrolizumab (five cycles, 200 mg) and neoadjuvant chemoradiotherapy using paclitaxel, carboplatin, and 44.1 Gy radiotherapy in 21 fractions followed by surgery. After surgery, pembrolizumab treatment was continued for 2 years or until progression, unacceptable toxicity, death, or patients' refusal. Most occurring adverse events were neutropenia (50%) in the neoadjuvant and liver enzyme elevation (31%) in the adjuvant setting. Some 46% of patients had a pathological complete response. After a median follow-up of 11.7 months, 6-month and 12-month overall survival was 89% and 82%, respectively. Currently, the exploration of end points and possible biomarker analyses are ongoing to subsequently proceed with a phase III trial.

An ongoing trial is currently recruiting patients with oesophageal adenocarcinoma randomizing between induction chemotherapy with carboplatin and paclitaxel followed by chemoradiotherapy consisting of carboplatin and paclitaxel concurrently with radiotherapy with versus without pembrolizumab (NCT02998268). The primary aim of the study is pathological complete response rate and secondary outcomes include R0 resection rate and median overall survival. Completion of the study is planned for April 2023.

Studies have shown promising results for treatment with monoclonal antibodies for advanced oesophageal cancer. At present, nivolumab is FDA approved as an adjuvant treatment for patients with locally advanced oesophageal cancer with incomplete pathological response after neoadjuvant chemoradiotherapy and radical surgery. More studies are currently underway to test monoclonal antibody treatment with or without chemotherapy for locally advanced resectable oesophageal cancer, increasingly claiming its role in clinical practice. An overview of the randomized trials that are currently ongoing for patients with locally advanced resectable oesophageal or oesophagogastric cancer using monoclonal antibodies is presented in Table 11.8.

Future perspectives

Oesophageal cancer still accounts for the sixth most cancer-related deaths overall, with 509,000 deaths worldwide in 2018.[113] Furthermore, the incidence of adenocarcinoma of the oesophagus is still rising in high-income countries, most probably with excess body weight and gastro-oesophageal reflux disease as key factors. Furthermore, the need for surgical resection is affecting patients' quality of life after treatment.

Further improving survival

Survival has improved from 12% to 35% after primary surgery over the last decades.[1,2,73] After addition of neoadjuvant chemo(radio)therapy, 5-year survival steadily increased to approximately 50%.[4,68,114] Subsequent analyses of the CROSS trial showed that locoregional recurrences developed in 14% of the patients after neoadjuvant chemoradiotherapy followed by surgery versus 34% in patients undergoing surgery alone.[115] Furthermore, only 1% of patients undergoing neoadjuvant chemoradiotherapy followed by surgery had an isolated recurrence within the radiotherapy field. However, after neoadjuvant therapy and surgery with curative intent, nearly 40% of patients develop distant metastases (vs 48% in patients undergoing surgery alone). Since patients who have distant metastases show a dismal 5-year survival of 5–10%, the prognosis in these patients is largely determined by the development of distant metastases.[4,68] These results indicate that neoadjuvant chemoradiotherapy is fairly efficient in locoregionally controlling the primary tumour but that this approach only has a modest systemic effect. In theory it could be beneficial to add chemotherapy before or after chemoradiotherapy in order to increase the systemic effects of the neoadjuvant therapy and to eliminate subclinical micrometastases already present at the time of diagnosis. An earlier phase II study randomized patients with oesophageal cancer between induction chemotherapy followed by chemoradiotherapy and surgery versus chemoradiotherapy alone followed by surgery.[116] The pathological complete response rate as well as the overall survival were not different between both groups. However, a secondary analysis of the data did reveal a survival advantage for a subgroup of patients with moderately or well-differentiated tumours.[117] The previously discussed FLOT regimen includes docetaxel which has already showed its efficacy in the metastatic setting, both first line and second line.[118,119] This suggests that the FLOT regimen could have a more prominent systemic effect than neoadjuvant chemoradiotherapy according to the CROSS regimen. Unfortunately, in the FLOT study the authors have not yet reported on the rate of distant metastases between both groups. The lower pathological complete response rate in FLOT versus CROSS (adenocarcinoma; 17% vs 23%) and the lower rates of microscopically margin-free resections in FLOT versus CROSS (85% vs 92%) suggest that locoregionally, FLOT might be less efficient than CROSS. However, these comparisons should be made with caution since CROSS included oesophageal cancer only and FLOT included mostly gastric cancer. Trials that are directly comparing both regimens are ongoing and results should be awaited.[70,71] In future, treatment with FLOT followed or preceded by CROSS could, possibly, combine the strengths of the locoregional efficacy of CROSS with the systemic efficacy of FLOT. The phase II TNT-OES-1 trial is currently investigating this combination in patients with oesophageal or junctional adenocarcinoma with oligometastases.[120] In head and neck cancer, a phase III trial has already shown the efficacy of induction docetaxel-containing chemotherapy followed by chemoradiotherapy over chemoradiotherapy alone, resulting in improved overall survival.[121] However, all these patients had squamous cell carcinoma and surgery was not routinely performed.

Several early preclinical studies suggested that aspirin could have an anti-metastatic effect in several cancers.[122,123] Later it has

Table 11.8 Currently ongoing randomized trials testing targeted therapy for primary treatment of patients with locally advanced resectable oesophageal cancer

NCT	mAb(s) used	Current status	Estimated completion	Planned inclusion	Histology	Experimental arm	Control arm	Primary outcome	Secondary outcomes
NCT02812641	Bevacizumab	Recruiting	December 2021	50	SCC	**Neoadjuvant:** cisplatin, fluorouracil, and bevacizumab with 40 Gy radiotherapy (20 × 2 Gy)	**Neoadjuvant:** cisplatin and fluorouracil with 40 Gy radiotherapy (20 × 2 Gy)	pCR	Acute/late toxicity, QOL, (metabolic) image response, PFS, OS
NCT03604991	Nivolumab/Ipilimumab	Recruiting	December 2023	278	AC	**Neoadjuvant:** carboplatin and paclitaxel with radiotherapy and nivolumab **Adjuvant:** nivolumab with or without ipilimumab	**Neoadjuvant:** carboplatin and paclitaxel with radiotherapy **Adjuvant:** nivolumab with or without ipilimumab	pCR	AE, OS, DFS
NCT02998268	Pembrolizumab	Recruiting	April 2023	46	AC	**Induction CT:** carboplatin and paclitaxel **CRT:** carboplatin and paclitaxel with radiotherapy and pembrolizumab	**Induction CT:** carboplatin and paclitaxel **CRT:** carboplatin and paclitaxel with radiotherapy	DFS	pCR, R0 resection rate, median survival, 1-yOS, reduction of local immune infiltration
NCT04280822	Toripalimab	Recruiting	March 2028	400	SCC	**Neoadjuvant:** cisplatin, paclitaxel, and toripalimab	**Neoadjuvant:** cisplatin and paclitaxel	EFS	pCR, DFS, OS, ORR, R0 resection rate, MPR, QoL
NCT04807673	Pembrolizumab	Recruiting	May 2028	342	SCC	**Neoadjuvant:** cisplatin, paclitaxel, and pembrolizumab **Adjuvant:** Pembrolizumab	**Neoadjuvant:** cisplatin and paclitaxel with radiotherapy	EFS	pCR, OS, DFS, MPR, ORR, R0 resection rate, peri- and postoperative complication
NCT04821843	Nimotuzumab	Recruiting	December 2025	2000	Both	**Neoadjuvant:** platinum-based or paclitaxel-based chemotherapy, with or without pembrolizumab	**Neoadjuvant:** platinum-based or paclitaxel-based chemotherapy and radiotherapy, with or without pembrolizumab	OS	DFS, pathological response, R0 resection rate, LRFS, DMFS
NCT04848753	Toripalimab	Recruiting	December 2026	500	SCC	**Neoadjuvant:** cisplatin, paclitaxel and toripalimab	**Neoadjuvant:** cisplatin, paclitaxel and placebo	EFS	pCR, OS

AC, adenocarcinoma; AE, adverse events; CRT, chemoradiotherapy; CT, chemotherapy; DFS, disease-free survival; DMFS, distant metastasis-free survival; EFS, event-free survival; LRFS, locoregional relapse-free survival; mAb, monoclonal antibody; MPR, major pathological response; NCT, national clinical trial; ORR, overall response rate; OS, overall survival; pCR, pathological complete response; PFS, progression-free survival; QOL, quality of life; SCC, squamous cell carcinoma; yOS, year overall survival.

been shown that aspirin has a protective effect for several cancers, including oesophageal cancer. The relative risk for developing oesophageal cancer was estimated to be 0.75 (95% CI 0.62–0.89) for aspirin users and a reduction in risk of death after 20 years was also seen for aspirin users (HR 0.42, 95% CI 0.25–0.71).[124,125] A Chinese study in which 1716 patients with oesophageal or gastric cancer were allocated to aspirin, placebo, or nothing at all reported survival rates of 51%, 41%, and 42%, respectively.[126] A double-blind phase III randomized trial is currently recruiting patients with oesophagogastric cancer to test the efficacy of aspirin in the adjuvant setting.[127]

Organ preservation after neoadjuvant treatment

After neoadjuvant chemotherapy, less than 16% of patients have a pathological complete response in the resection specimen.[41,42,46,52] After neoadjuvant chemoradiotherapy, however, this fraction is roughly one-third.[68,69] These patients can potentially be treated with (neoadjuvant) chemoradiotherapy without surgery, thus avoiding the risks of surgery. Moreover, patients who develop distant metastases after radical surgical resection (39% in the CROSS trial) could benefit from postponing surgery. The fact that the primary tumour has been completely removed indicates that undetectable micrometastases are already present at the time of diagnosis. However, to justify an organ-preserving treatment strategy, patients who have locoregional or distant residual or recurrent disease after neoadjuvant chemoradiotherapy have to be accurately identified. Before proceeding to surgery, patients without clinical evidence of residual or recurrent disease might then undergo active surveillance instead of surgery, consisting of frequent clinical response evaluations. In this way, surgery would be reserved for those patients who would really benefit from it.

Clinical response evaluation

If clinical response evaluations are falsely negative, a delay in detecting residual disease could potentially allow for tumour growth beyond resectability and for distant dissemination (Figure 11.8). Therefore, sensitivity seems the most important diagnostic parameter. However, a low corresponding specificity will cause overtreatment, since patients are falsely classified as having residual disease. For evaluating treatment response, several modalities have been investigated, including endoscopy with biopsies, endoscopic ultrasound (EUS) with fine-needle aspiration of suspected lymph nodes, computed tomography (CT), fluorodeoxyglucose positron emission tomography with CT (PET-CT), and magnetic resonance imaging.

In an early meta-analysis that included articles published before 2004, it was shown that the accuracy of CT is low for detecting residual disease after neoadjuvant chemotherapy or chemoradiotherapy, with a joint sensitivity and specificity of 54%.[128] Another meta-analysis that included all articles published before 2018 suggested that endoscopy with biopsies, EUS, and PET(-CT) as single modalities are also moderately accurate for detecting residual disease after neoadjuvant chemoradiotherapy.[129] For detecting residual disease at the primary tumour site, conventional biopsies had a pooled sensitivity of 33% and specificity of 95%, EUS had a pooled sensitivity of 96% and specificity of 8% and PET(-CT) yielded a pooled sensitivity of 69–74% and specificity of 52–72%. A systematic review on magnetic resonance imaging showed that residual tumour after neoadjuvant chemoradiotherapy can be identified with a sensitivity ranging from 60% to 87% and a specificity from 53% to 100% by using relative differences in apparent diffusion coefficient.[130] In another study, qualitative assessment of T2- and diffusion-weighted magnetic resonance imaging yielded a high sensitivity of 90–97%, but a poor specificity of 42–50%.[131]

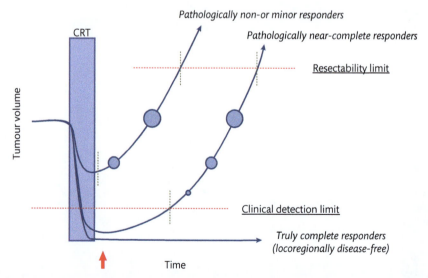

Figure 11.8 Tumour response after neoadjuvant chemoradiotherapy. CRT, chemoradiotherapy; Red arrow, time of clinical response evaluation (CRE); Vertical interrupted green lines, boundaries of theoretical time windows. First vertical interrupted green line on each curve refers to the first moment after CRT that a tumour becomes clinically detectable. Second vertical interrupted green line on each curve refers to the moment that a tumour becomes unresectable (T4b). Circles depict progression of locoregional tumour volume. The clinical detection limit is the minimal amount of disease that can be detected by the combination of symptoms, endoscopy with biopsies and imaging modalities.

Reproduced with permission from Noordman BJ, Wijnhoven BPL, Lagarde SM, Biermann K, van der Gaast A, Spaander MCW, et al. Active surveillance in clinically complete responders after neoadjuvant chemoradiotherapy for esophageal or junctional cancer. *Dis Esophagus*. 2017 Dec 1;30(12):1–8.

The accuracy of response evaluations can be increased if diagnostic modalities are combined. Guillem et al. showed that residual disease after chemoradiotherapy can be detected with a sensitivity of 89% and a specificity of 63% if a combination of clinical examination, endoscopic biopsies, EUS, barium oesophagography, and CT is used.[132] Noordman et al. investigated a combination of endoscopic bite-on-bite biopsies (double biopsy at the exact same location), EUS, and PET-CT for evaluating response to neoadjuvant chemoradiotherapy.[133] By using two response evaluations after completion of chemoradiotherapy, a sensitivity of 77% and a specificity of 72% were reached. The authors hypothesized that small amounts of residual tumour can be safely missed since in a strict active surveillance protocol these small amounts will regrow into a detectable but still resectable tumour. Based on this assumption, the authors showed that this set of diagnostics can detect greater than 10% residual tumour (i.e. tumour regression grade 3–4) with a sensitivity of 90%. Moreover, in 9% of patients unnecessary surgery could also be avoided since distant metastases were identified on PET-CT.

Active surveillance

A recent individual patient data meta-analysis included seven studies comprising a total of 788 patients with a clinically complete response after chemoradiotherapy.[134] Of these, 453 were randomized or propensity score matched; 196 who underwent active surveillance and 257 who underwent standard oesophagectomy. Overall survival was comparable between patients who underwent active surveillance and who underwent standard oesophagectomy in both an intention-to-treat analysis (HR 1.08, 95% CI 0.62–1.87; p = 0.75) and a per-protocol analysis (HR 0.93, 95% CI 0.56–1.54; p = 0.75). Of those patients who underwent a postponed oesophagectomy in the active surveillance group, 95% could undergo a radical resection. Only one of the included studies, however, was a randomized trial, which was terminated prematurely because of poor accrual. Moreover, all studies used different diagnostic modalities to assess whether a patient had a clinically complete response, including endoscopy with biopsies, EUS with fine needle aspiration, CT and PET-CT, and combinations of these. Also, active surveillance protocols varied in diagnostics modalities used and in surveillance frequency. Remarkably, postponed oesophagectomy was not performed in 43% of the patients who developed isolated locoregional recurrence during active surveillance, which was mostly due to the patient's condition or refusal. While this is a potential negative effect of active surveillance, in this meta-analysis it did not negatively affect survival. Two ongoing clinical trials, the French ESOSTRATE trial and Dutch SANO trial, are investigating an active surveillance strategy for patients with a clinically complete response to neoadjuvant chemoradiotherapy.[135,136] The SANO trial[136] uses a stepped-wedge cluster randomized trial design. With this design, not patients but institutions are being randomized, since randomized trials that compare a surgical treatment with a non-surgical treatment are often prematurely terminated due to poor participation. The SANO trial is expected to be report its first results at the end of 2023.

REFERENCES

1. Earlam R, Cunha-Melo JR. Oesophageal squamous cell carcinoma: I. A critical review of surgery. *Br J Surg*. 1980;**67**:381–390.
2. Hulscher JB, van Sandick JW, de Boer AG, et al. Extended transthoracic resection compared with limited transhiatal resection for adenocarcinoma of the esophagus. *N Engl J Med*. 2002;**347**:1662–1669.
3. Muller JM, Erasmi H, Stelzner M, Zieren U, Pichlmaier H. Surgical therapy of oesophageal carcinoma. *Br J Surg*. 1990;**77**:845–857.
4. Shapiro J, van Lanschot JJB, Hulshof M, et al. Neoadjuvant chemoradiotherapy plus surgery versus surgery alone for oesophageal or junctional cancer (CROSS): long-term results of a randomised controlled trial. *Lancet Oncol*. 2015;**16**:1090–1098.
5. Djarv T, Lagergren J, Blazeby JM, Lagergren P. Long-term health-related quality of life following surgery for oesophageal cancer. *Br J Surg*. 2008;**95**:1121–1126.
6. Noordman BJ, Verdam MGE, Lagarde SM, et al. Effect of neoadjuvant chemoradiotherapy on health-related quality of life in esophageal or junctional cancer: results from the randomized CROSS trial. *J Clin Oncol*. 2018;**36**:268–275.
7. Noordman BJ, Verdam MGE, Lagarde SM, et al. Impact of neoadjuvant chemoradiotherapy on health-related quality of life in long-term survivors of esophageal or junctional cancer: results from the randomized CROSS trial. *Ann Oncol*. 2018;**29**:445–451.
8. Delaney G, Jacob S, Featherstone C, Barton M. The role of radiotherapy in cancer treatment: estimating optimal utilization from a review of evidence-based clinical guidelines. *Cancer*. 2005;**104**:1129–1137.
9. Baskar R, Dai J, Wenlong N, Yeo R, Yeoh KW. Biological response of cancer cells to radiation treatment. *Front Mol Biosci*. 2014;**1**:24.
10. Thames HD Jr, Withers HR, Peters LJ, Fletcher GH. Changes in early and late radiation responses with altered dose fractionation: implications for dose-survival relationships. *Int J Radiat Oncol Biol Phys*. 1982;**8**:219–226.
11. Akakura I, Nakamura Y, Kakegawa T, Nakayama R, Watanabe H, Yamashita H. Surgery of carcinoma of the esophagus with preoperative radiation. *Chest*. 1970;**57**:47–57.
12. Sugimachi K, Matsufuji H, Kai H, et al. Preoperative irradiation for carcinoma of the esophagus. *Surg Gynecol Obstet*. 1986;**162**:174–176.
13. van Andel JG, Dees J, Dijkhuis CM, et al. Carcinoma of the esophagus: results of treatment. *Ann Surg*. 1979;**190**:684–689.
14. Arnott SJ, Duncan W, Kerr GR, et al. Low dose preoperative radiotherapy for carcinoma of the oesophagus: results of a randomized clinical trial. *Radiother Oncol*. 1992;**24**:108–113.
15. Gignoux M, Roussel A, Paillot B, et al. The value of preoperative radiotherapy in esophageal cancer: results of a study by the EORTC. *Recent Results Cancer Res*. 1988;**110**:1–13.
16. Launois B, Delarue D, Campion JP, Kerbaol M. Preoperative radiotherapy for carcinoma of the esophagus. *Surg Gynecol Obstet*. 1981;**153**:690–692.
17. Nygaard K, Hagen S, Hansen HS, et al. Pre-operative radiotherapy prolongs survival in operable esophageal carcinoma: a randomized, multicenter study of pre-operative radiotherapy and chemotherapy. The second Scandinavian trial in esophageal cancer. *World J Surg*. 1992;**16**:1104–1109.
18. Wang M, Gu XZ, Yin WB, Huang GJ, Wang LJ, Zhang DW. Randomized clinical trial on the combination of preoperative irradiation and surgery in the treatment of esophageal

carcinoma: report on 206 patients. *Int J Radiat Oncol Biol Phys.* 1989;**16**:325–327.
19. Arnott SJ, Duncan W, Gignoux M, et al. Preoperative radiotherapy for esophageal carcinoma. *Cochrane Database Syst Rev.* 2005;**4**:CD001799.
20. Fok M, Sham JS, Choy D, Cheng SW, Wong J. Postoperative radiotherapy for carcinoma of the esophagus: a prospective, randomized controlled study. *Surgery.* 1993;**113**:138–147.
21. Teniere P, Hay JM, Fingerhut A, Fagniez PL. Postoperative radiation therapy does not increase survival after curative resection for squamous cell carcinoma of the middle and lower esophagus as shown by a multicenter controlled trial. French University Association for Surgical Research. *Surg Gynecol Obstet.* 1991;**173**:123–130.
22. Xiao ZF, Yang ZY, Liang J, et al. Value of radiotherapy after radical surgery for esophageal carcinoma: a report of 495 patients. *Ann Thorac Surg.* 2003;**75**:331–336.
23. Zieren HU, Muller JM, Jacobi CA, Pichlmaier H, Muller RP, Staar S. Adjuvant postoperative radiation therapy after curative resection of squamous cell carcinoma of the thoracic esophagus: a prospective randomized study. *World J Surg.* 1995;**19**:444–449.
24. Malthaner RA, Wong RK, Rumble RB, Zuraw L; Members of the Gastrointestinal Cancer Disease Site Group of Cancer Care Ontario's Program in Evidence-based Care. Neoadjuvant or adjuvant therapy for resectable esophageal cancer: a systematic review and meta-analysis. *BMC Med.* 2004;**2**:35.
25. Lordick F, Mariette C, Haustermans K, Obermannova R, Arnold D, Committee EG. Oesophageal cancer: ESMO Clinical Practice Guidelines for diagnosis, treatment and follow-up. *Ann Oncol.* 2016;**27**(Suppl 5):v50–v57.
26. Ajani JA, D'Amico TA, Bentrem DJ, et al. Esophageal and Esophagogastric Junction Cancers, Version 2.2019, NCCN Clinical Practice Guidelines in Oncology. *J Natl Compr Canc Netw.* 2019;**17**:855–883.
27. Sjoquist KM, Burmeister BH, Smithers BM, et al. Survival after neoadjuvant chemotherapy or chemoradiotherapy for resectable oesophageal carcinoma: an updated meta-analysis. *Lancet Oncol.* 2011;**12**:681–692.
28. Dasari S, Tchounwou PB. Cisplatin in cancer therapy: molecular mechanisms of action. *Eur J Pharmacol.* 2014;**740**:364–378.
29. Jimenez P, Pathak A, Phan AT. The role of taxanes in the management of gastroesphageal cancer. *J Gastrointest Oncol.* 2011;**2**:240–249.
30. Longley DB, Harkin DP, Johnston PG. 5-fluorouracil: mechanisms of action and clinical strategies. *Nat Rev Cancer.* 2003;**3**:330–338.
31. Sagi JC, Kutszegi N, Kelemen A, et al. Pharmacogenetics of anthracyclines. *Pharmacogenomics.* 2016;**17**:1075–1087.
32. Chen J, Stubbe J. Bleomycins: towards better therapeutics. *Nat Rev Cancer.* 2005;**5**:102–112.
33. Hainsworth JD, Greco FA. Etoposide: twenty years later. *Ann Oncol.* 1995;**6**:325–341.
34. Moudi M, Go R, Yien CY, Nazre M. Vinca alkaloids. *Int J Prev Med.* 2013;**4**:1231–1235.
35. Ancona E, Ruol A, Santi S, et al. Only pathologic complete response to neoadjuvant chemotherapy improves significantly the long term survival of patients with resectable esophageal squamous cell carcinoma: final report of a randomized, controlled trial of preoperative chemotherapy versus surgery Alone. *Cancer.* 2001;**91**:2165–2174.
36. Law S, Fok M, Chow S, Chu K-M, Wong J. Preoperative chemotherapy versus surgical therapy alone for squamous cell carcinoma of the esophagus: a prospective randomized trial. *J Thorac Cardiovasc Surg.* 1997;**114**:210–217.
37. Maipang T, Vasinanukorn P, Petpichetchian C, et al. Induction chemotherapy in the treatment of patients with carcinoma of the esophagus. *J Surg Oncol.* 1994;**56**:191–197.
38. Roth JA, Pass HI, Flanagan MM, Graeber GM, Rosenberg JC, Steinberg S. Randomized clinical trial of preoperative and postoperative adjuvant chemotherapy with cisplatin, vindesine, and bleomycin for carcinoma of the esophagus. *J Thorac Cardiovasc Surg.* 1988;**96**:242–248.
39. Schlag PM. Randomized trial of preoperative chemotherapy for squamous cell cancer of the esophagus. *Arch Surg.* 1992;**127**:1446–1450.
40. Allum WH, Stenning SP, Bancewicz J, Clark PI, Langley RE. Long-term results of a randomized trial of surgery with or without preoperative chemotherapy in esophageal cancer. *J Clin Oncol.* 2009;**27**:5062–5067.
41. Medical Research Council Oesophageal Cancer Working Group. Surgical resection with or without preoperative chemotherapy in oesophageal cancer: a randomised controlled trial. *Lancet.* 2002;**359**:1727–1733.
42. Kelsen DP, Ginsberg R, Pajak TF, et al. Chemotherapy followed by surgery compared with surgery alone for localized esophageal cancer. *N Engl J Med.* 1998;**339**:1979–1984.
43. Kelsen DP, Winter KA, Gunderson LL, et al. Long-term results of RTOG trial 8911 (USA intergroup 113): a random assignment trial comparison of chemotherapy followed by surgery compared with surgery alone for esophageal cancer. *J Clin Oncol.* 2007;**25**:3719–3725.
44. Boonstra JJ, Kok TC, Wijnhoven BPL, et al. Chemotherapy followed by surgery versus surgery alone in patients with resectable oesophageal squamous cell carcinoma: long-term results of a randomized controlled trial. *BMC Cancer.* 2011;**11**:181.
45. Alderson D, Cunningham D, Nankivell M, et al. Neoadjuvant cisplatin and fluorouracil versus epirubicin, cisplatin, and capecitabine followed by resection in patients with oesophageal adenocarcinoma (UK MRC OE05): an open-label, randomised phase 3 trial. *Lancet Oncol.* 2017;**18**:1249–1260.
46. Yamasaki M, Yasuda T, Yano M, et al. Multicenter randomized phase II study of cisplatin and fluorouracil plus docetaxel (DCF) compared with cisplatin and fluorouracil plus Adriamycin (ACF) as preoperative chemotherapy for resectable esophageal squamous cell carcinoma (OGSG1003). *Ann Oncol.* 2017;**28**:116–120.
47. Shiraishi O, Yamasaki M, Makino T, et al. Feasibility of preoperative chemotherapy with docetaxel, cisplatin, and 5-fluorouracil versus adriamycin, cisplatin, and 5-fluorouracil for resectable advanced esophageal cancer. *Oncology.* 2017;**92**:101–108.
48. Wang T, Yu J, Liu M, et al. The benefit of taxane-based therapies over fluoropyrimidine plus platinum (FP) in the treatment of esophageal cancer: a meta-analysis of clinical studies. *Drug Des Devel Ther.* 2019;**13**:539–553.
49. Cunningham D, Allum WH, Stenning SP, et al. Perioperative chemotherapy versus surgery alone for resectable gastroesophageal cancer. *N Engl J Med.* 2006;**355**:11–20.
50. Ychou M, Boige V, Pignon JP, et al. Perioperative chemotherapy compared with surgery alone for resectable gastroesophageal adenocarcinoma: an FNCLCC and FFCD multicenter phase III trial. *J Clin Oncol.* 2011;**29**:1715–1721.
51. Al-Batran SE, Homann N, Pauligk C, et al. Perioperative chemotherapy with fluorouracil plus leucovorin, oxaliplatin,

and docetaxel versus fluorouracil or capecitabine plus cisplatin and epirubicin for locally advanced, resectable gastric or gastro-oesophageal junction adenocarcinoma (FLOT4): a randomised, phase 2/3 trial. *Lancet.* 2019;**393**:1948–1957.

52. Al-Batran SE, Hofheinz RD, Pauligk C, et al. Histopathological regression after neoadjuvant docetaxel, oxaliplatin, fluorouracil, and leucovorin versus epirubicin, cisplatin, and fluorouracil or capecitabine in patients with resectable gastric or gastro-oesophageal junction adenocarcinoma (FLOT4-AIO): results from the phase 2 part of a multicentre, open-label, randomised phase 2/3 trial. *Lancet Oncol.* 2016;**17**:1697–1708.

53. Ando N, Iizuka T, Kakegawa T, et al. A randomized trial of surgery with and without chemotherapy for localized squamous carcinoma of the thoracic esophagus: the Japan Clinical Oncology Group Study. *J Thorac Cardiovasc Surg.* 1997;**114**:205–209.

54. Ando N, Iizuka T, Ide H, et al. Surgery plus chemotherapy compared with surgery alone for localized squamous cell carcinoma of the thoracic esophagus: a Japan Clinical Oncology Group Study—JCOG9204. *J Clin Oncol.* 2003;**21**:4592–4596.

55. Ando N, Kato H, Igaki H, et al. A randomized trial comparing postoperative adjuvant chemotherapy with cisplatin and 5-fluorouracil versus preoperative chemotherapy for localized advanced squamous cell carcinoma of the thoracic esophagus (JCOG9907). *Ann Surg Oncol.* 2012;**19**:68–74.

56. Gebski V, Burmeister B, Smithers BM, Foo K, Zalcberg J, Simes J. Survival benefits from neoadjuvant chemoradiotherapy or chemotherapy in oesophageal carcinoma: a meta-analysis. *Lancet Oncol.* 2007;**8**:226–234.

57. Seiwert TY, Salama JK, Vokes EE. The concurrent chemoradiation paradigm—general principles. *Nat Clin Pract Oncol.* 2007;**4**:86.

58. Apinop C, Puttisak P, Preecha N. A prospective study of combined therapy in esophageal cancer. *Hepatogastroenterol.* 1994;**41**:391–393.

59. Le Prise E, Etienne PL, Meunier B, et al. A randomized study of chemotherapy, radiation therapy, and surgery versus surgery for localized squamous cell carcinoma of the esophagus. *Cancer.* 1994;**73**:1779–1784.

60. Bosset JF, Gignoux M, Triboulet JP, et al. Chemoradiotherapy followed by surgery compared with surgery alone in squamous-cell cancer of the esophagus. *N Engl J Med.* 1997;**337**:161–167.

61. Urba SG, Orringer MB, Turrisi A, Iannettoni M, Forastiere A, Strawderman M. Randomized trial of preoperative chemoradiation versus surgery alone in patients with locoregional esophageal carcinoma. *J Clin Oncol.* 2001;**19**:305–313.

62. Walsh TN, Noonan N, Hollywood D, Kelly A, Keeling N, Hennessy TP. A comparison of multimodal therapy and surgery for esophageal adenocarcinoma. *N Engl J Med.* 1996;**335**:462–467.

63. Burmeister B, Smithers M, Gebski V, et al. Surgery alone versus chemoradiotherapy followed by surgery for resectable cancer of the oesophagus: a randomised controlled phase III trial. *Lancet Oncol.* 2005;**6**:659–668.

64. Lv J, Cao XF, Zhu B, Ji L, Tao L, Wang DD. Long-term efficacy of perioperative chemoradiotherapy on esophageal squamous cell carcinoma. *World J Gastroenterol.* 2010;**16**:1649–1654.

65. Tepper J, Krasna MJ, Niedzwiecki D, et al. Phase III trial of trimodality therapy with cisplatin, fluorouracil, radiotherapy, and surgery compared with surgery alone for esophageal cancer: CALGB 9781. *J Clin Oncol.* 2008;**26**:1086–1092.

66. Lee JL, Park SI, Kim SB, et al. A single institutional phase III trial of preoperative chemotherapy with hyperfractionation radiotherapy plus surgery versus surgery alone for resectable esophageal squamous cell carcinoma. *Ann Oncol.* 2004;**15**:947–954.

67. Mariette C, Dahan L, Mornex F, et al. Surgery alone versus chemoradiotherapy followed by surgery for stage I and II esophageal cancer: final analysis of randomized controlled phase III trial FFCD 9901. *J Clin Oncol.* 2014;**32**:2416–2422.

68. van Hagen P, Hulshof MC, van Lanschot JJ, et al. Preoperative chemoradiotherapy for esophageal or junctional cancer. *N Engl J Med.* 2012;**366**:2074–2084.

69. Yang H, Liu H, Chen Y, et al. Neoadjuvant chemoradiotherapy followed by surgery versus surgery alone for locally advanced squamous cell carcinoma of the esophagus (NEOCRTEC5010): a phase III multicenter, randomized, open-label clinical trial. *J Clin Oncol.* 2018;**36**:2796–2803.

70. Reynolds JV, Preston SR, O'Neill B, et al. ICORG 10-14: NEOadjuvant trial in Adenocarcinoma of the oEsophagus and oesophagoGastric junction International Study (Neo-AEGIS). *BMC Cancer.* 2017;**17**:401.

71. Hoeppner J, Lordick F, Brunner T, et al. ESOPEC: prospective randomized controlled multicenter phase III trial comparing perioperative chemotherapy (FLOT protocol) to neoadjuvant chemoradiation (CROSS protocol) in patients with adenocarcinoma of the esophagus (NCT02509286). *BMC Cancer.* 2016;**16**:503.

72. Nakamura K, Kato K, Igaki H, et al. Three-arm phase III trial comparing cisplatin plus 5-FU (CF) versus docetaxel, cisplatin plus 5-FU (DCF) versus radiotherapy with CF (CF-RT) as preoperative therapy for locally advanced esophageal cancer (JCOG1109, NExT study). *Jpn J Clin Oncol.* 2013;**43**:752–755.

73. Earlam R, Cunha-Melo JR. Oesophageal squamous cell carcinoma: II. A critical view of radiotherapy. *Br J Surg.* 1980;**67**:457–461.

74. Herskovic A, Martz K, al-Sarraf M, et al. Combined chemotherapy and radiotherapy compared with radiotherapy alone in patients with cancer of the esophagus. *N Engl J Med.* 1992;**326**:1593–1598.

75. Cooper JS, Guo MD, Herskovic A, et al. Chemoradiotherapy of locally advanced esophageal cancer: long-term follow-up of a prospective randomized trial (RTOG 85-01). Radiation Therapy Oncology Group. *JAMA.* 1999;**281**:1623–1627.

76. Wong R, Malthaner R. Combined chemotherapy and radiotherapy (without surgery) compared with radiotherapy alone in localized carcinoma of the esophagus. *Cochrane Database Syst Rev.* 2006;**1**:CD002092.

77. Algan O, Coia LR, Keller SM, et al. Management of adenocarcinoma of the esophagus with chemoradiation alone or chemoradiation followed by esophagectomy: results of sequential nonrandomized phase II studies. *Int J Radiat Oncol Biol Phys.* 1995;**32**:753–761.

78. Stahl M, Stuschke M, Lehmann N, et al. Chemoradiation with and without surgery in patients with locally advanced squamous cell carcinoma of the esophagus. *J Clin Oncol.* 2005;**23**:2310–2317.

79. Bedenne L, Michel P, Bouche O, et al. Chemoradiation followed by surgery compared with chemoradiation alone in squamous cancer of the esophagus: FFCD 9102. *J Clin Oncol.* 2007;**25**:1160–1168.

80. Vincent J, Mariette C, Pezet D, et al. Early surgery for failure after chemoradiation in operable thoracic oesophageal cancer. Analysis of the non-randomised patients in FFCD 9102 phase III trial: chemoradiation followed by surgery versus chemoradiation alone. *Eur J Cancer*. 2015;**51**:1683–1693.
81. Minsky BD, Pajak TF, Ginsberg RJ, et al. INT 0123 (Radiation Therapy Oncology Group 94-05) phase III trial of combined-modality therapy for esophageal cancer: high-dose versus standard-dose radiation therapy. *J Clin Oncol*. 2002;**20**:1167–1174.
82. Hulshof M, Geijsen ED, Rozema T, et al. Randomized study on dose escalation in definitive chemoradiation for patients with locally advanced esophageal cancer (ARTDECO study). *J Clin Oncol*. 2021;**39**:2816–2824.
83. Swisher SG, Winter KA, Komaki RU, et al. A Phase II study of a paclitaxel-based chemoradiation regimen with selective surgical salvage for resectable locoregionally advanced esophageal cancer: initial reporting of RTOG 0246. *Int J Radiat Oncol Biol Phys*. 2012;**82**:1967–1972.
84. Miyata H, Yamasaki M, Takiguchi S, et al. Salvage esophagectomy after definitive chemoradiotherapy for thoracic esophageal cancer. *J Surg Oncol*. 2009;**100**:442–446.
85. Tachimori Y, Kanamori N, Uemura N, Hokamura N, Igaki H, Kato H. Salvage esophagectomy after high-dose chemoradiotherapy for esophageal squamous cell carcinoma. *J Thorac Cardiovasc Surg*. 2009;**137**:49–54.
86. Kroschinsky F, Stolzel F, von Bonin S, et al. New drugs, new toxicities: severe side effects of modern targeted and immunotherapy of cancer and their management. *Crit Care*. 2017;**21**:89.
87. Anvari K, Sima HR, Seilanian Toussi M, et al. EGFR expression in patients with esophageal squamous cell carcinoma and its association with pathologic response to preoperative chemoradiotherapy: a study in Northeastern Iran. *Arch Iran Med*. 2017;**20**:240–245.
88. Ekman S, Bergqvist M, Heldin CH, Lennartsson J. Activation of growth factor receptors in esophageal cancer—implications for therapy. *Oncologist*. 2007;**12**:1165–1177.
89. Homsi J, Daud AI. Spectrum of activity and mechanism of action of VEGF/PDGF inhibitors. *Cancer Control*. 2007;**14**:285–294.
90. Cunningham D, Stenning SP, Smyth EC, et al. Peri-operative chemotherapy with or without bevacizumab in operable oesophagogastric adenocarcinoma (UK Medical Research Council ST03): primary analysis results of a multicentre, open-label, randomised phase 2–3 trial. *Lancet Oncol*. 2017;**18**:357–370.
91. Fuchs CS, Tomasek J, Yong CJ, et al. Ramucirumab monotherapy for previously treated advanced gastric or gastro-oesophageal junction adenocarcinoma (REGARD): an international, randomised, multicentre, placebo-controlled, phase 3 trial. *Lancet*. 2014;**383**:31–39.
92. Wilke H, Muro K, Van Cutsem E, et al. Ramucirumab plus paclitaxel versus placebo plus paclitaxel in patients with previously treated advanced gastric or gastro-oesophageal junction adenocarcinoma (RAINBOW): a double-blind, randomised phase 3 trial. *Lancet Oncol*. 2014;**15**:1224–1235.
93. Vincenzi B, Zoccoli A, Pantano F, Venditti O, Galluzzo S. Cetuximab: from bench to bedside. *Curr Cancer Drug Targets*. 2010;**10**:80–95.
94. Ruhstaller T, Thuss-Patience P, Hayoz S, et al. Neoadjuvant chemotherapy followed by chemoradiation and surgery with and without cetuximab in patients with resectable esophageal cancer: a randomized, open-label, phase III trial (SAKK 75/08). *Ann Oncol*. 2018;**29**:1386–1393.
95. Suntharalingam M, Winter K, Ilson D, et al. Effect of the addition of cetuximab to paclitaxel, cisplatin, and radiation therapy for patients with esophageal cancer: the NRG Oncology RTOG 0436 phase 3 randomized clinical trial. *JAMA Oncol*. 2017;**3**:1520–1528.
96. Kordes S, van Berge Henegouwen MI, Hulshof MC, et al. Preoperative chemoradiation therapy in combination with panitumumab for patients with resectable esophageal cancer: the PACT study. *Int J Radiat Oncol Biol Phys*. 2014;**90**:190–196.
97. Lockhart AC, Reed CE, Decker PA, et al. Phase II study of neoadjuvant therapy with docetaxel, cisplatin, panitumumab, and radiation therapy followed by surgery in patients with locally advanced adenocarcinoma of the distal esophagus (ACOSOG Z4051). *Ann Oncol*. 2014;**25**:1039–1044.
98. Waddell T, Chau I, Cunningham D, et al. Epirubicin, oxaliplatin, and capecitabine with or without panitumumab for patients with previously untreated advanced oesophagogastric cancer (REAL3): a randomised, open-label phase 3 trial. *Lancet Oncol*. 2013;**14**:481–489.
99. Barok M, Joensuu H, Isola J. Trastuzumab emtansine: mechanisms of action and drug resistance. *Breast Cancer Res*. 2014;**16**:209.
100. Slamon DJ, Leyland-Jones B, Shak S, et al. Use of chemotherapy plus a monoclonal antibody against HER2 for metastatic breast cancer that overexpresses HER2. *N Engl J Med*. 2001;**344**:783–792.
101. Bang YJ, Van Cutsem E, Feyereislova A, et al. Trastuzumab in combination with chemotherapy versus chemotherapy alone for treatment of HER2-positive advanced gastric or gastro-oesophageal junction cancer (ToGA): a phase 3, open-label, randomised controlled trial. *Lancet*. 2010;**376**:687–697.
102. Safran HP, Winter K, Ilson DH, et al. Trastuzumab with trimodality treatment for oesophageal adenocarcinoma with HER2 overexpression (NRG Oncology/RTOG 1010): a multicentre, randomised, phase 3 trial. *Lancet Oncol*. 2022;**23**:259–269.
103. Stroes CI, Schokker S, Creemers A, et al. Phase II feasibility and biomarker study of neoadjuvant trastuzumab and pertuzumab with chemoradiotherapy for resectable human epidermal growth factor receptor 2-positive esophageal adenocarcinoma: TRAP study. *J Clin Oncol*. 2020;**38**:462–471.
104. Sharpe AH, Wherry EJ, Ahmed R, Freeman GJ. The function of programmed cell death 1 and its ligands in regulating autoimmunity and infection. *Nat Immunol*. 2007;**8**:239–245.
105. Ohigashi Y, Sho M, Yamada Y, et al. Clinical significance of programmed death-1 ligand-1 and programmed death-1 ligand-2 expression in human esophageal cancer. *Clin Cancer Res*. 2005;**11**:2947–2953.
106. Kato K, Cho BC, Takahashi M, et al. Nivolumab versus chemotherapy in patients with advanced oesophageal squamous cell carcinoma refractory or intolerant to previous chemotherapy (ATTRACTION-3): a multicentre, randomised, open-label, phase 3 trial. *Lancet Oncol*. 2019;**20**:1506–1517.
107. Janjigian YY, Shitara K, Moehler M, et al. First-line nivolumab plus chemotherapy versus chemotherapy alone for advanced gastric, gastro-oesophageal junction, and oesophageal adenocarcinoma (CheckMate 649): a randomised, open-label, phase 3 trial. *Lancet*. 2021;**398**:27–40.
108. Doki Y, Ajani JA, Kato K, et al. Nivolumab combination therapy in advanced esophageal squamous-cell carcinoma. *N Engl J Med*. 2022;**386**:449–462.

109. Shah MA, Adenis A, Enzinger PC, et al. Pembrolizumab versus chemotherapy as second-line therapy for advanced esophageal cancer: phase 3 KEYNOTE-181 study. *J Clin Oncol.* 2019;**37**(Suppl 4):2.
110. Sun JM, Shen L, Shah MA, et al. Pembrolizumab plus chemotherapy versus chemotherapy alone for first-line treatment of advanced oesophageal cancer (KEYNOTE-590): a randomised, placebo-controlled, phase 3 study. *Lancet.* 2021;**398**:759-771. Erratum in: *Lancet.* 2021;**398**:1874.
111. Kelly RJ, Ajani JA, Kuzdzal J, et al. Adjuvant nivolumab in resected esophageal or gastroesophageal junction cancer. *N Engl J Med.* 2021;**384**:1191-1203.
112. Hong MH, Kim HR, Park SY, et al. A phase II trial of preoperative chemoradiotherapy and pembrolizumab for locally advanced esophageal squamous cell carcinoma (ESCC). *J Clin Oncol.* 2019;**37**(15 Suppl):4027.
113. Bray F, Ferlay J, Soerjomataram I, Siegel RL, Torre LA, Jemal A. Global cancer statistics 2018: GLOBOCAN estimates of incidence and mortality worldwide for 36 cancers in 185 countries. *CA Cancer J Clin.* 2018;**68**:394-424.
114. Al-Batran SE, Homann N, Pauligk C, et al. Perioperative chemotherapy with fluorouracil plus leucovorin, oxaliplatin, and docetaxel versus fluorouracil or capecitabine plus cisplatin and epirubicin for locally advanced, resectable gastric or gastro-oesophageal junction adenocarcinoma (FLOT4): a randomised, phase 2/3 trial. *Lancet.* 2019;**393**:1948-1957.
115. Oppedijk V, van der Gaast A, van Lanschot JJ, et al. Patterns of recurrence after surgery alone versus preoperative chemoradiotherapy and surgery in the CROSS trials. *J Clin Oncol.* 2014;**32**:385-391.
116. Ajani JA, Xiao L, Roth JA, et al. A phase II randomized trial of induction chemotherapy versus no induction chemotherapy followed by preoperative chemoradiation in patients with esophageal cancer. *Ann Oncol.* 2013;**24**:2844-2849.
117. Shimodaira Y, Slack RS, Harada K, et al. Influence of induction chemotherapy in trimodality therapy-eligible oesophageal cancer patients: secondary analysis of a randomised trial. *Br J Cancer.* 2018;**118**:331-337.
118. Ford HE, Marshall A, Bridgewater JA, et al. Docetaxel versus active symptom control for refractory oesophagogastric adenocarcinoma (COUGAR-02): an open-label, phase 3 randomised controlled trial. *Lancet Oncol.* 2014;**15**:78-86.
119. Van Cutsem E, Moiseyenko VM, Tjulandin S, et al. Phase III study of docetaxel and cisplatin plus fluorouracil compared with cisplatin and fluorouracil as first-line therapy for advanced gastric cancer: a report of the V325 Study Group. *J Clin Oncol.* 2006;**24**:4991-4997.
120. van der Zijden CJ, Eyck BM, van der Gaast A, et al. ChemoTherapy aNd chemoradiotherapy for adenocarcinoma of the OESophagus and esophagogastric junction with oligometastases: Protocol of the TNT-OES-1 trial. *Contemp Clin Trials Commun.* 2022;**28**:100934.
121. Ghi MG, Paccagnella A, Ferrari D, et al. Induction TPF followed by concomitant treatment versus concomitant treatment alone in locally advanced head and neck cancer. A phase II–III trial. *Ann Oncol.* 2017;**28**:2206-2212.
122. Gasic GJ, Gasic TB, Murphy S. Anti-metastatic effect of aspirin. *Lancet.* 1972;**2**:932-933.
123. Gasic GJ, Gasic TB, Stewart CC. Antimetastatic effects associated with platelet reduction. *Proc Natl Acad Sci U S A.* 1968;**61**:46-52.
124. Corley DA, Kerlikowske K, Verma R, Buffler P. Protective association of aspirin/NSAIDs and esophageal cancer: a systematic review and meta-analysis. *Gastroenterol.* 2003;**124**:47-56.
125. Rothwell PM, Fowkes FG, Belch JF, Ogawa H, Warlow CP, Meade TW. Effect of daily aspirin on long-term risk of death due to cancer: analysis of individual patient data from randomised trials. *Lancet.* 2011;**377**:31-41.
126. Liu JF, Jamieson GG, Wu TC, Zhu GJ, Drew PA. A preliminary study on the postoperative survival of patients given aspirin after resection for squamous cell carcinoma of the esophagus or adenocarcinoma of the cardia. *Ann Surg Oncol.* 2009;**16**:1397-1402.
127. Coyle C, Cafferty FH, Rowley S, et al. ADD-ASPIRIN: a phase III, double-blind, placebo controlled, randomised trial assessing the effects of aspirin on disease recurrence and survival after primary therapy in common non-metastatic solid tumours. *Contemp Clin Trials.* 2016;**51**:56-64.
128. Westerterp M, van Westreenen HL, Reitsma JB, et al. Esophageal cancer: CT, endoscopic US, and FDG PET for assessment of response to neoadjuvant therapy—systematic review. *Radiology.* 2005;**236**:841-851.
129. Eyck BM, Onstenk BD, Noordman BJ, et al. Accuracy of detecting residual disease after neoadjuvant chemoradiotherapy for esophageal cancer: a systematic review and meta-analysis. *Ann Surg.* 2020;**271**:245-256.
130. Vollenbrock SE, Voncken FEM, Bartels LW, Beets-Tan RGH, Bartels-Rutten A. Diffusion-weighted MRI with ADC mapping for response prediction and assessment of oesophageal cancer: a systematic review. *Radiother Oncol.* 2020;**142**:17-26.
131. Vollenbrock SE, Voncken FEM, van Dieren JM, et al. Diagnostic performance of MRI for assessment of response to neoadjuvant chemoradiotherapy in oesophageal cancer. *Br J Surg.* 2019;**106**:596-605.
132. Guillem P, Fabre S, Mariette C, Triboulet JP. Surgery after induction chemoradiotherapy for oesophageal cancer. *Eur J Surg Oncol.* 2003;**29**:158-165.
133. Noordman BJ, Spaander MCW, Valkema R, et al. Detection of residual disease after neoadjuvant chemoradiotherapy for oesophageal cancer (preSANO): a prospective multicentre, diagnostic cohort study. *Lancet Oncol.* 2018;**19**:965-974.
134. van der Wilk BJ, Eyck BM, Hofstetter WL, et al. Chemoradiotherapy followed by active surveillance versus standard esophagectomy for esophageal cancer: a systematic review and individual patient data meta-analysis. *Ann Surg.* 2022;**275**:467-476.
135. ClinicalTrials.gov. Comparison of systematic surgery versus surveillance and rescue surgery in operable oesophageal cancer with a complete clinical response to radiochemotherapy (Esostrate). Identifier NCT02551458. National Library of Medicine; 2015. https://ClinicalTrials.gov/show/NCT02551458
136. Noordman BJ, Wijnhoven BPL, Lagarde SM, et al. Neoadjuvant chemoradiotherapy plus surgery versus active surveillance for oesophageal cancer: a stepped-wedge cluster randomised trial. *BMC Cancer.* 2018;**18**:142.
137. Schuhmacher C, Gretschel S, Lordick F, et al. Neoadjuvant chemotherapy compared with surgery alone for locally advanced cancer of the stomach and cardia: European Organisation for Research and Treatment of Cancer randomized trial 40954. *J Clin Oncol.* 2010;**28**:5210-5218.
138. Zhao Y, Dai Z, Min W, et al. Perioperative versus preoperative chemotherapy with surgery in patients with resectable squamous cell carcinoma of esophagus: a phase III randomized trial. *J Thorac Oncol.* 2015;**10**:1349-1356.

12

Oesophageal cancer
Endoscopic treatment

Thomas Rösch

Introduction

The incidence of oesophageal cancer, especially in relation to reflux disease and Barrett's oesophagus (BO), is rising in the Western world, while squamous cell carcinoma has a high incidence in certain other areas.[1–3] With the widespread use of gastrointestinal endoscopy for a variety of symptoms and conditions, and the increasing awareness and training level of endoscopists, the detection rate of early lesions is also increasing.[4,5] Apart from a few high-risk areas with formal screening programmes for squamous cell carcinoma, there are no established screening programmes for BO, but most countries have some recommendations for surveillance of known BO patients.[6–10]

Techniques of endoresection: endoscopic mucosal resection versus endoscopic submucosal dissection

The preparatory steps for patients in whom endoscopic resection is considered, are as follows (Figures 12.1–12.5):

1. Endoscopy of the lesion, mostly repeated in the centre which performs the resection, unless endoscopic images of sufficient quality are provided.
2. Endoscopic ultrasound (EUS) of the lesion and adjacent lymph nodes (optional)[11–13]; in flat lesions, EUS is often negative (Figure 12.6).
3. Computed tomography of the thorax and abdomen in case of questionable lesions (optional, see below), mainly useful to exclude larger lymph nodes and distant metastases, both of which are very rare in low-risk cancers.
4. Also, most importantly, the general condition of the patient should be taken into account; in contrast to gastrectomy, oesophagectomy is a procedure with a higher mortality and morbidity.

Only lesions with certain histological criteria should be considered for endoscopic resection.[8,14] The problem here is, however, that these criteria are derived from histopathological analyses of resection specimens and can only be accurately defined after resection. They include mucosal cancers, T1a (m), grading G1/2, absence of lymphatic (L0) and venous (V0) infiltration, as well as some others (tumour budding etc.). Whether slight submucosal infiltration (500 µm) should be considered to be a low-risk criterion in BO early neoplasia, is currently debated. This cut-off of defining low-risk lesions is usually a very low risk of lymph node metastases which has to be weighed against the mortality of surgery. Definitions and numbers can only be found in the Japanese literature from early gastric cancer with an assumed 0 risk for lymph node metastases[15–18] and a very low risk for gastrectomy. They seemed to have just been transferred to the oesophagus, where surgery has a different risk profile. So, we clearly need more data from Western countries to give evidence-based advice to our patients who are mostly elderly and often have an increased surgical risk.

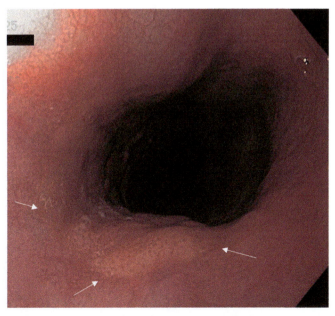

Figure 12.1 Early oesophageal squamous cell cancer, hardly visible (between arrows).

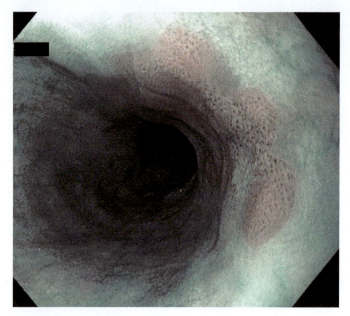

Figure 12.2 A subtle squamous cell lesion which can be better delineated with enhanced imaging (here narrow band imaging, Olympus) with pathological vessels.

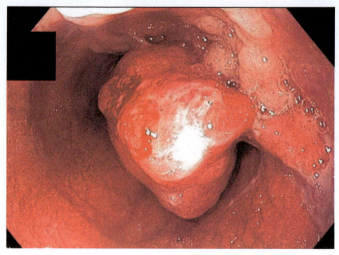

Figure 12.4 Bulky neoplastic lesion in BO, surprisingly T1a after ESD; this underlines the option of performing endoresection for primarily diagnostic purposes which can turn into a curative treatment as in this case.

The assessment or prediction of these risk criteria by means of endoscopy or EUS has been claimed in the Japanese literature, but the accuracy is still debated, and results could often not be reproduced in the West. Despite development of many criteria and scoring systems, accuracy in the real world seems to be low, even in Japan, in a study with a different focus in early oesophageal cancer. Thus, a practical approach would be that—given sufficient expertise and a very low complication rate—endoscopic resection is attempted or performed, and after results of histopathology (of course, showing complete R0 resection), further management is discussed, which could mean subsequent surgery. We perform only endoscopy in presumed early low-risk lesions, and add EUS or computed tomography in tumours of questionable infiltration depth or confirmed risk criteria after endoscopic resection.

Endoscopic resection[19,20] is then done with the following precautions and steps:

1. At least in elderly or frail patients, general anaesthesia should be considered for lengthy oesophageal procedures.
2. Endoscopy should define the lesion and its extent and marking is then done around the lesion; the markings should not be present after resection, irrespective of the technique (piecemeal or en bloc).
3. The classic technique described in detail in Chapter 20 has been endoscopic mucosal resection (EMR) (Figures 12.7 and 12.8),

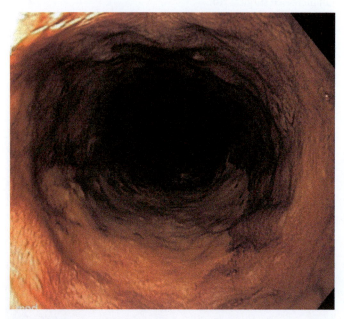

Figure 12.3 A more extensive squamous cell lesion which can be better delineated with enhanced imaging using direct staining with Lugol (iodine) solution which leaves the lesion unstained (yellow).

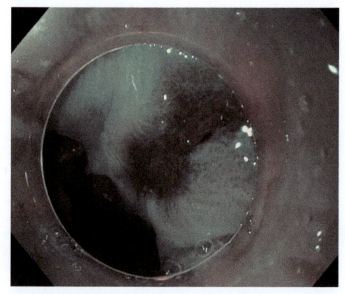

Figure 12.5 More discrete lesion above a BO, mimicking inflammation; histology showed mucosal cancer with partially subepithelial growth.

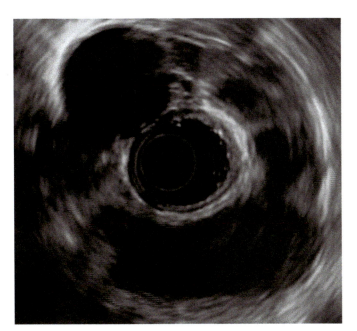

Figure 12.6 Normal oesophageal wall on EUS in a patient with flat mucosal cancer in the oesophagus.

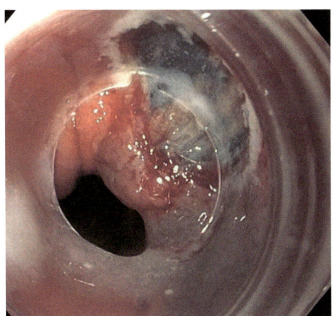

Figure 12.8 A similarly large area was resected in this patient also by piecemeal EMR; this image shows the first resection area, which is continued distally and laterally.

which is an injection, suck, and cut technique, and exists in several variations, such as the classic Inoue cap technique, or the banding and resection version. Both can be equally efficacious as shown in two randomized trials.[21–25] With multiple resections ('piecemeal'), also large areas and even a circumferential resection can be done. The technique is relatively simple and does not seem to have to have a long learning curve; the complication rate is low.

4. More recently, en bloc resection by means of endoscopic submucosal dissection (ESD) has been introduced (Figures 12.9–12.11), which uses several dedicated knives and, after marking and submucosal injection, consists of circumcision and the dissection from the underlying muscularis/remaining submucosa.[26] While the en bloc concept is of course more attractive especially for cancers (perhaps less so for precursors such as high-grade dysplasia), the technique is more complex and more difficult to teach and learn, and, perhaps partially due to the longer learning curve, seems to have a much higher complication rate, at least initially. Most of these complications seem to be manageable by endoscopy during or after the procedure.

5. Full-thickness resection has started also to slowly develop into endoscopic neoplasia management, but, unless a clumsy combination of transmural resection and then closure is used, one-step full-thickness devices are limited by lesion size. Results in selected case series are satisfactory, but not brilliant, and have mostly been gained in the colorectum.[27–29]

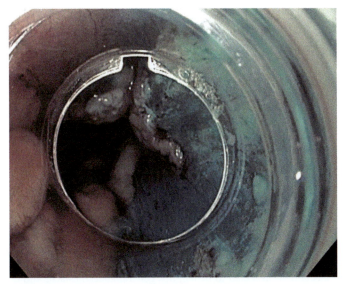

Figure 12.7 Large area piecemeal EMR of Barrett cancer; the bluish resection area shows fine remnants of remaining submucosa.

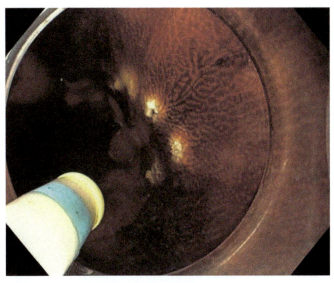

Figure 12.9 ESD using a short knife (DualKnife), starting with marking of the squamous cell lesion after staining with Lugol.

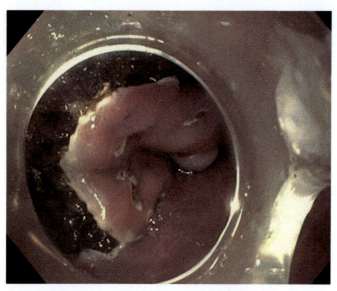

Figure 12.10 Start of ESD at the proximal margin at some distance to the prior markings.

Patients are admitted for one to a few days in hospital in most countries to be able to manage postprocedural complications effectively. In addition, this issue is, however, also dominated by the healthcare system and not only by medical necessities.

Barrett's oesophagus: current multimodal endoscopic eradication concepts

In patients with BO, the current endoscopic treatment concept is different from squamous cell carcinoma since together with removal of (visible) neoplastic lesions, the entire BO is eradicated, initially by means of stepwise resection, nowadays by a combination of resection of visible lesions and ablation of the remaining

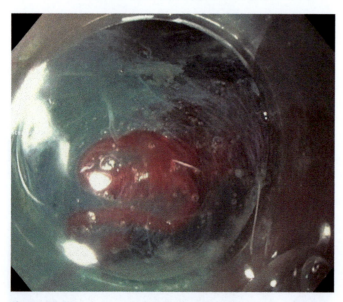

Figure 12.11 Submucosal space during ESD with blue-stained saline and some submucosal vessels to be coagulated.

BO, mainly due to a lower complication rate.[30-32] Although only supported by evidence from one small randomized trial,[33] this concept is believed to reduce the rate of recurrences and, even more importantly, metachronous lesions, which can amount to 30% or more over 3–5 years.[34,35] Thus, the contribution of endoresection is more to prevent neoplasia recurrence, and that of ablation to prevent BO recurrence (which then also predisposes to neoplasia) (Figure 12.12). Apart from the two resection techniques under discussion (see also 'Complications and their prevention'), ablation is mostly done by radiofrequency ablation in a mean of 3–3.5 sessions, which is the technique where we have the most scientific evidence.[7,36,37] Other thermal techniques such as argon beam coagulation,[38-40] or, more recently, cryotherapy,[41,42] may also find their way into the multimodality therapy of neoplastic BO. However, recurrence rates over time, even if mostly minor, histologically non-neoplastic BO, and often only evident on routine biopsy, can be substantial and amount to 30% over several years.[43-46]

Notably, the concept of eradication of non-neoplastic BO to prevent recurrences, by any of the ablation techniques, is not recommended, primarily due to a low risk of malignant degeneration (0.1–0.2% per patient year), moderate long-term success rates of ablation, and some (even if very low) risk of complications; in addition, after prophylactic coagulation, follow-up would still be necessary.

Pathology diagnosis

Pathological analysis of the resected specimen[16] (Figure 12.13) after endoscopic resection requires proper specimen handling (pinning on cork) and determines whether curative resection was achieved,[47,48] which includes the following parameters:

1. Complete (R0) resection; in case of en bloc resection by ESD, this relates to deep and lateral parameters, while in case of piecemeal resection by EMR, there is consensus that R0 only refers to basal margins while lateral margins can be affected, assuming that the entire area defined by the macroscopic aspect has been resected endoscopically. In these cases, one or two subsequent endoscopies with negative biopsies some weeks or months after the procedure can be taken as surrogate parameter for oncological therapeutic success.
2. Grading G1/2, absence of vascular (V0) and lymphatic involvement (L0).
3. Other parameters (absence of tumour budding) are less well established.

If all criteria are fulfilled, the resection is called curative and the patient can enter follow-up (or in case of BO, additional ablative treatment). This means that the risk of lymph node metastases is very low (for discussion, see above) and the long-term outcome favourable.

Complications and their prevention

Depending on patient risk factors and estimated procedure duration, for therapeutic endoscopic interventions in the oesophagus, especially if predicted to be lengthy, general anaesthesia should be considered. Although there are no data from randomized trials, this

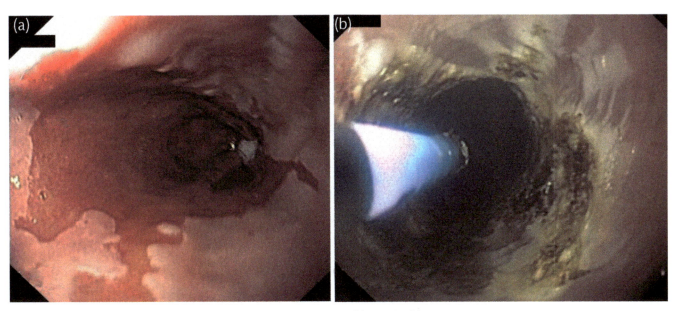

Figure 12.12 Ablation of remaining BO by argon plasma coagulation before (a) and after (b).

approach is likely to reduce sedation-associated complications, and in case of endoscopic complications such as perforation or severe bleeding, endoscopic complication management appears to be safer and easier.

Otherwise, the main complications (adverse events) of endoresection in the oesophagus are bleeding and perforation.[21,45,49,50] Bleeding during the procedure is usually not classified as a complication since in almost 100% of cases it can be managed endoscopically (it would be called a complication if transfusion or conversion to surgery is required). Only post-procedural bleeding requiring an intervention such as re-endoscopy, transfusion, or intensive care unit admission (or finally prolongation of hospital stay, although this varies between centres) should be called a complication. After oesophageal resections, this risk is usually well below 5% and probably higher with more extensive resections. Preventive measures such as prophylactic coagulation, clipping, or administration of haemostatic powders or gels, are partially established for other organs, like the colon, but there is no good evidence of their usefulness in the oesophagus.

The perforation rate of endoscopic resection is usually less than 3% (or in most centres <1%) and with the expansion of the endoscopic armamentarium of clipping or suturing, many of these can nowadays also be managed endoscopically if detected during the procedure (Figure 12.14). Air leakage into the mediastinum or abdomen usually quickly resolves if carbon dioxide is used instead of room air, which is strongly recommended; in some cases, abdominal air decompression by transabdominal puncture may be necessary. If the leak can be closed successfully, usually short-term antibiotics are administered, and the patient has to be admitted or stay in hospital a

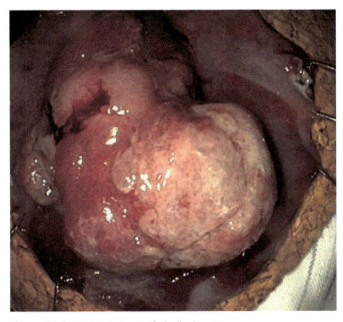

Figure 12.13 ESD specimen of a bulky Barrett cancer.

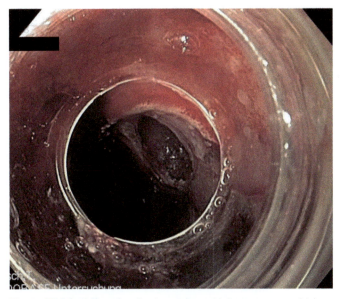

Figure 12.14 EMR perforation in a patient with Barrett cancer which could be closed conservatively.

bit longer, but no further measures are required. Clinical and laboratory monitoring is required.

After extensive resections in the oesophagus, a rise in leucocyte counts (often up to 15,000/uL) and C-reactive protein—with some delay (can be up to 100 mg/dL) can be observed without additional measures necessary, if the patient's clinical condition is stable. Severe pain is rare, but can occur in a few patients even without perforation (?burn syndrome), but in general, a prophylactic high-dose proton pump inhibitor for a few days is recommended for prevention. If the patient deteriorates after the resection, on the next day, with rising laboratory values, pain and/or fever, interdisciplinary consultation is recommended, as well as further diagnostic tests such as repeat endoscopy and/or computed tomography and/or an X-ray swallow, both with water-soluble contrast. Whether later closure by endoscopy is an option is determined by whether extraluminal collections are present and if so, whether and how these can be drained. Stenting (preferentially with a covered stent adapted to the luminal diameter and stent fixation) and/or intraluminal or defect sponge therapy has been reported to be successful, but close clinical monitoring by an interdisciplinary team is required.

The most frequent complication occurring in the weeks after endoresection is the development of an oesophageal stricture. Depending on the extent of resection, the stricture rate is greatly variable, ranging from 10% to 80%, and is certainly most frequent with circumferential resection in one session (almost 100%), with stepwise full resection having a stricture rate between 30% and 70%. Notably, strictures with less extensive or also stepwise full resection are much easier to treat and mostly require three to five dilatation sessions. Various measures for stricture prevention have been suggested such as oral or topical administration of steroids or other substances or application of cell sheaths, some with spectacular results in small series reported by the inventor.

Complications after ablation therapy are principally similar in nature, but the rate is even lower.[51] They mostly consist of strictures, with rates mostly well below 10%, also due to various recent modifications of the radiofrequency ablation technique.

Clinical results

Endoscopic resection therapy compares favourably with surgery in early oesophageal cancer with regard to oncological prognosis (similar) but mainly complication rate (mortality and morbidity are greatly reduced).[52] A comparative Cochrane analysis of endotherapy versus surgery interestingly concluded that none of the 13 comparative studies selected was randomized and would have fulfilled selection criteria,[53] so high-class evidence such as from a randomized trial is not available. The individual retrospective studies are listed in this review and all have limited patient numbers between 90 and 200 overall.[53] They all show very high survival rates (>90%) for both groups at 3–5 years, with substantially higher morbidity and higher mortality for surgery versus endoscopy.[54]

Among the various endotherapies, the decision whether to perform EMR or ESD in early oesophageal cancer, has been ongoing almost since the introduction of ESD. Despite a large number of cases being done in the far East, and increasingly in the West, a randomized trial has not been published, with one exception, a small multicentre study (n = 40) from Germany in Barrett's neoplasia, showing (as expected) higher R0 rates with ESD with similar complication rates[55]; however, even if recurrence rates were not different (one recurrence in the ESD group), this study was not powered for outcome. So, evidence rests on so-called meta-analyses of retrospective studies and case series.[24,56-58] They mostly state higher R0 and lower recurrence rates for ESD, which may be due to the fact that they all come from the far East, where squamous cell cancer is much more frequent than Barrett's neoplasia.

The situation in BO is different due to the multifocal nature of the disease and the current concept of resection and ablation to eradicate the entire Barrett's area (see above). Thus, lateral R0 resection rates with ESD in Barrett's neoplasia are often very high for cancer, but much less so for high-grade dysplasia; furthermore, results for EMR are also very good in the literature.[59] The addition of ablation is commonly believed to greatly reduce recurrence rates,[8] but this mostly rests on indirect evidence, since only one smaller randomized study exists.[33]

Currently, due to the unclear evidence, most advanced endoscopy centres probably treat early squamous cell cancer by means of ESD, also because of its higher aggressiveness. In Barrett's neoplasia, ESD may be more useful in visible and sessile/bulky cancers which may have a higher risk of being technically more challenging and may also show deeper tumour infiltration. For the concept of total Barrett's eradication, resection and ablation has been shown to be superior to multistep resection, mainly due to lower complication (stricture) rates.

Technical developments

While the use of EMR has been stable over the years—it started with simple snare resection, then was complemented by prior saline injection—it now rests on two main techniques, namely the original cap technique developed by H. Inoue, and the banding technique.[20,21] Both are fairly equivalent with regard to efficacy and complications.[22,23] The progress of EMR has been limited currently.

There has been recent progress with long-lasting injection fluids, which has been the subject of an ongoing search for a long time, but recent commercialization of different, more sticky solutions (which are also more expensive than saline or colloid solutions) has seen some papers with better technical success; overall outcome was not the topic of these studies.

ESD technology has been much more diverse,[60] and developments are rapid and multiple, ranging from new knives to simple tools to unfolding the specimens and making the dissection plane more accessible, to finally two-arm robot-like big apparatus. Their foremost application is seen in the colon, where it is probably needed the least in the vast majority of cases with benign lesions. In the oesophagus, these devices are too large, and therefore the current standard ESD technique is the tunnel resection method[61,62] which takes advantage of the lateral margins being left until the end and the submucosal tunnel providing a good and large resection plane.

Summary and indications

Currently, endoscopic resection has become the method of choice for low-risk early oesophageal lesions (for definitions see above). In cases where this may be considered doubtful, other imaging modalities are of limited help in decision-making. In case of doubt, endoscopic resection—here mostly in the form of ESD—is attempted and can be primarily regarded as a large biopsy which can be curative depending on histopathological analysis. Interdisciplinary consultation first with pathologists for ascertaining histological criteria and then with surgeons and the patient is necessary in borderline cases to find the right balance between oncological and procedural risk. We have developed an experimental concept of a transabdominal laparoscopic lymph node sampling for distal oesophageal adenocarcinoma which could be helpful in a further risk stratification.[63] Given the general tendency of multimodal oncological therapy encompassing surgery, medical oncology, and radiotherapy, it is foreseeable that endoscopic methods may also become part of such concepts in earlier stage lesions.

REFERENCES

1. Lagergren J, Smyth E, Cunningham D, Lagergren P. Oesophageal cancer. *Lancet*. 2017;**390**:2383–2396.
2. Uhlenhopp DJ, Then EO, Sunkara T, Gaduputi V. Epidemiology of esophageal cancer: update in global trends, etiology and risk factors. *Clin J Gastroenterol*. 2020;**13**:1010–1021.
3. Marques de Sá I, Marcos P, Sharma P, Dinis-Ribeiro M. The global prevalence of Barrett's esophagus: a systematic review of the published literature. *United European Gastroenterol J*. 2020;**8**:1086–1105.
4. Syed T, Doshi A, Guleria S, Syed S, Shah T. Artificial intelligence and its role in identifying esophageal neoplasia. *Dig Dis Sci*. 2020;**65**:3448–3455.
5. Tan MC, Mansour N, White DL, Sisson A, El-Serag HB, Thrift AP. Systematic review with meta-analysis: prevalence of prior and concurrent Barrett's oesophagus in oesophageal adenocarcinoma patients. *Aliment Pharmacol Ther*. 2020;**52**:20–36.
6. Maitra I, Date RS, Martin FL. Towards screening Barrett's oesophagus: current guidelines, imaging modalities and future developments. *Clin J Gastroenterol*. 2020;**13**:635–649.
7. McGoran JJ, Ragunath K. Endoscopic management of Barrett's esophagus: Western perspective of current status and future prospects. *Dig Endosc*. 2021;**33**:720–729.
8. Sharma P, Shaheen NJ, Katzka D, Bergman J. AGA clinical practice update on endoscopic treatment of Barrett's esophagus with dysplasia and/or early cancer: expert review. *Gastroenterology*. 2020;**158**:760–769.
9. Feuerstein JD, Castillo NE, Akbari M, et al. Systematic analysis and critical appraisal of the quality of the scientific evidence and conflicts of interest in practice guidelines (2005–2013) for Barrett's esophagus. *Dig Dis Sci*. 2016;**61**:2812–2822.
10. Nguyen TH, Thrift AP, Rugge M, El-Serag HB. Prevalence of Barrett's esophagus and performance of societal screening guidelines in an unreferred primary care population of U.S. veterans. *Gastrointest Endosc*. 2021;**93**:409–419.
11. DaVee T, Ajani JA, Lee JH. Is endoscopic ultrasound examination necessary in the management of esophageal cancer? *World J Gastroenterol*. 2017;**23**:751–762.
12. Hucl T. Role of endosonography prior to endoscopic treatment of esophageal cancer. *Minerva Chirur*. 2018;**73**:410–416.
13. Qumseya BJ, Bartel MJ, Gendy S, Bain P, Qumseya A, Wolfsen H. High rate of over-staging of Barrett's neoplasia with endoscopic ultrasound: systemic review and meta-analysis. *Dig Liver Dis*. 2018;**50**:438–445.
14. Kolb JM, Wani S. Endoscopic eradication therapy for Barrett's oesophagus: state of the art. *Curr Opin Gastroenterol*. 2020;**36**:351–358.
15. Hatta W, Gotoda T, Kanno T, et al. Prevalence and risk factors for lymph node metastasis after noncurative endoscopic resection for early gastric cancer: a systematic review and meta-analysis. *J Gastroenterol*. 2020;**55**:742–753.
16. Kumarasinghe MP, Bourke MJ, Brown I, et al. Pathological assessment of endoscopic resections of the gastrointestinal tract: a comprehensive clinicopathologic review. *Mod Pathol*. 2020;**33**:986–1006.
17. Zhang QW, Zhang XT, Gao YJ, Ge ZZ. Endoscopic management of patients with early gastric cancer before and after endoscopic resection: a review. *J Dig Dis*. 2019;**20**:223–228.
18. De Marco MO, Tustumi F, Brunaldi VO, et al. Prognostic factors for ESD of early gastric cancers: a systematic review and meta-analysis. *Endosc Int Open*. 2020;**8**:E1144–E1155.
19. Ahmed Y, Othman M. EMR/ESD: techniques, complications, and evidence. *Curr Gastroenterol Rep*. 2020;**22**:39.
20. Ishihara R, Arima M, Iizuka T, et al. Endoscopic submucosal dissection/endoscopic mucosal resection guidelines for esophageal cancer. *Dig Endosc*. 2020;**32**:452–493.
21. Dan X, Lv XH, San ZJ, et al. Efficacy and safety of multiband mucosectomy versus cap-assisted endoscopic resection for early esophageal cancer and precancerous lesions: a systematic review and meta-analysis. *Surg Laparosc Endosc Percutan Tech*. 2019;**29**:313–320.
22. Zhang YM, Boerwinkel DF, Qin X, et al. A randomized trial comparing multiband mucosectomy and cap-assisted endoscopic resection for endoscopic piecemeal resection of early squamous neoplasia of the esophagus. *Endoscopy*. 2016;**48**:330–338.
23. May A, Gossner L, Behrens A, et al. A prospective randomized trial of two different endoscopic resection techniques for early stage cancer of the esophagus. *Gastrointest Endosc*. 2003;**58**:167–175.
24. Han C, Sun Y. Efficacy and safety of endoscopic submucosal dissection versus endoscopic mucosal resection for superficial esophageal carcinoma: a systematic review and meta-analysis. *Dis Esophagus*. 2020;**34**:doaa081.
25. Yang D, Othman M, Draganov PV. Endoscopic mucosal resection vs endoscopic submucosal dissection for Barrett's esophagus and colorectal neoplasia. *Clin Gastroenterol Hepatol*. 2019;**17**:1019–1028.
26. Draganov PV, Wang AY, Othman MO, Fukami N. AGA Institute clinical practice update: endoscopic submucosal dissection in the United States. *Clin Gastroenterol Hepatol*. 2019;**17**:16–25.
27. Hajifathalian K, Ichkhanian Y, Dawod Q, et al. Full-thickness resection device (FTRD) for treatment of upper gastrointestinal tract lesions: the first international experience. *Endosc Int Open*. 2020;**8**:E1291–E1301.
28. Zwager LW, Bastiaansen BAJ, Bronzwaer MES, et al. Endoscopic full-thickness resection (eFTR) of colorectal lesions: results from the Dutch colorectal eFTR registry. *Endoscopy*. 2020;**52**:1014–1023.
29. Schmidt A, Beyna T, Schumacher B, et al. Colonoscopic full-thickness resection using an over-the-scope device: a prospective multicentre study in various indications. *Gut*. 2018;**67**:1280–1289.
30. Alderson D, Wijnhoven BP. Interventions for Barrett's oesophagus and early cancer. *Br J Surg*. 2016;**103**:475–476.
31. Desai M, Saligram S, Gupta N, et al. Efficacy and safety outcomes of multimodal endoscopic eradication therapy in Barrett's

esophagus-related neoplasia: a systematic review and pooled analysis. *Gastrointest Endosc*. 2017;**85**:482–495.
32. de Matos MV, da Ponte-Neto AM, de Moura DTH, et al. Treatment of high-grade dysplasia and intramucosal carcinoma using radiofrequency ablation or endoscopic mucosal resection + radiofrequency ablation: meta-analysis and systematic review. *World J Gastrointest Endosc*. 2019;**11**:239–248.
33. Manner H, Rabenstein T, Pech O, et al. Ablation of residual Barrett's epithelium after endoscopic resection: a randomized long-term follow-up study of argon plasma coagulation vs. surveillance (APE study). *Endoscopy*. 2014;**46**:6–12.
34. Belghazi K, Bergman J, Pouw RE. Endoscopic resection and radiofrequency ablation for early esophageal neoplasia. *Dig Dis*. 2016;**34**:469–475.
35. Pech O. Endoscopic treatment of early Barrett's neoplasia: expanding indications, new challenges. *Adv Exp Med Biol*. 2016;**908**:99–109.
36. Kahn A, Shaheen NJ, Iyer PG. Approach to the post-ablation Barrett's esophagus patient. *Am J Gastroenterol*. 2020;**115**:823–831.
37. Watts AE, Cotton CC, Shaheen NJ. Radiofrequency ablation of Barrett's esophagus: have we gone too far, or not far enough? *Curr Gastroenterol Rep*. 2020;**22**:29.
38. Pech O. Hybrid argon plasma coagulation in patients with Barrett esophagus. *Gastroenterol Hepatol*. 2017;**13**:610–612.
39. Peerally MF, Bhandari P, Ragunath K, et al. Radiofrequency ablation compared with argon plasma coagulation after endoscopic resection of high-grade dysplasia or stage T1 adenocarcinoma in Barrett's esophagus: a randomized pilot study (BRIDE). *Gastrointest Endosc*. 2019;**89**:680–689.
40. Wronska E, Polkowski M, Orlowska J, Mroz A, Wieszczy P, Regula J. Argon plasma coagulation for Barrett's esophagus with low-grade dysplasia: a randomized trial with long-term follow-up on the impact of power setting and proton pump inhibitor dose. *Endoscopy*. 2021;**53**:123–132.
41. Shaheen NJ, Greenwald BD, Peery AF, et al. Safety and efficacy of endoscopic spray cryotherapy for Barrett's esophagus with high-grade dysplasia. *Gastrointest Endosc*. 2010;**71**:680–685.
42. van Munster SN, Overwater A, Haidry R, Bisschops R, Bergman J, Weusten B. Focal cryoballoon versus radiofrequency ablation of dysplastic Barrett's esophagus: impact on treatment response and postprocedural pain. *Gastrointest Endosc*. 2018;**88**:795–803.
43. Anders M, Bahr C, El-Masry MA, et al. Long-term recurrence of neoplasia and Barrett's epithelium after complete endoscopic resection. *Gut*. 2014;**63**:1535–1543.
44. Caillol F, Godat S, Autret A, et al. Neoplastic Barrett's oesophagus and long-term follow-up after endoscopic therapy: complete histological eradication of Barrett associated with high-grade dysplasia significantly decreases neoplasia relapse. *Surg Endosc*. 2016;**30**:5410–5418.
45. Desai M, Saligram S, Gupta N, et al. Efficacy and safety outcomes of multimodal endoscopic eradication therapy in Barrett's esophagus-related neoplasia: a systematic review and pooled analysis. *Gastrointest Endosc*. 2017;**85**:482–495.
46. Haidry RJ, Dunn JM, Butt MA, et al. Radiofrequency ablation and endoscopic mucosal resection for dysplastic Barrett's esophagus and early esophageal adenocarcinoma: outcomes of the UK National Halo RFA Registry. *Gastroenterology*. 2013;**145**:87–95.
47. Marginean EC, Dhanpat J. Pathologic assessment of endoscopic resection specimens with superficial carcinoma of the esophagus: current practice and practical issues. *Ann N Y Acad Sci*. 2020;**1482**:130–145.
48. Overwater A, van der Meulen KE, Künzli HT, et al. Optimizing histopathologic evaluation of EMR specimens of Barrett's esophagus-related neoplasia: a randomized study of 3 specimen handling methods. *Gastrointest Endosc*. 2019;**90**:384–392.
49. Isomoto H, Yamaguchi N, Minami H, Nakao K. Management of complications associated with endoscopic submucosal dissection/endoscopic mucosal resection for esophageal cancer. *Dig Endosc*. 2013;**25**(Suppl 1):29–38.
50. Komeda Y, Bruno M, Koch A. EMR is not inferior to ESD for early Barrett's and EGJ neoplasia: an extensive review on outcome, recurrence and complication rates. *Endosc Int Open*. 2014;**2**:E58–E64.
51. Qumseya BJ, Wani S, Desai M, et al. Adverse events after radiofrequency ablation in patients with Barrett's esophagus: a systematic review and meta-analysis. *Clin Gastroenterol Hepatol*. 2016;**14**:1086–1095.
52. Smith I, Kahaleh M. Endoscopic versus surgical therapy for Barrett's esophagus neoplasia. *Expert Rev Gastroenterol Hepatol*. 2015;**9**:31–35.
53. Bennett C, Green S, DeCaestecker J, et al. Surgery versus radical endotherapies for early cancer and high-grade dysplasia in Barrett's oesophagus. *Cochrane Database Syst Rev*. 2020;**5**:CD007334.
54. Pech O, Bollschweiler E, Manner H, Leers J, Ell C, Holscher AH. Comparison between endoscopic and surgical resection of mucosal esophageal adenocarcinoma in Barrett's esophagus at two high-volume centers. *Ann Surg*. 2011;**254**:67–72.
55. Terheggen G, Horn EM, Vieth M, et al. A randomised trial of endoscopic submucosal dissection versus endoscopic mucosal resection for early Barrett's neoplasia. *Gut*. 2017;**66**:783–793.
56. Wang J, Ge J, Zhang XH, Liu JY, Yang CM, Zhao SL. Endoscopic submucosal dissection versus endoscopic mucosal resection for the treatment of early esophageal carcinoma: a meta-analysis. *Asian Pac J Cancer Prev*. 2014;**15**:1803–1806.
57. Guo HM, Zhang XQ, Chen M, Huang SL, Zou XP. Endoscopic submucosal dissection vs endoscopic mucosal resection for superficial esophageal cancer. *World J Gastroenterol*. 2014;**20**:5540–5547.
58. Cao Y, Liao C, Tan A, Gao Y, Mo Z, Gao F. Meta-analysis of endoscopic submucosal dissection versus endoscopic mucosal resection for tumors of the gastrointestinal tract. *Endoscopy*. 2009;**41**:751–757.
59. Pech O, May A, Manner H, et al. Long-term efficacy and safety of endoscopic resection for patients with mucosal adenocarcinoma of the esophagus. *Gastroenterology*. 2014;**146**:652–660.
60. Harlow C, Sivananthan A, Ayaru L, Patel K, Darzi A, Patel N. Endoscopic submucosal dissection: an update on tools and accessories. *Ther Adv Gastrointest Endosc*. 2020;**13**:2631774520957220.
61. Liu YZ, Lv XH, Deng K, Yang JL. Efficacy and safety of endoscopic submucosal tunnel dissection vs endoscopic submucosal dissection for early superficial upper gastrointestinal precancerous lesions and tumors: a meta-analysis. *J Dig Dis*. 2020;**21**:480–489.
62. Zhang T, Zhang H, Zhong F, Wang X. Efficacy of endoscopic submucosal tunnel dissection versus endoscopic submucosal dissection for superficial esophageal neoplastic lesions: a systematic review and meta-analysis. *Surg Endosc*. 2021;**35**:52–62.
63. Stüben BO, Duprée A, Mann O. Gastro-oesophageal reflux disease. In: . Oesophagus and Stomach. Volume Editors Matthias Reeh and Jacob Izbicki. pp 49–64. Oxford University Press UK. 2023. Submitted for publication

13

Oesophageal cancer
Surgery

Björn-Ole Stüben, Karl-Frederick Karstens, Michael Nentwich, Jakob R. Izbicki, and Matthias Reeh

History of surgery of the oesophagus

Surgery of the oesophagus is often seen as a rite of passage for many visceral surgeons, and is one of the most complex surgical procedures currently performed. Hence, we first wanted to give a brief overview of the historical landmarks in oesophageal surgery.

Due to its perilous localization in the cervical region and the thoracic cavity running between major vessels and air passages, the oesophagus was out of the surgeon's reach for a long time.

The earliest report of cervical oesophagotomy dates back to the 17th century. Cervical oesophagectomy was not performed for another 200 years, and the intrathoracic resection of the oesophagus was only made possible by the introduction of intratracheal anaesthesia.

In 1676, Richard Wiseman[1] advised that a tear in the oesophagus should be sutured, while Stoffel[2] stated that a stricture in the cervical oesophagus should be bypassed.

In 1701, John Baptiste Verduc[3] documented the surgical extraction of foreign bodies from the cervical oesophagus if they could not be removed by other means. A vertical incision of the oesophagus was performed following tracheostomy, with the patient sitting and the head firmly extended.

In 1880, Gross collected 39 cases of surgical removal of foreign bodies in the cervical oesophagus. With only three fatalities, Gross concluded that the removal of foreign objects from the cervical oesophagus was, in fact, a safe procedure.[4]

With the introduction of anaesthesia by Long and Morton,[5] the discovery of pathogenic bacteria (Pasteur)[6] and antisepsis (Lister),[7] and the development of gastrointestinal surgical techniques (Billroth among others),[8] actual resection of the cervical oesophagus became possible, and Czerny performed the first successful cervical oesophagectomy for oesophageal cancer in 1877.[9]

For centuries, treatment of oesophageal trauma was only possible in the cervical portion of the oesophagus. Between the 17th and 19th centuries, surgeons considered wounds of the thoracic oesophagus beyond treatment. In the US Civil War and World War I, most trauma to the thoracic oesophagus were fatal.

In the 20th century, oesophageal surgery advanced rapidly due to the introduction of intratracheal anaesthesia (Meltzer and Auer),[10] Fleming's[11] discovery of antibiotics, and improved radiological and gastrointestinal surgical techniques. World War II led to increased surgical experiences with a subsequent improvement in emergency medicine, especially emergency thoracotomy.

World War II also led to a better understanding of the physiology of shock and open pneumothorax, leading to wounds of the thoracic oesophagus becoming treatable. Studies performed in operating theatres during World War II showed that injury to the thoracic oesophagus presented an indication for emergent thoracic and abdominal exploration, and this has remained so ever since.[12]

In 1946, Barrett[13] made a notable advance in the management of oesophageal perforation when he performed the first successful repair of a spontaneous oesophagus perforation. Early oesophagus surgery was not marked by success, and few patients survived following surgery.

The first resection of the thoracic oesophagus was performed by Torek in 1913.[14] Between 1936 to 1939 Lanman[15] attempted to anastomose the two segments of the oesophagus. Among four patients there were no long-term survivors. Grey Turner[16] introduced resection of the thoracic oesophagus in 1931, blindly mobilizing it through cervical and abdominal incisions. Two years later, Oshawa[17] first reported resection of the thoracic oesophagus and immediate oesophagogastrostomy with eight out of 18 patients surviving following surgery.

During World War II, Richard Sweet[18] reported that by division of the left and short gastric arteries, the stomach can be used to provide a viable oesophageal replacement.

In 1946, Ivor Lewis[19] introduced oesophagectomy and oesophagogastrostomy through a right-sided thoracotomy, solving many problems that had faced surgeons attempting oesophagectomy by a left-sided thoracotomy.

Currently, thoracoabdominal oesophagectomy is a standardized and frequently performed procedure. The following chapter provides a surgical insight into the conventional operation techniques applied when resecting the oesophagus.

Transhiatal blunt oesophageal dissection and gastric pull-up

Indications

- Adenocarcinoma of the distal oesophagus (>T1 stage).
- Intraepithelial squamous cell neoplasia.
- Poor-risk patients.
- Extensive stricture (stenosis) due to erosion (chemical burns) unresponsive to non-surgical treatment including bougienage.
- Extensive peptic stricture (stenosis).
- Relapse of the megaoesophagus after surgical repair of cardiospasm combined with peptic strictures and failure of dilatation.
- Extensive benign oesophageal tumours (exceptional cases, usually local excision).
- Oesophageal rupture or iatrogenic perforation with mediastinitis (primary repair not feasible).

Contraindications

- Florid gastroduodenal ulcer.
- Infiltration of the aorta.
- Distant metastases.

Approach

- Upper transverse incision with a median T-shaped extension.
- Alternative: upper midline incision with left periumbilical incision.

Procedure

- Mobilization of the left lateral liver lobe by transection of the left triangular ligament, placing a pack under the left lobe of the liver to prevent injury to the adjacent structures (Figure 13.1).
  - This step ensures optimal visualization of the diaphragmatic oesophageal hiatus.
  - *Expert tip*: to prevent bile leak from an irregular bile duct, oversewn suture ligation of the tip of the triangular ligament should be performed.
- Skeletonization of the greater curvature, sparing the left and right gastroepiploic vessels up to the splenic hilum (Figure 13.2).
  - *Expert tip*: moderate traction on the transverse colon and countertraction at the stomach result in a proper exposure of the gastrocolic ligament.
- Transection of the left gastroepiploic artery directly at its origin, the splenic artery (Figure 13.3). This ensures that the existing anastomosis between the left and right epiploic artery is preserved.
- Transection and ligature of the short gastric vessels, mobilizing the fundus and the greater curvature.
- Incision of the parietal peritoneum at the upper pancreatic margin.
  - *Expert tip*: position the greater curvature cranially and anteriorly during this step.

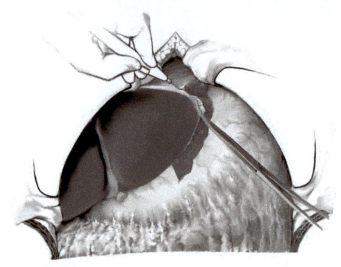

Figure 13.1 Mobilization of the left liver lobe. The left triangular ligament is transected with electrocautery.

Reproduced with permission from Reeh, M., Yekebas, E.F., Izbicki, J. (2016). Subtotal esophagectomy: transhiatal approach. In: Clavien, P.A., Sarr, M., Fong, Y., Miyazaki, M. (eds) *Atlas of Upper Gastrointestinal and Hepato-Pancreato-Biliary Surgery*. Springer, Berlin, Heidelberg. https://doi.org/10.1007/978-3-662-46546-2_11

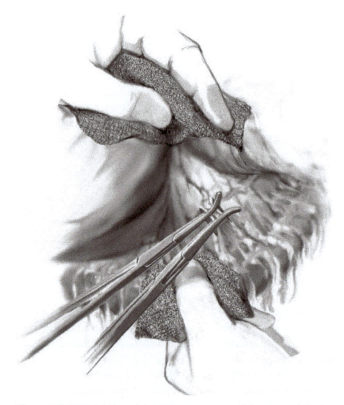

Figure 13.2 Dissection of the greater curvature of the stomach from below. The arcade between the left and right gastroepiploic vessels as well as the origin of the right gastroepiploic vessels are spared right up to the level of the splenic hilum.

Reproduced with permission from Reeh, M., Yekebas, E.F., Izbicki, J. (2016). Subtotal esophagectomy: transhiatal approach. In: Clavien, P.A., Sarr, M., Fong, Y., Miyazaki, M. (eds) *Atlas of Upper Gastrointestinal and Hepato-Pancreato-Biliary Surgery*. Springer, Berlin, Heidelberg. https://doi.org/10.1007/978-3-662-46546-2_11

Transhiatal blunt oesophageal dissection and gastric pull-up

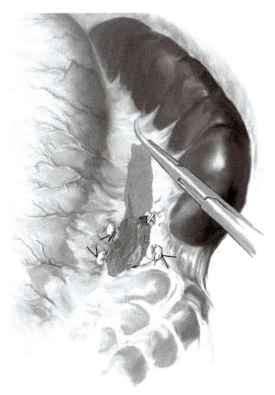

Figure 13.3 Dissection of the greater curvature towards the splenic hilum, with the left gastroepiploic artery in the picture having been transected directly at its origin.

Reproduced with permission from Reeh, M., Yekebas, E.F., Izbicki, J. (2016). Subtotal esophagectomy: transhiatal approach. In: Clavien, PA., Sarr, M., Fong, Y., Miyazaki, M. (eds) *Atlas of Upper Gastrointestinal and Hepato-Pancreato-Biliary Surgery*. Springer, Berlin, Heidelberg. https://doi.org/10.1007/978-3-662-46546-2_11

- Transection of the left gastric vein.
- Lymphadenectomy of the hepatoduodenal ligament and the hepatic artery up to the coeliac trunk. Include lymphatic tissue around the portal vein as well as the common bile duct (Figure 13.4a,b).
- Division of the right gastric artery close to its origin below the pylorus (Figure 13.4c).
- Transection of the left gastric artery. All lymph nodes along the left gastric artery, the splenic artery, the common hepatic artery, and the coeliac trunk as well as the para-aortic lymph nodes are removed.
  - The blood supply of the gastric tube is provided solely by the right gastroepiploic artery.
- Kocher manoeuvre: while medially retracting the duodenum, the peritoneum is incised close to the duodenum. Subsequently, blunt dissection of the avascular plane between duodenum, head of the pancreas, and the retroperitoneal vessels is performed until the anterior wall of the inferior vena cava is exposed.
  - The Kocher manoeuvre aids in providing a tension-free positioning of the gastric tube to the neck.
- Mobilization of the abdominal portion of the oesophagus.
- Dissection of the lesser omentum. The cranial part of the hepatogastric ligament is bluntly tunnelled with the finger and dissected from the diaphragm with electrocautery.
  - *Expert tip*: check for an accessory left hepatic artery, which should be preserved.

- The diaphragmatic crura are incised with electrocautery and both stumps ligated for better exposure of the oesophageal hiatus.
- Blunt mobilization of the oesophagus is performed with the index finger, carefully removing connective tissue fibres between the oesophagus, diaphragmatic crura, and the abdominal aorta (Figure 13.5).
- The abdominal oesophagus is mobilized and pulled caudally.
- Ventral incision of the hiatus following transection of the left inferior phrenic vein between ligatures (Figure 13.6).
- The retrocardial lymphatic tissue is removed en bloc with the specimen (Figure 13.7).
- Transhiatal oesophageal dissection by detaching its anterior surface from the pericardium.
- Sharp dissection anteriorly up to the tracheal bifurcation and posteriorly from the posterior mediastinum, completing the dissection bluntly by hand (Figure 13.8).
- The trachea and the brachiocephalic trunk are palpable anteriorly (Figure 13.9).
- After complete anterior and posterior mobilization, the oesophagus is pulled caudally. The so-called lateral oesophageal ligaments consisting of vagal branches, pulmonary ligaments, and oesophageal aortic branches should be transected sharply between clamps or clips (Figure 13.10).
- Excision of the parietal pleura, and if tumour infiltration exists, en bloc resection of adherent tissue, can be performed after enlargement of the diaphragmatic incision (Figure 13.11).
- Dissection up to the tracheal bifurcation by division of the lateral ligaments.
- Lymphadenectomy of the posterior mediastinum (Figure 13.12) and posterior portion of the tracheal bifurcation (Figure 13.13).
- Blunt dissection of the oesophagus proximally to the tracheal bifurcation by pulling the lateral ligaments caudally and ligating them.
- Complete blunt dissection up to the upper thoracic aperture (Figure 13.14).

Construction of the gastric tube

- Starting at the fundus, the lesser curvature is resected using a linear stapler device (Figure 13.15). It follows the direction of the pylorus.
  - Shortening of the gastric tube can be avoided by stretching the stomach longitudinally.
- The staple line is oversewn by interrupted seromuscular sutures (Figure 13.16).
  - The diameter of the gastric tube should be 2.5–3.0 cm

Mobilization of the cervical oesophagus

- Turn the patient's head to the right for better exposure.
- Make a skin incision along the anterior edge of the sternocleidomastoid muscle.
- Dissect the platysma and perform blunt dissection between the straight cervical muscles and the sternocleidomastoid muscle, followed by lateral retraction of the sternocleidomastoid muscle.
- Sharply dissect the omyhoid muscle (Figure 13.17). This exposes the lateral edge of the thyroid, the jugular vein, and the carotid artery by retracting the strap muscles medially (Figure 13.18).
- Displace the oesophagus using a curved instrument.

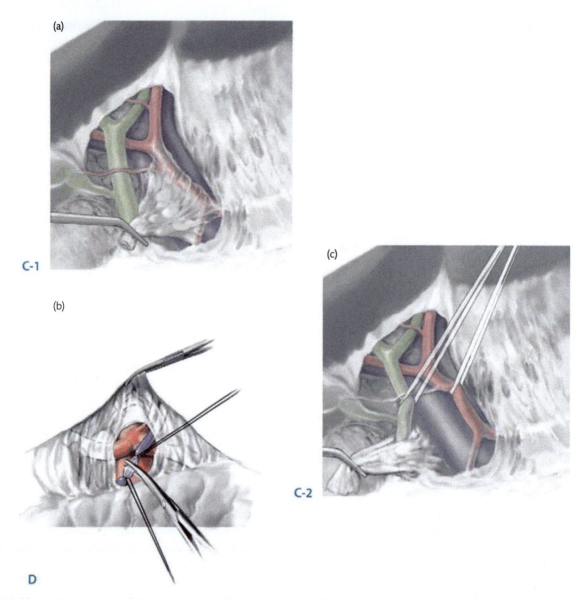

Figure 13.4 (a) Lymphadenectomy of the hepatoduodenal ligament, removing all lymph tissue around the hepatic artery, portal vein, and common bile duct. (b) Clear identification using vessel loops of the hepatic artery and common bile duct. (c) Transection of the left gastric artery.
Reproduced with permission from Reeh, M., Yekebas, E.F., Izbicki, J. (2016). Subtotal esophagectomy: transhiatal approach. In: Clavien, PA., Sarr, M., Fong, Y., Miyazaki, M. (eds) *Atlas of Upper Gastrointestinal and Hepato-Pancreato-Biliary Surgery*. Springer, Berlin, Heidelberg. https://doi.org/10.1007/978-3-662-46546-2_11

- The dissection of the cervical and upper thoracic oesophagus is completed bluntly with a finger or dissector.
- Transection of the oesophagus using a stapler (Figure 13.21) or scissors (Figure 13.19) after ligation of the aboral part of the oesophagus.
  - Prior removal of the nasogastric tube should not be forgotten.
- A strong thread (Figure 13.21) or rubber band (Figure 13.20) is fixed at the aboral stump of the oesophagus before the oesophagus is transposed into the abdominal cavity.
- Pull up of the gastric tube.
  - Oesophageal bed (Figure 13.22)/retrosternal (Figure 13.23)/ presternal (Figure 13.24) positioning is possible. In case of an R2 resection, the presternal pull-up should be preferred.
- Side-to-side two-layer anastomosis of the gastric tube and the oesophageal stump is performed. The first seromuscular suture line is done in an interrupted fashion (Figure 13.25). The protruding parts of the oesophagus and the gastric tube are resected (Figure 13.26). The second inner suture line of the posterior wall can be performed as a running suture (Figure 13.27); if the cervical oesophagus remains long enough, a stapler anastomosis can also be performed (28.0 mm circular stapler).
- An enteral three-lumen feeding tube is then inserted over the anastomosis and placed into the first jejunal loop for postoperative enteral nutrition (Figure 13.28).
- The anterior wall is completed with interrupted or running sutures (Figure 13.29). The second suture line can be performed in

Transhiatal blunt oesophageal dissection and gastric pull-up

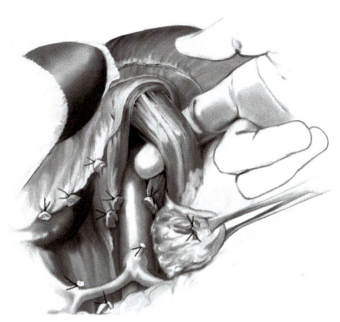

Figure 13.5 The diaphragmatic crura have been incised with electrocautery and the stumps ligated. The oesophagus is mobilized with the index finger, carefully removing connective tissue between the oesophagus and the diaphragmatic crura and abdominal aorta.

Reproduced with permission from Reeh, M., Yekebas, E.F., Izbicki, J. (2016). Subtotal esophagectomy: transhiatal approach. In: Clavien, PA., Sarr, M., Fong, Y., Miyazaki, M. (eds) *Atlas of Upper Gastrointestinal and Hepato-Pancreato-Biliary Surgery*. Springer, Berlin, Heidelberg. https://doi.org/10.1007/978-3-662-46546-2_11

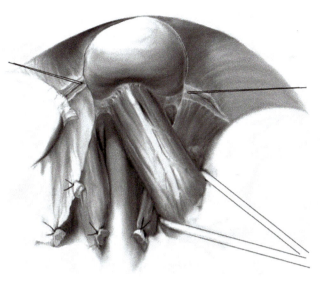

Figure 13.7 Retrocardial lymphatic tissue is removed with the specimen en bloc. Retractors may aid in visualization.

Reproduced with permission from Reeh, M., Yekebas, E.F., Izbicki, J. (2016). Subtotal esophagectomy: transhiatal approach. In: Clavien, PA., Sarr, M., Fong, Y., Miyazaki, M. (eds) *Atlas of Upper Gastrointestinal and Hepato-Pancreato-Biliary Surgery*. Springer, Berlin, Heidelberg. https://doi.org/10.1007/978-3-662-46546-2_11

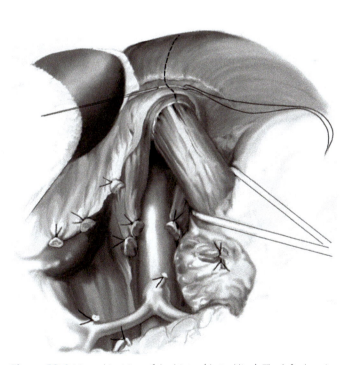

Figure 13.6 Ventral incision of the hiatus (dotted line). The left phrenic vein is transected between ligatures.

Reproduced with permission from Reeh, M., Yekebas, E.F., Izbicki, J. (2016). Subtotal esophagectomy: transhiatal approach. In: Clavien, PA., Sarr, M., Fong, Y., Miyazaki, M. (eds) *Atlas of Upper Gastrointestinal and Hepato-Pancreato-Biliary Surgery*. Springer, Berlin, Heidelberg. https://doi.org/10.1007/978-3-662-46546-2_11

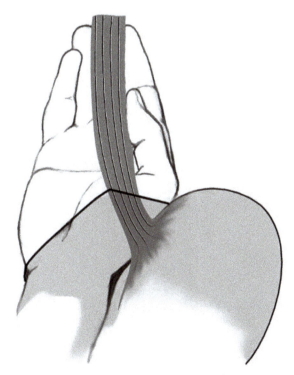

Figure 13.8 Blunt mobilization of the oesophagus from the posterior mediastinum.

Reproduced with permission from Reeh, M., Yekebas, E.F., Izbicki, J. (2016). Subtotal esophagectomy: transhiatal approach. In: Clavien, PA., Sarr, M., Fong, Y., Miyazaki, M. (eds) *Atlas of Upper Gastrointestinal and Hepato-Pancreato-Biliary Surgery*. Springer, Berlin, Heidelberg. https://doi.org/10.1007/978-3-662-46546-2_11

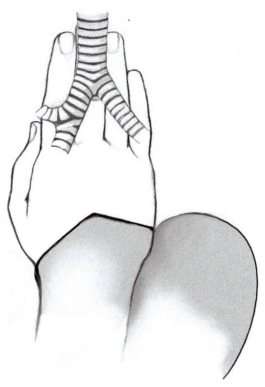

Figure 13.9 Ensure adequate mobilization of the oesophagus by palpating the trachea anteriorly.
Reproduced with permission from Reeh, M., Yekebas, E.F., Izbicki, J. (2016). Subtotal esophagectomy: transhiatal approach. In: Clavien, PA., Sarr, M., Fong, Y., Miyazaki, M. (eds) *Atlas of Upper Gastrointestinal and Hepato-Pancreato-Biliary Surgery*. Springer, Berlin, Heidelberg. https://doi.org/10.1007/978-3-662-46546-2_11

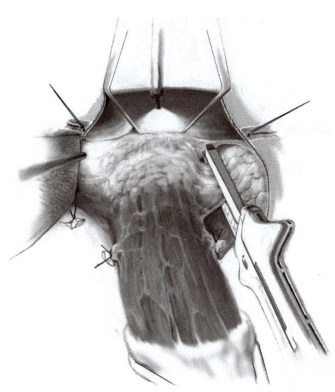

Figure 13.11 Excision of the parietal pleura.
Reproduced with permission from Reeh, M., Yekebas, E.F., Izbicki, J. (2016). Subtotal esophagectomy: transhiatal approach. In: Clavien, PA., Sarr, M., Fong, Y., Miyazaki, M. (eds) *Atlas of Upper Gastrointestinal and Hepato-Pancreato-Biliary Surgery*. Springer, Berlin, Heidelberg. https://doi.org/10.1007/978-3-662-46546-2_11

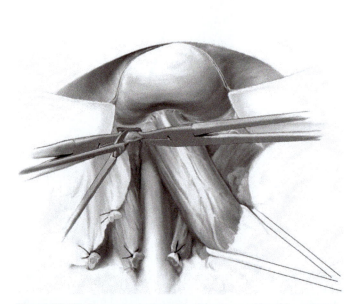

Figure 13.10 Sharp transection of the lateral oesophageal ligaments.
Reproduced with permission from Reeh, M., Yekebas, E.F., Izbicki, J. (2016). Subtotal esophagectomy: transhiatal approach. In: Clavien, PA., Sarr, M., Fong, Y., Miyazaki, M. (eds) *Atlas of Upper Gastrointestinal and Hepato-Pancreato-Biliary Surgery*. Springer, Berlin, Heidelberg. https://doi.org/10.1007/978-3-662-46546-2_11

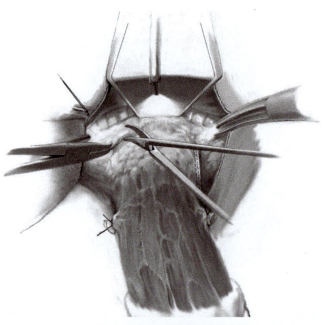

Figure 13.12 Dissection up to the tracheal bifurcation including lymphadenectomy of the posterior mediastinum.
Reproduced with permission from Reeh, M., Yekebas, E.F., Izbicki, J. (2016). Subtotal esophagectomy: transhiatal approach. In: Clavien, PA., Sarr, M., Fong, Y., Miyazaki, M. (eds) *Atlas of Upper Gastrointestinal and Hepato-Pancreato-Biliary Surgery*. Springer, Berlin, Heidelberg. https://doi.org/10.1007/978-3-662-46546-2_11

Transhiatal blunt oesophageal dissection and gastric pull-up

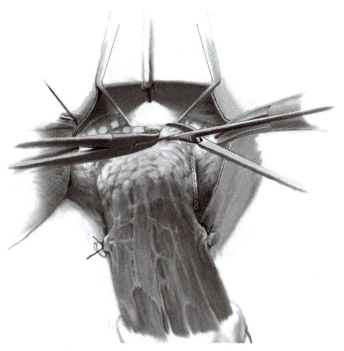

Figure 13.13 Lymphadenectomy posterior to the tracheal bifurcation.
Reproduced with permission from Reeh, M., Yekebas, E.F., Izbicki, J. (2016). Subtotal esophagectomy: transhiatal approach. In: Clavien, PA., Sarr, M., Fong, Y., Miyazaki, M. (eds) *Atlas of Upper Gastrointestinal and Hepato-Pancreato-Biliary Surgery*. Springer, Berlin, Heidelberg. https://doi.org/10.1007/978-3-662-46546-2_11

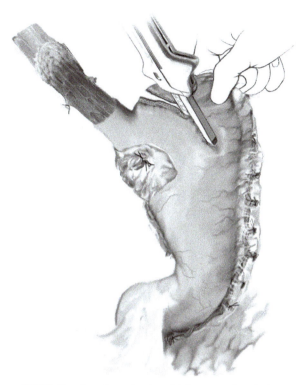

Figure 13.15 Creation of gastric tube with linear stapling device.
Reproduced with permission from Reeh, M., Yekebas, E.F., Izbicki, J. (2016). Subtotal esophagectomy: transhiatal approach. In: Clavien, PA., Sarr, M., Fong, Y., Miyazaki, M. (eds) *Atlas of Upper Gastrointestinal and Hepato-Pancreato-Biliary Surgery*. Springer, Berlin, Heidelberg. https://doi.org/10.1007/978-3-662-46546-2_11

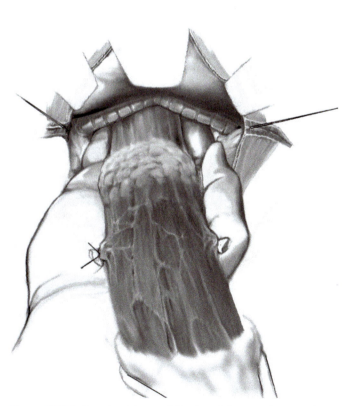

Figure 13.14 Complete blunt mobilization of the oesophagus to the upper thoracic aperture.
Reproduced with permission from Reeh, M., Yekebas, E.F., Izbicki, J. (2016). Subtotal esophagectomy: transhiatal approach. In: Clavien, PA., Sarr, M., Fong, Y., Miyazaki, M. (eds) *Atlas of Upper Gastrointestinal and Hepato-Pancreato-Biliary Surgery*. Springer, Berlin, Heidelberg. https://doi.org/10.1007/978-3-662-46546-2_11

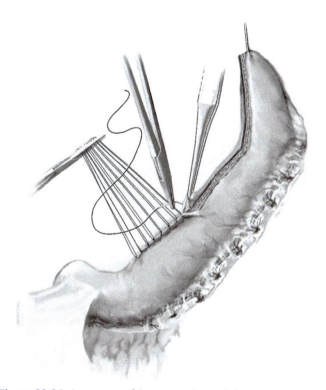

Figure 13.16 Oversewing of the gastric tube staple line.
Reproduced with permission from Reeh, M., Yekebas, E.F., Izbicki, J. (2016). Subtotal esophagectomy: transhiatal approach. In: Clavien, PA., Sarr, M., Fong, Y., Miyazaki, M. (eds) *Atlas of Upper Gastrointestinal and Hepato-Pancreato-Biliary Surgery*. Springer, Berlin, Heidelberg. https://doi.org/10.1007/978-3-662-46546-2_11

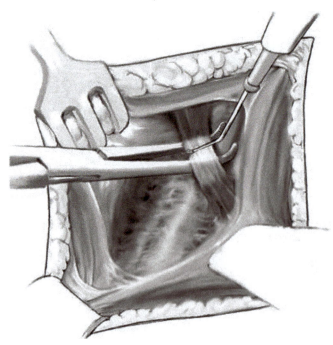

Figure 13.17 Sharp dissection of the omohyoid muscle.
Reproduced with permission from Reeh, M., Yekebas, E.F., Izbicki, J. (2016). Subtotal esophagectomy: transhiatal approach. In: Clavien, PA., Sarr, M., Fong, Y., Miyazaki, M. (eds) *Atlas of Upper Gastrointestinal and Hepato-Pancreato-Biliary Surgery*. Springer, Berlin, Heidelberg. https://doi.org/10.1007/978-3-662-46546-2_11

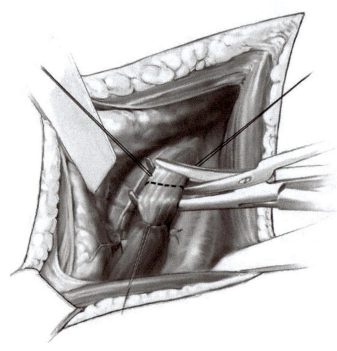

Figure 13.19 Transection of the oesophagus using scissors.
Reproduced with permission from Reeh, M., Yekebas, E.F., Izbicki, J. (2016). Subtotal esophagectomy: transhiatal approach. In: Clavien, PA., Sarr, M., Fong, Y., Miyazaki, M. (eds) *Atlas of Upper Gastrointestinal and Hepato-Pancreato-Biliary Surgery*. Springer, Berlin, Heidelberg. https://doi.org/10.1007/978-3-662-46546-2_11

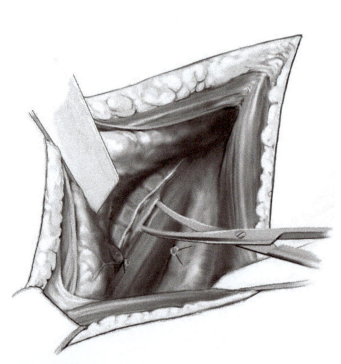

Figure 13.18 Retraction of the strap muscles medially exposes the internal jugular vein and the carotid sheath.
Reproduced with permission from Reeh, M., Yekebas, E.F., Izbicki, J. (2016). Subtotal esophagectomy: transhiatal approach. In: Clavien, PA., Sarr, M., Fong, Y., Miyazaki, M. (eds) *Atlas of Upper Gastrointestinal and Hepato-Pancreato-Biliary Surgery*. Springer, Berlin, Heidelberg. https://doi.org/10.1007/978-3-662-46546-2_11

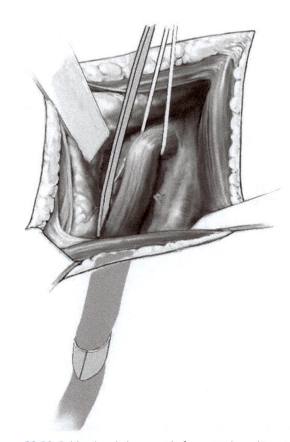

Figure 13.20 Rubber band placement before oesophageal transection.
Reproduced with permission from Reeh, M., Yekebas, E.F., Izbicki, J. (2016). Subtotal esophagectomy: transhiatal approach. In: Clavien, PA., Sarr, M., Fong, Y., Miyazaki, M. (eds) *Atlas of Upper Gastrointestinal and Hepato-Pancreato-Biliary Surgery*. Springer, Berlin, Heidelberg. https://doi.org/10.1007/978-3-662-46546-2_11

Transhiatal blunt oesophageal dissection and gastric pull-up

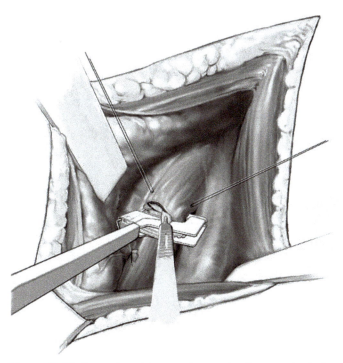

Figure 13.21 Transection of the oesophagus using linear stapler device. A thread has been placed prior to transection.
Reproduced with permission from Reeh, M., Yekebas, E.F., Izbicki, J. (2016). Subtotal esophagectomy: transhiatal approach. In: Clavien, PA., Sarr, M., Fong, Y., Miyazaki, M. (eds) *Atlas of Upper Gastrointestinal and Hepato-Pancreato-Biliary Surgery*. Springer, Berlin, Heidelberg. https://doi.org/10.1007/978-3-662-46546-2_11

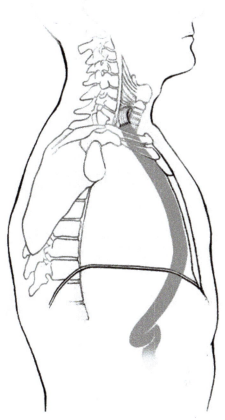

Figure 13.23 Retrosternal placement of the gastric tube.
Reproduced with permission from Reeh, M., Yekebas, E.F., Izbicki, J. (2016). Subtotal esophagectomy: transhiatal approach. In: Clavien, PA., Sarr, M., Fong, Y., Miyazaki, M. (eds) *Atlas of Upper Gastrointestinal and Hepato-Pancreato-Biliary Surgery*. Springer, Berlin, Heidelberg. https://doi.org/10.1007/978-3-662-46546-2_11

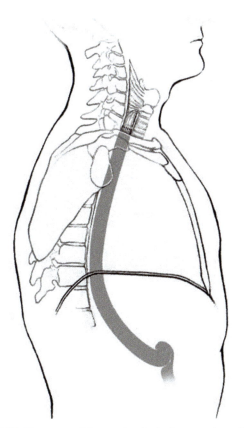

Figure 13.22 Placement of the gastric tube in the oesophageal bed.
Reproduced with permission from Reeh, M., Yekebas, E.F., Izbicki, J. (2016). Subtotal esophagectomy: transhiatal approach. In: Clavien, PA., Sarr, M., Fong, Y., Miyazaki, M. (eds) *Atlas of Upper Gastrointestinal and Hepato-Pancreato-Biliary Surgery*. Springer, Berlin, Heidelberg. https://doi.org/10.1007/978-3-662-46546-2_11

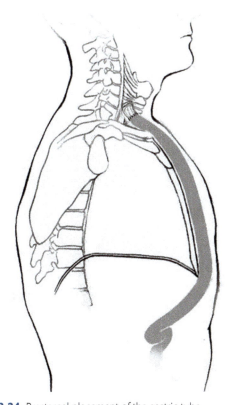

Figure 13.24 Presternal placement of the gastric tube.
Reproduced with permission from Reeh, M., Yekebas, E.F., Izbicki, J. (2016). Subtotal esophagectomy: transhiatal approach. In: Clavien, PA., Sarr, M., Fong, Y., Miyazaki, M. (eds) *Atlas of Upper Gastrointestinal and Hepato-Pancreato-Biliary Surgery*. Springer, Berlin, Heidelberg. https://doi.org/10.1007/978-3-662-46546-2_11

13 Oesophageal cancer: surgery

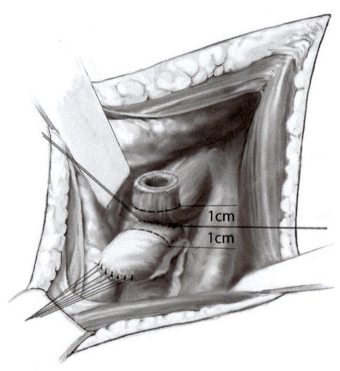

Figure 13.25 Side-to-side anastomosis of the gastric tube and the oesophageal stump.
Reproduced with permission from Reeh, M., Yekebas, E.F., Izbicki, J. (2016). Subtotal esophagectomy: transhiatal approach. In: Clavien, PA., Sarr, M., Fong, Y., Miyazaki, M. (eds) *Atlas of Upper Gastrointestinal and Hepato-Pancreato-Biliary Surgery*. Springer, Berlin, Heidelberg. https://doi.org/10.1007/978-3-662-46546-2_11

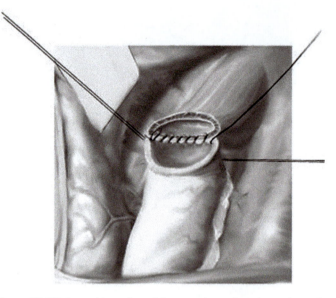

Figure 13.27 Second inner line of the posterior wall can be performed as a running suture.
Reproduced with permission from Reeh, M., Yekebas, E.F., Izbicki, J. (2016). Subtotal esophagectomy: transhiatal approach. In: Clavien, PA., Sarr, M., Fong, Y., Miyazaki, M. (eds) *Atlas of Upper Gastrointestinal and Hepato-Pancreato-Biliary Surgery*. Springer, Berlin, Heidelberg. https://doi.org/10.1007/978-3-662-46546-2_11

a U-shaped fashion. This may provide an inversion of the anastomosis into the gastric tube (Figure 13.30).
- A soft drainage is placed dorsal to the anastomosis, followed by closure of the skin.
- Drainage of the mediastinum is performed by two soft drains placed through the abdominal incision (Figure 13.31).

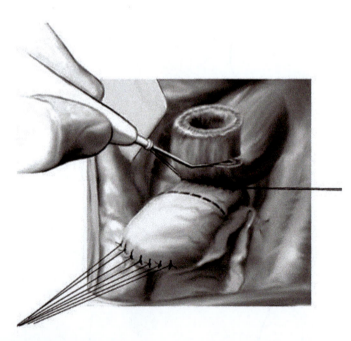

Figure 13.26 Resection of protruding parts of the oesophagus and the gastric tube.
Reproduced with permission from Reeh, M., Yekebas, E.F., Izbicki, J. (2016). Subtotal esophagectomy: transhiatal approach. In: Clavien, PA., Sarr, M., Fong, Y., Miyazaki, M. (eds) *Atlas of Upper Gastrointestinal and Hepato-Pancreato-Biliary Surgery*. Springer, Berlin, Heidelberg. https://doi.org/10.1007/978-3-662-46546-2_11

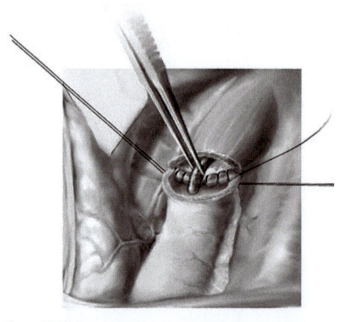

Figure 13.28 Enteral tube placement.
Reproduced with permission from Reeh, M., Yekebas, E.F., Izbicki, J. (2016). Subtotal esophagectomy: transhiatal approach. In: Clavien, PA., Sarr, M., Fong, Y., Miyazaki, M. (eds) *Atlas of Upper Gastrointestinal and Hepato-Pancreato-Biliary Surgery*. Springer, Berlin, Heidelberg. https://doi.org/10.1007/978-3-662-46546-2_11

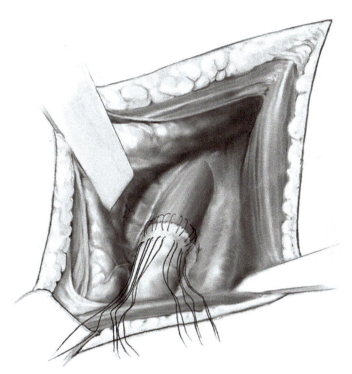

Figure 13.29 Anterior wall is completed with interrupted or running sutures.
Reproduced with permission from Reeh, M., Yekebas, E.F., Izbicki, J. (2016). Subtotal esophagectomy: transhiatal approach. In: Clavien, PA., Sarr, M., Fong, Y., Miyazaki, M. (eds) *Atlas of Upper Gastrointestinal and Hepato-Pancreato-Biliary Surgery*. Springer, Berlin, Heidelberg. https://doi.org/10.1007/978-3-662-46546-2_11

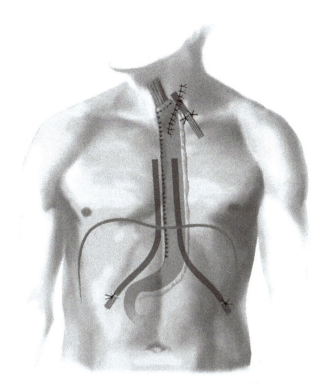

Figure 13.31 Transhiatal and cervical drainage placement.
Reproduced with permission from Reeh, M., Yekebas, E.F., Izbicki, J. (2016). Subtotal esophagectomy: transhiatal approach. In: Clavien, PA., Sarr, M., Fong, Y., Miyazaki, M. (eds) *Atlas of Upper Gastrointestinal and Hepato-Pancreato-Biliary Surgery*. Springer, Berlin, Heidelberg. https://doi.org/10.1007/978-3-662-46546-2_11

Subtotal en bloc oesophagectomy: abdominothoracic approach

Introduction

The goal of this operation is to remove an oesophageal cancer with the widest possible lymphatic clearance (two-field lymphadenectomy) which comprises upper abdominal lymphadenectomy and lymphatic clearance of the posterior and mid mediastinum.

Indications

- Thoracic oesophageal carcinoma.
- Benign stricture, if the transhiatal approach is not advised (adherence to trachea, aorta).

Contraindications

See 'Contraindications' for the transhiatal approach.

Approach

- Patient in the left lateral position for the thoracic part of the operation (Figure 13.32).
- Anterolateral thoracotomy through the fifth intercostal space.
- Repositioning to the supine position.
- Upper transverse incision with a median extension.

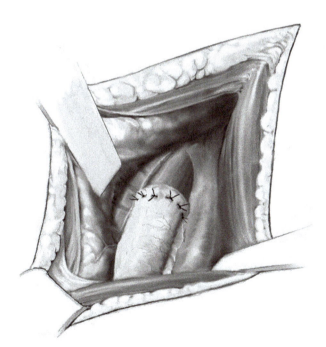

Figure 13.30 U-shaped interrupted sutures provide an inversion of the oesophagus into the gastric tube.
Reproduced with permission from Reeh, M., Yekebas, E.F., Izbicki, J. (2016). Subtotal esophagectomy: transhiatal approach. In: Clavien, PA., Sarr, M., Fong, Y., Miyazaki, M. (eds) *Atlas of Upper Gastrointestinal and Hepato-Pancreato-Biliary Surgery*. Springer, Berlin, Heidelberg. https://doi.org/10.1007/978-3-662-46546-2_11

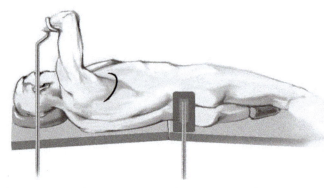

Figure 13.32 Left lateral positioning for thoracic part of operation.
Reproduced with permission from Nentwich, M., Kutup, A. (2016). Subtotal esophagectomy: abdominothoracic approach. In: Clavien, PA., Sarr, M., Fong, Y., Miyazaki, M. (eds) *Atlas of Upper Gastrointestinal and Hepato-Pancreato-Biliary Surgery*. Springer, Berlin, Heidelberg. https://doi.org/10.1007/978-3-662-46546-2_12

Procedure

Thoracic part

- Thoracotomy through the fifth intercostal space from the apex of the scapula to the submammary fold (Figure 13.32).
- Positioning of two retractors. Single left lung ventilation.
- The mediastinal pleura is incised along the resection line for the en bloc oesophagectomy.
- The incision begins at the pulmonary ligament, circumcising the dorsal part of the hilum of the lung and along the right bronchus (Figure 13.33). It follows the right main bronchus at the lateral margin of the superior vena cava up to the thoracic aperture.
  - Exposure of the pulmonary ligament is improved if the lung is pushed cranially and laterally. Care must be taken not to injure the vein of the lower lobe of the right lung.

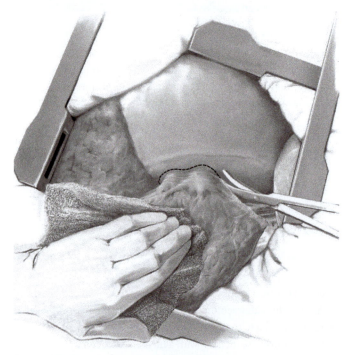

Figure 13.33 Division of the pulmonary ligament.
Reproduced with permission from Nentwich, M., Kutup, A. (2016). Subtotal esophagectomy: abdominothoracic approach. In: Clavien, PA., Sarr, M., Fong, Y., Miyazaki, M. (eds) *Atlas of Upper Gastrointestinal and Hepato-Pancreato-Biliary Surgery*. Springer, Berlin, Heidelberg. https://doi.org/10.1007/978-3-662-46546-2_12

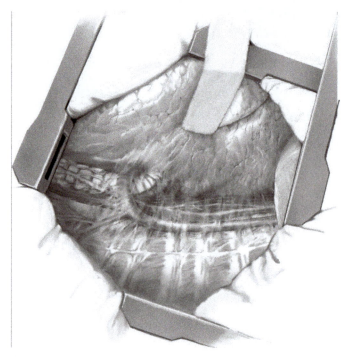

Figure 13.34 Identification of the right phrenic nerve.
Reproduced with permission from Nentwich, M., Kutup, A. (2016). Subtotal esophagectomy: abdominothoracic approach. In: Clavien, PA., Sarr, M., Fong, Y., Miyazaki, M. (eds) *Atlas of Upper Gastrointestinal and Hepato-Pancreato-Biliary Surgery*. Springer, Berlin, Heidelberg. https://doi.org/10.1007/978-3-662-46546-2_12

- Change the direction of the incision line caudally along the right margin of the spine down to the diaphragm along the azygos vein.
  - Always identify the right phrenic nerve (Figure 13.34).
- The superior vena cava and the azygos vein are dissected. Suture ligation towards the vena cava and ligation of the azygos venal stump are performed (Figure 13.35).
- Lymphadenectomy starts from the superior vena cava up to the confluence of the two venae anonymae. Dissection of the brachiocephalic trunk and right subclavian artery is followed by dissection of the right vagus nerve and identification of the right recurrent laryngeal nerve.

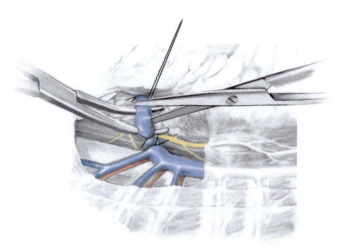

Figure 13.35 Ligation of the azygos vein.
Reproduced with permission from Nentwich, M., Kutup, A. (2016). Subtotal esophagectomy: abdominothoracic approach. In: Clavien, PA., Sarr, M., Fong, Y., Miyazaki, M. (eds) *Atlas of Upper Gastrointestinal and Hepato-Pancreato-Biliary Surgery*. Springer, Berlin, Heidelberg. https://doi.org/10.1007/978-3-662-46546-2_12

Subtotal en bloc oesophagectomy: abdominothoracic approach

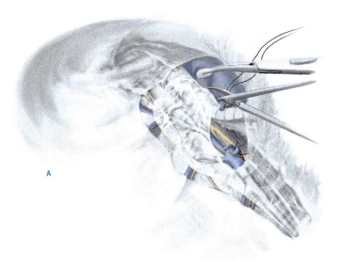

Figure 13.36 Radical lymphadenectomy along the dorsal wall of the superior vena cava.

Reproduced with permission from Nentwich, M., Kutup, A. (2016). Subtotal esophagectomy: abdominothoracic approach. In: Clavien, PA., Sarr, M., Fong, Y., Miyazaki, M. (eds) *Atlas of Upper Gastrointestinal and Hepato-Pancreato-Biliary Surgery*. Springer, Berlin, Heidelberg. https://doi.org/10.1007/978-3-662-46546-2_12

- Caudal to the branching of the recurrent laryngeal nerve, the vagus nerve is transected and the distal part pushed towards the en bloc specimen.
- Lymphadenectomy is performed along the dorsal wall of the superior vena cava (Figure 13.36).
- After completing the preparation of the superior vena cava, the trachea and the right-sided main bronchus are completely freed from lymphatic tissue.
- Dissection of the pre- and paratracheal fat and lymphatic tissue towards the oesophagus is performed (Figure 13.37).

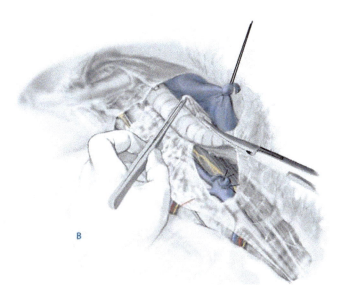

Figure 13.37 Pre- and paratracheal fat and lymphatic tissue dissected towards the oesophagus.

Reproduced with permission from Nentwich, M., Kutup, A. (2016). Subtotal esophagectomy: abdominothoracic approach. In: Clavien, PA., Sarr, M., Fong, Y., Miyazaki, M. (eds) *Atlas of Upper Gastrointestinal and Hepato-Pancreato-Biliary Surgery*. Springer, Berlin, Heidelberg. https://doi.org/10.1007/978-3-662-46546-2_12

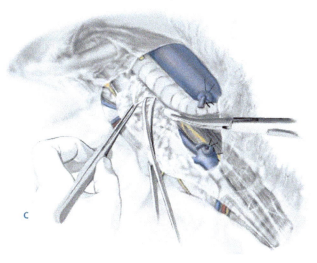

Figure 13.38 Dissection of the retrotracheal lymph nodes.

Reproduced with permission from Nentwich, M., Kutup, A. (2016). Subtotal esophagectomy: abdominothoracic approach. In: Clavien, PA., Sarr, M., Fong, Y., Miyazaki, M. (eds) *Atlas of Upper Gastrointestinal and Hepato-Pancreato-Biliary Surgery*. Springer, Berlin, Heidelberg. https://doi.org/10.1007/978-3-662-46546-2_12

- Dissection of the retrotracheal lymph nodes (Figure 13.38).
  - During this step, care should be taken not to injure the membranaceous part of the trachea.
  - *Expert tip*: direct suture or pericardial flap should be used in case of injury to the trachea.
- Lymph node dissection continues with the upper paraoesophageal lymph nodes (Figure 13.39). All intercostal veins draining into the azygos vein are ligated and divided (Figure 13.40).
- Lymphadenectomy of the subcarinal lymph nodes is performed with dissection of the left main bronchus (Figure 13.40).
- Para-aortic lymphadenectomy is performed (Figure 13.41), dissecting the oesophageal branches of the thoracic aorta and ligating these (Figure 13.42).

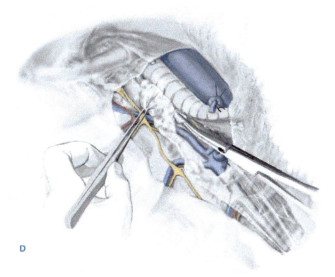

Figure 13.39 Dissection of the upper para-oeosophageal nodes.

Reproduced with permission from Nentwich, M., Kutup, A. (2016). Subtotal esophagectomy: abdominothoracic approach. In: Clavien, PA., Sarr, M., Fong, Y., Miyazaki, M. (eds) *Atlas of Upper Gastrointestinal and Hepato-Pancreato-Biliary Surgery*. Springer, Berlin, Heidelberg. https://doi.org/10.1007/978-3-662-46546-2_12

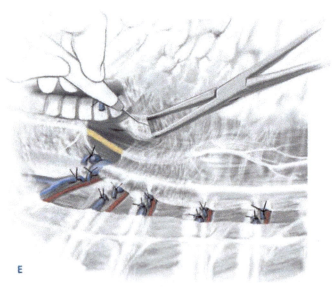

Figure 13.40 Lymph node dissection along the left main bronchus.
Reproduced with permission from Nentwich, M., Kutup, A. (2016). Subtotal esophagectomy: abdominothoracic approach. In: Clavien, PA., Sarr, M., Fong, Y., Miyazaki, M. (eds) *Atlas of Upper Gastrointestinal and Hepato-Pancreato-Biliary Surgery*. Springer, Berlin, Heidelberg. https://doi.org/10.1007/978-3-662-46546-2_12

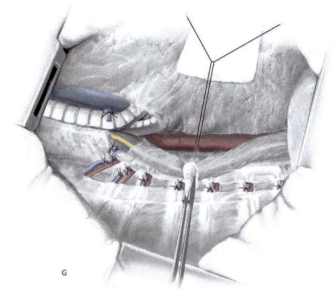

Figure 13.42 Ligation of the aortic oesophageal branches.
Reproduced with permission from Nentwich, M., Kutup, A. (2016). Subtotal esophagectomy: abdominothoracic approach. In: Clavien, PA., Sarr, M., Fong, Y., Miyazaki, M. (eds) *Atlas of Upper Gastrointestinal and Hepato-Pancreato-Biliary Surgery*. Springer, Berlin, Heidelberg. https://doi.org/10.1007/978-3-662-46546-2_12

- Identification and dissection of the thoracic duct with double ligatures directly above the diaphragm and at the level of the main carina (Figure 13.43).
- Completion of mediastinal lymphadenectomy with removal of the left-sided para-aortic and retropericardial lymph nodes as well as the intermediate and lower lobe bronchus down to the oesophageal hiatus.
- After complete mobilization of the oesophageal specimen, thoracic drains are placed in the right thoracic cavity.
- Closure of the thoracic incision and repositioning for abdominal part.

Abdominal part

See transhiatal approach.

Abdominothoracic en bloc oesophagectomy with high intrathoracic anastomosis

High intrathoracic anastomosis may be performed without compromising the oncological requirements as an alternative to collar anastomosis for the treatment of intrathoracic tumours.

- *Benefits*: shorter operating time.

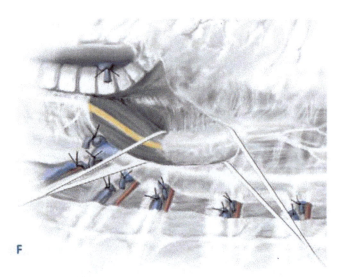

Figure 13.41 Para-aortal lymphadenectomy (oesophagus lateralized by rubber band placement).
Reproduced with permission from Nentwich, M., Kutup, A. (2016). Subtotal esophagectomy: abdominothoracic approach. In: Clavien, PA., Sarr, M., Fong, Y., Miyazaki, M. (eds) *Atlas of Upper Gastrointestinal and Hepato-Pancreato-Biliary Surgery*. Springer, Berlin, Heidelberg. https://doi.org/10.1007/978-3-662-46546-2_12

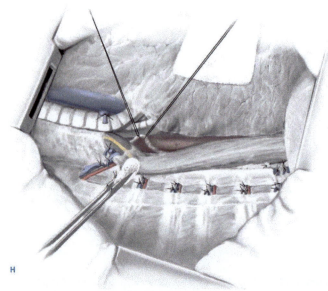

Figure 13.43 Identification of the thoracic duct and double ligation.
Reproduced with permission from Nentwich, M., Kutup, A. (2016). Subtotal esophagectomy: abdominothoracic approach. In: Clavien, PA., Sarr, M., Fong, Y., Miyazaki, M. (eds) *Atlas of Upper Gastrointestinal and Hepato-Pancreato-Biliary Surgery*. Springer, Berlin, Heidelberg. https://doi.org/10.1007/978-3-662-46546-2_12

- *Risk*: developing significant mediastinitis when anastomotic leakage occurs.

Approach

- Helical positioning of the patient with 45° elevation of the right thorax and elevated arm.
- Supine positioning by turning the table for the abdominal part.
- Turn the table to the left for the thoracic part.

Procedure

Abdominal part and mobilization of the oesophagus

See transhiatal approach.

High intrathoracic anastomosis

- Transection of the oesophagus 5 cm below the upper thoracic aperture over a purse-string 45 clamp. Alternatively, the oesophagus can be transected and a monofilament running suture applied as a purse-string suture.
- Dilatation of the proximal oesophageal stump with a blunt clamp. The anvil of a circular stapler (28 mm preferably) is introduced into the oesophageal stump and fixation performed using the purse-string suture.
- Mobilization of the gastric tube through the diaphragmatic oesophageal hiatus is performed followed by resection of the apex of the gastric tube. Introduce the stapler into the gastric tube and perforate the wall at the prospective anastomotic site with the head of the stapling device (Figure 13.44).

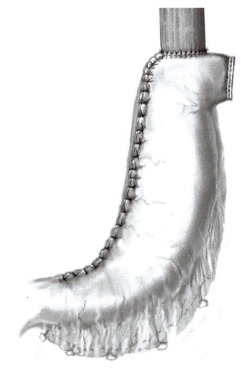

Figure 13.45 End-to-side gastro-oesophagostomy.
Reproduced with permission from Nentwich, M., Kutup, A. (2016). Subtotal esophagectomy: abdominothoracic approach. In: Clavien, PA., Sarr, M., Fong, Y., Miyazaki, M. (eds) *Atlas of Upper Gastrointestinal and Hepato-Pancreato-Biliary Surgery*. Springer, Berlin, Heidelberg. https://doi.org/10.1007/978-3-662-46546-2_12

- In case of a limited length of the gastric tube, the stapling device is inserted through a ventral gastrotomy, and an end-to-end gastro-oesophagostomy is performed.
- Connection of the anvil is followed by firing the instrument (Figure 13.45).
- Check for completeness of the anastomotic rings by removing the stapler and disconnecting the anvil from the stapler head.
- Closure and resection of the protruding part of the anastomosis are done using a linear stapler.
- Insertion of a nasogastric feeding tube over the anastomosis and placed into the first jejunal loop for decompression and postoperative enteral feeding.
- Placement of a thoracic drainage in the right thoracic cavity.

Limited resection of the gastro-oesophageal junction with isoperistaltic jejunal interposition

Limited resection of the gastro-oesophageal junction includes complete removal of the oesophageal segment containing metaplastic mucosa, the lower oesophageal sphincter, and part of the lesser gastric curvature, after which a neofundus is created.

Even early-stage adenocarcinomas of the distal oesophagus (T1b) seed lymph node metastases in up to 20% of patients, making removal of the lymph nodes of the lesser curvature, the hepatic and splenic arteries, the coeliac trunk, the para-aortal region, and the inferior mediastinum an essential part of the operation. In patients with early tumours, staged as uT1a on preoperative endosonography

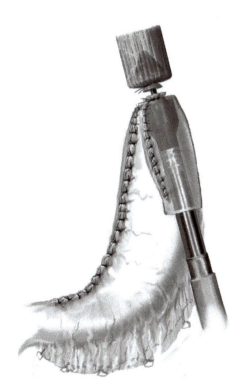

Figure 13.44 Introduction of the stapler into the gastric tube.
Reproduced with permission from Nentwich, M., Kutup, A. (2016). Subtotal esophagectomy: abdominothoracic approach. In: Clavien, PA., Sarr, M., Fong, Y., Miyazaki, M. (eds) *Atlas of Upper Gastrointestinal and Hepato-Pancreato-Biliary Surgery*. Springer, Berlin, Heidelberg. https://doi.org/10.1007/978-3-662-46546-2_12

or severe dysplasia in the distal oesophagus (Barrett's oesophagus), a limited resection of the proximal stomach, cardia, and distal oesophagus with interposition of a pedicled isoperistaltic jejunal segment offers excellent functional and oncological results.

Indications

- Severe dysplasia in the distal oesophagus (Barrett's oesophagus).
- Distal adenocarcinoma of the oesophagus (stage T1a and b) (Union for International Cancer Control (UICC) 2005 classification).
- For palliation (stenotic tumour with severe dysphagia or profuse haemorrhage in selected patients).

Contraindications

- Oesophageal carcinoma staged T2 and higher.
- Long Barrett's segment above the carina.

Approach

- Upper transverse incision with median T-shaped.
- Insertion of a Rochard retractor to elevate costal margin.

Procedure

- The left liver lobe is completely mobilized and the lesser omentum is incised medial to the anterior and posterior gastric vagal branches. A longitudinal median diaphragmatic incision enables exposure of the inferior posterior mediastinum.
- The distal oesophagus is then mobilized including the paraoesophageal tissue. The vagal nerves are divided.
- Intraoperative oesophagoscopy identifies the cranial limit of the Barrett's segment by diaphanoscopy. This marks the proximal resection margin (Figure 13.46).
- Lymphadenectomy around the splenic and hepatic artery is performed, the left gastric vein is divided, and the left gastric artery is

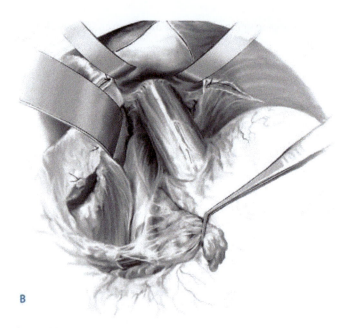

Figure 13.47 Lymphadenectomy.
Reproduced with permission from Dohrmann, T., Mann, O., Izbicki, J. (2016). Laparoscopic and conventional limited resection of the gastroesophageal junction with isoperistaltic jejunal interposition. In: Clavien, PA., Sarr, M., Fong, Y., Miyazaki, M. (eds) *Atlas of Upper Gastrointestinal and Hepato-Pancreato-Biliary Surgery*. Springer, Berlin, Heidelberg. https://doi.org/10.1007/978-3-662-46546-2_13

divided at the coeliac trunk. The coeliac trunk and the para-aortic region above the coeliac trunk are then cleared from lymphatic tissue (Figure 13.47).

- Approximately 1 cm proximal to the cranial limit of the Barrett's segment or carcinoma, a purse-string clamp is placed and the oesophagus divided (Figure 13.48).

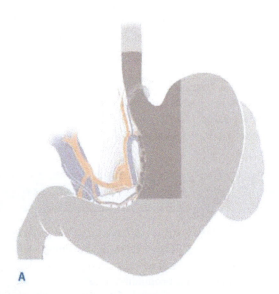

Figure 13.46 Diaphanoscopy identifies the cranial extent of Barrettnial extent
Reproduced with permission from Dohrmann, T., Mann, O., Izbicki, J. (2016). Laparoscopic and conventional limited resection of the gastroesophageal junction with isoperistaltic jejunal interposition. In: Clavien, PA., Sarr, M., Fong, Y., Miyazaki, M. (eds) *Atlas of Upper Gastrointestinal and Hepato-Pancreato-Biliary Surgery*. Springer, Berlin, Heidelberg. https://doi.org/10.1007/978-3-662-46546-2_13

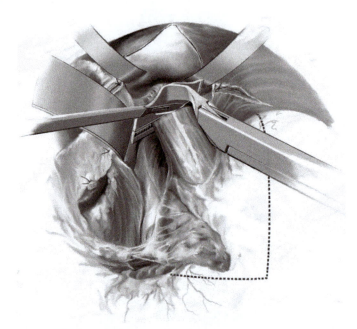

Figure 13.48 Oesophageal transection.
Reproduced with permission from Dohrmann, T., Mann, O., Izbicki, J. (2016). Laparoscopic and conventional limited resection of the gastroesophageal junction with isoperistaltic jejunal interposition. In: Clavien, PA., Sarr, M., Fong, Y., Miyazaki, M. (eds) *Atlas of Upper Gastrointestinal and Hepato-Pancreato-Biliary Surgery*. Springer, Berlin, Heidelberg. https://doi.org/10.1007/978-3-662-46546-2_13

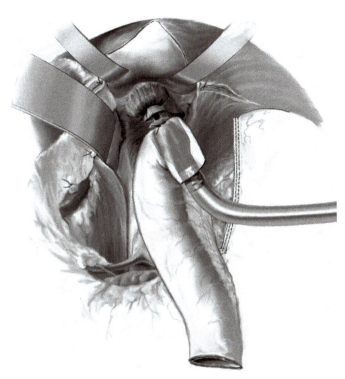

Figure 13.49 Stapler introduction into the jejunal interponate.
Reproduced with permission from Dohrmann, T., Mann, O., Izbicki, J. (2016). Laparoscopic and conventional limited resection of the gastroesophageal junction with isoperistaltic jejunal interposition. In: Clavien, PA., Sarr, M., Fong, Y., Miyazaki, M. (eds) *Atlas of Upper Gastrointestinal and Hepato-Pancreato-Biliary Surgery*. Springer, Berlin, Heidelberg. https://doi.org/10.1007/978-3-662-46546-2_13

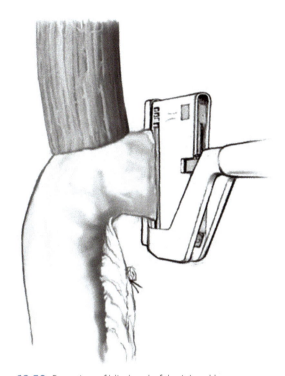

Figure 13.50 Resection of blind end of the jejunal loop.
Reproduced with permission from Dohrmann, T., Mann, O., Izbicki, J. (2016). Laparoscopic and conventional limited resection of the gastroesophageal junction with isoperistaltic jejunal interposition. In: Clavien, PA., Sarr, M., Fong, Y., Miyazaki, M. (eds) *Atlas of Upper Gastrointestinal and Hepato-Pancreato-Biliary Surgery*. Springer, Berlin, Heidelberg. https://doi.org/10.1007/978-3-662-46546-2_13

- Removal of the cardia and lesser curvature is performed by placing multiple linear staplers down to the border between antrum and body. Thus, a neofundus is formed.
  - In case an advanced tumour stage is encountered, possible extension of the operation including transhiatal oesophagectomy or oesophagogastrectomy should be performed.
- A 15–20 cm long segment of the proximal jejunum is isolated and transposed with its mesenteric root to the diaphragmatic region through the mesocolon and behind the stomach.
  - Care must be taken while dissecting the vascular pedicle of this jejunal interposition to provide adequate length. It is imperative to form an isoperistaltic jejunal interposition which can be pulled up retrogastrically and retrocolically.
- The proximal anastomosis is performed using a circular stapling device (28.0 mm) as a terminolateral oesophagojejunostomy.
- The stapler is introduced into the end of the jejunal interponate (Figure 13.49). After firing of the anastomosis, the blind end of the loop is then resected and closed by a linear stapler and oversewn (Figure 13.50).
- Close to the base of the neofundus the gastric stapler line is removed over a distance of 3.0–4.0 cm and a terminolateral or laterolateral jejunogastrostomy performed (Figure 13.51).
- The remaining gastric suture line is oversewn. A terminoterminal jejunojejunostomy reconstructs the enteric passage. Drainage of the mediastinum is warranted by two soft drains from the abdomen. Finally, an anterior and/or posterior hiatal repair is performed.

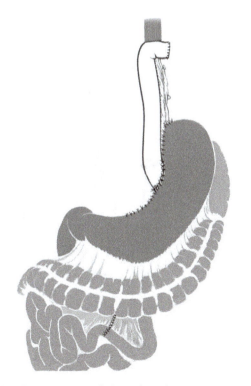

Figure 13.51 Construction of a latero-lateral jejunogastrostomy.
Reproduced with permission from Dohrmann, T., Mann, O., Izbicki, J. (2016). Laparoscopic and conventional limited resection of the gastroesophageal junction with isoperistaltic jejunal interposition. In: Clavien, PA., Sarr, M., Fong, Y., Miyazaki, M. (eds) *Atlas of Upper Gastrointestinal and Hepato-Pancreato-Biliary Surgery*. Springer, Berlin, Heidelberg. https://doi.org/10.1007/978-3-662-46546-2_13

REFERENCES

1. Wiseman R. *Several Chirurgicall Treatises*. London: R. Royston; 1676.
2. Stoffel. Quoted in Hochberg LA. *Thoracic Surgery Before the 20th Century*. New York: Vantage Press; 1960.
3. Verduc J. *Traite des Operations de Chirurgie*. Paris: Laurent d'Houry; 1701.
4. Gross SW. American gastrostomy, oesophagostomy, internal oesophagotomy, combined oesophagotomy, oesophagectomy and retrograde divulsion in the treatment of stricture of the oesophagus. *Am J Med Sci*. 1884;**88**:58–69.
5. Morton WTG. *On the Physiological Effects of Sulphuric Ether, and its Superiority to Chloroform*. Boston, MA: David Clapp; 1850.
6. Pasteur L. *Etudes sur le Vin. Imprimenss Imperials-Gauthier-Villars*. Paris: Masson; 1866.
7. Lister J. On the antiseptic principle in the practice of surgery. *Br Med J*. 1867;**2**:246.
8. Billroth T. Quoted in Hurwitz A, Degenshein GA, Hoeber PB, James M. Milestones in modern surgery. *Ann Surg*. 1958;**148**:866.
9. Czerny V. Neue operationen. *Zentralbl Chir*. 1877;**4**:433–434.
10. Meltzer SJ, Auer J. Continuous respiration without respiratory movements. *J Exp Med*. 1909;**11**:622.
11. Flemming A. On the antibacterial action of cultures of penicillin with special reference to their use in the isolation of B. influenzae. *Br J Exp Pathol*. 1929;**10**:226.
12. Brewer LA. History of surgery of the esophagus. *Am J Surg*. 1980;**139**:730–743.
13. Barrett N. Spontaneous perforation of the oesophagus: review of the literature and report of three new cases. *Thorax*. 1946;**1**:48.
14. Torek F. The first successful resection of the thoracic portion of the esophagus for carcinoma: preliminary report. *JAMA*. 1913;**60**:1533.
15. Lanman TH. Congenital atresia of the esophagus: a study of thirty-two cases. *Arch Surg*. 1940;**41**:1060–1083.
16. Turner G. *The Esophagus*. London: Cassell and Company; 1946.
17. Oshawa T. The surgery of the oesophagus. *Arch Jpn Chir*. 1933;**10**:605.
18. Sweet R. Surgical management of cancer of the mid-esophagus. Preliminary report. *N Engl J Med*. 1945;**233**:1–7.
19. Lewis I. The surgical treatment of carcinoma of the oesophagus with special reference to a new operation for growths of the middle third. *Br J Surg*. 1946;**34**:18–31.

14

Oesophageal cancer
Minimally invasive surgery and robotic surgery

Gijsbert van Boxel, Pieter C. van der Sluis, Peter P. Grimminger, and Richard van Hillegersberg

Introduction

The oesophagus and its surrounding lymphatic tissue can be resected en bloc through several surgical approaches in the treatment of oesophageal cancer: (1) transhiatal, (2) Ivor Lewis (abdominal and right thoracic approach), (3) McKeown (abdominal, right thoracic, and cervical approach), or (4) left thoracoabdominal (thoraco-phrenico-laparotomy incision). The variety of approaches brings with it multiple permutations within which minimally invasive methods can be applied. The term 'minimally invasive oesophagectomy' (MIO) is therefore, at times confusingly, used to describe the spectrum of minimally invasive methods applied to the variety of surgical approaches to the treatment of cancer of the oesophagus. For example, a laparoscopic transhiatal oesophagectomy is a form of MIO, but does not include a formal two-field lymphadenectomy. Equally, an Ivor Lewis procedure performed by means of a laparoscopic abdominal phase and a right (open) thoracotomy could be considered a form of MIO, but still requires a large thoracic incision.

In general, MIO by means of a transthoracic approach (transthoracic oesophagectomy (TTO)) is now probably the most common modality of oesophageal resection; the term MIO should be considered to refer to a totally minimally invasive Ivor Lewis (two-stage, intrathoracic anastomosis) or McKeown (three-stage, cervical anastomosis) oesophagectomy.[1] In instances where either the abdominal or thoracic phase is performed by open surgery, the procedure should be referred to as 'hybrid' oesophagectomy (commonly laparoscopic abdomen and right thoracotomy). Minimally invasive left-sided approaches to the oesophagus are not routinely performed due to its right-sided position and are only described in the context of specific pathology in case report format.

The rationale behind the development of MIO mirrors that of most other minimally invasive approaches in surgery: expected faster recovery, reduced blood loss, less pain, earlier mobilization and a reduction in perioperative complications, smaller scars, and improved quality of life. Of course, this has to be matched by equal (or better) functional and oncological outcomes, both in the short and long term. This chapter reviews the history, technical aspects, and evidence for MIO. More recently, the introduction of robotic systems for MIO, robot-assisted minimally invasive oesophagectomy (RAMIO), has dramatically increased the uptake of this procedure. The value of robotics, technical considerations, and available evidence will be considered.

History of minimally invasive oesophagectomy

A minimally invasive approach to part of an Ivor Lewis oesophagectomy was first described in 1992.[2] In this case series of five patients, the oesophagus was mobilized by video-assisted thoracoscopic surgery combined with laparotomy for the abdominal phase. The first step towards a complete MIO was by means of a laparoscopic transhiatal approach, although this approach omits a formal two-field lymphadenectomy, which has since become the standard of care in the treatment of oesophageal cancer.[3] Subsequently, minimally invasive Ivor Lewis and McKeown procedures were developed involving a laparoscopic abdominal phase combined with a thoracoscopic thoracic phase. Concerns about the thoracoscopic component with regard to its safety, standardization, and reproducibility across centres led to the development of the 'hybrid' oesophagectomy consisting of an open thoracotomy while maintaining a laparoscopic abdominal phase.

In 2003, Luketich et al. reported the first substantial series of true MIO (thoracoscopy plus laparoscopy) showing low morbidity and mortality in 222 patients. Postoperative outcomes were good, although there were some concerns about oncological radicality at the time.[4]

MIO was performed with the patient in the left lateral decubitus position during the thoracic phase of the operation. However, this approach required single-lung ventilation with a double-lumen tube and was therefore proposed to be accompanied by potentially more significant pulmonary complications. In order to standardize the technique of MIO, and consequently overcome the associated technical difficulties, MIO in a prone position was reported in a large patient cohort.[5] Several groups adopted this approach and a systematic review showed that the prone position for the thoracic phase of the operation was feasible, indeed had lower respiratory complications compared to open surgery, and reduced operative time likely because of the superior exposure of the operative field and the better ergonomics of the surgeon's stance.[6] Conversely, urgent conversion to a classic right-sided lateral thoracotomy, if needed, is more difficult in the prone position. Oesophageal resection in a modified semi-prone position was thus adopted by surgeons around the world, as a solution to overcome this potential surgical challenge, while retaining the majority of the benefits of the prone position.[7]

A recent survey of worldwide practice showed that the uptake of MIO has increased dramatically; in 2007, 14% of patients were operated by MIO, compared to 43% in 2015.[8] Dutch cancer registries, for example, now show that greater than 85% of oesophagectomies are performed and completed by minimally invasive methods.[9]

Surgical techniques

Ivor Lewis oesophagectomy is a two-phase operation requiring repositioning of the patient during the procedure. Typically, the procedure commences with the abdominal phase, unless there is, for example, concern about resectability of the tumour in the thorax.

Abdominal phase

Patient positioning

The abdominal phase is performed with the patient in the supine position. The surgeons either positions themselves on the right side of the patient, or between the legs ('French position'). Depending on the phase of the operation, the operation table can be tilted in an anti-Trendelenburg position (head-end up) and/or left side up during the mobilization of the greater curve and division of the short gastric vessels. Both arms should be secured by the side of the patient to allow for easy access by the surgical team and avoid overstretching the arm by table position.

Port positioning and resectional approach

Port positioning varies according to individual surgeon's preference, but all aim to create adequate triangulation in the supraumbilical area, liver retraction (static or dynamic), and assistance. Typically, a 12 mm camera port is placed about 8–10 cm below the xiphisternum (two-thirds along a vertical line from the xiphisternum to the umbilicus). A further two 12 mm ports are placed on either side of the camera ports in a roughly horizontal line. An assistant port is placed in the left flank and a liver retractor is either introduced from the xiphisternum (Nathanson) or from the right flank (liver paddle (Medtronic, Minneapolis, MN, USA) or static snake liver retractor; Artisan Medical Devices, Medford, NJ, USA). An advantage of the handheld liver retractor is that its position can be easily changed to allow for retraction of the stomach during the coeliac trunk lymphadenectomy.

A variety of approaches have been described with regard to the abdominal dissection and lymphadenectomy during an oesophagectomy. The oncological principles established during open surgery remain and radical lymphadenectomy has been shown to be vital in long-term survival. Most surgeons will advocate a 'no grasp technique' with regard to the stomach as this will become the gastric conduit and any disruption to its submucosal blood supply can be catastrophic. Equally, great care should be taken not to cause thermal damage during the dissection of the greater curve by keeping a distance from the right gastroepiploic artery which will form the main blood supply of the gastric conduit. During the dissection, the right gastric, left gastric, and short gastric arteries and veins are all ligated and associated lymph tissue resected according to D2 principles. A gastric conduit is commonly formed intracorporeally using a stapling device (more details below).

Hiatal dissection inevitably produces a significant defect through which the gastric conduit will be pulled up. Nonetheless, consideration needs to be given to partial closure of the hiatus, although most surgeons choose to do this once the conduit has been pulled up (during the thoracic phase). Sutures can also be placed during the abdominal phase which can be tied from the thorax once the appropriate calibre of the hiatus has been established. Alternatively, these sutures are placed thoracoscopically, although traditional straight (non-articulated) instrumentation makes this challenging. Once the dissection is completed, a feeding jejunostomy may be created and the wounds closed. The patient is then turned onto their left side (right side up) for the thoracic phase of the procedure.

Gastric conduit formation

It has become uniform practice throughout the world to form a conduit from the stomach following resection of the oesophagus. The blood supply of the conduit is notoriously precarious, running singly on the right gastroepiploic artery and its submucosal arterioles. Linear cutting staplers are commonly used (either 45 or 60 mm) to form a tube starting at the angulus, following the greater curve of the stomach. The best width of the tube is still a topic of discussion, but most groups adopt 4 cm to not cause stenosis, but to retain good neo-oesophageal function. Advances in stapler technology (such as tri-staplers) have resulted in fewer surgeons opting to oversew the staple line of the conduit.

Routine use of indocyanine green to assess gastric conduit blood supply is not standard practice, but the technology is rapidly becoming more commonplace in resectional oesophageal surgery. The fluoroscopic dye allows visualization of poorly perfused areas, which are particularly relevant if present at the tip of the conduit as this is the site of the oesophagogastric anastomosis.

Practice with regard to managing the gastric pylorus varies greatly. The use of botulinum toxin injections, endoscopic balloon dilatation, or pyloromyotomy are all practised in MIO but convincing evidence on which approach is best is lacking.[10,11]

Thoracic phase

Patient positioning

Patient positioning is crucial in all surgery, but particularly relevant in the thoracic phase of an oesophagectomy. The objectives are to have good access to the posterior mediastinum to permit careful dissection of the oesophagus and its associated lymphatic tissue. The right lung and vertebral column hinder direct access and the use of the prone position may make this worse. The semi-prone position can aid in gaining access and has therefore been adopted more frequently in the past few years. The intercostal spaces are relatively small and 12 mm port insertion can be challenging as a consequence.

The spaces can be enlarged by extending the right shoulder to 90° and 'breaking' the table in the mid-thoracic region.

Semi-prone

Figure 14.1 shows the patient in the semi-prone position. Typically, four ports are placed in the intercostal spaces 5, 7, 8, 6/5 forming an arc. After decompression of the right lung (either by means of a double-lumen tube or a bronchial blocker), CO_2 at 6–8 mmHg is insufflated through one of the assistant ports to keep the lung out of the operative field. Following division of the right pulmonary ligament, an extensive en bloc mediastinal lymph node dissection is performed (para-oesophageal, infra-carinal, aortic pulmonary window, subcarinal, with or without paratracheal). The azygos arch is ligated and the thoracic duct clipped about 5 cm above the level of the diaphragm where it is more likely to have no further tributaries and thus reducing the chance of chylothorax.[12] Hereafter, the oesophagus is mobilized and resected en bloc with the surrounding mediastinal and subcarinal lymph nodes, and the thoracic duct.

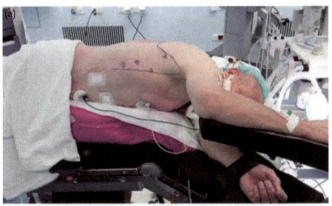
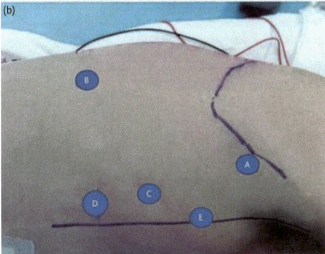

Figure 14.1 Semi-prone patient positioning for thoracic phase of RAMIO. Four robotic trochars are used (A-D) with a further assistant port (E).
Reproduced from Seesing MF, Goense L, Ruurda JP, Luyer MD, Nieuwenhuijzen GA, van Hillegersberg R. Minimally invasive esophagectomy: propensity score-matched analysis of semi-prone versus prone position. Surg Endosc. 2018; 32 (6):2758–65 under a Creative Commons Attribution 4.0 International License (http://creativecommons.org/licenses/by/4.0/)

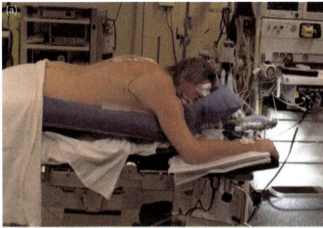
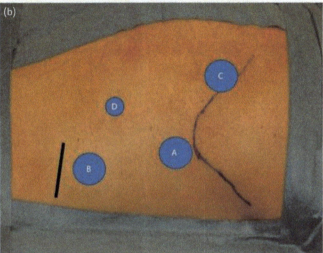

Figure 14.2 Prone position patient for MIO. Three 10mm ports (A-C) and a further 5mm port.
Reproduced from Seesing MF, Goense L, Ruurda JP, Luyer MD, Nieuwenhuijzen GA, van Hillegersberg R. Minimally invasive esophagectomy: propensity score-matched analysis of semi-prone versus prone position. Surg Endosc. 2018; 32 (6):2758–65 under a Creative Commons Attribution 4.0 International License (http://creativecommons.org/licenses/by/4.0/)

Prone

During prone positioning for MIO (Figure 14.2), a 12 mm camera port is commonly placed posterior to the tip of the scapula and CO_2 is insufflated to a pressure of 6–8 mmHg. The second and third 12 mm ports are placed in the eighth intercostal space in the right posterior axillary line and medial to the scapula, respectively. A 5 mm port is placed halfway between the spine and the original eighth intercostal port. The resectional strategy is nearly identical to that described in the prone position, although the orientation is different from the semi-prone position.

Specimen extraction

The standard Ivor Lewis oesophagectomy commences in the abdomen and the patient is turned to permit the thoracic phase thereafter. As a result, the specimen is most commonly extracted through a mini-thoracotomy created by extending one of the thoracoscopic port sites. In some situations (e.g. where there is a question about operability in the thorax; stage 4B tumour), the surgeon may opt the to start with the thoracoscopic part of the operation and the specimen is extracted at the end of the abdominal phase. Equally, in the context of transhiatal MIO, the specimen is extracted through the abdominal wall. Here, extraction of the specimen typically requires a 4–5 cm incision (dependent on the bulk of the tumour) and practice varies between units. The midline incision can be extended to form a mini-laparotomy. Alternatively, the left-sided 12 mm port can be widened to create a small transverse incision. The incidence of port/extraction site metastases in laparoscopic oncological surgery has been a topic of extensive research and the aetiology remains unclear. Despite any evidence, the use of wound protectors is advocated to reduce wound infections and, potentially, reduce the risk of tumour seeding.

Oesophagogastric anastomosis

The oesophagogastric anastomosis constructed following oesophagectomy has many variations. It can be formed in the chest or in the neck; be handsewn, stapled, or a combination of both; and end to end, end to side, or side to side. In the context of MIO, all these varieties exist. Although handsewn anastomoses have become more commonplace in the context of RAMIO, in the absence of wristed instruments, most MIO anastomosis will encompass a stapled element. Typically, a linear stapling device is used and the remaining enterotomy closed with a barbed suture, or a circular stapling device (e.g. OrVil, Medtronic) can be used with the anker introduced through the mouth. The main considerations are anastomotic integrity and functionality including low benign stricture rates. A recent meta-analysis showed that stapled anastomoses are associated with reduced leak rates and reduced stricture rates.[13] However, this study included cervical, intrathoracic, linear, and circular stapled techniques and did not specifically investigate this question in the context of MIO.

Learning curve

Training in complex minimally invasive surgical techniques such as a two-stage oesophagectomy is a long process with learning curves from 50 to 119 cases described.[14,15] A recent meta-analysis suggested as many as 36 anastomotic leaks in a series of 646 should be directly attributed to the learning curve.[14] Equally, early series in MIO have reported higher rates of acute gastric conduit necrosis, which in some cases were attributed to technique and to the learning curve effect.[15]

Evidence for minimally invasive oesophagectomy

Trials and studies

The number of randomized controlled trials comparing minimally invasive methods to open surgery for oesophagectomy are small. In fact, a lot of the current evidence base is dependent on reported case series and subsequent meta-analyses. With this in mind, current evidence should be recognized to reflect a heterogeneous population and a technique which is by no means standardized.

The first published randomized control trial comparing outcomes after minimally invasive TTO and open TTO was the Traditional Invasive vs. Minimally invasive Esophagectomy (TIME) trial in 2012.[16] To date, this study remains the only randomized controlled trial comparing MIO to open TTO. It assessed several perioperative outcomes, oncological outcomes, and quality of life measurements, even though the study was primarily powered to assess perioperative pulmonary complications. Beyond the TIME trial, there are multiple meta-analyses completed between 2009 and 2019, which have compared perioperative and oncological outcomes of MIO and open oesophagectomy (OO). These studies are primarily based on case series, although the increased uptake of MIO over the past decade has led to studies including over 15,000 patients.[17,18]

The MIRO trial was the first to compare open TTO with hybrid two-stage oesophagectomy (laparoscopic abdominal phase and open thoracic phase).[19] The primary end point was 30-day morbidity (grade II–IV on the Clavien–Dindo system). This trial recruited 207 patients from 12 centres and showed a reduction in major postoperative morbidity (odds ratio 0.31, 95% confidence interval (CI) 0.18–0.55; p <0·001) with equivalent 3-year oncological outcomes.[20]

Perioperative outcomes and complications

Operative time and intraoperative blood loss are commonly used in studies as surrogate markers for the quality and ease of surgery. In MIO, the total operative time has been shown to be consistently longer compared to OO. The TIME trial reported the average operative time to be 330 minutes for MIO compared to 300 minutes for OO (p = 0.002). These findings have been mirrored in multiple meta-analyses. A reduction in intraoperative blood loss was reported in the TIME trial: 200 mL for MIO patients compared to 475 mL for OO patients.[16] Again, this observation was mirrored in the majority of meta-analyses.

The most recent meta-analysis assessing perioperative complications in MIO compared to OO included nearly 6000 cases of oesophageal resections and reported a complication rate of 41.5% for the MIO group, compared to 48.2% for the OO group (p <0.05).[21] This finding was similar to that reported previously showing significant differences in total complications between the open group and MIO group.[22,23] Surgical technique-related complications such as splenic laceration, tracheal laceration, pneumothorax, chylothorax, and haemorrhage appear reduced in MIO patients once the surgeon has passed the learning curve.[24]

The primary outcomes of the TIME trial were pulmonary complications, although definitions, particularly of pneumonia, were not standardized and the relatively high rate of reported pulmonary complications, particularly in the open group (36%), was questioned.[16] Although controversial, the TIME trial showed that MIO was superior to OO in terms of postoperative pulmonary infections (relative risk (RR) 0.30, 95% CI 0.12–0.76; p = 0.005).[16] Meta-analyses by Nagpal et al.,[22] Guo et al.,[23] and Ly et al.[25] showed that patients had less respiratory complications (RR 0.74, 95% CI 0.58–0.94; p = 0.01) following MIO compared to OO.

Cardiovascular complications such as arrhythmia, acute myocardial infarction, and subsequent heart failure are not uncommon following oesophagectomy. There are no meta-analyses that specifically compare the incidence of these complications between MIO and OO. In the TIME trial, however, these were less common in MIO group of patients compared to those who underwent the open procedure (odds ratio 0.770, 95% CI 0.681–0.872; p <0.05).[16]

Anastomotic leak following oesophagectomy is a dreaded complication because it is associated with significant morbidity and mortality. The rate of this complication ranges from 4% to 17% and has proved to be similar between MIO and OO groups.[26]. Zhou et al. performed a meta-analysis specifically investigating the incidence of anastomotic leak in MIO compared to OO.[27] This study included 5537 patients from 43 separate studies and showed an incidence of anastomotic leak of 8.3% in the MIO group compared to 9.7% in OO; this was not statistically significant.[27] It is worth noting that the study population was heterogeneous reflecting the various locations and techniques of anastomosis construction; ultimately this question can only be answered in a randomized controlled trial.

The incidence of recurrent laryngeal nerve palsy has been reported in previous studies to range between 3.6% and 7%.[4] Despite the fact that the TIME trial and Xiong et al.[28] showed a significantly lower rate of vocal cord palsies and recurrent laryngeal nerve injuries in MIO, meta-analyses conducted by Nagpal et al.,[22] Guo et al.,[23] and Sgourakis et al.[29] have failed to show any significance difference between MIO and OO.

The reduced surgical trauma associated with minimally invasive surgery has led to reduced hospital stays following major resectional surgery in a variety of specialties. The desire to reduce physiological insult, reduce complications, and increase early ambulation was anticipated to reduce hospital stay for MIO patients following oesophagectomy and improve the early quality of life. The TIME trial showed that the average hospital stay for MIO is 11 days compared to 14 days for OO (p 0.044). A study by Rodham et al.[30] reviewed the available case series and trials in 2015 and concluded that all bar one study showed either reduced or equal length of stay for MIO. It should be noted that the introduction of MIO significantly overlaps with 'enhanced recovery' pathways which will potentially be a confounding factor in many of these comparative studies.

While the results of MIO are promising, population-based studies in the UK, Japan, the US, and the Netherlands have demonstrated increased reintervention rates after MIO.[24,31–33] Some authors postulated that this was possibly an effect of the learning curve that was experienced by surgeons and centres during the early adaptation phase. This may be a plausible explanation, as the MIO learning curve can be associated with additional morbidity and takes 50–119 cases, depending on the chosen parameters of proficiency.[14] Regardless, these data represent the outcomes in the countries of inclusion and should therefore be carefully considered. As such, follow-up studies are warranted to investigate whether the reintervention rate has normalized in the more recent years.

Oncological outcomes

Oncological outcomes include rate of R0 resection, lymph node retrieval, and disease-free and overall survival.

A R0 resection rate was reported in 92% of MIO and 84% of OO in the TIME trial. It is worth noting that R0 resection rates appear to be affected by the type of neoadjuvant therapy given and, unless compared in the context of a prospective trial, comparative case series may be misleading.

The studies comparing the number of lymph nodes harvested in MIO compared to OO show that the resection is at least equal in MIO patients. The TIME trial showed no significant difference in lymph node yield.[16] Equally, meta-analyses by Osugi et al.[34] and Smithers et al.[35] reported an equal number of lymph nodes. Conversely, Dantoc et al.[36] found an increased number of harvested lymph nodes during MIO compared to OO (16 vs 10; $p = 0.025$).

Although earlier it was suggested that there was a possible early survival benefit for MIO compared with OO, analysis of long-term disease-free and overall survival appear equivalent in MIO compared to OO.[37,38] The TIME trial reported on 3-year outcomes and showed no significant difference between the groups.[39] A recent meta-analysis, however, which included 14,592 patients, concluded that long-term survival in MIO compares 'well' with OO and 'may even be better' on the grounds that the pooled analysis showed a 18% reduction in all-cause mortality for MIO compared to OO.[40]

The future of minimally invasive oesophagectomy

Advances in minimally invasive technology and expertise have seen a rapid increase in the uptake of MIO. The evidence to date supports this technique to be oncologically equivalent and likely to cause a reduction in postoperative complications. Advances in robotic technology and the expected increase in available systems over the coming years will increase further the use of minimally invasive methods.

Several trials are currently recruiting patients comparing MIO to open (robotic—see later) oesophagectomy to further assess safety, perioperative morbidity, and long-term outcomes. A multicentre, prospective, randomized, open, and parallel controlled trial in China aims to compare the effectiveness of MIO to open McKeown oesophagectomy for resectable oesophageal cancer. It is expecting to recruit 324 patients in each arm over a 3-year period.[41] The use of RAMIO as a treatment for oesophageal cancer will be discussed in the next section.

Robot-assisted minimally invasive thoraco-laparoscopic oesophagectomy

History

RAMIO (also known as RAMIE) was developed in the UMC Utrecht in the Netherlands in 2003.[42] Compared to conventional minimally invasive surgery, robotic surgery benefits from a stable ten times magnified three-dimensional view. The articulated instruments enable precise tissue handling and dissection with seven degrees of freedom of movement.[43] These technical advantages are helpful in the difficult mediastinal (lymph node) dissection around vital organs, such as the heart, aorta, pulmonary vein, trachea, and bronchi.[42,43] Conventional MIO is a technically difficult procedure and learning curves from 50 to 119 cases have been described.[14,15] For this reason, MIO is not routinely applied as a standard approach for oesophageal cancer worldwide.[32] RAMIO might overcome these difficulties by the superior view and articulated instruments. For the development of RAMIO by our group, a five-stage development process for the assessment of surgical innovation (*IDEAL*) was followed.[44]

Our first experience, with 21 patients with resectable oesophageal cancer undergoing RAMIO (stage 1, *Idea*), was described in a prospective cohort study in 2006.[42] Technical feasibility and early technical modifications were described in 2009 in a prospective cohort study including 47 patients (stage 2a, *Development*).[45] In 2015, the oncological long-term follow-up was described in a prospective cohort study including 108 patients.[46] (stage 2b, *Exploration*). Stage 1–2b focused on the development of a new technique and the description of its outcomes. Stage 3 (*Assessment*) aims to assess effectiveness against current standards. For resectable oesophageal cancer, the open TTO is considered to be the gold standard worldwide.[8] Therefore we decided to compare RAMIO to open TTO in a single-centre randomized controlled trial.[47]

Before analysis of a novel surgical technique with the current standards can be performed, the learning curve of the novel technique has to be completed. In 2012, when the trial was initiated, our centre was the only centre worldwide that had clearly passed the learning phase with a joint experience of more than 170 RAMIO procedures.[48] As no other institution worldwide had comparable surgical expertise, it was decided to perform a single-centre randomized controlled trial. The trial design, rationale, and the protocol were published in 2012.[47]

Between January 2012 and August 2016, 236 patients with resectable intrathoracic oesophageal cancer were screened in the UMC Utrecht, of whom 138 patients were considered eligible for the ROBOT trial. Finally, 112 patients (allocation ratio 81%) were randomized in a 1:1 fashion to undergo either RAMIO or open TTO and 109 patients were included in the intention-to-treat analysis.[49] The primary end point of the occurrence of overall surgery-related postoperative complications (MCDC grade ≥2) occurred in 32 of 54 patients after RAMIO (59%) and in 44 of 55 patients after open TTO (80%) (RR with RAMIO 0.74, 95% CI 0.57–0.96; $p = 0.02$). Pulmonary complications were the most frequently observed secondary end point and occurred in 17 of 54 patients in the RAMIO group (32%) and in 32 of 55 patients in the open TTO group (58%) (RR 0.54, 95% CI 0.34–0.85; $p = 0.005$). Cardiac complications were observed in 17 of 45 patients in the RAMIO group (22%) and in 26 of 55 patients in the open TTO group (47%) (RR 0.47, 95% CI 0.27–0.83; $p = 0.006$). Functional recovery at postoperative day 14 was significantly better in the RAMIO group: 38 of 54 patients (70%) compared to the open TTO group (28 of 55 patients, 51%) (RR 1.48, 95% CI 1.03–2.13; $p = 0.04$). Mean postoperative pain (visual analogue scale) during the first 14 days was significantly lower after RAMIO compared to open TTO (1.86 vs 2.62; $p < 0.001$). Both at discharge as well as 6 weeks after discharge, quality of life was higher after RAMIO compared to open TTO (mean difference 13.4 (95% CI 2.0–24.7; $p = 0.02$) and 11.1 (95% CI 1.0–21.1; $p = 0.03$), respectively).[49]

It was concluded that RAMIO was associated with a significantly lower percentage of postoperative complications compared to open TTO. RAMIO was also associated with less blood loss, a lower percentage of pulmonary complications and cardiac complications compared to open TTO, lower postoperative pain, and better functional recovery and short-term quality of life. Oncological outcomes, such as the percentage of radical resections (R0), the number of resected lymph nodes, and disease-free and overall survival were comparable between groups and in concordance with the highest standards worldwide nowadays. Together with the previous randomized trial comparing MIO to open TTO (TIME trial),[13] results of this randomized controlled trial provide evidence to use minimally invasive surgery for patients with resectable oesophageal cancer aiming at improving postoperative outcomes and quality of life.[12]

Stage 4 (*Long-term study*) of the IDEAL recommendations is currently assessed with the extension of indications for RAMIO in upper oesophageal cancer with upper mediastinal lymph node metastases, cT4b oesophageal cancer following downstaging with neoadjuvant therapy or other types of salvage surgery, and registration of cases in the national registry database, the Dutch Upper Gastrointestinal Cancer Audit, and the worldwide Upper GI International Robotic Association online platform.

Operation technique

Robotic abdominal phase: preparation, positioning, and trocar placement

All patients receive a thoracic epidural catheter preoperatively to decrease the risk of postoperative pulmonary failure and to improve analgesic quality. Currently, a multicentre randomized controlled trial is being performed in the Netherlands in which the epidural catheter is compared to paravertebral anaesthesia in order to establish which anaesthetic management is the best for patients undergoing oesophagectomy.[50]

Patients receive two large-bore peripheral cannulae, a central venous line in the right internal jugular vein, an arterial line, a urinary catheter, and a nasogastric tube. Currently, the role of the central venous line is assessed in order to facilitate faster postoperative recovery. Antibiotic prophylaxis is provided by intravenous administration of 2000 mg cefazolin and 500 mg metronidazole. Patients are intubated using a double-lumen tube, using both lumens in the abdominal phase.

For the Ivor Lewis approach with an intrathoracic anastomosis, the patient is first put in a supine anti-Trendelenburg position, tilted to the right for the robotic abdominal phase using the da Vinci Xi robotic system (Intuitive Surgical Inc., Sunnyvale, CA, USA).[51] Figure 14.1 shows the position of the robotic trocars. The camera is inserted through the umbilical 12 mm assistant port. In this way, all robotic trocars can be introduced under direct vision. Pneumoperitoneum is created with CO_2 insufflation of 12 mm Hg. The 8 mm robotic ports are placed in the following positions: left lateral, left and right pararectal, and right lateral (Figure 14.1). The robotic patient side cart is placed at the right side of the patient The trocars are docked and the robotic instruments are installed in the following order: arm 1, cadiere forceps; arm 2, robotic vessel sealer; arm 3, camera; and arm 4, monopolar cautery hook. The snake liver retractor (Artisan Medical Devices) is placed through a 5 mm port in the right flank (Figure 14.1).

Robotic abdominal phase: operative procedure

A left pleural Jackson–Pratt drain is placed in the left pleural sinus through the eighth intercostal space to facilitate the release of a possible pneumothorax. First, the abdominal cavity and the liver are inspected for possible metastases followed by opening of the hepatogastric ligament. The liver is retracted upwards to get a good view of the gastro-oesophageal junction using the snake liver retractor. The lesser omentum/hepatogastric ligament is transected at the level of the pars flaccida, close to the liver (Figure 14.3). Hereafter the peritoneum of the left and right crus of the diaphragm are opened. The greater curvature is dissected in the direction of the duodenum and spleen with special attention given to preserve the right gastroepiploic arcade using the robotic vessel sealer

Robot-assisted minimally invasive thoraco-laparoscopic oesophagectomy

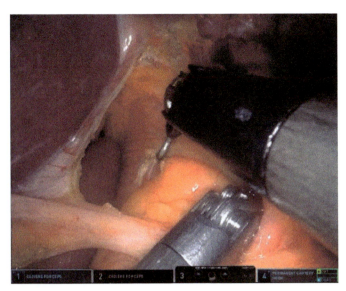

Figure 14.3 Dissection of the hepatogastric ligament to the hiatus.

(Figure 14.4). The colonic hepatic flexure is mobilized from the duodenum and adhesions to the gallbladder are transected. The stomach is lifted upwards, enabling transection of retrogastric adhesions. Using the robotic vessel sealer, the short gastric vessels are transected at the level of the gastric wall to prevent involvement of the retroperitoneal splenic vessels (Figure 14.5).

The left gastric vein and artery are isolated by using the monopolar cautery hook. The left gastric vein is transected with the robotic vessel sealer and the left gastric artery is transected after ligation with robotic Hem-o-Lok clips (Weck Closure Systems, Research Triangle Park, NC, USA) (Figure 14.6). Abdominal lymphadenectomy includes lymph nodes surrounding the left gastric artery, the splenic artery, common hepatic artery, and the lesser omental lymph nodes (stations 1–3, 7–9, and 11) (Figure 14.7). The distal oesophagus is dissected at the level of the crus, with special attention to the aorta and intrathoracic part of the inferior vena cava. The right gastric artery and vein are transected at the level just above the crow's foot whereafter the gastric conduit of about 3–4 cm in width is formed using a robotic 60 mm linear stapler (SureForm, Intuitive Surgical Inc., Sunnyvale). The tip of the gastric conduit is reattached to the resection specimen with 3-0 Vicryl sutures, in line with the resection specimen, to facilitate pull-up to the mediastinum during the thoracic phase. The hiatal dissection is hereafter completed (Figure 14.8). The trocars are removed under vision and the wounds are closed with a Monocryl and the assistant port with Vicryl and Monocryl sutures.[51] A jejunostomy feeding tube is placed robotically in the second jejunal loop after Treitz's ligament.

Robotic thoracic phase: preparation, positioning, and trocar placement

To enable selective single-lung ventilation of the right lung during the thoracic phase, patients are intubated with a left-sided double-lumen tube. Adequate positioning of the double-lumen tube is achieved with a fibreoptic bronchoscope. Patients are positioned in the left lateral decubitus position, tilted 45° towards the prone position (semi-prone) to keep the collapsed lung from the operating field (Figure 14.9). To minimize postoperative pulmonary complications, 10 mg/kg methylprednisolone is administered. The operating table is flexed, lowering the legs and upper thorax to extend the

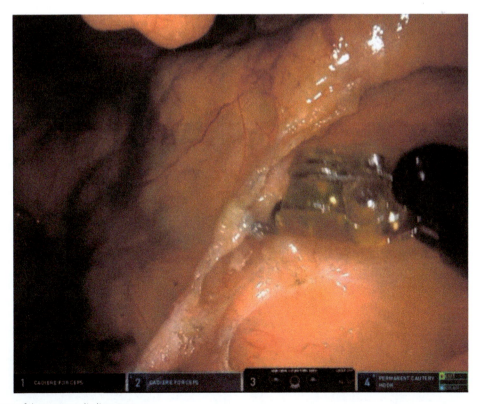

Figure 14.4 Dissection of the gastrocolic ligament.

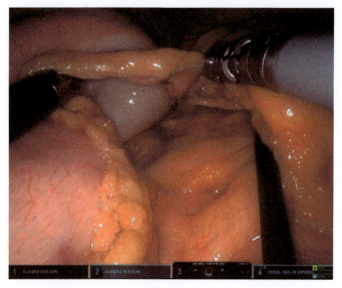

Figure 14.5 Dissection of the short gastric vessels.

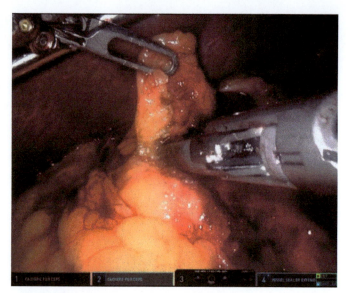

Figure 14.7 Dissection of the hepatic artery.

thorax maximally and to widen the intercostal space for introduction of the trocars. The trocar positions are marked relative to the scapula following a curved line in order to avoid collision (Figure 14.9). The robotic system is placed at the right side of the patient (Figure 14.4). Before incision, the right lung is collapsed. A robotic trocar is placed in the sixth intercostal space. CO_2 is insufflated up to a level of 8 mmHg to enhance desufflation of the right lung. Under vision, robotic trocars are placed in the fourth, eighth, and tenth intercostal spaces. A 12 mm assistant trocar is placed in the fifth intercostal space (Figure 14.9). The robotic patient side cart is placed at the right side of the patient and targeted. The oesophagus at the level of the left main bronchus is used as the target point. The trocars are docked and the robotic instruments are installed in the following order: arm 1, cadiere forceps; arm 2, vessel sealer; arm 3, 30° endoscope (camera); and arm 4, permanent monopolar cautery hook.

Robotic thoracic phase: operative procedure

By use of the cautery hook, the pulmonary ligament is divided and the parietal pleura at the right side of the oesophagus is dissected. The azygos arc is divided using robotic Hem-o-lok clips (Figure 14.10). The parietal pleura is dissected up to the level above the azygos arc and the oesophagus is dissected from the trachea. The vagal nerve is identified and spared at this level. A right paratracheal lymph node dissection is performed (Figure 14.11). The trachea, the right main bronchus and the superior caval vein are used as borders for dissection. The oesophagus is lifted with the second arm and the trachea and left main bronchus are exposed. A lymph node dissection along the left recurrent nerve is performed (Figure 14.12). The right vagal nerve is transected at the level of the caudal border of the right main bronchus, sparing the bronchial branches.

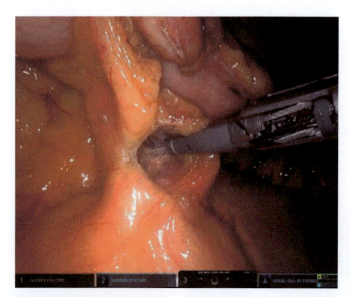

Figure 14.6 Left gastric division.

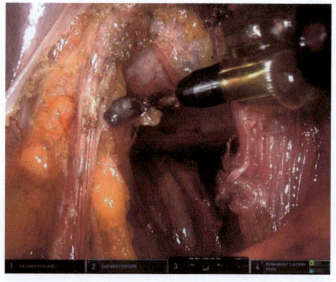

Figure 14.8 Hiatal dissection.

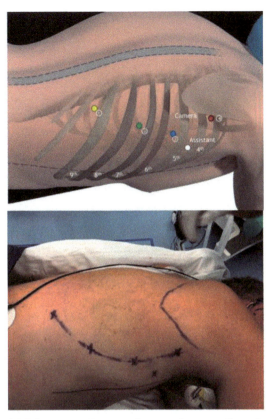

Figure 14.9 Patient positioning and trocars placement (thoracic phase).

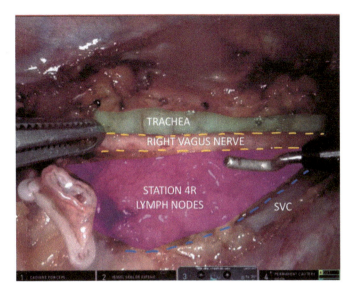

Figure 14.11 Right paratracheal dissection.

Hereafter the parietal pleura on the left side of the oesophagus is opened cranially to caudally along the azygos vein and the oesophagus with para oesophageal lymph nodes are dissected up to the level of the aorta. The aorta-oesophageal vessels are divided with a sealer and the dorsal aortic branches preserved (Figure 14.13). The thoracic duct is clipped with a Hem-o-Lok at the level of the diaphragm and included in the resection specimen (Figure 14.14). The oesophagus is dissected from the pericardium (Figure 14.15) and lifted with the second arm, followed by dissection over the pulmonary vein up to the level of the subcarinal nodes, which are dissected en bloc (Figure 14.16). Finally, the oesophagus is mobilized at the level of the crus and the gastric conduit pulled in to the chest using the cadiere and the small grasper forceps.

The oesophagus is transected with the cautery hook, above the level of the azygos arc. The incision for the trocar in the eighth intercostal space is widened and an Alexis port (Applied Medical, Rancho Santa Margarita, CA, USA) is placed, which serves as a wound protector. The resection specimen is removed through the Alexis port and hereafter, the robotic trocar is re-placed. With a Vicryl 4-0 suture, the muscular and mucosal layer of the oesophagus are relined to prevent muscular slip of the oesophageal wall during the construction of the anastomosis and stay sutures placed at each quadrant. Indocyanine green is used to find the level of demarcation of the gastric conduit tip (Figure 14.6). The excess gastric conduit is removed by robotic 65 mm stapling at the level of demarcation. After alignment of the gastric conduit in the former oesophageal tract, the cautery hook is used to open the gastric

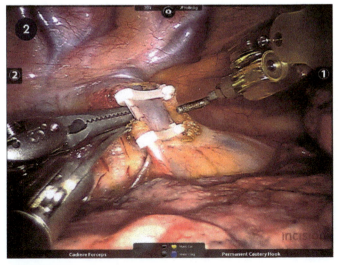

Figure 14.10 Division of the azygos vein.

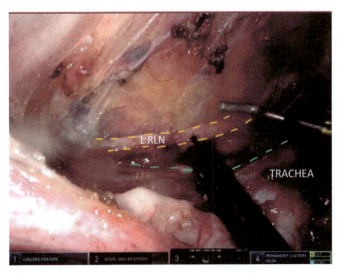

Figure 14.12 Left paratracheal dissection.

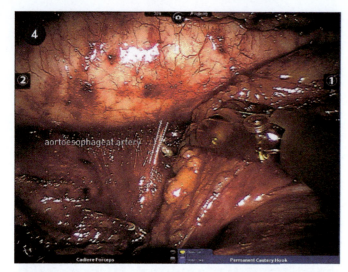

Figure 14.13 Dissection of the aorta and aorto-oesophageal branches.

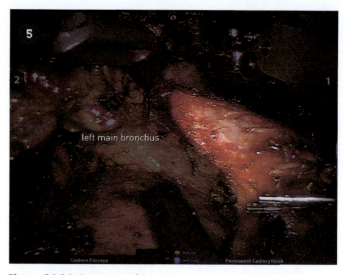

Figure 14.16 Dissection of the carina.

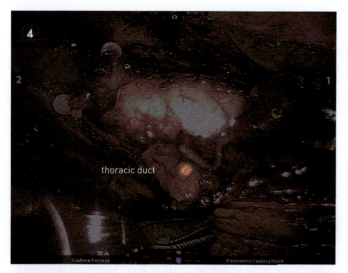

Figure 14.14 Dissection of the thoracic duct.

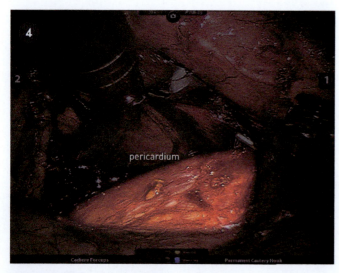

Figure 14.15 Pericardial dissection.

tube. V-Loc 4-0 (Medtronic) is used for a handsewn running end-to-side oesophagogastric anastomosis (Figure 14.8). Vicryl 3-0 is used for four anti-traction sutures, covering the anastomosis with a layer of gastric conduit (Figure 14.9). Hereafter, an omental wrap is placed, covering the anastomosis completely and fixed with sutures (Figure 14.10). The diaphragm is closed with a crural plasty using Mersilene 0.

It is also possible to perform the oesophagogastric anastomosis with a circular stapler. After full mobilization and dissection of the specimen, the assistant trocar port is widened in the direction towards the middle axillary line, similar to a mini-thoracotomy. A medium-sized Alexis wound retractor is inserted. The 28 mm stapler head of the circular stapler (DST Series EEA, Medtronic) is inserted though the mini-thoracotomy into the oesophageal stump and a Prolene 2.0 purse-sting suture is knotted manually using the knot pusher. The 8 mm 30° endoscope is inserted via trocar number 1 and hand guided. The oesophageal specimen is pulled out extracorporeally through the mini-thoracotomy, which results in the pulling up of the prepared gastric conduit into the chest. The lesser curvature is opened to insert the circular stapler into the stomach. The stapler is then pushed into the chest and positioned manually for the best suited position for the anastomosis. After the circular anastomosis is performed, the da Vinci Xi is docked onto the patient again with the following set-up: 8 mm 30° endoscope in trocar 1 (intercostal space 10), robotic EndoWrist stapler 45 mm in trocar 2 (intercostal space 8), and the vessel sealer in trocar 3 (intercostal space 6). The camera is on the far left; the stapler can be guided using the left hand, and the vessel sealer using the right hand. A thick 38-French gastric tube is inserted into the gastric conduit to prevent narrowing the conduit during the final step in stapling the rest of the gastric conduit (Figure 14.4). After the specimen is completely stapled apart and recovered, the position for the V-Loc running suture around the circular anastomosis is performed using the tip-up fenestrated grasper in trocar 1, the fenestrated bipolar forceps in trocar 2, the da Vinci 8 mm 30° endoscope in trocar 3, and the needle driver in trocar 4. Hereafter, an omental wrap is placed, covering the anastomosis completely and fixed with sutures and anti-tension pleural stitches are placed.[51]

After placement of a chest tube the right lung is insufflated. The wounds are closed with a Vicryl 1 and a Monocryl suture Both the oesophagus and cardia resection specimen and the excess gastric conduit are sent for pathological examination and the paratracheal, subcarinal, peri-oesophageal, and left gastric artery are marked in the resection specimen.

When there is an indication for a cervical anastomosis, the robotic thoracic phase is performed first followed by the robotic abdominal phase and an open cervical phase for a handsewn end-to-side oesophagogastrostomy (McKeown).[42]

Conclusion

The ROBOT trial showed that RAMIO resulted in a lower percentage of overall surgery-related and cardiopulmonary complications with less postoperative pain, better short-term quality of life, and a better postoperative functional recovery compared to open TTO.[49] Oncological outcomes were equal and in concordance with the highest standards at present. This randomized controlled trial provided evidence for the use of RAMIO to improve short-term postoperative outcomes in patients with resectable oesophageal cancer.[49]

The question remains whether RAMIO is superior to conventional MIO, which has shown comparable benefits compared to OTE in a randomized trial (TIME trial).[16] There is considerable evidence that both MIO and RAMIO are alternatives to the standard OO for oesophageal cancer. However, it remains to be shown whether the technical advantages of RAMIO contribute to better results compared to conventional MIO.

In Asian studies, where RAMIO was compared to MIO, a higher mean lymph node yield along the recurrent laryngeal nerve was observed in favour of RAMIO.[52–54] Furthermore, RAMIO showed a reduced rate of recurrent laryngeal nerve injury compared to MIO.[55] In a retrospective cohort analysis, 50 RAMIO procedures were compared to 50 MIO procedures.[56] Compared to MIO, RAMIO showed improved lymphadenectomy compared to conventional MIO (27 vs 23 lymph nodes; $p = 0.043$).[56] The technical superiority of RAMIO over MIO due to the three-dimensional, ten times enlarged image combined with the excellent dexterity might results in an improved lymph node dissection and possibly less recurrent laryngeal nerve injuries.[57]

A population-based cohort study in the Netherlands, including 2698 patients, showed that a higher lymph node yield was significantly associated with improved overall survival, indicating a therapeutic value of extended lymphadenectomy during oesophagectomy.[58] With possible better lymphadenectomy with RAMIO, overall and disease-free survival might be superior after RAMIO.

The difference between RAMIO and MIO might also be found in the postoperative fatigue of the surgeon. With RAMIO, the surgeon sits behind the console in an ergonomic better position than with MIO where the surgeon stands at the table. Furthermore, the four-arm technique allows the console surgeon to be in full control of the instruments, camera, and tissue retraction with the fourth arm. With reduced postoperative fatigue after RAMIO, the surgeon might be able to perform at a higher level during the rest of the week.

The aforementioned scientific evidence shows the need for randomized controlled trials comparing RAMIO to conventional MIO. Such randomized controlled trials can only be performed in high-volume centres of oesophageal surgery, in which both RAMIO and MIO are performed on a regular basis with standardized protocols. Furthermore, surgeons in these hospital trials should have passed the learning curve both for MIO and RAMIO.[48]

Currently, there are two Asian multicentre randomized controlled trials recruiting oesophageal squamous cell carcinoma patients comparing RAMIO to conventional MIO: the REVATE trial (ClinicalTrials.gov Identifier: NCT03713749)[57] and the RAMIE trial (ClinicalTrials.gov Identifier: NCT03094351).[59] Results for these trials are awaited with great interest and might answer the question whether RAMIO is superior to MIO for patients with oesophageal squamous cell carcinoma in the Asian population. Together with the results of the ROBOT-2 trial (ClinicalTrials.gov Identifier: NCT04306458), which started in Mainz, Germany, in 2021, the aforementioned trials might elucidate the role of RAMIO compared to MIO in the treatment of oesophageal cancer.

REFERENCES

1. Giugliano DN, Berger AC, Rosato EL, Palazzo F. Total minimally invasive esophagectomy for esophageal cancer: approaches and outcomes. *Langenbecks Arch Surg.* 2016;**401**:747–756.
2. Cuschieri A, Shimi S, Banting S. Endoscopic oesophagectomy through a right thoracoscopic approach. *J R Coll Surg Edinb*. 1992;**37**:7–11.
3. Luketich JD, Nguyen NT, Schauer PR. Laparoscopic transhiatal esophagectomy for Barrett's esophagus with high grade dysplasia. *JSLS*. 1998;**2**:75–77.
4. Luketich JD, Alvelo-Rivera M, Buenaventura PO, et al. Minimally invasive esophagectomy: outcomes in 222 patients. *Ann Surg.* 2003;**238**:486–494.
5. Palanivelu C, Prakash A, Senthilkumar R, et al. Minimally invasive esophagectomy: thoracoscopic mobilization of the esophagus and mediastinal lymphadenectomy in prone position—experience of 130 patients. *J Am Coll Surg.* 2006;**203**:7–16.
6. Koyanagi K, Ozawa S, Tachimori Y. Minimally invasive esophagectomy performed with the patient in a prone position: a systematic review. *Surg Today.* 2016;**46**:275–284.
7. Seesing MF, Goense L, Ruurda JP, Luyer MD, Nieuwenhuijzen GA, van Hillegersberg R. Minimally invasive esophagectomy: propensity score-matched analysis of semi-prone versus prone position. *Surg Endosc.* 2018;**32**:2758–2765.
8. Haverkamp L, Seesing MF, Ruurda JP, et al. Worldwide trends in surgical techniques in the treatment of esophageal and gastroesophageal junction cancer. *Dis Esophagus* 2017;**30**:1–7.
9. DUCA annual report or publication (https://dica.nl/duca/home) accessed on 29/01/2023.
10. Akkerman RD, Haverkamp L, van Hillegersberg R, Ruurda JP. Surgical techniques to prevent delayed gastric emptying after esophagectomy with gastric interposition: a systematic review. *Ann Thorac Surg.* 2014;**98**:1512–1519.
11. Hadzijusufovic E, Tagkalos E, Neumann H, et al. Preoperative endoscopic pyloric balloon dilatation decreases the rate of delayed gastric emptying after Ivor-Lewis esophagectomy. *Dis Esophagus.* 2019;**32**:doy097.
12. Schurink B, Defize IL, Mazza E, et al. Two-field lymphadenectomy during esophagectomy: the presence of thoracic duct lymph nodes. *Ann Thorac Surg.* 2018;**106**:435–439.

13. Zhang X, Yu Q, Tian H, Lv D. Meta-analysis of stapled versus hand-sewn esophagogastric anastomosis *Int J Clin Exp Med*. 2018;**11**:11606–11618.
14. van Workum F, Stenstra MHBC, Berkelmans GHK, et al. Learning curve and associated morbidity of minimally invasive esophagectomy: a retrospective multi-center study. *Ann Surg*. 2019;**269**:88–94.
15. Ramage L, Deguara J, Davies A, et al. Gastric tube necrosis following minimally invasive oesophagectomy is a learning curve issue. *Ann R Coll Surg Engl*. 2013;**95**:329–334.
16. Biere SS, van Berge Henegouwen MI, Maas KW, et al. Minimally invasive versus open oesophagectomy for patients with oesophageal cancer: a multicentre, open-label, randomised controlled trial. *Lancet*. 2012;**379**:1887–1892.
17. Verhage RJ, Hazebroek EJ, Boone J, Van Hillegersberg R. Minimally invasive surgery compared to open procedures in esophagectomy for cancer: a systematic review of the literature. *Minerva Chir*. 2009;**64**:135–146.
18. Biere SS, Cuesta MA, van der Peet DL. Minimally invasive versus open esophagectomy for cancer: a systematic review and meta-analysis. *Minerva Chir*. 2009;**64**:121–133.
19. Briez N, Piessen G, Bonnetain F, et al. Open versus laparoscopically-assisted oesophagectomy for cancer: a multicentre randomised controlled phase III trial—the MIRO trial. *BMC Cancer*. 2011;**11**:310.
20. Mariette C, Markar SR, Dabakuyo-Yonli TS, et al. Hybrid minimally invasive esophagectomy for esophageal cancer. *N Engl J Med*. 2019;**380**:152–162.
21. Yibulayin W, Abulizi S, Lv H, Sun W. Minimally invasive oesophagectomy versus open esophagectomy for resectable esophageal cancer: a meta-analysis. *World J Surg Oncol*. 2016;**14**:304.
22. Nagpal K, Ahmed K, Vats A, et al. Is minimally invasive surgery beneficial in the management of esophageal cancer? A meta-analysis. *Surg Endosc*. 2010;**24**:1621–1629.
23. Guo W, Ma X, Yang S, et al. Combined thoracoscopic-laparoscopic esophagectomy versus open esophagectomy: a meta-analysis of outcomes. *Surg Endosc*. 2016;**30**:3873–3881.
24. Seesing MFJ, Gisbertz SS, Goense L, et al. A propensity score matched analysis of open versus minimally invasive transthoracic esophagectomy in the Netherlands. *Ann Surg*. 2017;**266**:839–846.
25. Lv L, Hu W, Ren Y, Wei X. Minimally invasive esophagectomy versus open esophagectomy for esophageal cancer: a meta-analysis. *Onco Targets Ther*. 2016;**9**:6751–6762.
26. Giugliano DN, Berger AC, Rosato EL, Palazzo F. Total minimally invasive esophagectomy for esophageal cancer: approaches and outcomes. *Langenbecks Arch Surg*. 2016;**401**:747–756.
27. Zhou C, Ma G, Li X, Li J, Yan Y, Liu P, et al. Is minimally invasive esophagectomy effective for preventing anastomotic leakages after esophagectomy for cancer? A systematic review and meta-analysis. *World J Surg Oncol*. 2015;**13**:269.
28. Xiong WL, Li R, Lei HK, Jiang ZY. Comparison of outcomes between minimally invasive oesophagectomy and open oesophagectomy for oesophageal cancer. *ANZ J Surg*. 2017;**87**:165–170.
29. Sgourakis G, Gockel I, Radtke A, et al. Minimally invasive versus open esophagectomy: meta-analysis of outcomes. *Dig Dis Sci*. 2010;**55**:3031–3040.
30. Rodham P, Batty JA, McElnay PJ, Immanuel A. Does minimally invasive oesophagectomy provide a benefit in hospital length of stay when compared with open oesophagectomy? *Interact Cardiovasc Thorac Surg*. 2016;**22**:360–367.
31. Sihag S, Kosinski AS, Gaissert HA, et al. Minimally invasive versus open esophagectomy for esophageal cancer: a comparison of early surgical outcomes from the society of thoracic surgeons national database. *Ann Thorac Surg*. 2016;**101**:1281–1288.
32. Mamidanna R, Bottle A, Aylin P, et al. Short-term outcomes following open versus minimally invasive esophagectomy for cancer in England: a population-based national study. *Ann Surg*. 2012;**255**:197–203.
33. Takeuchi H, Miyata H, Ozawa S, et al. Comparison of short-term outcomes between open and minimally invasive esophagectomy for esophageal cancer using a nationwide database in Japan. *Ann Surg Oncol*. 2017;**24**:1821–1827.
34. Osugi H, Takemura M, Higashino M, Takada N, Lee S, Kinoshita H. A comparison of video-assisted thoracoscopic oesophagectomy and radical lymph node dissection for squamous cell cancer of the oesophagus with open operation. *Br J Surg*. 2003;**90**:108–113.
35. Smithers BM, Gotley DC, Martin I, Thomas JM. Comparison of the outcomes between open and minimally invasive esophagectomy. *Ann Surg*. 2007;**245**:232–240.
36. Dantoc M, Cox MR, Eslick GD. Evidence to support the use of minimally invasive esophagectomy for esophageal cancer: a meta-analysis. *Arch Surg*. 2012;**147**:768–776.
37. Dantoc MM, Cox MR, Eslick GD. Does minimally invasive esophagectomy (MIE) provide for comparable oncologic outcomes to open techniques? A systematic review. *J Gastrointest Surg*. 2012;**16**:486–494.
38. Lazzarino AI, Nagpal K, Bottle A, Faiz O, Moorthy K, Aylin P. Open versus minimally invasive esophagectomy: trends of utilization and associated outcomes in England. *Ann Surg*. 2010;**252**:292–298.
39. Straatman J, van der Wielen N, Cuesta MA, et al. Minimally invasive versus open esophageal resection: three-year follow-up of the previously reported randomized controlled trial: the TIME Trial. *Ann Surg*. 2017;**266**:232–236.
40. Gottlieb-Vedi E, Kauppila JH, Malietzis G, Nilsson M, Markar SR, Lagergren J. Long-term survival in esophageal cancer after minimally invasive compared to open esophagectomy: a systematic review and meta-analysis. *Ann Surg*. 2019;**270**:1005–1017.
41. Mu J, Gao S, Mao Y, et al. Open three-stage transthoracic oesophagectomy versus minimally invasive thoraco-laparoscopic oesophagectomy for oesophageal cancer: protocol for a multicentre prospective, open and parallel, randomised controlled trial. *BMJ Open*. 2015;**5**:e008328.
42. van Hillegersberg R, Boone J, Draaisma WA, Broeders IA, Giezeman MJ, Borel Rinkes IH. First experience with robot-assisted thoracoscopic esophagolymphadenectomy for esophageal cancer. *Surg Endosc*. 2006;**20**:1435–1439.
43. Ruurda JP, Draaisma WA, van Hillegersberg R, et al. Robot-assisted endoscopic surgery: a four-year single-center experience. *Dig Surg*. 2005;**22**:313–320.
44. McCulloch P, Altman DG, Campbell WB, et al. No surgical innovation without evaluation: the IDEAL recommendations. *Lancet*. 2009;**374**:1105–1112.
45. Boone J, Schipper ME, Moojen WA, et al. Robot-assisted thoracoscopic oesophagectomy for cancer. *Br J Surg*. 2009;**96**:878–886.
46. Van der Sluis PC, Ruurda JP, Verhage RJ, et al. Oncologic long-term results of robot-assisted minimally invasive thoraco-laparoscopic esophagectomy with two-field lymphadenectomy for esophageal cancer. *Ann Surg Oncol*. 2015;**22**:1350–1356.

47. Van der Sluis PC, Ruurda JP, Van der Horst S, et al. Robot-assisted minimally invasive thoraco-laparoscopic esophagectomy versus open transthoracic esophagectomy for resectable esophageal cancer, a randomized controlled trial (ROBOT trial). *Trials*. 2012;**13**:230.
48. Van der Sluis PC, Ruurda JP, Van der Horst S, et al. The learning curve for robot-assisted minimally invasive thoraco-laparoscopic esophagectomy for esophageal cancer: results from 312 cases. *Ann Thorac Surg*. 2018;**106**:264–271.
49. van der Sluis PC, van der Horst S, May AM, et al. Robot-assisted minimally invasive thoracolaparoscopic esophagectomy versus open transthoracic esophagectomy for resectable esophageal cancer: a randomized controlled trial. *Ann Surg*. 2019;**269**:621–630.
50. Kingma BF, Eshuis WJ, de Groot EM, et al. Paravertebral catheter versus EPidural analgesia in Minimally invasive Esophageal resectioN: a randomized controlled multicenter trial (PEPMEN trial). *BMC Cancer*. 2020;**20**:142.
51. Grimminger PP, Hadzijusufovic E, Babic B, van der Sluis PC, Lang H. Innovative fully robotic 4-arm Ivor Lewis esophagectomy for esophageal cancer (RAMIE4). *Dis Esophagus*. 2020;**16**:33.
52. Park S, Hwang Y, Lee HJ, Park IK, Kim YT, Kang CH. Comparison of robot-assisted esophagectomy and thoracoscopic esophagectomy in esophageal squamous cell carcinoma. *J Thorac Dis*. 2016;**8**:2853–2861.
53. Chao YK, Hsieh MJ, Liu YH, Liu HP. Lymph node evaluation in robot assisted versus video-assisted thoracoscopic esophagectomy for esophageal squamous cell carcinoma: a propensity-matched analysis. *World J Surg*. 2018;**42**:590–598.
54. Deng HY, Huang WX, Li G, et al. Comparison of short-term outcomes between robot-assisted minimally invasive esophagectomy and video assisted minimally invasive esophagectomy in treating middle thoracic esophageal cancer. *Dis Esophagus*. 2018;**31**:1–7.
55. Jin D, Yao L, Yu J, et al. Robotic-assisted minimally invasive esophagectomy versus the conventional minimally invasive one: a meta-analysis and systematic review. *Int J Med Robot*. 2019;**15**:e1988.
56. Tagkalos E, Goense L, Hoppe-Lotichius M, et al. Robot-assisted minimally invasive esophagectomy (RAMIE) compared to conventional minimally invasive esophagectomy (MIE) for esophageal cancer: a propensity-matched analysis. *Dis Esophagus*. 2020;**33**:doz060.
57. Chao YK, Li ZG, Wen YW, et al. Robotic-assisted Esophagectomy vs Video-Assisted Thoracoscopic Esophagectomy (REVATE): study protocol for a randomized controlled trial. *Trials*. 2019;**20**:346.
58. Visser E, van Rossum PSN, Ruurda JP, van Hillegersberg R. Impact of lymph node yield on overall survival in patients treated with neoadjuvant chemoradiotherapy followed by esophagectomy for cancer: a population-based cohort study in the Netherlands. *Ann Surg*. 2017;**266**:863–869.
59. Yang Y, Zhang X, Li B, et al. Robot-assisted esophagectomy (RAE) versus conventional minimally invasive esophagectomy (MIE) for resectable esophageal squamous cell carcinoma: protocol for a multicenter prospective randomized controlled trial (RAMIE trial, robot-assisted minimally invasive Esophagectomy). *BMC Cancer*. 2019;**19**:60.

15

Oesophageal cancer
Future aspects of treatment

Thorsten Oliver Goetze and Salah-Eddin Al-Batran

Introduction

Gastric and oesophageal carcinomas, including adenocarcinomas of the oesophagogastric junction (OGJ), were responsible for more than 1 million deaths worldwide in 2018. The primary curative treatment method for gastric and OGJ carcinomas is surgical resection, but with surgery alone the 5-year survival rates are unsatisfactory. Therefore, perioperative systemic therapy combinations are becoming increasingly used and are effective for both stomach and junctional tumours. Neoadjuvant radiotherapy or radiochemotherapy is also an option. To date, there have been no direct comparisons between perioperative chemotherapy and neoadjuvant radiochemotherapy. That is why the decision regarding which strategy is the best for the individual patient is often not easy to make.

Gastro-oesophageal carcinomas include squamous cell carcinomas (SCCs) of the oesophagus, proximal adenocarcinomas of the OGJ (oesophageal to subcardiac adenocarcinomas), and distal gastric adenocarcinomas. According to estimates, this group of carcinomas was responsible for more than 1.6 million new cases worldwide and more than 1 million deaths in 2018, and thus is an important public health problem.[1] The incidence of OGJ carcinomas has risen mainly in Western countries. Population-based analyses report an increase in incidence of nearly 2.5-fold since the 1970s in the United States.[2,3] So the main problem and challenge in the Western world when talking about oesophageal cancer in the future concerns adenocarcinomas of the OGJ.

Classification of oesophagogastric junction tumours

A standard system is still missing for classifying junctional tumours. The Siewert classification subdivides junctional tumours into three types, based on the endoscopic assessment of the location of the tumour epicentre and its relationship to the Z-line. This enables tailored surgery as well as a uniform documentation of endoscopic findings and interventions, but depends on the expertise of the endoscopist.[4,5]

- Type I tumours are up to 5 cm proximal of the anatomical transition, the Z-line.
- Type II tumours span the anatomical transition and have their epicentre up to 2 cm below and 1 cm above the Z-line.
- Type III tumours range up to 5 cm below the Z-line into the stomach.[6]

The classification system of the American Joint Committee on Cancer (8th edition) classifies a tumour as an OGJ tumour if its epicentre lies in the distal oesophagus, or reaches less than 2 cm into the proximal stomach (Siewert type I and II) based on surgical resection specimens.[7]

However, sometimes it is difficult for endoscopists to identify the exact epicentre of the tumour, since the intraluminal mass often extends the artificial boundaries of type I to type III. In addition, new molecular profiling studies[8,9] make clear that SCCs of the oesophagus are biologically more similar to SCCs of other organs, for example, head and neck tumours, and differ significantly from type I adenocarcinomas, but are treated with the same surgical technique—an oesophageal resection.

These are all aspects to be addressed in future research on oesophageal and esophagogastric cancers.

Surgery as primary therapy

Surgery remains the primary curative treatment method for these carcinomas. The overall prognosis for this condition with surgery alone includes unsatisfactory 5-year survival rates at an average of 30%, caused by distant and locoregional recurrences.[10] Consequently, neoadjuvant as well as perioperative multimodal concepts (strategies using chemotherapy or radiation or the combination of both) are used, with the intent to address occult micrometastatic seeding and improve the overall survival (OS).

What poses a problem is that gastric, OGJ, and distal oesophageal carcinomas are often treated together within trials as are oesophageal adenocarcinomas and SCCs. While in curative treatment the assignment of perioperative chemotherapy to distal gastric carcinomas and neoadjuvant radiochemotherapy to oesophageal SCC seems to be clear, the area of adenocarcinomas of the OGJ remains controversial. However, considering current data and earlier landmark studies in detail, there is growing evidence based on analysing subgroups of these trials that perioperative chemotherapy seems to be effective.

Multimodal approaches at a glance

Several pioneering studies have established paradigms for multimodal therapy of locally advanced gastro-oesophageal carcinomas with perioperative chemotherapy or preoperative chemoradiotherapy. The Dutch landmark ChemoRadiotherapy for Oesophageal cancer followed by Surgery Study (CROSS) in the year 2012 showed superior R0 resection rates and a significantly improvement of long-term survival with neoadjuvant radiotherapy in combination with simultaneous weekly chemotherapy with carboplatin and paclitaxel in comparison to surgery only. The CROSS trial included mostly type I oesophageal adenocarcinomas, some type II adenocarcinomas of the OGJ, as well as 23% oesophageal SCCs. Accordingly, the CROSS regimen became the standard of care.[11]

Recently, increasingly effective perioperative systemic therapy combinations for both gastric and OGJ carcinomas are also being investigated. The German FLOT4 trial included OGJ carcinomas (56%) and distal gastric adenocarcinomas (44%) and compared docetaxel-based triplet chemotherapy FLOT (5-fluorouracil (5-FU), leucovorin, oxaliplatin, docetaxel) with standard anthracycline-based triplet therapy ECF/ECX (epirubicin, cisplatin, and 5-FU or capecitabine) from the Medical Research Council Adjuvant Gastric Infusional Chemotherapy (MAGIC) trial. The evaluation showed superior results in OS with the FLOT compared to the MAGIC protocol.[12,13]

So far, however, there have been no direct studies comparing perioperative chemotherapy and neoadjuvant radiochemotherapy in locally advanced OGJ carcinomas. Therefore, it is difficult to decide which is the most effective strategy for these patients although for distal gastric carcinomas and SCCs of the oesophagus, the answer is clear.

For the OGJ, the answer remains controversial and future investigations are needed, but analyses of the data especially of subgroups of the already available trials show there are currently some options available. In the following section, we will discuss current data for optimal management of locally advanced adenocarcinomas of the OGJ.

Curative approaches

The prognosis of patients with local advanced OGJ carcinoma is poor with surgery alone. The concepts of perioperative chemotherapy and of neoadjuvant chemoradiotherapy, which have improved survival compared to surgery only, have been variously implemented in the Western world. A detailed analysis shows that data for perioperative chemotherapy are more consistent than those for neoadjuvant chemoradiotherapy.

ACCORD trial

One of the first studies focusing on OGJ carcinomas was the French FNCLCC ACCORD 07-FFCD 9703 study. Surgery alone was compared to two or three cycles of cisplatin/5-FU followed by surgery and the same systemic therapy postoperatively.[14] Of 224 patients in the study, 75% had a OGJ carcinoma (11% type I, 64% type II or type III). Only 24% of the included patients had distal gastric carcinoma.

The perioperative chemotherapy arm led to a significantly improved OS (5-year OS rate 38% vs 24%; hazard ratio (HR) 0.69, 95% confidence interval (CI) 0.50–0.95; $p = 0.02$). OGJ type II/III tumours showed the greatest benefit from the perioperative chemotherapy (HR 0.57, 95% CI 0.39–0.83).

MAGIC trial

The British landmark phase III study, MAGIC,[15] with perioperative ECF versus surgery alone included mainly patients with gastric cancer but also OGJ carcinomas. However, the focus was on distal gastric carcinomas:

- Of the 503 participants, 74% were patients with adenocarcinoma of the stomach (including type III carcinoma).
- 11.5% of patients had OGJ carcinomas type II.
- 14.5% of patients had type I adenocarcinomas of the OGJ.

Like the FNCLCC study, perioperative chemotherapy significantly improved the progression-free survival and the OS (5-year OS rates 36% vs 23%, HR 0.75, 95% CI 0.60–0.93; $p = 0.009$) compared with surgery alone. All patients, regardless of the anatomical localization of the tumour (type I, type II OGJ, and type III/stomach), benefited from perioperative chemotherapy. The subgroup who benefited the most were the patients with junctional tumours (HR for death in the OGJ subgroup 0.49, 95% CI 0.28–0.88)—comparable results to the previously mentioned French study with a focus on OGJ tumours.

FLOT4-AIO trial

The results of the most recent German FLOT4 trial of the AIO (Working Group Internal Oncology)[12,13] favoured the treatment of OGJ tumours with perioperative chemotherapy. In 716 patients with locally advanced, resectable gastric or OGJ carcinomas, four cycles of the FLOT regimen (5-FU, oxaliplatin, docetaxel pre- and postoperatively) with three cycles of the MAGIC regimen (ECF/ECX pre- and postoperatively) were compared. Most patients (56%) had adenocarcinomas of the OGJ (24% type I, 32% type II/III, and 15% with Barrett's); 44% of the patients had distal gastric carcinomas. For comparison, the FLOT4 trial included numerically more OGJ carcinoma patients than in the whole CROSS trial (see following section); 80% of the patients in FLOT4 were node positive, in CROSS, this occurred in only 65% of the patients. The FLOT regimen improved the mean OS significantly. The OS of 35 months in the ECF/ECX group of the FLOT4 trial was exactly the same outcome as the MAGIC trial. The ECF/ECX group has not underperformed in the FLOT4 trial, showing the strength of the study. In the FLOT group, the OS was approximately 50 months (HR 0.77, 95% CI 0.63–0.94; $p = 0.02$), which is a significant OS improvement compared to the standard arm and even a doubling of the survival time compared to purely surgical intervention (standard in all other mentioned landmark trials). According to the phase II study part of the FLOT4 trial, the arm using the FLOT regimen showed significantly higher rates of pathological complete regression rates according to Becker 1a (16% (95% CI 10–23%) vs 6% (95% CI: 3–11%); $p = 0.02$). This was especially pronounced in the presence of the intestinal-type histology (23%). This is important in the context of proximal adenocarcinomas because most OGJ tumours according to the work of The Cancer Genome Atlas research network are chromosomal unstable (CIN), whereas most diffuse/mixed types are distal gastric carcinomas.[8,9] So the highest rate of pathological complete response by FLOT was shown in the CROSS-sensitive anatomical location, where CROSS shows the same pathological complete response rates.

The results of the third landmark trial, the FLOT4-AIO trial, support the treatment of junctional tumours with a perioperative chemotherapy approach.

CROSS trial

The wide use of neoadjuvant chemoradiotherapy for OGJ and most importantly SCCs of the oesophagus is based mainly on the results of the CROSS trial.[11] This randomized phase III study showed a benefit of neoadjuvant chemoradiation (weekly paclitaxel and carboplatin in combination with radiation (41.4 Gy) followed by surgery) compared with surgery without neoadjuvant therapy. The study included a total of 366 patients, a mix of oesophageal SCCs and adenocarcinomas. Although 76% of patients had oesophageal carcinomas and only 24% junctional tumours, three-quarters of all tumours were adenocarcinomas and only 23% showed a squamous cell histology. Of the adenocarcinomas, 73.2% corresponded to OGJ type I and 24% OGJ type II. The median OS in the intention to-treat population showed a definite benefit for the neoadjuvant therapy with a delta of 13% in the 5-year survival of the total population—similar, for example, to the result of the MAGIC trial (HR 0.66, 95% CI 0.495–0.871; $p = 0.003$). Patients with the more common adenocarcinomas benefited to a much lesser extent (HR 0.741, 95% CI 0.536–1.024; $p = 0.07$) compared with patients of the SCC group (HR 0.422, 95% CI 0.226–0.788; $p = 0.007$).

The multivariate analysis showed that the survival benefit in the adenocarcinoma group was statistically not significant (HR 0.741, 95% CI 0.536–1.024; $p = 0.07$). The specific results of the adenocarcinoma subgroups type I and type II are not known to date. Further subgroup analyses of the CROSS trial demonstrated that the relative benefit of neoadjuvant chemoradiotherapy was limited to the node-negative patients while patients with node-positive disease did not significantly benefit from neoadjuvant chemoradiation (HR 0.807, 95% CI 0.576–1.130; $p = 0.21$).[16]

The greatest survival advantage, and the best pathological remission in CROSS, was for SCC patients with a pathological complete response rate of 49% ($p = 0.008$). Three-quarters of all carcinomas included in CROSS, however, were adenocarcinomas.

Consideration should also be given to the R0 resection rate of 92% in the radiochemotherapy group versus 69% in the group without neoadjuvant therapy (surgical intervention only). This shows, according to the authors, the good response of chemoradiotherapy. The R0 resection rate of only 69% in the standard arm, however, indicates inadequate surgery that may have been compensated for by the addition of chemoradiation in the interventional arm.

The fact that only 364 patients were analysed indicates that CROSS was a relatively small and heterogeneous study. When comparing neoadjuvant chemoradiotherapy according to CROSS and chemotherapy with FLOT it is often ignored that the CROSS trial compared surgery alone with neoadjuvant chemoradiation plus surgery, while in the FLOT4 trial perioperative FLOT plus surgery was compared with the former standard for perioperative systemic therapy (ECF/ECX) and the FLOT regimen showed a benefit for the patients in all subgroups. The benefit for perioperative FLOT therapy was independent of the localization of the primary tumour, the histological subgroup, and the nodal status.

According to current data, FLOT is the most effective perioperative therapy for locally advanced operable adenocarcinoma of both the stomach and the OGJ.

Cure: trends and perspectives

Several ongoing clinical trials are investigating these problems.

- The multicentre German ESOPEC study is a randomized phase III study comparing perioperative chemotherapy with FLOT versus the preoperative chemoradiotherapy CROSS in patients with adenocarcinoma of the OGJ (NCT02509286).
- A similar German AIO-RACE study is comparing the use of two cycles of FLOT induction chemotherapy followed by neoadjuvant radiochemotherapy with 5-FU/oxaliplatin adjuvant FLOT therapy in OGJ tumours types I–III versus perioperative FLOT therapy alone.
- The Neo-AEGIS study by the Irish Clinical Research Group (ICORG; Protocol 10-14) randomizes patients with adenocarcinoma of the oesophagus or of the OGJ to preoperative chemoradiotherapy according to the CROSS protocol or perioperative chemotherapy with ECF/ECX according to the MAGIC protocol (NCT01726452).
- The TOPGEAR study, an international phase III study, is treating patients with adenocarcinoma of the stomach or OGJ with either perioperative chemotherapy (ECF, recently amended to FLOT) or with preoperative chemotherapy (ECF or FLOT) followed by preoperative chemoradiotherapy with 5-FU or capecitabine (NCT01924819).

In the study landscape with a perioperative curative approach, an addition to the treatment with a cytotoxic standard chemotherapy using immune checkpoint inhibitors is currently under evaluation. Several randomized phase III studies are examining the role of immunotherapy in the preoperative situation in gastro-oesophageal tumours.

- In the ICONIC trial, the anti-programmed cell death protein 1 ligand (PD-L1) antibody avelumab in combination with the FLOT regimen will be evaluated in the perioperative setting (NCT03399071).
- Another phase II/III study examines nivolumab and ipilimumab in patients with oesophageal and OGJ tumours. Patients are divided into groups with preoperative chemoradiotherapy with or without nivolumab; this is followed by a second randomization to either adjuvant nivolumab or nivolumab/ipilimumab after resection (NCT03604991).

- In the German AIO-DANTE study, FLOT with or without atezolizumab perioperatively is currently being evaluated in gastric and OGJ carcinomas (NCT03421288).
- The PANDA study uses neoadjuvant capecitabine, oxaliplatin, and docetaxel in combination with atezolizumab in resectable stomach or OGJ tumours (NCT03448835).

Palliation: trends and perspectives

There have been some innovations and changes in the conventional treatment, as well as in immunotherapy, in the palliation of gastric and OGJ carcinomas. According to the randomized, double-blind placebo-controlled phase III study TAGS,[17] TAS-102 (trifluridine/tipiracil) improved OS significantly compared to placebo. Patients could be included with histologically confirmed, metastatic adenocarcinoma in the stomach, including adenocarcinoma of the OGJ. The approval of TAS-102 by the European Medicines Agency for this indication was given in September 2019.

Checkpoint inhibitor therapy

The phase III trial ATTRACTION-2[18] published in 2017 showed a significant survival benefit for nivolumab and is a new treatment option for previously treated patients with adenocarcinoma of the stomach or OGJ.

Ongoing studies with non-Asian patients are examining nivolumab in advanced stomach or OGJ cancer in different settings as well as in earlier lines of therapy. Data from the KEYNOTE-059 and KEYNOTE-012 studies[19,20] were responsible for the approval of pembrolizumab by the US Food and Drug Administration for patients with gastric and OGJ carcinomas with a PD-L1 combined positive score (CPS) of at least 1. In the area of gastric carcinomas, there were also studies with a negative result for immunotherapy, for example, pembrolizumab as a second-line therapy in KEYNOTE-061,[21] or avelumab as a third-line therapy in the Javelin-300 study.[22]

In practice, certain subgroups appear to benefit from immune oncological therapy. Important parameters for possible response to immune oncological therapy are hot tumours with, for example, Epstein–Barr virus positivity, high-level microsatellite instability, and PD-L1 CPS of 1 or greater or even 10 in gastric carcinoma. A current publication by Kim et al. provides a good overview of this.[23]

Tabernero et al. at ASCO 2019 presented the phase III study KEYNOTE-062,[24] with pembrolizumab monotherapy versus pembrolizumab in combination with chemotherapy versus chemotherapy alone in first-line therapy in adenocarcinomas of the stomach and the OGJ. The results showed a non-inferiority for pembrolizumab monotherapy compared to standard-of-care chemotherapy in patients with CPS of at least 1. At a CPS of at least 10, there was a clear survival advantage under pembrolizumab compared with chemotherapy, with a better compatibility from pembrolizumab. Surprisingly the combination of chemotherapy plus pembrolizumab showed no superiority over standard-of-care chemotherapy. A sweeping change in the present daily routine therapy, however, is not expected.

There are two positive studies for oesophageal cancer in second-line therapy with checkpoint inhibition. In KEYNOTE-181, pembrolizumab significantly improved OS versus chemotherapy as second-line therapy for advanced oesophageal cancer with PD-L1 CPS of 10 or greater, with a more favourable safety profile and stable and similar quality of life.[25] These data support pembrolizumab as a new second-line standard of care for oesophageal cancer with PD-L1 CPS of at least 10, especially in the SCC population. In the ATTRACTION-3 trial, nivolumab demonstrated a superior OS and a favourable safety profile versus CT in patients with previously treated advanced oesophageal SCC, with survival benefit observed regardless of tumour PD-L1 expression.[26] Therefore, nivolumab may represent a new standard second-line treatment option for patients with advanced oesophageal SCC. However, this trial mainly studied Asian subjects because only 18 patients out of the total of 419 were non-Asians.

Due to the positive date of Checkmate 649 and Keynote—590 the combination of platinum and 5 Fu based chemotherapy in combination with nivolumab is approved for gastric cancer and plus pembrolizumab for squamous and adenocarcinoma oesophageal cancer in 1st line setting.

REFERENCES

1. Bray F, Ferlay J, Soerjomataram I, et al. Global cancer statistics 2018: GLOBOCAN estimates of incidence and mortality worldwide for 36 cancers in 185 countries. *CA Cancer J Clin*. 2018;**68**:394–424.
2. Blot WJ, Devesa SS, Kneller RW, et al. Rising incidence of adenocarcinoma of the esophagus and gastric cardia. *JAMA*. 1991;**265**:1287–1289.
3. Buas MF, Vaughan TL. Epidemiology and risk factors for gastroesophageal junction tumors: understanding the rising incidence of this disease. *Semin Radiat Oncol*. 2013;**23**:3–9.
4. Siewert RJ, Hölscher AH, Becker K, et al. Cardia cancer: attempt at a therapeutically relevant classification. *Chirurg*. 1987;**58**:25–32.
5. Siewert RJ, Feith M, Werner M, et al. Adenocarcinoma of the esophagogastric junction: results of surgical therapy based on anatomical/topographic classification in 1,002 consecutive patients. *Ann Surg*. 2000;**232**:353–361.
6. Siewert JR, Stein HJ. Classification of adenocarcinoma of the oesophagogastric junction. *Br J Surg*. 1998;**85**:1457–1459.
7. Amin MB, Edge SB, Greene FL, et al. *AJCC Cancer Staging Manual*. 8th ed. New York: Springer; 2017.
8. Cancer Genome Atlas Research Network. Comprehensive molecular characterization of gastric adenocarcinoma. *Nature*.2014;**513**:202–209.
9. Cancer Genome Atlas Research Network; Analysis Working Group: Asan University; et al. Integrated genomic characterization of oesophageal carcinoma. *Nature*. 2017;**541**:169–175.
10. Njei B, McCarty TR, Birk JW. Trends in esophageal cancer survival in United States adults from 1973 to 2009: a SEER database analysis. *J Gastroenterol Hepatol*. 2016;**31**:1141–1146.
11. van Hagen P, Hulshof MC, van Lanschot JJ, et al. Preoperative chemoradiotherapy for esophageal or junctional cancer. *N Engl J Med*. 2012;**366**:2074–2084.
12. Al-Batran SE, Hofheinz RD, Pauligk C, et al. Histopathological regression after neoadjuvant docetaxel, oxaliplatin, fluorouracil, and leucovorin versus epirubicin, cisplatin, and fluorouracil or capecitabine in patients with resectable gastric or gastro-oesophageal junction adenocarcinoma (FLOT4-AIO): results from the phase 2 part of a multicentre, open-label, randomised phase 2/3 trial. *Lancet Oncol*. 2016;**17**:1697–1708.

13. Al-Batran SE, Homann N, Pauligk C, et al. Perioperative chemotherapy with fluorouracil plus leucovorin, oxaliplatin, and docetaxel versus fluorouracil or capecitabine plus cisplatin and epirubicin for locally advanced, resectable gastric or gastro-oesophageal junction adenocarcinoma (FLOT4): a multicentre, open-label, randomised, phase 2/3 trial. *Lancet.* 2019;**393**:1948–1957.

14. Ychou M, Boige V, Pignon JP, et al. Perioperative chemotherapy compared with surgery alone for resectable gastroesophageal adenocarcinoma: an FNCLCC and FFCD multicenter phase III trial. *J Clin Oncol.* 2011;**29**:1715–1721.

15. Cunningham D, Allum WH, Stenning SP, et al. Perioperative chemotherapy versus surgery alone for resectable gastroesophageal cancer. *N Engl J Med.* 2006;**355**:11–20.

16. Shapiro J, van Lanschot JJB, Hulshof MCCM, et al. Neoadjuvant chemoradiotherapy plus surgery versus surgery alone for oesophageal or junctional cancer (CROSS): long-term results of a randomised controlled trial. *Lancet Oncol.* 2015;**16**:1090–1098.

17. Shitara K, Doi T, Dvorkin M, et al. Trifluridine/tipiracil versus placebo in patients with heavily pretreated metastatic gastric cancer (TAGS): a randomised, double-blind, placebo-controlled, phase 3 trial. *Lancet Oncol.* 2018;**19**:1437–1448.

18. Kang YK, Boku N, Satoh T, et al. Nivolumab in patients with advanced gastric or gastrooesophageal junction cancer refractory to, or intolerant of, at least two previous chemotherapy regimens (ONO-4538-12, ATTRACTION-2): a randomised, double-blind, placebo-controlled, phase 3 trial. *Lancet.* 2017;**390**:2461–2471.

19. Bang YJ, Muro K, Fuchs CS, et al. KEYNOTE-059 cohort 2: safety and efficacy of pembrolizumab (pembro) plus 5-fluorouracil (5-FU) and cisplatin for first-line (1L) treatment of advanced gastric cancer. *J Clin Oncol.* 2017;**35** (Suppl 15):4012.

20. Muro K, Chung HC, Shankaran V, et al. Pembrolizumab for patients with PD-L1-positive advanced gastric cancer (KEYNOTE-012): a multicentre, open-label, phase 1b trial. *Lancet Oncol.* 2016;**17**:717–726.

21. Shitara K, Özgüroğlu M, Bang YJ, et al. Pembrolizumab versus paclitaxel for previously treated, advanced gastric or gastro-oesophageal junction cancer (KEYNOTE-061): a randomised, open-label, controlled, phase 3 trial. *Lancet.* 2018;**392**:123–133.

22. Bang YJ, Ruiz EY, van Cutsem E et al. Phase III, randomised trial of avelumab versus physician's choice of chemotherapy as third-line treatment of patients with advanced gastric or gastro-oesophageal junction cancer: primary analysis of JAVELIN Gastric 300. *Ann Oncol.* 2018;**29**:2052–2060.

23. Kim ST, Cristescu R, Bass AJ, et al. Comprehensive molecular characterization of clinical responses to PD-1 inhibition in metastatic gastric cancer. *Nat Med.* 2018;**24**:1449–1458.

24. Tabernero J, van Cutsem E, Bang YJ, et al. Pembrolizumab with or without chemotherapy versus chemotherapy for advanced gastric or gastroesophageal junction (G/GEJ) adenocarcinoma: the phase III KEYNOTE-062 study. *J Clin Oncol.* 2019;**37**(18 Suppl):LBA4007.

25. Kojima T, Muro K, Francois E. Pembrolizumab versus chemotherapy as second-line therapy for advanced esophageal cancer: phase III KEYNOTE-181 study. *J Clin Oncol.* 2019;**37**(4 Suppl):2.

26. Kato K, Cho BC, Takahashi M. Nivolumab versus chemotherapy in patients with advanced oesophageal squamous cell carcinoma refractory or intolerant to previous chemotherapy (ATTRACTION-3): a multicentre, randomised, open-label, phase 3 trial *Lancet Oncol.* 2019;**20**:1506–1517.

PART 3
Gastric cancer

16. Gastric cancer: epidemiology, symptoms, diagnosis, and staging 177
    Takaaki Arigami and Shoji Natsugoe

17. Gastric cancer: multimodal treatment 187
    Mickael Chevallay, Thorsten Oliver Goetze, Salah-Eddin Al-Batran, and Stefan Mönig

18. Gastric cancer: endoscopic treatment 199
    Chang Seok Bang

19. Gastric cancer: surgery 209
    Matthias Biebl, Dino Kröll, Sascha Chopra, and Johann Pratschke

20. Gastric cancer: minimally invasive surgery and robotic surgery 217
    Makoto Hikage and Masanori Terashima

21. Gastric cancer: future aspects of treatment 231
    Alexander B.J. Borgstein, Suzanne S. Gisbertz, and Mark I. van Berge Henegouwen

16

Gastric cancer
Epidemiology, symptoms, diagnosis, and staging

Takaaki Arigami and Shoji Natsugoe

Introduction

The diagnostic tools and techniques for gastric cancer identification and treatment have made remarkable progress. These developments have resulted in a high incidence of patients with early gastric cancer. Therefore, endoscopic treatments, such as endoscopic mucosal resection and endoscopic submucosal dissection, have been extensively performed on them. Furthermore, the eighth edition of the *TNM Classification of Malignant Tumours* was recently published in which the stage groupings for gastric cancer have been revised to include a lymph node metastatic status.[1] This classification is presently used in clinical management and supports the diagnosis and treatment of gastric cancer. This chapter focuses on the epidemiology, symptoms, diagnostics, and staging in patients with gastric cancer.

Epidemiology

Incidence

Currently, gastric cancer is the fifth most common malignancy in the world.[2] In 2008, 989,600 new patients with gastric cancer were identified worldwide.[3] The number of patients with newly diagnosed gastric cancer was 984,000 in 2013.[4] Moreover, geographical differences are relevant in the incidence of gastric cancer and indicate a 15–20 times difference between high- and low-risk countries.[5] For instance, the high-risk areas for gastric cancer include Japan, Korea, China, Central and South America, and Eastern Europe. By contrast, the low-risk areas include North America, Southern Asia, North and East Africa, Australia, and New Zealand.[5] Interestingly, the incidence of gastric cancer has gradually decreased in East Asia, particularly in Japan and Korea. Age-standardized occurrence rates of gastric cancer per 100,000 people in 1999 and 2015 decreased from 40.0 to 33.2, respectively, in Japan.[6] Similarly, age-standardized occurrence rates per 100,000 people in 1999 and 2015 decreased from 43.6 to 33.8, respectively, in Korea.[7]

Mortality

Gastric cancer is the second leading cause of cancer-related death worldwide. In 2008 and 2013, 738,000 and 841,000 patients died of gastric cancer, respectively.[3,4] Not surprisingly, mortality rates caused by gastric cancer in East Asia and South America are high. Mortality rates per 100,000 for the US were 2.0 in 2012.[8] However, in Korea, mortality rates per 100,000 after adjustment for the global population were 13.0 and 9.7 (15.1 among males and 5.7 among females) in 2012 and 2014, respectively.[7] In Japan, the rates per 100,000 were 16.8, 12.8, and 9.2 in 2001, 2009, and 2017, respectively.[6] Accordingly, these data demonstrate the reduced mortality in countries with high-risk populations for gastric cancer. These findings may be caused by recent advances in diagnostic tools, surgical approach, and chemotherapy.

Survival

According to prognostic analyses in 71 countries with populations at high risk of gastric cancer, the 5-year survival rate was 48.6% between 2000 and 2004 and 68.9% between 2010 and 2014.[9] In Korea, the 5-year survival rate has dramatically improved from 42.8% in 1993–1995 to 75.4% in 2011–2015.[7] In Japan, the 5-year overall survival rate of patients with distant metastasis was 16.4%.[10] In the US, the 5-year survival rate has been reported to be 31%.[11] Furthermore, stage-related prognostic data indicate that the 5-year survival rate after surgery in patients with stage IA, IB, and IIIC is 94%, 88%, and 18%, respectively.[12] In the UK, the 5- and 10-year survival rates are 19% and 15%, respectively.[13] The average 5-year survival rate is 26% in Europe.[13]

Risk factors and prevention of gastric cancer

The International Agency for Research on Cancer has investigated chemicals, occupations, physical agents, biological agents, and other agents for the risk assessment of human carcinogens. These carcinogenic agents have been classified into two groups, based on evidence, as follows: carcinogenic agents with sufficient evidence in humans and agents with limited evidence in humans.[14] The International Agency for Research on Cancer classification proposes

Table 16.1 Preventable exposure associated with gastric cancer

Agents with sufficient evidence	Agents with limited evidence
Helicobacter pylori	Asbestos
Rubber production	Epstein–Barr virus
Tobacco smoking	Lead compounds
X-radiation	Inorganic nitrate
Gamma radiation	Pickled vegetables
	Salted fish
	Chinese style

Source: data from Cogliano VJ, Baan R, Straif K, et al. Preventable exposures associated with human cancers. J Natl Cancer Inst. 2011;103:1827–1839.

that Helicobacter pylori, rubber production, tobacco smoking, and X-ray and gamma radiation are carcinogenic agents in gastric cancer with sufficient evidence (Table 16.1).[14] This information is essential for the prevention of carcinogenesis in gastric cancer.

Helicobacter pylori

Barry Marshall and Robin Warren discovered a close relationship between H. pylori and gastritis in 1982.[15] Further studies have indicated H. pylori infections are a key risk factor for the development of peptic ulcers and gastric carcinogenesis.[16] In a study of 1526 Japanese patients, Uemura et al. reported that the occurrence of gastric cancer was 2.9% in 1246 patients with an H. pylori infection over 7.8 years and 0% in 280 non-infected control patients.[17] Furthermore, gastric cancer was not identified in 253 infected patients receiving eradication therapy.[17]

Recently, Korean investigators have reported that the incidence of H. pylori infections in adults has decreased from more than 80% in the 1980s to less than 55% in 2011.[18,19] In a study of 170,752 Japanese people, Wang et al. indicated that the predicted prevalence of an H. pylori infection was 60.9%, 64.1%, 34.9%, and 6.6% among people who were born in 1910, 1940, 1970, and 2000, respectively.[20] In future, these findings may have an impact on the clinical management of patients with gastric cancer.

Tobacco smoking

To date, many studies have demonstrated that tobacco smoking increases the risk of gastric cancer. In Europe, smoking is associated with 17% of gastric cancer cases (11% globally).[21] A systematic review and meta-analysis of 42 cohort studies suggested that the relative risk (RR) estimates between current smokers and non-smokers were 1.62 in males and 1.20 in females.[22] Furthermore, the RR ranged from 1.3 in smokers with the lowest consumptions to 1.7 in smokers using approximately 30 cigarettes per day.[22] Smoking has been significantly related with both cardia (RR = 1.87) and non-cardia (RR = 1.60) cancers.[22]

Alcohol

Alcohol is closely related to gastric carcinogenesis, although the risks in association with the actual amount of consumption remain unclear. According to a meta-analysis based on 44 case–control and 15 cohort studies, the pooled RR was 1.07 between alcohol drinkers and non-drinkers and 1.20 between heavy alcohol drinkers (four or more drinks per day) and non-drinkers.[23] These results suggest that heavy alcohol consumption increases the risk of gastric cancer. Several studies have reported that alcohol causes inflammation in the stomach, resulting in gastritis.[24]

Obesity

Obesity has been ranked as a risk factor for several gastrointestinal cancers, such as in the pancreas, liver, oesophagus, colorectum, and gall bladder.[25] A meta-analysis based on 16 studies showed obesity (body mass index ≥30 kg/m^2) was related to an increased risk of gastric cancer (odds ratio (OR) = 1.13), compared with patients at a healthy weight (body mass index = 18.5–<25 kg/m^2).[26] Additionally, a stratified analysis indicated males (OR = 1.27) and non-Asians (OR = 1.14) have a close link between obesity and the risk of gastric cancer.[26] Recent studies have focused on obesity-induced tumour necrosis factor alpha and interleukin-6 signalling during carcinogenesis and tumour progression.[27]

Epstein–Barr virus (EBV)

EBV has been reported to be present in tumour cells in approximately 9% of gastric carcinomas.[28] A meta-analysis consisting of 70 studies demonstrated that the incidence of EBV-associated gastric cancer is two times higher in males (11.1%) than in females (5.2%).[29] Furthermore, tumours in a postsurgical gastric stump or remnant stomach had a high incidence of being EBV positive (35.1%), compared with tumours in the gastric cardia (13.6%), corpus (13.1%), or antrum (5.2%).[29] The country-related occurrence of EBV-associated gastric cancer was 8.3% in Asia, 9.2% in Europe, and 9.9% in the US.[29] Interestingly, several investigators have indicated that patients with EBV-positive gastric cancer have a better prognosis than those with EBV-negative gastric cancer.[30] However, the reasons remain uncertain.

Socioeconomic status

A low socioeconomic status has been reported to be related to an increased risk of gastric cancer and lower survival rates,[31] whereas populations with high socioeconomic status have a reduced risk of gastric cancer. A meta-analysis that reviewed 25 studies, including 9773 patients with gastric cancer and 24,373 controls, indicated that the pooled OR for the highest compared with the lowest socioeconomic status was 0.60.[31]

Non-steroidal anti-inflammatory drugs (NSAIDs)

Cyclooxygenase (COX)-2 is overexpressed in patients with several malignancies, including gastric cancer.[32] Moreover, previous studies have shown the vital role of COX-2 in carcinogenesis.[32] On the other hand, NSAIDs are well known to suppress the production of COX-1 and COX-2 via prostaglandin-dependent and -independent pathways. A systematic review and meta-analysis extracted from 2831 patients with gastric cancer indicated that NSAID use was correlated with a reduced risk of gastric cancer in a dose-dependent manner (OR = 0.78).[33] Then, a subgroup analysis demonstrated that NSAID use was significantly associated with a risk reduction for non-cardia gastric cancer (OR = 0.72).[33]

Symptoms

The majority of patients with early-stage gastric cancer have no signs or symptoms of the disease. Accordingly, symptoms caused by gastric cancer often do not appear until tumours are advanced. For instance, the incidence of gastric outlet obstruction ranges between 14.9% and 35.0% in patients with antral gastric cancer.[34] These findings are the key issue in the pre-therapeutic management of patients with gastric cancer. Signs and symptoms of gastric cancer may include fatigue, poor appetite, feeling full, heartburn, nausea, vomiting, unexplained weight loss, stomach pain, and bloody stools.

Diagnosis

Screening for gastric cancer has been changing dramatically in the world. This screening generally involves several diagnostic examinations, such as upper gastrointestinal barium X-ray radiography (UGI-XR), oesophagogastroduodenoscopy (OGD), and serum pepsinogen testing. Furthermore, patients initially identified by screening need further examinations, such as endoscopic ultrasonography (EUS), computed tomography (CT), and fluorodeoxyglucose positron emission tomography (FDG-PET). It is important to understand an accurate staging system to formulate a therapeutic plan in patients with gastric cancer.

Upper gastrointestinal barium X-ray radiography

UGI-XR was introduced in Japan in the 1960s as an effective mass screening programme for gastric cancer. The sensitivity of UGI-XR ranged from 60% to 80%.[35] Then, the specificity and true positive rates were 90% and 0.7–2.0%, respectively.[35] The overall results of Japanese cancer screenings in 2007 showed that 5600 patients with gastric cancer were identified in 6,390,000 people receiving medical screenings using UGI-XR.[35] However, half of the screen-detected gastric cancers had tumours at a different site according to the OGD.[35] These results suggest that UGI-XR has low accuracy in the true detection rate of early gastric cancer.

Oesophagogastroduodenoscopy

OGD was introduced as a screening platform for gastric cancer in Japan in 2015. OGD has clinical utility as a direct visual tool for assessing the gastric mucosa. Additionally, pathological examination can be performed using tissue specimens biopsied using OGD. A Japanese cohort study between 2002 and 2004 indicated that the detection rate of gastric cancer was approximately 2.7 and 4.6 times higher in OGD than in UGI-XR.[36] Moreover, a population-based cohort study, including 14,274 subjects, demonstrated that OGD screenings could reduce gastric cancer mortality by 67% compared with UGI-XR screenings.[37]

Magnifying endoscopy is a useful tool for the real-time visualization of microscopic images in the mucosal surface. Furthermore, narrow-band imaging (NBI) has been developed and incorporated into the magnifying endoscopic system. Currently, magnifying NBI (M-NBI) has been widely disseminated and has made a significant contribution to the clinical management of patients with gastric cancer. Yao et al. constructed the vessel plus surface (VS) classification system using M-NBI for the diagnosis of early gastric cancer (Figure 16.1).[38] In particular, this system can support an accurate assessment, including the delineation of tumour margins, in patients with superficial (0–II) gastric cancer. Currently, this VS classification system has been accepted as a promising systematic method

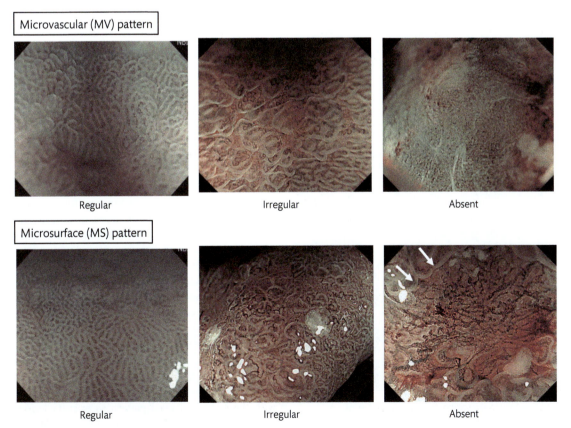

Figure 16.1 VS classification. Demarcation lines (arrow).

worldwide and is practical for the diagnosis of early gastric cancer using M-NBI.

According to the VS classification system, microvascular and microsurface patterns are divided into three categories, including regular, irregular, and absent.[38] Then, M-NBI findings have a clear demarcation line between cancerous and non-cancerous mucosa. Consequently, if a tumour has an irregular microvascular pattern with a demarcation line or irregular microsurface pattern with a demarcation line, this lesion can be diagnosed as a cancerous mucosa.[38] In the diagnosis of small depressed lesions measuring 10 mm or less in diameter, the accuracy, sensitivity, and specificity in conventional white light imaging (C-WLI) were 65%, 40%, and 68%, respectively.[38] On the other hand, the accuracy, sensitivity, and specificity in M-NBI were 90%, 60%, and 94%, respectively.[38] These results suggest a high accuracy and specificity of M-NBI compared with C-WLI. Interestingly, the combined assessment of C-WLI and M-NBI produced a further significant improvement of the diagnostic performance (accuracy 97%, sensitivity 95%, and specificity 97%).[38] In the clinical management of OGD for detecting early gastric cancer, M-NBI findings after a detailed observation under C-WLI are essential to prevent cancerous lesions from being overlooked.

Endoscopic ultrasonography

EUS has been used clinically as an imaging modality to predict the depth of tumour invasion and regional lymph node metastasis since the early 1980s (Figures 16.2 and 16.3). A meta-analysis that reviewed eight studies comprising 1736 patients with gastric cancer showed that the sensitivity of EUS for T1, T2, T3, and T4 staging was 82%, 72%, 68%, and 52%, respectively.[39] Then, the

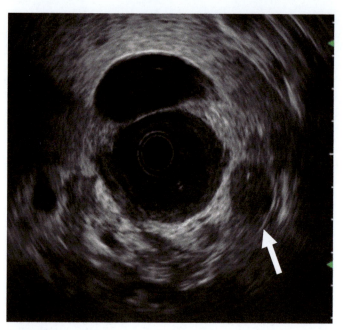

Figure 16.3 EUS. This case had lymph node swelling in station No. 4d (arrow).

specificity of EUS for T1, T2, T3, and T4 staging was 89%, 84%, 87%, and 97%, respectively.[39] In the diagnosis of lymph node metastases, the sensitivity and specificity of EUS were 91% and 49%, respectively.[39] Another meta-analysis indicated that the sensitivity and specificity of EUS for mucosal cancer were 76% and 72%, respectively.[40] Moreover, this meta-analysis showed that the sensitivity and specificity of EUS for submucosal cancer were 62% and 78%, respectively.[40] Consequently, the authors concluded that EUS has a relatively low accuracy for staging the depth of tumour invasion in early gastric cancer.

EUS has several disadvantages in the clinical management of patients with gastric cancer. Akashi et al. reported that ulcerous changes within tumours decrease the accuracy of a EUS-based diagnosis in patients with early gastric cancer.[41] The most significant defect of EUS may be that its imaging assessment depends on the expertise of the operator.

Computed tomography

CT is the most common examination for assessing the depth of tumour invasion and lymph node metastasis, as well as EUS (Figures 16.4 and 16.5). In addition, CT has the clinical utility to detect distant metastasis, such as liver and lung metastasis (Figure 16.6). However, it is clinically difficult to diagnose peritoneal dissemination by CT. Therefore, peritoneal dissemination is assumed through secondary CT findings, such as ascites, peritoneal nodules, and a high density of adipose tissue in the greater omentum or mesentery (Figures 16.7–16.9).

Bando et al. defined lymph node metastasis when CT scanning was performed with 2 mm slices and images were obtained at 5 mm intervals as follows: lymph nodes measuring at least 10 mm at the longest diameter, convergent lymph nodes, or lymph nodes with the same enhanced pattern as primary lesions.[42] According to these criteria for determining clinical nodal involvement, the

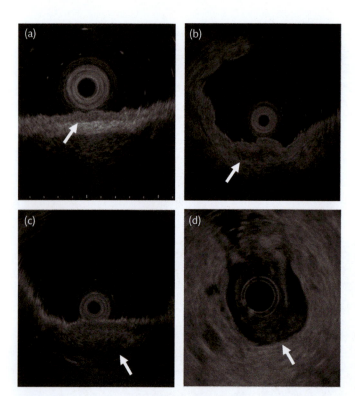

Figure 16.2 EUS. (a) Mucosal invasion. (b) Submucosal invasion. (c) Invasion of muscularis propria. (d) Invasion of subserosa.

Diagnosis 181

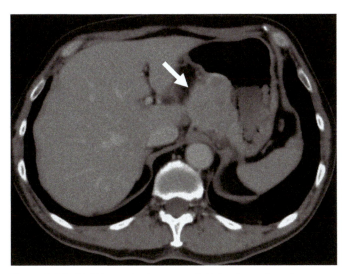

Figure 16.4 CT. This case had gastric wall thickening at the primary tumour site (arrow).

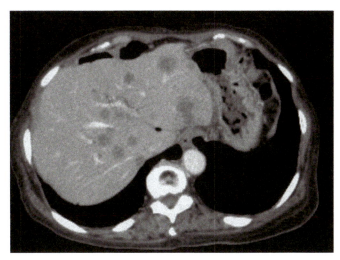

Figure 16.6 CT. This case had multiple liver metastases.

overall concordance rate in a study of 3033 patients was 63.5% (1713/2699).[42] Even among 2047 patients who were determined to be clinically N0, 554 patients (27.8%) had pathological lymph node metastasis.[42] They reported that the rate of underdiagnosed nodal metastases reached 29.8% (805/2699), whereas the rate of overdiagnosis was only 6.7% (181/2699).[42] Further developments in CT imaging will significantly contribute to high diagnostic accuracy in patients with gastric cancer.

Fluorodeoxyglucose positron emission tomography

FDG-PET has a high specificity for detecting lymph node metastasis and distant metastasis identified by CT scanning (Figures 16.10–16.12). A systematic review indicated that the sensitivity and specificity of FDG-PET for metastatic lymph node detection were 21–40% and 89–100%, respectively.[43] Furthermore, the sensitivity

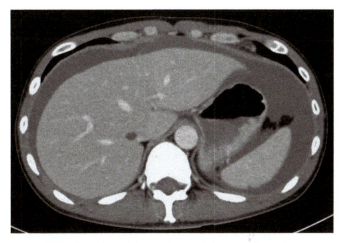

Figure 16.7 CT. This case had ascites and shows peritoneal dissemination.

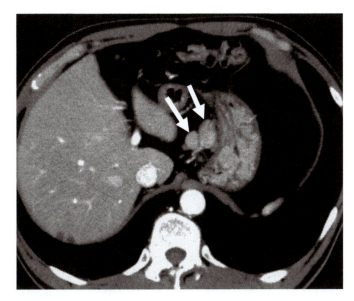

Figure 16.5 CT. This case had lymph node metastasis in station No. 3 (arrow).

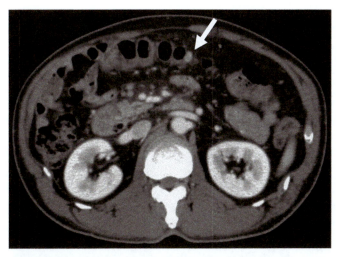

Figure 16.8 CT. This case had a peritoneal nodule and showed peritoneal dissemination (arrow).

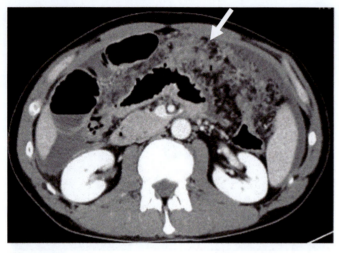

Figure 16.9 CT. This case had a high density of adipose tissue in the greater omentum (arrow) and showed peritoneal dissemination.

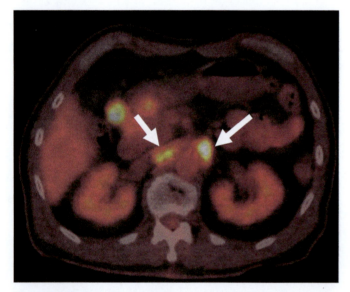

Figure 16.10 FDG-PET. This case had an abnormal FDG uptake in the para-aortic lymph nodes (arrow) and showed distant metastasis.

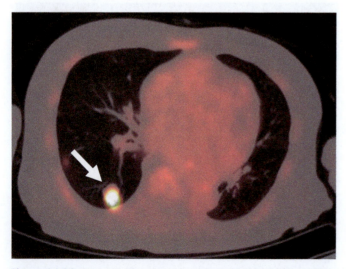

Figure 16.11 FDG-PET. This case had an abnormal FDG uptake in the lung (arrow) and shows lung metastasis.

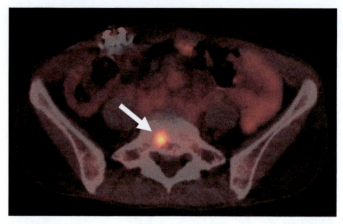

Figure 16.12 FDG-PET. This case had an abnormal FDG uptake in the lumbar vertebra (arrow) and shows bone metastasis.

and specificity for distant metastasis detection were 35–74% and 74–99%, respectively.[43] In addition, this report showed that the tumour response by chemotherapy could be detected at an earlier phase by FDG-PET than with CT (Figure 16.13).[43]

In the clinical application of FDG-PET for gastric cancer management, several key issues have been determined. Initially, a normal gastric mucosa has a physiological FDG uptake.[44] In particular, the standard uptake value in the upper third of the stomach has been reported to be significantly higher than in the lower third. Secondly, since undifferentiated adenocarcinomas have a low FDG uptake, it is clinically hard to detect these tumours using FDG-PET.[45] This finding may cause frequent false-negative cases in similar histological types. Thirdly, FDG uptake depends on the primary tumour size. A systematic review reported that the detectability of FDG-PET in tumours measuring greater than 30 mm and those less than or equal to 30 mm was 70.8% and 26%, respectively.[46] Currently, clinical trials associated with treatments using a dynamic property of FDG are in progress.

Staging

In 2016, the Union for International Cancer Control (UICC) published a new version of the TNM classification of stomach cancer as the eighth edition (Table 16.2).[1] In 2017, the Japanese Gastric Cancer Association published the 15th edition of the Japanese Classification of Gastric Carcinoma. This Japanese classification is consistent with the eighth edition of the UICC/TNM.

In the eighth edition of the TNM classification, tumours involving the oesophagogastric junction whose epicentre is located within the proximal 2 cm of the cardia (Siewert types I/II) are treated and staged as oesophageal cancers.[1] However, tumours whose epicentre is located more than 2 cm distal from the oesophagogastric junction (Siewert type III) are treated and staged by the TNM classification of stomach cancer.[1] Furthermore, the eighth edition of the TNM classification shows two different staging systems based on clinical and pathological diagnosis, respectively (Table 16.3 and Table 16.4).[1] The establishment of clinical stage grouping before treatments are supported by the spread of neoadjuvant chemotherapy in the strategic management of patients with advanced gastric cancer.

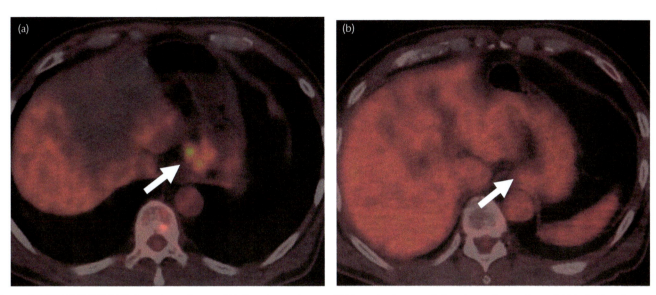

Figure 16.13 FDG-PET. (a) Before chemotherapy. (b) After chemotherapy. FDG uptake decreased after chemotherapy (arrow). This finding shows a partial response from chemotherapy.

Table 16.2 TNM classification of stomach cancer

T–primary tumour	
TX	Primary tumour cannot be assessed
T0	No evidence of primary tumour
Tis	Carcinoma *in situ*: intraepithelial tumour without invasion of the lamina propria, high-grade dysplasia
T1	Tumour invades lamina propria, muscularis mucosae, or submucosa
T1a	Tumour invades lamina propria or muscularis mucosae
T1b	Tumour invades submucosa
T2	Tumour invades muscularis propria
T3	Tumour invades subserosa
T4	Tumour perforates serosa (visceral peritoneum) or invades adjacent structures[a,b,c]
T4a	Tumour perforates serosa
T4b	Tumour invades adjacent structures[a,b]

Notes
[a] The adjacent structures of the stomach are the spleen, transverse colon, liver, diaphragm, pancreas, abdominal wall, adrenal gland, kidney, small intestine, and retroperitoneum.
[b] Intramural extension to the duodenum or oesophagus is classified by the depth of greatest invasion in any of these sites including stomach.
[c] Tumour that extends into gastrocolic or gastrohepatic ligaments or into greater or lesser omentum, without perforation of visceral peritoneum, is T3.

N–regional lymph nodes	
NX	Regional lymph nodes cannot be assessed
N0	No regional lymph node metastasis
N1	Metastasis in 1 to 2 regional lymph nodes
N2	Metastasis in 3 to 6 regional lymph nodes
N3	Metastasis in 7 or more regional lymph nodes
N3a	Metastasis in 7 to 15 regional lymph nodes
N3b	Metastasis in 16 or more regional lymph nodes

M–distant metastasis	
M0	No distant metastasis
M1	Distant metastasis

Note: distant metastasis includes peritoneal seeding, positive peritoneal cytology, and omental tumour not part of continuous extension.

Reproduced with permission from Brierley JD, Gospodarowicz MK, Wittekind C, *TNM Classification of Malignant Tumours*, 8th Edition, John Wiley & Sons, 2017.

Table 16.3 Clinical stages of stomach cancer

Stage I	T1, T2	N0	M0
Stage IIA	T1, T2	N1, N2, N3	M0
Stage IIB	T3, T4a	N0	M0
Stage III	T3, T4a	N1, N2, N3	M0
Stage IVA	T4b	Any N	M0
Stage IVB	Any T	Any N	M1

Reproduced with permission from Brierley JD, Gospodarowicz MK, Wittekind C, *TNM Classification of Malignant Tumours*, 8th Edition, John Wiley & Sons, 2017.

The International Gastric Cancer Association Staging Project proposed a new stage grouping of gastric cancer for the eighth edition of the TNM classification.[47] According to the criteria for the pathological stage of the TNM classification, patients with N3 were classified into two groups of N3a and N3b. N3a and N3b were defined as having a metastatic status in 7–15 regional lymph nodes and in 16 or more regional lymph nodes, respectively.[1] A validation study based on the National Cancer Database obtained from 12,041 patients demonstrated the clear separation of the prognostic analysis.[48] The eighth edition of the TNM classification would be expected to support the clinical management of tumour diagnosis and treatment in patients with gastric cancer.

Table 16.4 Pathological stages of stomach cancer

Stage I	Tis	N0	M0
Stage IA	T1	N0	M0
Stage IB	T1	N1	M0
	T2	N0	M0
Stage IIA	T1	N2	M0
	T2	N1	M0
	T3	N0	M0
Stage IIB	T1	N3a	M0
	T2	N2	M0
	T3	N1	M0
	T4a	N0	M0
Stage IIIA	T2	N3a	M0
	T3	N2	M0
	T4a	N1, N2	M0
	T4b	N0	M0
Stage IIIB	T1, T2	N3b	M0
	T3, T4a	N3a	M0
	T4b	N1, N2	M0
Stage IIIC	T3, T4a	N3b	M0
	T4b	N3a, N3b	M0
Stage IV	Any T	Any N	M1

Note: the AJCC publishes prognostic groups for after neoadjuvant therapy (categories with the prefix 'y').
Reproduced with permission from Brierley JD, Gospodarowicz MK, Wittekind C, *TNM Classification of Malignant Tumours*, 8th Edition, John Wiley & Sons, 2017.

REFERENCES

1. Brierley JD, Gospodarowicz MK, Wittekind C, eds. *TNM Classification of Malignant Tumours*. 8th ed. Oxford: John Wiley & Sons; 2017.
2. Global Burden of Disease Cancer Collaboration, Fitzmaurice C, Allen C, et al. Global, regional, and national cancer incidence, mortality, years of life lost, years lived with disability, and disability-adjusted life-years for 32 cancer groups, 1990 to 2015: a systematic analysis for the Global Burden of Disease Study. *JAMA Oncol*. 2017;**3**:524–548.
3. Jemal A, Bray F, Center MM, Ferlay J, Ward E, Forman D. Global cancer statistics. *CA Cancer J Clin*. 2011;**61**:69–90.
4. Global Burden of Disease Cancer Collaboration, Fitzmaurice C, Dicker D, et al. The global burden of cancer 2013. *JAMA Oncol*. 2015;**1**:505–527.
5. Stock M, Otto F. Gene deregulation in gastric cancer. *Gene*. 2005;**360**:1–19.
6. Foundation for Promotion of Cancer Research. Cancer statistics in Japan. 2017. https://ganjoho.jp/public/qa_links/report/statistics/2017_en.html
7. Kweon SS. Updates on cancer epidemiology in Korea, 2018. *Chonnam Med J*. 2018;**54**:90–100.
8. Ang TL, Fock KM. Clinical epidemiology of gastric cancer. *Singapore Med J*. 2014;**55**:621–628.
9. Allemani C, Matsuda T, Di Carlo V, et al. Global surveillance of trends in cancer survival 2000–14 (CONCORD-3): analysis of individual records for 37 513 025 patients diagnosed with one of 18 cancers from 322 population-based registries in 71 countries. *Lancet*. 2018;**391**:1023–1075.
10. Katai H, Ishikawa T, Akazawa K, et al. Five-year survival analysis of surgically resected gastric cancer cases in Japan: a retrospective analysis of more than 100,000 patients from the nationwide registry of the Japanese Gastric Cancer Association (2001–2007). *Gastric Cancer*. 2018;**21**:144–154.
11. Rawla P, Barsouk A. Epidemiology of gastric cancer: global trends, risk factors and prevention. *Prz Gastroenterol*. 2019;**14**:26–38.
12. Howlader NA, Krapcho M, Miller D, et al. *SEER Cancer Statistics Review, 1975–2014*. Bethesda, MD: National Cancer Institute https://seer.cancer.gov/csr/1975_2014/
13. Cancer Research UK. Stomach cancer survival trends over time. 2018. https://www.cancerresearchuk.org/health-professional/cancer-statistics/statistics-by-cancer-type/stomach-cancer/survival#heading-Two
14. Cogliano VJ, Baan R, Straif K, et al. Preventable exposures associated with human cancers. *J Natl Cancer Inst*. 2011;**103**:1827–1839.
15. Warren JR, Marshall B. Unidentified curved bacilli on gastric epithelium in active chronic gastritis. *Lancet*. 1983;**1**:1273–1275.
16. Suerbaum S, Michetti P. Helicobacter pylori infection. *N Engl J Med*. 2002;**347**:1175–1186.
17. Uemura N, Okamoto S, Yamamoto S, et al. Helicobacter pylori infection and the development of gastric cancer. *N Engl J Med*. 2001;**345**:784–789.
18. Kim HS, Lee YC, Lee HW, et al. Seroepidemiologic study of Helicobacter pylori infection in Korea. *Korean J Gastroenterol*. 1999;**33**:170–182.
19. Lim SH, Kwon JW, Kim N, et al. Prevalence and risk factors of Helicobacter pylori infection in Korea: nationwide multicenter study over 13 years. *BMC Gastroenterol*. 2013;**13**:104.

20. Wang C, Nishiyama T, Kikuchi S, et al. Changing trends in the prevalence of H. pylori infection in Japan (1908–2003): a systematic review and meta-regression analysis of 170,752 individuals. *Sci Rep*. 2017;**7**:15491.
21. World Cancer Research Fund/American Institute for Cancer Research (WCRF/AICR). *Continuous Update Project Report: Diet, Nutrition, Physical Activity and Stomach Cancer 2016* [Revised 2018]. London: World Cancer Research Fund International; 2018.
22. Ladeiras-Lopes R, Pereira AK, Nogueira A, et al. Smoking and gastric cancer: systematic review and meta-analysis of cohort studies. *Cancer Causes Control*. 2008;**19**:689–701.
23. Tramacere I, Negri E, Pelucchi C, et al. A meta-analysis on alcohol drinking and gastric cancer risk. *Ann Oncol*. 2012;**23**:28–36.
24. Tsugane S, Sasazuki S. Diet and the risk of gastric cancer: review of epidemiological evidence. *Gastric Cancer*. 2007;**10**:75–83.
25. Avgerinos KI, Spyrou N, Mantzoros CS, Dalamaga M. Obesity and cancer risk: emerging biological mechanisms and perspectives. *Metabolism*. 2019;**92**:121–135.
26. Lin XJ, Wang CP, Liu XD, et al. Body mass index and risk of gastric cancer: a meta-analysis. *Jpn J Clin Oncol*. 2014;**44**:783–791.
27. Yoon YS, Kwon AR, Lee YK, Oh SW. Circulating adipokines and risk of obesity related cancers: a systematic review and meta-analysis. *Obes Res Clin Pract*. 2019;**13**:329–339.
28. Boysen T, Mohammadi M, Melbye M, et al. EBV-associated gastric carcinoma in high- and low-incidence areas for nasopharyngeal carcinoma. *Br J Cancer*. 2009;**101**:530–533.
29. Murphy G, Pfeiffer R, Camargo MC, Rabkin CS. Meta-analysis shows that prevalence of Epstein-Barr virus-positive gastric cancer differs based on sex and anatomic location. *Gastroenterology*. 2009;**137**:824–833.
30. Liu X, Liu J, Qiu H, et al. Prognostic significance of Epstein-Barr virus infection in gastric cancer: a meta-analysis. *BMC Cancer*. 2015;**15**:782.
31. Rota M, Alicandro G, Pelucchi C, et al. Education and gastric cancer risk—an individual participant data meta-analysis in the StoP project consortium. *Int J Cancer*. 2020;**146**:671–681.
32. Song J, Su H, Zhou YY, Guo LL. Cyclooxygenase-2 expression is associated with poor overall survival of patients with gastric cancer: a meta-analysis. *Dig Dis Sci*. 2014;**59**:436–445.
33. Wang WH, Huang JQ, Zheng GF, Lam SK, Karlberg J, Wong BC. Non-steroidal anti-inflammatory drug use and the risk of gastric cancer: a systematic review and meta-analysis. *J Natl Cancer Inst*. 2003;**95**:1784–1791.
34. Watanabe A, Maehara Y, Okuyama T, Kakeji Y, Korenaga D, Sugimachi K. Gastric carcinoma with pyloric stenosis. *Surgery*. 1998;**123**:330–334.
35. Kato M, Asaka M. Recent development of gastric cancer prevention. *Jpn J Clin Oncol*. 2012;**42**:987–994.
36. Tashiro A, Sano M, Kinameri K, Fujita K, Takeuchi Y. Comparing mass screening techniques for gastric cancer in Japan. *World J Gastroenterol*. 2006;**12**:4873–4874.
37. Hamashima C, Shabana M, Okada K, Okamoto M, Osaki Y. Mortality reduction from gastric cancer by endoscopic and radiographic screening. *Cancer Sci*. 2015;**106**:1744–1749.
38. Yao K. Clinical application of magnifying endoscopy with narrow-band imaging in the stomach. *Clin Endosc*. 2015;**48**:481–490.
39. Nie RC, Yuan SQ, Chen XJ, et al. Endoscopic ultrasonography compared with multidetector computed tomography for the preoperative staging of gastric cancer: a meta-analysis. *World J Surg Oncol*. 2017;**15**:113.
40. Pei Q, Wang L, Pan J, Ling T, Lv Y, Zou X. Endoscopic ultrasonography for staging depth of invasion in early gastric cancer: a meta-analysis. *J Gastroenterol Hepatol*. 2015;**30**:1566–1573.
41. Akashi K, Yanai H, Nishikawa J, et al. Ulcerous change decreases the accuracy of endoscopic ultrasonography diagnosis for the invasive depth of early gastric cancer. *Int J Gastrointest Cancer*. 2006;**37**:133–138.
42. Bando E, Makuuchi R, Tokunaga M, Tanizawa Y, Kawamura T, Terashima M. Impact of clinical tumor-node-metastasis staging on survival in gastric carcinoma patients receiving surgery. *Gastric Cancer*. 2017;**20**:448–456.
43. Shimada H, Okazumi S, Koyama M, Murakami K. Japanese Gastric Cancer Association Task Force for Research Promotion: clinical utility of ^{18}F-fluoro-2-deoxyglucose positron emission tomography in gastric cancer. A systematic review of the literature. *Gastric Cancer*. 2011;**14**:13–21.
44. Coupe NA, Karikios D, Chong S, et al. Metabolic information on staging FDG-PET-CT as a prognostic tool in the evaluation of 97 patients with gastric cancer. *Ann Nucl Med*. 2014;**28**:128–135.
45. Małkowski B, Staniuk T, Srutek E, Gorycki T, Zegarski W, Studniarek M. (18)F-FLT PET/CT in patients with gastric carcinoma. *Gastroenterol Res Pract*. 2013;**2013**:696423.
46. Kaneko Y, Murray WK, Link E, Hicks RJ, Duong C. Improving patient selection for 18F-FDG PET scanning in the staging of gastric cancer. *J Nucl Med*. 2015;**56**:523–529.
47. Sano T, Coit DG, Kim HH, et al. Proposal of a new stage grouping of gastric cancer for TNM classification: International Gastric Cancer Association staging project. *Gastric Cancer*. 2017;**20**:217–225.
48. In H, Solsky I, Palis B, Langdon-Embry M, Ajani J, Sano T. Validation of the 8th edition of the AJCC TNM Staging System for Gastric Cancer using the National Cancer Database. *Ann Surg Oncol*. 2017;**24**:3683–3691.

17

Gastric cancer
Multimodal treatment

Mickael Chevallay, Thorsten Oliver Goetze, Salah-Eddin Al-Batran, and Stefan Mönig

Introduction

Gastric cancer is one of the leading causes of cancer-related deaths worldwide. It has an aggressive local and distant spread due to its rich vascularization, the accompanying lymphatics, and the venous drainage directly into the liver. Two principal histological subtypes of gastric cancer are the intestinal and diffuse types. The latter carries a worse prognosis and represents 20% of all gastric cancers with a growing incidence worldwide.[1] Gastric cancer also seems to be occurring higher anatomically in the stomach with lesions in the cardia becoming more prevalent.[2] In Western countries, this disease is usually discovered at an advanced stage. Using their national screening programmes, Eastern countries have been able to diagnose gastric cancer at an earlier stage. In this situation, treatment is mainly resection. It is accepted that surgery is the only curative treatment and should be offered to all patients eligible for operation.

Gastric cancer can be divided into four categories according to its spread: early (involving the stomach only), locally advanced (stomach and local lymph nodes), oligometastatic (stomach and limited distant organs affected but potentially curatively resectable), and metastatic (widespread distant disease). The overall outcomes of gastric treatment are still disappointing with high recurrence rates and low 5-year survivals with 70% of patients diagnosed with gastric cancer not being alive 5 years after the diagnosis.[3] Even for the subgroup of patients who present with localized disease without regional lymph node metastases, the 5-year relative survival rate is unsatisfactory. This high recurrence rate and poor results make the disease difficult to control by surgery alone and this approach is no longer the only treatment available. Multimodal management is the key to improvement of survival and local control.

Attempts have been made to explore neoadjuvant, adjuvant, and perioperative therapy, such as radiation therapy, chemotherapy, chemoradiotherapy, and immunotherapy in the treatment of gastric cancer after surgical resection. We summarize in this chapter the place of each part of the multimodal treatment for gastric cancer: surgery, chemotherapy, radiotherapy, and immunotherapy.

Surgery

Curative treatment

For locally controllable disease by resection, surgery is the only curative treatment. Subtotal or total gastrectomy with systematic regional lymphadenectomy is considered adequate. The goal of the operation is to ensure adequate local clearance, appropriate lymphadenectomy, and an uncomplicated anastomosis with low morbidity. The surgeon should decide between a total or subtotal gastrectomy and this decision is mainly based on the localization of the tumour. Residual disease at the resection margin is one of the feared outcomes after oncological surgery and it has been shown to adversely affect survival in gastric cancer patients. An R0 resection, defined by en bloc resection of the primary tumour without microscopic or macroscopic residual disease, should be the objective for each procedure. According to Lauren, the diffuse histological subtype tends to spread further superficially to the mucosal and submucosal layers and generally requires a total gastrectomy. The official German S3 guidelines[4,5] propose a resection margin of 5 cm for intestinal and 8 cm for the diffuse subtype. If an 8 cm margin is not possible, a frozen section should be part of the procedure to ensure free resection margins. The optimal resection margin is still under discussion and additional studies are required to find a balance between oncological safety and surgical morbidity.[6]

Nodal involvement is also another prognostic factor. Surgeons have always given importance to lymphadenectomy and its extension. It has been an important source of debate during the last decades. Two different points of view have emerged. In Eastern countries, D2 lymphadenectomy has been considered the standard procedure since the 1960s, particularly in Japan.[7] In Asian countries, extended lymphadenectomy seems to give superior results in terms of survival and recurrence. This could be explained by the greater Asian surgical experience with this dissection, by the younger age of Asian patients, and by less abdominal fat resulting in the higher feasibility of the procedure.[8] A criticism that Western surgeons have advocated is that Asian results were often provided by retrospective and non-randomized studies.[9] By contrast, in Western countries D2 lymphadenectomy was for a long time not considered a standard procedure in clinical practice because D2 was a complicated and challenging surgical technique. In addition, according to former studies, in Western randomized clinical trials,[9,10] D2 seemed associated with a higher rate of surgical complications and higher perioperative mortality, without a real survival benefit. Driven by these results, Western surgeons preferred during the 1990s to perform limited dissections.

This preference for limited lymphadenectomy by Western surgeons changed with the long-term results of the 'Dutch trial'.[11] The authors randomized 1078 patients with gastric adenocarcinoma to D1 or D2 lymphadenectomy; 11% of the D1 patients and 38% of the D2 patients had a splenectomy. Among them, 3% of the D1 patients and 30% of the D2 patients had a pancreatico-splenectomy. The short-term results showed an increase in mortality, morbidity, and reoperation rates in the extended lymphadenectomy group. However, the long-term results[12] after 15 years showed that the D2 group had lower locoregional recurrence and gastric cancer-related death rates than D1 surgery. Based on these long-term results, the authors concluded that a spleen-preserving D2 resection was currently a safer procedure than the original D2 lymphadenectomy (which required splenectomy). This lymphadenectomy should be recommended as a surgical approach for patients with curable gastric cancer. Upfront surgery is, however, rare in Western countries as the disease tends to be discovered in a more advanced stage and surgery is generally incorporated into a multimodal treatment.

The standard surgical treatment for gastric cancer is subtotal or total gastrectomy with D2 lymphadenectomy. A minimally invasive approach (robotic or laparoscopic) can be considered for early stages.[13,14] Figure 17.1 summarizes the recommended treatment according to the gastric cancer stage in Western countries.

Oligometastatic cancer

Patients are often found to have distant disease which may not be suitable for direct surgery. However, surgery is still the only curative treatment for them, even in these advanced cases. To obtain a cure, all tumour tissue must be removed. Chemotherapy is the standard treatment for incurable advanced gastric or gastro-oesophageal junction (GOJ) adenocarcinomas and the role of surgery for patients with limited or so-called oligometastatic disease is for the moment not clear.

Whether the addition of gastrectomy to chemotherapy improves the prognosis for patients with a single non-curable factor was examined in the REGATTA trial.[15] This randomized phase III trial included oligometastatic gastric cancer and was conducted in Japan, South Korea, and Singapore. Patients were randomized to palliative systemic chemotherapy alone or to surgery including gastrectomy in the form of only a D1 resection, followed by adjuvant systemic chemotherapy. To note, no curative approach was proposed in either the systemic or the surgical arm. The REGATTA study failed to show a benefit for D1 gastrectomy followed by chemotherapy for gastric cancer patients with a single non-curable factor. Due to the study concept, REGATTA was not able to define the role of surgery in the oligometastatic setting of gastric cancer. The main criticism of this study was that metastases were not removed during the gastrectomy procedure.

This principle has been called into question by the German prospective FLOT3 trial.[16] In this non-randomized trial, patients with a limited metastatic disease who received neoadjuvant fluorouracil, leucovorin, oxaliplatin, and docetaxel (FLOT) therapy proceeded to radical tumour surgery including resection of all metastatic sites. The results showed favourable survival compared to the other metastatic patients with palliative surgery or systemic therapy only. Limitations of this trial included the non-randomized character but it provided a strong rationale for the currently recruiting German FLOT5-RENAISSANCE trial.[17] This trial addresses potential benefits of surgical intervention in the stomach or GOJ adenocarcinomas with oligometastatic diseases. FLOT5 is a prospective, multicentre, randomized phase III trial. Previously untreated patients with oligometastatic disease (retroperitoneal lymph node metastases only or a maximum of one incurable organ site that is potentially resectable or locally controllable with or without retroperitoneal

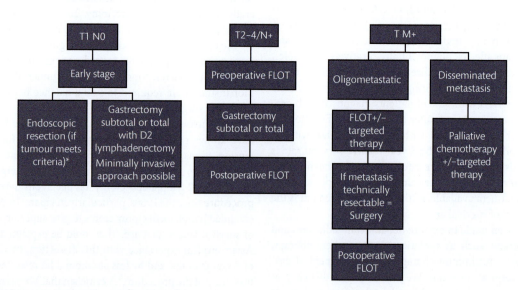

Figure 17.1 Gastric cancer treatment according to staging.

* Lesion criteria to be treated with an endoscopic resection (lesions of <2 cm in size in raised type, lesions of <1 cm in size in flat types, degree of histological differentiation: good or moderate (G1/G2), no macroscopic ulceration, invasion limited to the mucosa, no residual invasive disease after endoscopic resection).

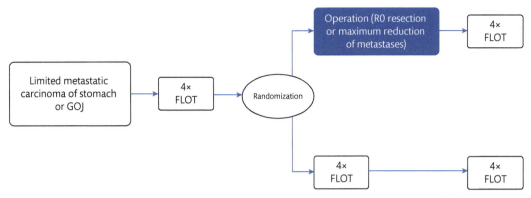

Figure 17.2 Diagram of the FLOT5-RENAISSANCE trial comparing chemotherapy alone versus surgical resection for oligometastatic gastric cancer. FLOT, fluorouracil, leucovorin, oxaliplatin, and docetaxel. While waiting for the FLOT5 results, radical surgical resection of metastatic gastric cancer is, at the moment, not recommended.

lymph nodes) receive four cycles of FLOT therapy. Patients without disease progression after four cycles are randomized to receive either an additional four to eight cycles of FLOT or radical surgical resection of primary and all metastatic sites followed by subsequent FLOT cycles. Figure 17.2 summarizes the study diagram. The results of this study should be able to determine the exact role of surgery in limited metastatic gastric cancer. This could potentially lead to a new standard of therapy and answer a long-standing question. If the outcome for the surgical arm is negative, patients with adenocarcinoma of the stomach or GOJ with oligometastatic lesions will be no longer be considered for curative surgery.

Chemotherapy

Major advances in the multimodal treatment strategy for gastric cancer have changed clinical management of the disease over the last 15 years. Initially, surgical resection alone in the advanced stage showed poor long-term results. The addition of chemotherapy allowed better local and distant control. Questions regarding the timing and the optimal therapy are still unresolved. Local standards exist according to the region and local gastric cancer profile. There are possibilities for improvement in the standardization of perioperative management. A US retrospective study[18] from 1999 to 2009 showed that the number of patients given adjuvant treatment compared to radical surgery was very low. Only 19.1% of patients received postoperative chemoradiation therapy, and 1.9% received perioperative chemotherapy. Most of the patients underwent surgery alone (60.9%) which is suboptimal management for an aggressive tumour such as a gastric cancer.

Perioperative chemotherapy

The first study that revolutionized the oncological treatment of gastric cancer was the Medical Research Council Adjuvant Gastric Infusional Chemotherapy (MAGIC) trial in 2006.[19] This trial has established evidence for the perioperative approach. A total of 503 patients with gastric, GOJ, and oesophageal adenocarcinomas were enrolled and then randomized to either perioperative chemotherapy (epirubicin, cisplatin, and fluorouracil (ECF)) plus surgery or surgery alone. The results showed that the 5-year survival for patients randomized to perioperative ECF was significantly better compared to those undergoing surgery alone (36% vs 23%; $p = 0.009$). Of note, 40% of these patients underwent D2 lymphadenectomy and only 42% of patients were able to complete the six planned cycles of chemotherapy. Only 68% of patients proceeded with surgery. The French Action Clinique Coordonnees en Cancerologie Digestive (ACCORD-07)[20] study also concluded in favour of perioperative chemotherapy compared to surgery alone. With their 224 patients with resectable adenocarcinoma of the lower oesophagus, GOJ, or stomach, the group randomized to the perioperative chemotherapy and surgery had a better overall survival (5-year rate 38% vs 24%; $p = 0.02$) and a better disease-free survival (5-year rate 34% vs 19%; $p = 0.003$). The specific group with gastric cancer consisted of 55 patients (25% of the total cohort) and also showed an improvement of overall survival. The main criticism in both trials is that fewer than 50% of the patients received postoperative chemotherapy. After the results of these two randomized trials, a perioperative treatment strategy has emerged as an alternate standard of care.

Given the modest efficacy of adjuvant chemotherapy and the infrequency with which chemotherapy can be administered postoperatively, a purely preoperative chemotherapy regimen is an attractive option. The European Organization for Research and Treatment of Cancer (EORTC) 40954 trial[21] tried to evaluate if the neoadjuvant treatment might be better than the perioperative treatment with inconsistent postoperative chemotherapy. Unfortunately, the authors had to prematurely close the study due to poor accrual after reaching 40% of its 180 patients required per arm. The results available for the included patients showed that preoperative chemotherapy was feasible in most cases in the neoadjuvant arm as 69 (95.8%) of 72 patients received both modalities. While a number of important findings significantly favoured the neoadjuvant approach (higher complete resection rate, smaller primary tumour size, and less lymph node metastases) compared with surgery alone, this study did not demonstrate a statistically significant survival benefit for neoadjuvant therapy in locally advanced gastric cancer. After a median follow-up of 4.4 years and 67 deaths, a survival benefit could not be shown (hazard ratio (HR) 0.84, 95% confidence interval (CI) 0.52–1.35; $p = 0.466$). The lack of a survival advantage, except for the fact that the trial was not powered enough, could be also attributed to the much higher rates of D2 resection (>92% in both arms in contrast to 43% in the MAGIC trial), which could mitigate the benefit of preoperative chemotherapy. The main evidence for the efficacy of preoperative chemotherapy results from a series of patients who mainly had a suboptimal lymphadenectomy leading to the hypothesis that preoperative chemotherapy could fill the gap of a limited surgery.

In Eastern regions, the standard of care is adjuvant treatment particularly S-1 (an oral fluoropyrimidine) chemotherapy. A Japanese trial, the JCOG0210 trial[22], was designed to evaluate the efficacy and safety of preoperative chemotherapy with S-1 and cisplatin followed by gastrectomy with D2 lymph node dissection for gastric cancer. The completion rate of the protocol treatment was 73.5% (80% CI 63.7–81.7%). In addition, the rate of treatment-related deaths, which was another end point, was 2.0% (1/49).

This safety and feasibility study set the basis for the JCOG0501 trial[23] which subsequently compared the neoadjuvant S-1 and cisplatin followed by D2 gastrectomy over a control arm of upfront surgery for patients with aggressive tumours (linitis plastica or large (≥8 cm) ulcero-invasive-type tumours) Postoperative adjuvant chemotherapy was offered to all patients after the first protocol. The trial included 150 patients in each arm and published the short-term results. Neoadjuvant treatment was completed in 79% of the patients. Major grade 3/4 adverse events during neoadjuvant treatment were observed in 30 patients (19.7%). Gastrectomy was performed in 147 patients (99%) in the control group and 139 patients (92%) in the neoadjuvant group. There were no significant differences in Clavien–Dindo[24] grade 2–4 morbidity and mortality (25.2% and 1.3% in control and 15.8% and 0.7% in neoadjuvant group, respectively). The authors concluded that neoadjuvant treatment for aggressive gastric cancer (linitis plastica or the large diffuse type) followed by D2 gastrectomy could be performed without reducing the chances of resection or increasing the morbidity or mortality. The long-term results of this trial are not yet available and might hopefully answer the question about the overall survival and oncological advantage of a neoadjuvant treatment.

Chemotherapy regimens are evolving in order to find the one with the highest response rate and the lowest toxicity. The FLOT combination has been shown to be successful for the treatment of stage IV oesophageal, GOJ, and gastric cancer.[25] The toxicity of FLOT appears to be moderate and the regimen is tolerated, even in the elderly population.[26] Subsequent studies have shown similar results with the recent FLOT trial reporting a superior advantage of a docetaxel-based regimen over the established regimens used in MAGIC. The multicentre, randomized FLOT4-AIO phase III trial[27] compared perioperative chemotherapy with the taxane-based triplet FLOT to the anthracycline-based triplet ECF/epirubicin, cisplatin, and capecitabine (ECX) in 716 patients with localized gastric or GOJ adenocarcinoma. Thirty-seven per cent of patients with ECF/ECX versus 50% with FLOT completed planned perioperative chemotherapy. FLOT improved median overall survival (35 months with ECF/ECX vs 50 months with FLOT; HR 0.77, 95% CI 0.63–0.94; p = 0.012) and nearly doubled the overall survival compared with pure surgery in the surgery-only arm in the MAGIC study (23% vs 45%). FLOT also showed a significantly higher rate of complete pathological remissions compared to ECF/ECX (16%, 95% CI 10–23% vs 6%, 95% CI 3–11%; p = 0.02). The phase III data show, moreover, that FLOT significantly improves 3-year overall survival (57% vs 48%) and the progression-free survival (30 vs 18 months) compared to the former standard ECF/ECX. Based on this data, the FLOT regimen is the new standard in perioperative therapy of gastric or oesophagogastric adenocarcinomas.

In these studies, only a fraction of the patients received the planned postoperative therapy, raising the question whether the benefit rested mainly on the preoperative part of the treatment.

The German NeoFLOT trial[28] was designed to compare an intensified, prolonged neoadjuvant treatment regimen in patients with gastric or GOJ adenocarcinoma at the T3, T4, and/or N1 stages. The patients received six cycles of neoadjuvant FLOT and application of adjuvant chemotherapy was explicitly not part of the protocol. Surgical resection, including D2 lymphadenectomy, was scheduled within 2–6 weeks after the completion of the last cycle. R0 resection rate was evaluated as the primary end point. Secondary end points included the complete pathological response rate.

The authors recruited 59 patients. Nine were not able to undergo surgical resection after the neoadjuvant chemotherapy. The primary end point, R0 resection rate, was 86%. Ten patients (20%) achieved complete pathological remission. Most of the good responders had an intestinal type tumour. The median disease-free survival was 32.9 months. Adjuvant therapy was administered in 39 patients (67.2%). The R0 resection rate of 86% relates to a rate of 79% in the MAGIC trial and 87% in the ACCORD trial obtained after preoperative therapy. In the NeoFLOT trial, the Lauren classification was evaluable in all patients achieving complete pathological remission showing the impact of histological tumour type on response and prognosis. This study indicates that intensified six cycles of FLOT is effective and tolerable in resectable gastric cancer. The hypothetical advantages of preoperative treatment could be the early treatment of micrometastases, higher dose intensity of delivered chemotherapy prior to the morbidity of surgery, and improved chance of complete pathological response and curative resection.

In Europe, perioperative chemotherapy using the FLOT regimen is the standard for T stage greater than 2 or N+ gastric cancer.

Postoperative chemotherapy

The US INT 0116 trial[29] demonstrated a significantly improved overall survival and 3-year recurrence-free survival in patients receiving bolus fluorouracil plus leucovorin with radiation therapy after surgical resection compared to those receiving surgery alone. Because this trial was conducted at a time when modified D2 lymphadenectomy was not routinely performed in the US, 90% of the patients underwent D0 or D1 lymphadenectomy. This led to routine criticism that the improved survival observed in the chemoradiation group was due to multimodal therapy compensating for inadequate surgical clearance of involved lymph nodes. While the median 10-year follow-up data from the study showed continued benefit in the chemoradiation group irrespective of extent of lymphadenectomy,[30] the advantage of adjuvant chemotherapy in combination with radiation was proven, but this approach is more or less recommendable after inadequate surgery.

In the East, two major trials—the Japanese ACTS-GC trial[31] and the Korean CLASSIC trial[32]—have shown survival benefit for postoperative chemotherapy. In the ACT-GC trial, patients with stage II or III gastric cancer who underwent gastrectomy with D2 lymph node dissection were randomly assigned to undergo surgery followed by adjuvant therapy with S-1 during a year or surgery alone.

They included 530 patients in each group and showed that the 3-year overall survival rate was 80.1% in the S-1 group and 70.1% in the surgery-only group favouring the chemotherapy group.

The JACCRO GC-07[33] phase III trial combined S-1 with docetaxel versus S-1 alone and showed that addition of a taxane was effective in patients with stage III gastric cancer. This trial indicated that taxanes are effective and could be safely introduced as a complement in the postoperative situation in gastric cancer patients.

The CLASSIC trial randomly assigned 1035 patients to receive capecitabine and oxaliplatin (CapeOx) for 6 months after gastrectomy with D2 lymphadenectomy or only observation. A disease-free survival benefit was shown in the chemotherapy group with at 3 years, a HR of 0.56 (95% CI 0.44–0.72; p <0.0001). The 5-year overall survival was 78% in the adjuvant arm versus 69% in the observation arm (p = 0.0029). This represented a 34% reduction in the risk of death with CapeOx versus surgery alone (HR 0.66, 95% CI 0.51–0.85; p = 0.0015).

In Asian countries, only adjuvant chemotherapy is proposed due to the results of these well-conducted studies. The difference of tumour localization and stage at diagnosis prevent the application of these conclusions to the Western population.

Metastatic disease

The prognosis of advanced or metastatic gastric cancer is poor with a 5-year overall survival rate of only 4%.[3] The standard of care therapy for patients with advanced disease is systemic chemotherapy. Treatment of gastric cancer in this setting has not changed dramatically over the last decades, and is primarily palliative. A meta-analysis from 2019[34] has retrieved the randomized controlled trials comparing different first-line systemic treatments against advanced gastric cancer. A total of 119 studies were eligible. The authors concluded that the fluoropyrimidine plus oxaliplatin doublet (especially capecitabine or S-1) should be considered as the preferred first-line regimen due to the acceptable survival benefits and lower toxicity. Other active agents include taxanes, anthracyclines, irinotecan, and biological agents such as trastuzumab for HER2-overexpressing gastric cancers.

For advanced disease, a frontline regimen should include a fluoropyrimidine and oxaliplatin doublet.

Intraperitoneal chemotherapy

Gastric cancer cells diffuse mainly through lymphatic flow and via cell seeding after serosal invasion. About 53–60% of patients affected by advanced gastric cancer present with peritoneal carcinomatosis (stage III–IV) which is more than the 40% of patients with liver metastases.[35]

At an intraoperative abdominal examination, peritoneal seeding is found in 10–20% of patients scheduled for potentially curative resection.[36] Cancer dissemination within the peritoneal cavity is a clear obstacle to radical resection. In contrast to lymphatic and haematogenous dissemination, peritoneal spread is a locoregional extension rather than a sign of systemic metastasis. However, preoperative recognition of peritoneal involvement is difficult as all imaging techniques have major limitations because of the low-volume density of peritoneal nodules.[37]

Intraperitoneal chemotherapy was proposed as an alternative to systemic chemotherapy as it allows a high intraperitoneal drug concentration to directly act on the free tumour cells and peritoneal nodules. This direct instillation perioperatively of chemotherapy into the abdominal cavity is heated as the raised temperature extends the locoregional effects with increased penetration into malignant nodules and an increased antimitotic effect.[38] The common contraindications for hyperthermic intraperitoneal chemotherapy (HIPEC) are age greater than 70 years, important comorbidities, clinical aggravation with systemic chemotherapy, malnutrition, extra-abdominal metastases, and liver metastases when unresectable.[38]

The use of HIPEC in gastric cancer was studied in a retrospective multicentric French study undertaken between February 1989 and August 2007. Glehen et al.[39] evaluated 159 patients who underwent cytoreductive surgery and perioperative intraperitoneal chemotherapy (HIPEC) and showed 1-, 3-, and 5-year survival rates of 43%, 18%, and 13%, respectively, that increased up to 61%, 30%, and 23%, respectively, in patients with a complete cytoreduction. The authors reported the completeness of cytoreduction as being the principal independent prognostic factor. The study showed that if cytoreductive surgery does not allow enough downstaging, the survival rates are poor with a median survival of 6–8 months.

Another approach to peritoneal carcinomatosis is bidirectional chemotherapy, a concept introduced by Yonemura et al.[40,41] involving a neoadjuvant intraperitoneal and systemic chemotherapy that can act on peritoneal carcinomatosis from the inside of the peritoneum and from the subperitoneal blood vessels. They proposed a drug regimen with oral S-1, Taxotere, and cisplatin and intraperitoneal cisplatin and docetaxel. In their study, they included 194 patients who received this regimen. At the end, patients were re-evaluated with a laparoscopy. If no sign of peritoneal involvement (cytology or macroscopic) was noted, the patients proceeded to cytoreductive surgery and HIPEC. Of the 194 patients, 152 (78.3%) underwent surgery and HIPEC. A complete response was observed in 24.3% of patients. Median survival time of the remaining 42 patients was 9.2 months. Overall survival was 32, 14.1, 5.9, 5.9, and 0% for 1, 2, 3, 4, and 5 years, respectively. The authors concluded that bidirectional chemotherapy with cytoreductive surgery and HIPEC for patients with peritoneal carcinomatosis can be performed safely, with acceptable morbidity and mortality. The response to bidirectional chemotherapy, optimal cytoreductive surgery, and limited peritoneal dissemination seem to be essential to achieve the best outcomes in these patients.

Patients with signet ring cell cancer are at a higher risk of peritoneal seeding. The place for prophylactic HIPEC for this particularly aggressive tumour is being evaluated by the currently starting German FLOT9 trial.[42] This multicentric trial is including patients with signet ring cell cancer at a curative stage without metastases. Patients will receive neoadjuvant FLOT cycles and then be randomized into curative surgery with adjuvant FLOT or curative surgery combined with intraoperative prophylactic HIPEC and adjuvant FLOT. Results of this study will provide evidence for the role of prophylactic intraoperative chemotherapy.

Surgery combined with intraperitoneal chemotherapy could improve survival and reduce the recurrence rates compared with surgery alone in selected cases. Intraperitoneal chemotherapy could be proposed for peritoneal carcinomatosis with a peritoneal cancer index less than 7. However, safety outcomes should be further evaluated by larger samples and the use of this specific technique is for the moment reserved to be included in trial protocols.

Radiotherapy

Radiotherapy is commonly used to control the local spread of tumours and has been a major advance in the oncological field. Gastric cancer has an aggressive local spread and radiotherapy has been employed for its local control.

In the case of gastric cancer, the history of radiotherapy began with the comparison of adjuvant chemotherapy and radiotherapy following surgical resection. The results of the British Stomach Cancer Group[43] failed to demonstrate an overall survival benefit. Outcomes were generally discouraging with patient 5-year overall survival of 17% in any treatment group. This preliminary study argued against adjuvant treatment and radiotherapy. The conclusion was that surgery remains the standard treatment for this condition and the use of adjuvant therapy was restricted.

Four years later, a study from China[44] compared 370 patients who either underwent surgery alone or received a preoperative dose of 40 Gy to the gastric cardia, GOJ, and limited regional lymph nodes. A significant overall survival advantage (absolute risk reduction of ~10% at 5 years) was noted in the group receiving the neoadjuvant radiotherapy. This survival benefit set the basis for the potential benefit of radiotherapy in gastric cancer.

Adjuvant treatment

The benefits of adjuvant radiotherapy in the management of gastric cancer became more clearly defined in 2001 after the publication of the Intergroup 0116 trial[29,30] from the US. Patients included in this study had at least stage Ib adenocarcinoma of the stomach or GOJ although most tumours were in the distal stomach, were T3 or T4 stage, and had associated nodal disease. The patients were randomized to undergo observation or adjuvant chemoradiotherapy following surgical resection. Chemotherapy consisted of fluorouracil with leucovorin, and radiation therapy with a 45 Gy dose to the tumour bed and regional lymph nodes. The overall survival was improved in the chemoradiotherapy group with a median survival of 36 months compared with 27 months in the surgery-alone group. The local recurrence rate (29% vs 19%) and regional recurrence rate (65% vs 72%) were also better following adjuvant chemoradiotherapy. Distant metastatic disease rates were similar between the two arms: 16% following chemoradiotherapy plus surgery and 18% following surgery alone. The limited extent of lymph node dissection performed in most patients enrolled in the trial has been the principal criticism. Although a full D2 lymph node dissection was recommended by the investigators, only 10% of enrolled patients underwent this procedure. Furthermore, only 36% of patients underwent a D1 resection, while the remaining 54% of patients were treated with a D0 resection. Given the high rate of lymph node involvement, many experts have argued that chemoradiotherapy may have compensated for suboptimal lymph node dissection and may be unnecessary in patients who undergo more extensive surgery. However, in total, these data confirmed the benefit of adjuvant chemoradiotherapy in the postoperative setting, particularly in node-positive patients who received no neoadjuvant therapy.

To overcome these criticisms, a Korean randomized phase III trial (ARTIST)[45] evaluated adjuvant chemoradiotherapy in patients with stage IB–IIIC who had undergone R0 resection with complete D2 lymphadenectomy. The authors randomized patients into chemotherapy and chemoradiotherapy groups. The patients received two cycles of capecitabine and cisplatin together prior to chemoradiotherapy with capecitabine, followed by another two cycles. The chemotherapy group was chosen as the control arm. The median follow-up was 5 years, after which time there were no significant differences in disease-free survival or overall survival. There was a trend towards improved disease-free survival following the use of chemoradiotherapy (HR 0.74; $p = 0.09$), which was the primary end point of the trial. On initial reporting, 3-year disease-free survival was similar between groups. However, an advantage in intestinal type tumours and positive node subgroup was found with a better disease-free survival at 3 years ($p = 0.0365$). This suggests that radiotherapy helped for the locoregional control in advanced gastric tumours.

The ARTIST 2 trial[46] randomized patients with node-positive gastric cancer after D2 lymphadenectomy to three different adjuvant treatments, stratified according to stage, type of surgery, and Lauren classification: adjuvant S-1 for 1 year, S-1 plus oxaliplatin (SOX) for 6 months, or SOX plus chemoradiotherapy 45 Gy (SOXRT). A total of 538 patients were included in the interim efficacy analysis. Stage II and III consisted of 31% and 69%, respectively, of all patients. The disease-free survival in the control arm (S-1) was significantly shorter than in SOX and SOXRT arms: S-1 versus SOX, 0.617 ($p = 0.016$) and S-1 versus SOXRT, 0.686 ($p = 0.057$). The disease-free survival at 3-years was found to be 65%, 78%, and 73% in S-1, SOX, and SOXRT arms, respectively. The authors did not find any difference in disease-free survival between the multi-regimen chemotherapy and chemoradiotherapy. Based on the results after the observation of 145 recurrence events, the independent data monitoring committee considered the results enough to meet the end point of the trial and recommended early stopping. The authors concluded that in patients with curatively D2 resected, stage II/III, node-positive gastric cancer, both adjuvant multiple regimen chemotherapy or chemoradiotherapy are effective in prolonging disease-free survival when compared to S-1 monotherapy. However, when compared to the multiple regimen postoperatively, the adjunction of radiotherapy in the postoperative period did not appear to add an advantage in term of disease-free survival and survival.

The debate regarding whether adjuvant chemoradiotherapy or perioperative chemotherapy in terms of patient outcomes for locally advanced gastric cancer was still pending but the CRITICS[47] trial has helped guide treatment decisions. In this European international study, all patients received three cycles of neoadjuvant epirubicin, oxaliplatin or cisplatin, and capecitabine prior to undergoing definitive surgical resection. Following surgery, patients were treated according to preoperative randomization, which consisted of an additional three cycles of epirubicin, cisplatin, and capecitabine or of epirubicin, oxaliplatin, and capecitabine, or chemoradiotherapy with 45 Gy combined with capecitabine and cisplatin. A total of 788 patients were enrolled and randomly assigned to chemotherapy ($n = 393$) or chemoradiotherapy ($n = 395$). At a median follow-up of 61.4 months, the median overall survival was 43 months in the chemotherapy group and 37 months in the chemoradiotherapy group (HR 1.01, 95% CI 0.84–1.22; $p = 0.90$). The extent of surgical resection was greater than in the Intergroup 0116 study, with nearly 90% of patients receiving at least D1 lymphadenectomy and a median of 20 lymph nodes removed. The 5-year overall survival was approximately 41% in both arms, and although these results appear to compare favourably to both the MAGIC and Intergroup 0116 trials, there was no evidence of superiority for either arm. The conclusion of this study is that chemoradiotherapy is not recommended for patients with a R0 resection after neoadjuvant treatment unless the patient is unable to tolerate a multiagent chemotherapy in the postoperative setting.

The role of chemoradiotherapy is less well defined for patients who undergo surgical resection with either positive margins or gross residual disease, because no prospective data exist to guide treatment decisions in this setting. A retrospective review[48] including patients from the Dutch lymphadenectomy trial revealed both a locoregional recurrence benefit (6% vs 26%) and an overall survival benefit (66% vs 29%) at 2 years following the addition of chemoradiotherapy to R1 resection. In a randomized trial examining neoadjuvant chemotherapy for patients with oesophageal cancer, long-term survival following R1 resection was achieved only in patients who received adjuvant chemoradiotherapy.

Adjuvant chemoradiotherapy is the standard care in the US according to the Intergroup 0116 trial despite methodological flaws. In other countries, the adjunction of radiotherapy to chemotherapy can be considered in patients with positive margins or gross residual disease.

Neoadjuvant treatment

For many sites throughout the gastrointestinal tract, neoadjuvant chemoradiotherapy is gaining acceptance as a bridge to surgical resection. A neoadjuvant chemoradiotherapy approach has been suggested to be beneficial by the German POET trial.[49] This study aimed to establish if the addition of neoadjuvant chemoradiotherapy to neoadjuvant chemotherapy improves survival outcomes for patients with adenocarcinomas of the GOJ. The POET trial randomized patients with Siewert type I–III adenocarcinoma of the GOJ to neoadjuvant chemotherapy or chemoradiotherapy. Neoadjuvant chemotherapy consisted of cisplatin, leucovorin, and fluorouracil in combination, while neoadjuvant chemoradiotherapy included this regimen followed by radiotherapy administered with concurrent cisplatin and etoposide. The chemoradiotherapy group demonstrated an improvement in median survival compared to the chemotherapy alone group (3-year survival 47.4% vs 27.7%) but with no statistical significance. Although the study was closed early and statistical significance was not achieved, results point to a survival advantage for preoperative chemoradiotherapy compared with preoperative chemotherapy in adenocarcinomas of the GOJ. Despite only randomizing 126 patients out of its target accrual of 354 patients, there was a higher rate of post-therapy pathologically complete response in the surgical specimens (15.6% vs 2%). The node positivity rate was also improved with chemoradiotherapy despite a dose of only 30 Gy.

Long-term results[50] reported at the 2016 Annual Meeting of the American Society of Clinical Oncology (ASCO) again noted an apparent overall survival advantage with chemoradiotherapy (39.5% vs 24.4% at 5 years), but these results failed to achieve statistical significance ($p = 0.055$).

The randomized phase III TOPGEAR[51] study was designed with the hope of elucidating the role of neoadjuvant chemoradiotherapy. The investigational arm of this trial employs a perioperative regimen as in the MAGIC trial, except chemoradiotherapy is substituted for the third neoadjuvant cycle of chemotherapy. Chemoradiotherapy consists of a 45 Gy dose to the entire stomach, any perigastric tumour extension, and regional lymph nodes. A recently published interim analysis suggests similar rates of surgical complications and treatment compliance in the investigational and control arms of this trial, but oncological outcomes are not yet available. Results from the TOPGEAR study should help clarify the role of radiotherapy in the setting of perioperative chemotherapy. After the publication of phase III data of the FLOT4 trial, TOPGEAR amended the protocol and enabled FLOT within the trial.

Neoadjuvant chemoradiotherapy confers several benefits relative to the postoperative setting, including smaller target volumes, improved patient compliance, and removal of the irradiated normal tissue at the time of resection.

Unresectable cancer

In contrast to data regarding patients with resectable gastric cancer, there are limited data to guide the treatment of patients with non-metastatic, unresectable gastric cancers. Nonetheless, chemoradiotherapy may have a role in achieving resectable durable palliation and conversion to resectable disease. A Japanese study[52] that employed chemoradiotherapy for patients with unresectable locally advanced gastric cancer demonstrated an eventual resection rate of 33.3% and an overall pathologically complete response rate of 13.3%. In this study, 40 Gy in 2 Gy daily fractions were delivered to the primary tumour and regional lymph nodes with concurrent S-1 and cisplatin. The authors also reported that all 30 patients required hospitalization due to disease-related symptoms at the time of diagnosis. In patients with good performance status and minimal comorbidity, incorporation of radiotherapy into gastric cancer treatment regimens could provide the highest likelihood of conversion to oncological resectability and disease control.

Targeted and immunotherapy

The poor results of the conventional treatment in case of advanced gastric cancer have prompted the search for alternative solutions. The erythroblastic leukaemia viral oncogene homolog 2 (ERBB2, also known as HER2) belongs to the family of epidermal growth factor receptor tyrosine kinases. This receptor is overexpressed in 10–20% of gastric cancer.[53,54] It is a negative prognostic factor in breast cancer, showing more aggressive biological behaviour and higher rate of recurrence. In gastric cancer, Her2 is only a predictive marker. Molecular targeted therapy against HER2 was developed to improve the prognosis of this tumour subtype. The mechanism of the immunotherapy is to administer antibodies against HER2 or one of its ligands to force its internalization and antagonize its recycling.

Trastuzumab was the first therapeutic antibody developed for the treatment of HER2-positive carcinomas. Its efficacy was first described in patients with breast cancer and demonstrated responses both as a single agent and in combination with chemotherapy.[55,56] Given the success in breast cancer in metastatic and adjuvant settings, evaluation of trastuzumab in gastric and oesophageal cancers was necessary.

The randomized international Trastuzumab for Gastric Cancer ToGA trial[57] evaluated trastuzumab in combination with a standard platinum/fluoropyrimidine combination versus platinum/fluoropyrimidine chemotherapy alone in inoperable locally advanced, recurrent, or metastatic HER2-positive GOJ or gastric adenocarcinoma. The addition of trastuzumab to chemotherapy improved median overall survival (13.8 months with the combination vs 11.1 months for chemotherapy alone, HR 0.74; $p = 0.0046$). The patients with higher HER2 expression seemed to obtain an even greater survival advantage (16.0 vs 11.8 months, HR 0.65). Kurokawa et al.[58] showed also promising efficacy and safety in combination with S-1 and cisplatin in combination for patients with HER2-positive unresectable gastric cancer. They recruited 56 patients with a response rate of 68% (95% CI 54–80%), and a disease control rate of 94% (95% CI 84–99%). The median overall survival was 16 months. Since the publication of these trials, the use of trastuzumab has become a standard option for patients with inoperable gastric cancer that is HER2 positive.

The role of monoclonal antibodies in the neoadjuvant setting is currently being investigated by the TRIGGER trial.[59] This Japanese study is comparing cisplatin, S-1, and trastuzumab to cisplatin and S-1 alone in the neoadjuvant setting followed by 1 year of adjuvant therapy after surgical resection. This randomized study should clarify the place of trastuzumab in the preoperative treatment of HER2-positive advanced gastric cancer.

The clinical utility of continuing trastuzumab beyond progression is still a research question. A study[60] conducted in China in patients with advanced HER2-positive gastric cancer showed slightly better survival on trastuzumab beyond progression (3 months vs 2 months without trastuzumab). This poor advantage of second-line therapy can be in part due to the heterogeneity of gastro-oesophageal cancers, which have less uniform expression of HER2 than breast cancer cells. Discordance in HER2 status between primary tumours and metastatic lesions may also bias the efficacy of HER2-directed agents.[61] HER2 expression can change at the time of disease progression and cancerous cells can lose the HER2 expression, becoming resistant to monoclonal antibodies. Retesting of HER2 expression is justified if trastuzumab is to be considered after progression on the first-line chemotherapy.

Despite HER2 copy number and high expression predicting the benefit of trastuzumab in clinical trials in breast and oesophagogastric cancers, only a minority of tumours respond to HER2 blockade with trastuzumab monotherapy. Other monoclonal antibodies have been studied such as pertuzumab, which recognizes a different epitope of HER2 than trastuzumab. The early clinical testing of pertuzumab showed very limited activity as a single agent but its combination with trastuzumab showed promising results.[62] Two ongoing, recruiting trials will clarify the utility to add pertuzumab in the treatment of resectable and metastatic gastric cancer.

The INNOVATION trial,[63] an international, randomized trial is addressing the place of adding two different antibodies, pertuzumab and trastuzumab, in the neoadjuvant setting. The authors will evaluate if neoadjuvant dual HER2 blockade with chemotherapy may lead to higher pathological complete response rates than trastuzumab and chemotherapy or chemotherapy alone in resectable gastric cancer. For the metastatic disease, the JACOB trial[64] has recruited patients with HER2-positive metastatic GOJ or gastric cancer and randomize them to pertuzumab in combination with trastuzumab, fluoropyrimidine, and cisplatin versus placebo, trastuzumab, and fluoropyrimidine. The overall results from JACOB were negative. Despite a 3.3-month absolute benefit in overall survival for the pertuzumab arm, no statistically significant benefit in overall survival for the addition of pertuzumab was shown.

The German phase II PETRARCA[65] trial has reached its primary end point. This randomized trial included patients with HER2-positive resectable oesophagogastric adenocarcinoma. Patients were randomized to a perioperative standard FLOT protocol versus FLOT and trastuzumab plus pertuzumab. The results showed a pathological complete response of 35% versus 12% in favour of the experimental arm. Therefore, the addition of trastuzumab and pertuzumab in the perioperative regimen improved local control. The results were presented at the ASCO meeting in 2020.

The sister study of PETRACA was the RAMSES trial[66] for HER2-negative patients in the perioperative setting (FLOT with or without ramucirumab) with results of the phase II data presented at the ASCO meeting 2020. The trial was negative regarding its primary end point which was the rate of complete or nearly complete pathological response; nevertheless, RAMSES was able to show that the combination of FLOT and ramucirumab showed an increase in the R0 resection rate from 83% to 97%.

Currently the DANTE phase II trial (FLOT8)[67] is evaluating the role of the programmed cell death protein 1 ligand (PD-L1) antibody atezolizumab in combination with FLOT in a randomized fashion for patients with locally advanced gastric or GOJ tumour.

The complex genetic landscape of oesophageal and gastric cancers has been extensively characterized in a genetic profiling effort by several research groups and The Cancer Genome Atlas consortium.[68] This major work gave much information and help in classifying gastric cancers into four major subtypes on their molecular and genetic data. Many tumours in these subcategories harbour targetable genetic mutations, providing opportunity for the development of new drugs.

Conclusion

Gastric cancer is an aggressive tumour, often discovered at an advanced stage. Its management by a single specialist is impossible and the expertise from different departments is mandatory.

Patients should be evaluated in the multidisciplinary setting with appropriate input from surgeons, medical oncologists, and radiation oncologists with extensive experience in the treatment of gastric malignancies. Ongoing prospective randomized trials will help to determine timing of chemotherapy and radiation in relation to surgery for gastric cancer. A better understanding of the gastric cancer biology has permitted adding to the therapeutic arsenal new precise antibodies that target specific steps of the oncological pathway in gastric cancer. Multiple trials will clarify the place of each new treatment and may improve the poor prognosis of gastric cancer.

REFERENCES

1. Stiekema J, Cats A, Kuijpers A, et al. Surgical treatment results of intestinal and diffuse type gastric cancer. Implications for a differentiated therapeutic approach? *Eur J Surg Oncol.* 2013;**39**:686–693.
2. Kaneko S, Yoshimura T. Time trend analysis of gastric cancer incidence in Japan by histological types, 1975–1989. *Br J Cancer.* 2001;**84**:400–405.
3. National Cancer Institute. Cancer stat facts: stomach cancer. 2020. https://seer.cancer.gov/statfacts/html/stomach.html
4. Mönig S, Ott K, Gockel I, et al. S3 guidelines on gastric cancer-diagnosis and treatment of adenocarcinoma of the stomach and esophagogastric junction. *Chirurg.* 2020;**91**:37–40.
5. Moehler M, Al-Batran SE, Andus T, et al. German S3-guideline 'Diagnosis and treatment of esophagogastric cancer'. *Z Gastroenterol.* 2011;**49**:461–531.
6. Niclauss N, Jung MK, Chevallay M, Mönig SP. Minimal length of proximal resection margin in adenocarcinoma of the esophagogastric junction: a systematic review of the literature. *Updates Surg.* 2019;**71**:401–409.
7. Murakami T. The general rules for the gastric cancer study in surgery. *Jpn J Surg.* 1973;**3**:61–71.
8. Bonenkamp J, van de Velde C, Kampschöer G, et al. Comparison of factors influencing the prognosis of Japanese, German, and Dutch gastric cancer patients. *World J Surg.* 1993;**17**:410–414.
9. Cuschieri A, Joypaul V, Fayers P, et al. Postoperative morbidity and mortality after D1 and D2 resections for gastric cancer: preliminary results of the MRC randomised controlled surgical trial. *Lancet.* 1996;**347**:995–999.
10. Cuschieri A, Weeden S, Fielding J, et al. Patient survival after D1 and D2 resections for gastric cancer: long-term results of the MRC randomized surgical trial. Surgical Co-operative Group. *Br J Cancer.* 1999;**79**:1522–1530.
11. Bonenkamp JJ, Songun I, Hermans J, et al. Randomised comparison of morbidity after D1 and D2 dissection for gastric cancer in 996 Dutch patients. *Lancet.* 1995;**345**:745–748.
12. Songun I, Putter H, Kranenbarg EM, Sasako M, van de Velde CJ. Surgical treatment of gastric cancer: 15-year follow-up results of the randomised nationwide Dutch D1D2 trial. *Lancet Oncol.* 2010;**11**:439–449.
13. Chevallay M, Jung M, Berlth F, Seung-Hun C, Morel P, Mönig S. Laparoscopic surgery for gastric cancer: the European point of view. *J Oncol.* 2019;**2019**:8738502.
14. Chevallay M, Bollschweiler E, Chandramohan SM, et al. Cancer of the gastroesophageal junction: a diagnosis, classification, and management review. *Ann N Y Acad Sci.* 2018;**1434**:132–138.
15. Fujitani K, Yang H, Mizusawa J, et al. Gastrectomy plus chemotherapy versus chemotherapy alone for advanced gastric cancer with a single non-curable factor (REGATTA): a phase 3, randomised controlled trial. *Lancet Oncol.* 2016;**17**:309–318.
16. Al-Batran SE, Homann N, Pauligk C, et al. Effect of neoadjuvant chemotherapy followed by surgical resection on survival in patients with limited metastatic gastric or gastroesophageal junction cancer: the AIO-FLOT3 Trial. *JAMA Oncol.* 2017;**3**:1237–1244.
17. Al-Batran SE, Goetze TO, Mueller DW, et al. The RENAISSANCE (AIO-FLOT5) trial: effect of chemotherapy alone vs. chemotherapy followed by surgical resection on survival and quality of life in patients with limited-metastatic adenocarcinoma of the stomach or esophagogastric junction—a phase III trial of the German AIO/CAO-V/CAOGI. *BMC Cancer.* 2017;**17**:893.
18. Snyder RA, Penson DF, Ni S, Koyama T, Merchant NB. Trends in the use of evidence-based therapy for resectable gastric cancer. *J Surg Oncol.* 2014;**110**:285–290.
19. Cunningham D, Allum WH, Stenning SP, et al. Perioperative chemotherapy versus surgery alone for resectable gastroesophageal cancer. *N Engl J Med.* 2006;**355**:11–20.
20. Ychou M, Boige V, Pignon JP, et al. Perioperative chemotherapy compared with surgery alone for resectable gastroesophageal adenocarcinoma: an FNCLCC and FFCD multicenter phase III trial. *J Clin Oncol.* 2011;**29**:1715–1721.
21. Schuhmacher C, Gretschel S, Lordick F, et al. Neoadjuvant chemotherapy compared with surgery alone for locally advanced cancer of the stomach and cardia: European Organisation for Research and Treatment of Cancer randomized trial 40954. *J Clin Oncol.* 2010;**28**:5210–5218.
22. Iwasaki Y, Sasako M, Yamamoto S, et al. Phase II study of preoperative chemotherapy with S-1 and cisplatin followed by gastrectomy for clinically resectable type 4 and large type 3 gastric cancers (JCOG0210). *J Surg Oncol.* 2013;**107**:741–745.
23. Terashima M, Iwasaki Y, Mizusawa J, et al. Randomized phase III trial of gastrectomy with or without neoadjuvant S-1 plus cisplatin for type 4 or large type 3 gastric cancer, the short-term safety and surgical results: Japan Clinical Oncology Group Study (JCOG0501). *Gastric Cancer.* 2019;**22**:1044–1052.
24. Dindo D, Demartines N, Clavien PA. Classification of surgical complications: a new proposal with evaluation in a cohort of 6336 patients and results of a survey. *Ann Surg.* 2004;**240**:205–213.
25. Al-Batran SE, Hartmann JT, Hofheinz R, et al. Biweekly fluorouracil, leucovorin, oxaliplatin, and docetaxel (FLOT) for patients with metastatic adenocarcinoma of the stomach or esophagogastric junction: a phase II trial of the Arbeitsgemeinschaft Internistische Onkologie. *Ann Oncol.* 2008;**19**:1882–1887.
26. Lorenzen S, Pauligk C, Homann N, Schmalenberg H, Jäger E, Al-Batran SE. Feasibility of perioperative chemotherapy with infusional 5-FU, leucovorin, and oxaliplatin with (FLOT) or without (FLO) docetaxel in elderly patients with locally advanced esophagogastric cancer. *Br J Cancer.* 2013;**108**:519–526.
27. Al-Batran SE, Homann N, Pauligk C, et al. Perioperative chemotherapy with fluorouracil plus leucovorin, oxaliplatin, and docetaxel versus fluorouracil or capecitabine plus cisplatin and epirubicin for locally advanced, resectable gastric or gastro-oesophageal junction adenocarcinoma (FLOT4): a randomised, phase 2/3 trial. *Lancet.* 2019;**393**:1948–1957.
28. Schulz C, Kullmann F, Kunzmann V, et al. NeoFLOT: multicenter phase II study of perioperative chemotherapy in resectable adenocarcinoma of the gastroesophageal junction or gastric adenocarcinoma—very good response predominantly in patients with intestinal type tumors. *Int J Cancer.* 2015;**137**:678–685.
29. Macdonald JS, Smalley SR, Benedetti J, et al. Chemoradiotherapy after surgery compared with surgery alone for adenocarcinoma of the stomach or gastroesophageal junction. *N Engl J Med.* 2001;**345**:725–730.
30. Smalley S, Benedetti J, Haller D, et al. Updated analysis of SWOG-directed Intergroup Study 0116: a phase III trial of adjuvant radiochemotherapy versus observation after curative gastric cancer resection. *J Clin Oncol.* 2012;**30**:2327–2333.
31. Sakuramoto S, Sasako M, Yamaguchi T, et al. Adjuvant chemotherapy for gastric cancer with S-1, an oral fluoropyrimidine. *N Engl J Med.* 2007;**357**:1810–1820.
32. Bang Y, Kim Y, Yang H, et al. Adjuvant capecitabine and oxaliplatin for gastric cancer after D2 gastrectomy

(CLASSIC): a phase 3 open-label, randomised controlled trial. *Lancet*. 2012;**379**:315–321.

33. Yoshida K, Kodera Y, Kochi M, et al. Addition of docetaxel to oral fluoropyrimidine improves efficacy in patients with stage III gastric cancer: interim analysis of JACCRO GC-07, a randomized controlled trial. *J Clin Oncol*. 2019;**37**:1296–1304.
34. Cheng J, Cai M, Shuai X, Gao J, Wang G, Tao K. First-line systemic therapy for advanced gastric cancer: a systematic review and network meta-analysis. *Ther Adv Med Oncol*. 2019;**11**:1758835919877726.
35. Roviello F, Caruso S, Marrelli D, et al. Treatment of peritoneal carcinomatosis with cytoreductive surgery and hyperthermic intraperitoneal chemotherapy: state of the art and future developments. *Surg Oncol*. 2011;**20**:e38–e54.
36. Hioki M, Gotohda N, Konishi M, Nakagohri T, Takahashi S, Kinoshita T. Predictive factors improving survival after gastrectomy in gastric cancer patients with peritoneal carcinomatosis. *World J Surg*. 2010;**34**:555–562.
37. McMullen J, Selleck M, Wall N, Senthil M. Peritoneal carcinomatosis: limits of diagnosis and the case for liquid biopsy. *Oncotarget*. 2017;**8**:43481–43490.
38. Feingold PL, Kwong ML, Sabesan A, Sorber R, Rudloff U. Cytoreductive surgery and hyperthermic intraperitoneal chemotherapy for gastric cancer and other less common disease histologies: is it time? *J Gastrointest Oncol*. 2016;**7**:87–98.
39. Glehen O, Gilly FN, Arvieux C, et al. Peritoneal carcinomatosis from gastric cancer: a multi-institutional study of 159 patients treated by cytoreductive surgery combined with perioperative intraperitoneal chemotherapy. *Ann Surg Oncol*. 2010;**17**:2370–2377.
40. Canbay E, Mizumoto A, Ichinose M, et al. Outcome data of patients with peritoneal carcinomatosis from gastric origin treated by a strategy of bidirectional chemotherapy prior to cytoreductive surgery and hyperthermic intraperitoneal chemotherapy in a single specialized center in Japan. *Ann Surg Oncol*. 2014;**21**:1147–1152.
41. Yonemura Y, Elnemr A, Endou Y, et al. Effects of neoadjuvant intraperitoneal/systemic chemotherapy (bidirectional chemotherapy) for the treatment of patients with peritoneal metastasis from gastric cancer. *Int J Surg Oncol*. 2012;**2012**:148420.
42. ClinicalTrials.gov. HIPEC + FLOT vs. FLOT alone in patients with gastric cancer and GEJ (PREVENT). 2020. https://clinicaltrials.gov/ct2/show/NCT04447352
43. Hallissey MT, Dunn JA, Ward LC, Allum WH. The second British Stomach Cancer Group trial of adjuvant radiotherapy or chemotherapy in resectable gastric cancer: five-year follow-up. *Lancet*. 1994;**343**:1309–1312.
44. Zhang ZX, Gu XZ, Yin WB, et al. Randomized clinical trial on the combination of preoperative irradiation and surgery in the treatment of adenocarcinoma of gastric cardia (AGC)—report on 370 patients. *Int J Radiat Oncol Biol Phys*. 1998;**42**:929–934.
45. Park SH, Sohn TS, Lee J, et al. Phase III trial to compare adjuvant chemotherapy with capecitabine and cisplatin versus concurrent chemoradiotherapy in gastric cancer: final report of the Adjuvant Chemoradiotherapy in Stomach Tumors Trial, including survival and subset analyses. *J Clin Oncol*. 2015;**33**:3130–3136.
46. Park S, Zang D, Han B, et al. ARTIST 2: interim results of a phase III trial involving adjuvant chemotherapy and/or chemoradiotherapy after D2-gastrectomy in stage II/III gastric cancer (GC). *J Clin Oncol*. 2019;**37**(15 Suppl):4001.
47. Cats A, Jansen EPM, van Grieken NCT, et al. Chemotherapy versus chemoradiotherapy after surgery and preoperative chemotherapy for resectable gastric cancer (CRITICS): an international, open-label, randomised phase 3 trial. *Lancet Oncol*. 2018;**19**:616–628.
48. Stiekema J, Trip AK, Jansen EP, et al. The prognostic significance of an R1 resection in gastric cancer patients treated with adjuvant chemoradiotherapy. *Ann Surg Oncol*. 2014;**21**:1107–1114.
49. Stahl M, Walz MK, Stuschke M, et al. Phase III comparison of preoperative chemotherapy compared with chemoradiotherapy in patients with locally advanced adenocarcinoma of the esophagogastric junction. *J Clin Oncol*. 2009;**27**:851–856.
50. Stahl M, Riera-Knorrenschild J, Stuschke M, et al. Preoperative chemoradiotherapy and the long-term run in curative treatment of locally advanced oesophagogastric junction adenocarcinoma: update of the POET phase III study. *J Clin Oncol*. 2016;**34**(15 Suppl):4031.
51. Leong T, Smithers BM, Haustermans K, et al. TOPGEAR: a randomized, phase III trial of perioperative ECF chemotherapy with or without preoperative chemoradiation for resectable gastric cancer: interim results from an international, intergroup trial of the AGITG, TROG, EORTC and CCTG. *Ann Surg Oncol*. 2017;**24**:2252–2258.
52. Saikawa Y, Kubota T, Kumagai K, et al. Phase II study of chemoradiotherapy with S-1 and low-dose cisplatin for inoperable advanced gastric cancer. *Int J Radiat Oncol Biol Phys*. 2008;**71**:173–179.
53. He C, Bian XY, Ni XZ, et al. Correlation of human epidermal growth factor receptor 2 expression with clinicopathological characteristics and prognosis in gastric cancer. *World J Gastroenterol*. 2013;**19**:2171–2178.
54. Jørgensen JT, Hersom M. HER2 as a prognostic marker in gastric cancer—a systematic analysis of data from the literature. *J Cancer*. 2012;**3**:137–144.
55. Slamon D, Eiermann W, Robert N, et al. Adjuvant trastuzumab in HER2-positive breast cancer. *N Engl J Med*. 2011;**365**:1273–1283.
56. Kast K, Schoffer O, Link T, et al. Trastuzumab and survival of patients with metastatic breast cancer. *Arch Gynecol Obstet*. 2017;**296**:303–312.
57. Bang YJ, Van Cutsem E, Feyereislova A, et al. Trastuzumab in combination with chemotherapy versus chemotherapy alone for treatment of HER2-positive advanced gastric or gastro-oesophageal junction cancer (ToGA): a phase 3, open-label, randomised controlled trial *Lancet*. 2010;**376**:687–697.
58. Kurokawa Y, Sugimoto N, Miwa H, et al. Phase II study of trastuzumab in combination with S-1 plus cisplatin in HER2-positive gastric cancer (HERBIS-1). *Br J Cancer* 2014;**110**:1163–1168.
59. Kataoka K, Tokunaga M, Mizusawa J, et al. A randomized phase II trial of systemic chemotherapy with and without trastuzumab followed by surgery in HER2-positive advanced gastric or esophagogastric junction adenocarcinoma with extensive lymph node metastasis: Japan Clinical Oncology Group study JCOG1301 (Trigger Study). *Jpn J Clin Oncol*. 2015;**45**:1082–1086.
60. Li Q, Jiang H, Li H, et al. Efficacy of trastuzumab beyond progression in HER2 positive advanced gastric cancer: a multicenter prospective observational cohort study. *Oncotarget*. 2016;**7**:50656–50665.
61. Gumusay O, Benekli M, Ekinci O, et al. Discordances in HER2 status between primary gastric cancer and corresponding metastatic sites. *Jpn J Clin Oncol*. 2015;**45**:416–421.

62. Gianni L, Lladó A, Bianchi G, et al. Open-label, phase II, multicenter, randomized study of the efficacy and safety of two dose levels of pertuzumab, a human epidermal growth factor receptor 2 dimerization inhibitor, in patients with human epidermal growth factor receptor 2-negative metastatic breast cancer. *J Clin Oncol*. 2010;**28**:1131–1137.
63. Wagner AD, Grabsch HI, Mauer M, et al. EORTC-1203-GITCG—the 'INNOVATION'-trial: effect of chemotherapy alone versus chemotherapy plus trastuzumab, versus chemotherapy plus trastuzumab plus pertuzumab, in the perioperative treatment of HER2 positive, gastric and gastroesophageal junction adenocarcinoma on pathologic response rate: a randomized phase II-intergroup trial of the EORTC-Gastrointestinal Tract Cancer Group, Korean Cancer Study Group and Dutch Upper GI-Cancer group. *BMC Cancer*. 2019;**19**:494.
64. Liu T, Qin Y, Li J, et al. Pertuzumab in combination with trastuzumab and chemotherapy for Chinese patients with HER2-positive metastatic gastric or gastroesophageal junction cancer: a subpopulation analysis of the JACOB trial. *Cancer Commun (Lond)*. 2019;**39**:38.
65. Hofheinz R, Haag G, Ettrich T, et al. Perioperative trastuzumab and pertuzumab in combination with FLOT versus FLOT alone for HER2-positive resectable esophagogastric adenocarcinoma: final results of the PETRARCA multicenter randomized phase II trial of the AIO. *J Clin Oncol*. 2020;**38**(15 Suppl):4502.
66. Al-Batran S, Hofheinz R, Schmalenberg H, et al. Perioperative ramucirumab in combination with FLOT versus FLOT alone for resectable esophagogastric adenocarcinoma (RAMSES/FLOT7): results of the phase II-portion—a multicenter, randomized phase II/III trial of the German AIO and Italian GOIM. *J Clin Oncol*. 2020;**38**(15 Suppl):4501.
67. Al-Batran, S, Pauligk C, Hofheinz R, et al. Perioperative atezolizumab in combination with FLOT versus FLOT alone in patients with resectable esophagogastric adenocarcinoma: DANTE, a randomized, open-label phase II trial of the German Gastric Group of the AIO and the SAKK. *J Clin Oncol*. 2019;**37**(15 Suppl):TPS4142.
68. Cancer Genome Atlas Research Network. Comprehensive molecular characterization of gastric adenocarcinoma. *Nature*. 2014;**513**:202–209.

18

Gastric cancer
Endoscopic treatment

Chang Seok Bang

Introduction

Gastric cancer remains a health-related burden worldwide and is the third leading cause of cancer-related mortality.[1] With the widespread implementation of endoscopic screening programmes in high-risk regions for gastric cancer, the proportion of patients diagnosed with early gastric cancers (EGCs) has increased.[2-4] Although previous studies have shown that endoscopic screening programmes reduced mortality rates of gastric cancer by 42–47%,[2,4,5] these results would not have been guaranteed without excellent therapeutic outcomes for EGCs.[6]

Endoscopic submucosal dissection (ESD) is indicated for superficial gastrointestinal neoplasms with negligible risk of lymph node metastasis (LNM).[7-9] This procedure has an advantage of achieving en bloc resection (removal of the lesion in a single piece) of mucosal and submucosal tumours irrespective of the size and location of the lesions, enabling the retrieval of a pathological specimen to determine whether or not a curative resection was achieved. The stomach is preserved and surgery avoided. The procedure has evolved through an improvement in endoscopic skills, expertise, and equipment, and a better understanding of the indications, short-term and long-term outcomes, and management of adverse events.[6,10] ESD technique is being applied and developed into different procedures aiming to restore function of organs such as peroral endoscopic myotomy (POEM) for the treatment of achalasia or gastric POEM (G-POEM) for the treatment of gastroparesis as well as neoplasms. Natural orifice transluminal endoscopic surgery (NOTES) or third space endoscopy is a new field which may be used in the future.

In this chapter, the indications, procedural details, therapeutic outcomes, management of adverse events of ESD, and post-ESD surveillance strategy will be discussed.

Endoscopic mucosal resection

After the introduction of the endoscopic mucosal resection (EMR) technique in 1984, this simple and convenient method has offered the means for both diagnosis and therapy.[11] The procedure involves submucosal fluid injection under the lesion (lifting it), snaring, and resection (Figure 18.1). However, the most important pitfall was difficulty in trapping lesions which had a flat morphology.[11] The steel wire slips easily when trapping the flat lesion, which leads to failure of en bloc resection and incomplete resection was associated with local recurrence.[8,11] Moreover, this procedure was not indicated for lesions larger than 2 cm owing to the limited size of the snare. Suctioning methods (cap-assisted EMR or EMR with band ligation) which are modified EMRs were also tried, but it was also difficult to apply for large lesions. Therefore, EMR after circumferential precutting with a specialized endoscopic knife was introduced in 1988 and this was evolved through the ESD technique.[12]

Endoscopic submucosal dissection procedure

Performing ESD is not limited to its technical aspects. An assessment of the lesions and the patient's age, preference, and surgical comorbidities should be considered. In terms of the lesion assessment, size, histology, ulceration (histological), and depth of invasion should be predicted prior to ESD because these factors are associated with the risk of LNMs. The diagnosis should be accurate and the indication precise prior to ESD. A standardized ESD procedure should be established and an evaluation of curability should be made (satisfying post-ESD criteria) after ESD. Proper management of adverse events and long-term post-endoscopic resection surveillance is also important. If a similar result is guaranteed in the short- and long-term outcomes compared to surgery, ESD can be implemented.[13]

The ESD technique comprises marking around the lesion, submucosal fluid injection, circumferential mucosal incision, dissection through the submucosa, and post-ESD wound management (Figure 18.2).

Margin delineation and assessment of depth of invasion

After detection of EGC which has morphological changes of neoplastic lesions, such as mucosal colour alterations, irregular surface contour, or loss of dynamic response to air insufflation, endoscopic

18 Gastric cancer

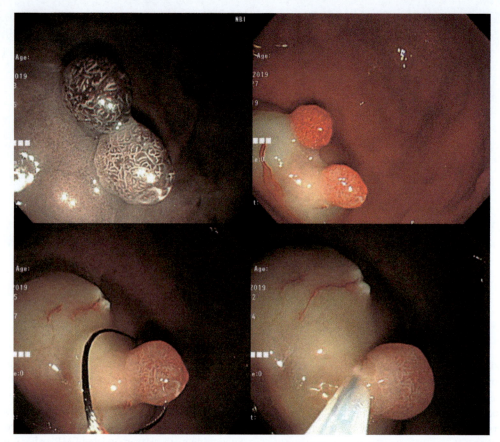

Figure 18.1 EMR. Submucosal fluid injection under the lesion (lifting the lesion), snaring, and resection of the lesion in sequence.

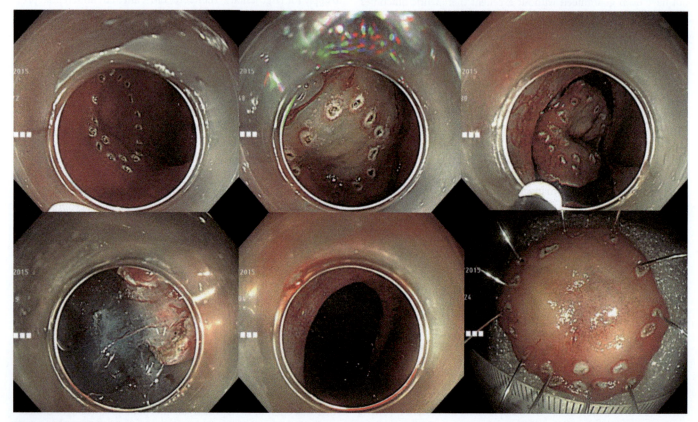

Figure 18.2 ESD. Marking around the lesion, submucosal fluid injection, circumferential mucosal incision, dissection through the submucosa in sequence.

ultrasonography (EUS) is usually performed to check the depth of invasion (securing the vertical margin) and regional LN enlargement. However, some studies have shown that EUS is not helpful to predict the depth of invasion compared to endoscopic visual inspection alone or along with a computed tomography scan to predict the depth of invasion of the lesion and to check the regional LNM[14–16]; therefore, performing EUS before ESD for EGC remains controversial.[17]

The application of endoscopic imaging technologies such as narrow-band imaging, confocal imaging, or magnifying techniques (so-called image-enhanced endoscopy) is also known to enhance diagnostic yield. The history of chromoendoscopy is old, but it is still a useful tool for characterization and margin delineation of the lesions (i.e. securing the lateral margin). Among the several dyes which have different mechanisms and contrast agents, indigo carmine has been most widely tried for the margin delineation of EGCs. It is not absorbed and makes the mucosal irregularities more visible.[18] The dye fills the depressed mucosal sites, thus highlighting the surface irregularities and such characteristics can help in estimating the depth of invasion of the lesions and determining the range of resection.[17] Therefore, it can be used before marking around the lesion. Methylene blue can also be used as a contrast agent in the stomach. However, it is also selectively absorbed in the specialized intestinal metaplasia.

Marking

The markings are generally placed 2–3 mm apart or more from the estimated border of the lesion in ESD of EGC with differentiated-type histology (EGC-DH) using an electrocautery device, such as argon plasma coagulation or the tip of the ESD knife.[19] However, EGC with undifferentiated-type histology (EGC-UH) is known to extend laterally along the proliferative zone in the intermediate layer of mucosa (subepithelial spreading) and the development pattern from the intermediate layer could make it not exposed to the surface mucosa.[3,20] Therefore, making a larger safety margin is recommended, although the exact extent has not been described. Previous clinical studies used markings 5–10 mm apart from the estimated borders of the lesion in ESD of EGC-UH.[19] Subepithelial spreading signet ring cell carcinoma (SRC) is more prevalent than the epithelial spreading type in cases with atrophy and intestinal metaplasia.[21–23] Therefore, making larger safety margins has been recommended in ESD for SRC with surrounding mucosa exhibiting atrophy and/or intestinal metaplasia.[21–23]

Submucosal fluid injection

Submucosal fluid injection via a needle creates a potential space as a dissection plane beneath the lesion.[24] Non-lifting means that the lesion invaded the muscularis propria, or that the injection needle is located in the muscularis propria, or possibly that submucosal fibrosis exists around the lesion. The injected fluid is eventually absorbed. A long-lasting submucosal fluid cushion is thought to be associated with increased safety and efficacy of ESD procedures, although evidence is lacking.[24]

Because the osmotic pressure of normal saline (and/or epinephrine (adrenaline)/indigo carmine) and tissue fluid is the same, it is absorbed quickly and repeated injections are required during the procedure.[25] Therefore, a variety of injectable fluids have been tried, such as hyaluronic acid, hydroxyethyl starch, hydroxypropyl methylcellulose, hypertonic saline, 50% dextrose, and glycerol. There is no single best injectable submucosal fluid currently.

Circumferential mucosal incision and dissection through the submucosal space

In this step of ESD, a transparent cap or hood attachment at the tip of the endoscope is essential. This can maintain a 3–4 mm distance of the endoscope tip from the lesion, providing visibility to the procedure. A circumferential mucosal incision with an endoscopic knife is performed outside the marking. The mucosal incision should be made deep enough so that the submucosal layer is fully visible. If a shallow incision is made, it might result in brisk haemorrhage and make the subsequent submucosal dissection difficult. The most important thing in submucosal dissection is to maintain the submucosal dissection plane visible and parallel to the muscularis propria, and carry out meticulous dissection using electrocautery. It should be noted that if deep blind dissection is done without endoscopic vision, brisk haemorrhage may make haemostasis difficult and extend the procedure time or result in perforation.

Pathological confirmation

Pathological confirmation of the resected specimen after ESD determines whether curative resection was achieved (satisfying ESD criteria), which implies a favourable long-term outcome.[23] If evaluation of the resected specimen does not demonstrate ulceration, penetration of the muscularis mucosa, or lymphovascular invasion (LVI), the risk of LNM is less than 1% (satisfying absolute ESD criteria). When the pathology shows a positive margin of the resected specimen, deep submucosal invasion, or LVI, gastrectomy should be performed. (If there was a positive horizontal margin or piecemeal resection was done, endoscopic surveillance or re-treatment is recommended rather than surgery.)

Post-endoscopic submucosal dissection wound management

To achieve clear resection margins, ESD inevitably leaves a large and deep ulcer, which can lead to major adverse events.[26] Haemorrhage of the ESD-induced ulcer is immediately treated during the procedure using various haemostatic devices. However, delayed haemorrhage is one of the drawbacks of ESD.[26] Previous reports suggested about 2.6–7% of patients showed delayed haemorrhage.[26] Careful coagulation of the exposed blood vessels at the resection site after ESD may reduce the risk of delayed haemorrhage.[27] However, a meta-analysis in 2017 revealed that delayed post-ESD haemorrhage was more common in patients who underwent prophylactic haemostasis than in those who did not.[28] Second-look endoscopy after ESD also did not reduce the risk of delayed post-ESD haemorrhage.[28]

Proton pump inhibitors (PPIs) are the most widely used anti-ulcer medication and are currently the standard treatment, not only in patients with peptic ulcers but also in patients with ESD-induced artificial gastric ulcers.[26] However, the optimal treatment regimen (intravenous vs oral, continuous infusion vs intermittent injections, once daily vs twice daily, etc.) or duration of treatment for ESD-induced gastric ulcers has not been established.[26] The mechanism of healing in ESD-induced gastric ulcers is different from that of a peptic ulcer. The pathogenic mechanism is completely mechanical; therefore, the mucosal damage is not by gastric acid or digestive enzymes, or cellular apoptosis by *Helicobacter pylori*.[26,29] The stomach usually contains little acid due to the periprocedural PPI injections and the normal mucosal protective mechanism is intact in patients who undergo gastric ESD. Therefore, ESD-induced artificial gastric ulcers usually heal within 8 weeks regardless of their size and location, H. pylori infection status, or the extent of gastric atrophy.[26,29,30] Considering that most of the ESD-induced episodes of haemorrhage occur within 28 days after the procedure, the recommended duration of the PPI therapy should be at least 4 weeks.[26,31] A recent randomized controlled trial also revealed that there was no difference in the healing rate of ESD-induced artificial gastric ulcers between the different PPIs used.[26]

Management of adverse events in endoscopic submucosal dissection

With the advances in their skills and expertise, endoscopists have focused on ensuring the quality of recovery of patients as well as reducing procedure-related adverse events.[32] A recent multicentre prospective study showed that 2.6–7% of patients underwent delayed haemorrhage and 1.7% underwent ESD-induced gastric perforation.[26] However, most of the delayed haemorrhage cases were treated with endoscopic haemostasis or conservative management without surgery or transarterial embolization. Surgical management is generally recommended for the treatment of ESD-induced gastric perforation. However, small perforations have recently been closed using endoscopic clip closure techniques.[33]

Procedure-related gastric perforation or haemorrhage might be less important, because it is usually managed by endoscopic haemostasis or clipping without additional surgical treatment. However, procedure-related abdominal pain or discomfort might lower the quality of recovery of patients after gastric ESD.[32]

Room air is the most commonly used material during diagnostic and therapeutic endoscopic procedures. However, it can cause abdominal pain, because it is poorly absorbed in the intestines and is mostly excreted by belching or passage of flatus.[32,34] Moreover, abdominal discomfort or pain due to retained gas is common. When gastric perforation occurs, the leaked air increases the intra-abdominal pressure and can induce a pneumoperitoneum. Although rarely observed, air embolism is another adverse event related to ESD-induced gastric perforation.[35–37] To overcome these potentially fatal adverse events, carbon dioxide (CO_2) instead of room air has been proposed as the insufflating agent, because CO_2 is rapidly absorbed by tissues.[32,34] CO_2 is 160 times more rapidly absorbed than nitrogen is and 13 times more rapidly absorbed than oxygen.[32,34,38] It is passively absorbed through the gastrointestinal mucosa into the bloodstream and eventually exhaled through the lungs.[32] Therefore, rapid absorption of CO_2 can minimize the barotrauma and can rapidly reduce luminal distension.[34]

The superior efficacy of CO_2 (vs room air) in reducing postoperative pain or discomfort during laparoscopic surgery has been established.[38] However, this has not been extensively evaluated in the field of gastric ESD.[32] Despite its theoretical safety, the superior recovery after CO_2 insufflation (vs room air insufflation) is uncertain after various endoscopic procedures, except for colonoscopy.[32,39] In addition, the superior recovery quality of CO_2 insufflation might not be applicable in gastric ESD, because most of the insufflated agents are excreted by belching or endoscopic suction immediately after a certain amount of air has accumulated in the stomach.[32] Therefore, the influence of insufflated agents on abdominal discomfort might be less significant than that of colonoscopy. Moreover, abdominal discomfort does not depend entirely on the use of insufflated agents, but is also associated with the sedation level of the patient.[32] The ESD-induced ulcer itself can cause abdominal discomfort regardless of the insufflating agents used. CO_2 insufflation may offer advantages over air with respect to unexpected serious adverse events of ESD, especially in gastric perforation.[32] However, it is not urgently necessary to relieve abdominal pain or discomfort in gastric ESD, especially for skilled endoscopists.[32]

Definition of therapeutic outcomes of endoscopic submucosal dissection

En bloc resection means removal of the lesion in a single piece and complete resection (R0 resection) means complete en bloc resection with negative lateral and vertical margins. Curative resection (satisfying ESD criteria) means R0 resection with absence of LVI and submucosal invasion less than 500 μm in gastric ESD.

Indications for endoscopic submucosal dissection

The proper selection of the ESD candidate is essential before performing ESD. The most fundamental hypothesis is that endoscopic resection can be done with curative intent in EGCs without LNM. Therefore, indications for ESD are made using the combination of factors that are associated with negligible LNM rates from the retrospective analysis of surgically resected specimens. These indications are categorized by EGC-DH and EGC-UH according to the differentiation of the lesion and specific size, morphology, and histology.[7,8,40]

The absolute indications for ESD for EGC include intramucosal EGC-DH of less than 2 cm in the absence of ulceration.[8,41] ESD is now accepted as standard treatment if the gastric cancer fulfils these criteria (intramucosal EGC-DH of <2 cm in the absence of ulceration without LVI).[42] The survival rate after ESD for EGCs for these indications was comparable to that achieved after surgery.[43] Although metachronous cancers were more common after ESD, they were usually treatable and did not affect survival.[43]

The indications for ESD have been expanded and these now include mucosal EGC-DH without ulceration irrespective of tumour size; mucosal EGC-DH with ulceration measuring less than 3 cm; mucosal EGC-UH measuring less than 2 cm without ulceration; and EGC-DH with minute submucosal invasion (≤500 μm depth of invasion) measuring less than 3 cm, without evidence of LVI.[17,41,42,44,45]

The current guidelines recommend adopting expanded indications as an investigational treatment because of insufficient evidence for them to be a curative treatment modality.[17,42,46] The risk of LNM when ESD is performed for these indications is higher than when it is performed for absolute indications but still remains acceptably low.[27] However, there are still unsolved questions, such as whether separate indications are needed according to the type of EGC-UH (poorly differentiated tubular vs poorly cohesive (including signet ring cell) carcinoma) or EGC with mixed-type histology (EGC-MH).[23] However, it is still necessary to examine the subdivisions of the indications and validate the expanded indication and standardization of the procedure and its precise application. Still, the occasional patient with higher-risk stigmata may be managed endoscopically, particularly in the presence of comorbidities that preclude safe operation.[47]

Recently published studies have shown comparable long-term outcomes between ESD under absolute and expanded indications.[48–50] Moreover, recent meta-analyses reporting the incidence of LNM according to the expanded criteria in comparison with the absolute criteria showed a comparable LNM rate in the subset of expanded criteria—the incidence of LNM was 0.2% for patients with absolute criteria, and for expanded criteria, 0.57% for mucosal EGC-DH with ulceration measuring less than 3 cm and 0.27% for mucosal EGC-DH without ulceration greater than 2 cm.[51] Based on recent studies, the absolute indication for gastric ESD was expanded to include these categories in revised Japanese gastric cancer treatment guidelines.[52] However, in Korean guidelines from the Korean Gastric Cancer Association, ESD is strongly recommended only for absolute criteria and ESD under expanded criteria is recommended weakly with moderate evidence.[53]

Adopting indications and criteria

Candidates for ESD are decided using predetermined indications. After ESD, the resected specimen is determined satisfying post-ESD criteria. Although the contents of indications and criteria is the same, adopting indications before ESD might be inaccurate.

Preoperative evaluation of EGCs in terms of size, depth, presence of ulceration, and LVI status are difficult and have inevitable discrepancies.[46] Although endoscopists have tried to adopt precise indications before ESD, there is always a possibility of an outside indications rate. This means that the resected specimen after ESD does not satisfy the post-ESD criteria and additional surgery or ESD should be carried out. Because it is difficult to accurately predict the depth of invasion and LVI of the lesion prior to ESD, patients should be informed that additional surgery or ESD may be needed after the procedure.[54]

Korean studies revealed that about one-third of ESD cases for absolute indications were shifted to beyond absolute criteria after ESD. Moreover, 42.8% of these out-of-indication cases were included in the beyond expanded criteria, which means there is difficulty in adopting precise indications prior to ESD.[55] Most published studies about therapeutic outcomes of ESD have focused on post-ESD criteria, which means a substantial portion of expanded criteria lesions might be originally considered as absolute indication lesions before ESD.[55]

In the study of the Korean multicentre registry of ESD for EGC-UH, there was also a discrepancy between pre-ESD indications and post-ESD criteria in 36.7% of all lesions.[56] Underestimation of the size was the most common reason of non-curative resection (71.4%), followed by underestimation of the depth of invasion (32%), and unpredictability of LVI (14.9%).[56]

Adopting precise indications is important; however, EGC-UH or EGC-MH itself might be a risk factor for out-of-indication rate, leading to non-curative resection.[57] More strict and separate indications might be necessary for the ESD of EGC-UH or EGC-MH.

Histology

Current indications for ESD are focused on tubular adenocarcinomas and divided by the differentiation of EGC based on a Japanese classification that categorizes gastric adenocarcinoma into differentiated and undifferentiated types.[23,42,58] The differentiated group in the Japanese classification for ESD refers to well- or moderately differentiated tubular adenocarcinoma or papillary adenocarcinoma (PAC), and the undifferentiated group refers to poorly differentiated adenocarcinoma, SRC, or mucinous adenocarcinoma.[23,42,58] Among the four predominant histological types in the World Health Organization classification, PAC is usually categorized into the differentiated group and SRC into the undifferentiated group; however, tubular adenocarcinoma is categorized according to differentiation and mucinous adenocarcinoma according to predominant components in either the differentiated or undifferentiated group.[23,42,59]

Histological discrepancies

A precise histological diagnosis is important before ESD, especially for EGC-UH. EGC-DH on biopsy before ESD can be changed to EGC-UH after ESD, leading to a change in overall treatment strategy.[23] Endoscopists usually adopt indications based on the pathological results of endoscopic biopsy before ESD. Therefore, there is a possibility of a discrepancy between the pre-ESD biopsy of the lesion and post-ESD biopsy of the resected specimen. In practice data for gastric dysplasia, EGC, or advanced gastric cancer, the final pathology was upgraded in 15.9% of cases and downgraded in 6.9% after ESD or surgery, compared to that on the initial endoscopic biopsy.[23,60] In a Korean ESD multicentre study including only EGC-UH cases after ESD, 54.9% showed a discrepancy between the pre- and post-ESD histology.[56] Other studies also reported rates of histological discrepancy of up to 84.7% in EGC-UH, compared to 16.3–53.7% for EGC-DH.[61] The difference in discrepancy rates among studies can be explained by the difference in the number of biopsy specimens, selection of biopsy sites in each study, and histological heterogeneity.[62] A previous study with histological mapping showed that the zone of transition from a differentiated to an undifferentiated histology was frequently found at one or two peripheral sites of the lesion.[62] Therefore, biopsy of peripheral sites may aid in an accurate diagnosis.[21] Inaccurate initial determination of differentiation leads to inappropriate application of the indications and occurs more frequently in EGC-UH than in EGC-DH. However, this factor was often not considered and the majority of studies on therapeutic outcomes of ESD for EGC-UH focused on post-ESD histology.[3,56] Among 14 studies included in the previous meta-analysis,[3] only two evaluated pre-ESD diagnosed cases of EGC-UH.[63,64] EGC-UH showing differentiated histology on pre-ESD biopsy is associated with a lower curative resection rate than that for undifferentiated histology on pre-ESD biopsy, and inaccurate initial diagnosis could affect the therapeutic outcomes of ESD.[21,23,62]

EGC-UH

EGC-UH including poorly differentiated adenocarcinoma or SRC, has distinctive growth patterns, and ESD for these lesions is still controversial, especially because the defining indications are unclear.[3] Although small (<2 cm) intramucosal EGC-UH without ulceration is included in the expanded criteria, controversies remain due to different biology and characteristics compared to EGC with differentiated-type histology (EGC-DH).[13,17,23,42,56] There is also little long-term outcome data to support ESD of EGC-UH.[55]

EGC-MH

Currently, differentiated-type predominant EGC mixed with an undifferentiated component (EGC-MD) is considered EGC-DH, whereas undifferentiated-type predominant EGC mixed with a differentiated component (EGC-MU) is considered EGC-UH in the Japanese classification of gastric carcinoma.[42,59] However, gastric cancer is histologically heterogeneous and a diagnosis of EGC-MH (EGC with histological heterogeneity) is challenging. It is only diagnosed after ESD or surgery as a pure-type gastric cancer and the determination can change from the initial biopsy to evaluation after therapeutic resection.[65] There have been no specific criteria developed for ESD for EGC-MH. Moreover, therapeutic outcomes of ESD for EGC-MH have not been clearly described.[66]

EGC-MH cases have been considered to be candidates for surgery because of a higher rate of LVI or LNM, larger lesion size, deeper depth of invasion, and higher rate of recurrence compared to pure-type gastric cancers in surgical series. Therefore, accurate diagnosis before endoscopic resection is important to avoid unnecessary procedures. However, histological discrepancy between biopsy and resected specimen is higher in EGC-MHs than pure-type gastric cancers.[67] Also, outcomes suggesting invasiveness seem to be more concerning because of the enrolment of larger lesions and deeper depth of invasion in surgical series compared to lesions undergoing endoscopic resection.[66]

ESD series of EGC-MH showed that EGC-MH cases have a larger size, deeper invasion, and higher rates of LVI and LNM than pure-type EGC cases. However, there was no LNM or extra-gastric recurrence after ESD if EGC-MD met the current curative resection criteria.[68] This was also consistent in several retrospective studies with surgically resected specimens and these studies commonly indicated that EGC-MD cases satisfying current ESD criteria showed no LNM.[69–71] However, a major issue is the difficulty in achieving curative resection in EGC-MH. Low curative resection rates of EGC-MH suggest that it is difficult to make a diagnosis prior to ESD and that EGC-MD itself was a risk factor for non-curative resection in studies of ESD specimens.[57,66]

To overcome these therapeutic pitfalls, pre-ESD biopsy of the surrounding region for an accurate diagnosis or for taking larger free lateral margins from the tumour in the ESD has been recommended.[66,72,73] A previous study with histological mapping also showed that the zone of transition from differentiated- to undifferentiated-type histology was frequently found at one or two peripheral sites of the lesion.[62] Therefore, biopsy of the peripheral sites may aid in accurate diagnosis, although currently there is no perfect approach.[21,66]

Papillary adenocarcinoma of the stomach

Among the five main histological types (tubular, papillary, mucinous, poorly cohesive, and mixed) of gastric adenocarcinoma in the World Health Organization classification, PAC of the stomach is a rare variant and it is histologically characterized by finger-like papillary epithelial processes lined with columnar neoplastic cells with a central fibrovascular core.[40,74,75] It is categorized into EGC-DH; however, aggressive features such as higher LVI or submucosal invasion rate have been reported,[76,77] whereas comparable LNM rate to the lesions meeting the current ESD criteria also has been reported.[78] PAC is generally defined as a tumour in which more than 50% of the involved area contains papillary structures across studies.[76–78] Although it is categorized into the differentiated group in the Japanese classification,[42] PAC mixed with other differentiated-type EGC, or mixed with undifferentiated-type EGC, is also classified according to the predominant component in the entire cancer. Surgical data on EGCs with PAC showed an LNM rate of 17.9% for all lesions included in this study, an LNM rate of 11.8% and an LVI rate of 17.6% for lesions that met the current ESD criteria, indicating adoption of the same ESD criteria for EGC-DH is unlikely.[40,77] Retrospective analysis of endoscopically resected EGCs with PAC also showed that the presence of a papillary structure was an independent risk factor for lymphatic involvement (odds ratio 8.1, 95% confidence interval 3.2–20.6).[79] However, another study with surgical data on EGC with PAC showed LNM rates comparable to those in differentiated tubular adenocarcinoma (1.5%, 1.1%, and 4.0% for mucosal EGCs and 9.45%, 11.9%, and 17.6% for submucosal EGCs, in EGC with PAC, differentiated tubular EGC, or EGC-UH, respectively), despite persistent aggressive features of higher LVI or submucosal invasion rates.[78] Moreover, no LNM occurred in lesions that met the current ESD criteria for PAC.[78] In terms of the long-term outcomes, metachronous recurrence occurred in 5.2% of the cases; however, there were no extra-gastric recurrences in patients who achieved curative resection for EGC with PAC during a median follow-up of 58 months.[80] Further research is needed to explain this discrepancy between studies, and the results of this study will provide evidence for the validity of current ESD criteria in addition to the technical feasibility of ESD for EGC with PAC.[40]

Short-term outcomes of endoscopic submucosal dissection

In terms of the en bloc resection rates, Chung et al. enrolled 1000 EGCs in six university hospitals from 2006 to 2007 and showed a rate of 95.3%.[81] However, this was a retrospective analysis. In another previous Korean study, the en bloc resection rate from 2005 to 2009 was 80.5%, but the outcome from 2009 to 2015 was 89.1%, indicating an improvement over time.[82] A 2018 prospective multicentre cohort study enrolled 697 patients in 12 nationwide hospitals from 2010 to 2011 and showed a 99.1% en bloc resection rate, irrespective of indications.[6,83]

In terms of the complete resection (an R0 negative lateral and vertical margin rate), previous reports have shown better therapeutic outcomes in lesions with absolute criteria (95.9–97.8%) than in lesions with expanded criteria (88.4–94.7%).[84,85] However, a 2015 multicentre study of 1105 consecutive EGCs in six university hospitals from 2003 to 2010 showed that there was no statistical difference in complete resection rate between lesions with absolute criteria (98.3%) and with expanded criteria (97.4%) in Korea.[86] However, this study was performed in a retrospective manner and more recently, two prospective multicentre cohort studies showed 81.3–81.7% complete resection rates, irrespective of indications.[33,83]

For curative resection, prospective multicentre cohort studies showed rates of 86.1–86.8%, irrespective of indications.[33,83] Non-curative resection cases were categorized as follows: group 1 (incomplete resection and met the ESD criteria), group 2 (complete resection and exceeded the ESD criteria), group 3 (incomplete resection and exceeded the ESD criteria), and group 4 (LVI regardless of complete resection). Group 3 and group 4 had higher rates of local recurrence after non-curative resection.[87] Non-curative resection is strongly associated with a higher incidence of local recurrence after EGC. Therefore, identification of the reason for non-curative resection is important. Considering that the prediction of LVI is more difficult than the depth of invasion or size of the lesion, efforts to adopt precise indications of the size, histology, or morphology and prediction of depth of invasion is important to reduce the risk of local recurrence or LNM of EGC.

Long-term outcomes of endoscopic submucosal dissection

The prognosis of EGC is known to be excellent with a 5-year survival rate of over 90% and a recent meta-analysis also revealed that there was no difference of overall survival and disease-specific survival between ESD and surgical treatment.[88]

However, many of the patients with out-of-indication cases refused to undergo an additional operation and had lower survival rates than those who were initially treated with surgery.[89] Retrospective studies usually excluded these patients because they were lost to follow-up. This might have resulted in a selection bias by excluding patients who were expected to have a poor prognosis. Thus, the comparable long-term outcomes after ESD based on the post-treatment pathology cannot provide direct evidence of comparable outcomes for preoperative expanded indications.[46] These can be supplemented by reporting the overall survival and disease-specific survival rates, separately.[46]

A recent Japanese nationwide registry analysis revealed that long-term outcomes including 5-year overall and disease-specific survival rates reached nearly 100% if curative resection was achieved irrespective of an absolute or expanded ESD indication.[90] In the lesions with ESD for expanded indications, cancer-related mortality in curatively resected lesions was 0.16% and this was comparable to the mortality rate of 0.35% in patients who underwent gastrectomy due to EGC.[90] However, there was only 1.6% of poorly differentiated adenocarcinoma, 1.9% of SRC, and 3.4% of PAC in this cohort and the results of this study could not explain the issue related to the histology explained above.

Post-endoscopic submucosal dissection surveillance strategy

Even if the curative resection criteria were satisfied for EGCs, close follow-up is mandatory. ESD can preserve nearly all the gastric mucosa.[91] Therefore, metachronous recurrence could develop in the background mucosa with an incidence of approximately 3% per year.[91,92] The median time to metachronous recurrence was 18 months (range: 7–75 months) in a meta-analysis.[91] Moreover, there is always a possibility for missed synchronous multiple gastric cancers in patients already treated by ESD.

However, there is no definite established surveillance interval after curative resection of EGC. Considering that most of the detected synchronous or metachronous EGCs are successfully treated by an additional ESD, the impact of local recurrence or missed cancers might be negligible if intensive surveillance were followed.[93] Although endoscopists adopt different surveillance intervals, intensive surveillance is preferred in the first to second year after ESD (such as 2 months after ESD and every 6 months) and annual surveillance has been recommended for at least 5 years after ESD.[93] The surveillance method includes endoscopy with or without computed tomography and chest X-ray. The National Comprehensive Cancer Network guideline recommended that follow-up after gastric cancer treatment should be conducted every 3–6 months for the first 3 years after R0 resection. For 3–5 years, the follow-up interval should be 6 months, and thereafter yearly.[17] However, this recommendation was not different between patients who underwent gastrectomy or ESD.

H. pylori is regarded as the most important pathogen in the development of gastric cancer and meta-analysis or randomized trials have clearly shown that *H. pylori* eradication prevents the development of metachronous gastric cancer after ESD of EGCs.[91,94] Therefore, *H. pylori* eradication should be recommended for patients who have undergone ESD for EGCs.

Conclusion

With the advances in expertise, the indication for ESD in the treatment of EGCs is expanding. However, there are also unanswered questions in the application of ESD such as whether separate indications are needed according to the type of EGC-UH, EGC-MH, or PAC and if expansion of indications is safe. Not only the technical aspects of ESD, but also the proper selection of the ESD candidates, considering their general condition, and the preferences of the patients are important. Long-term surveillance with risk factor management for metachronous recurrence should also be followed for the successful management of EGCs.

Acknowledgements

This research was supported by the Bio & Medical Technology Development Program of the National Research Foundation (NRF) and by the Korean government, Ministry of Science and ICT (MSIT) (grant number NRF2017M3A9E8033253).

REFERENCES

1. World Health Organization. Fact sheets on cancer. 2019. https://www.who.int/news-room/fact-sheets/detail/cancer
2. Jun JK, Choi KS, Lee HY, et al. Effectiveness of the Korean National Cancer Screening Program in reducing gastric cancer mortality. *Gastroenterology*. 2017;**152**:1319–1328.
3. Bang CS, Baik GH, Shin IS, et al. Endoscopic submucosal dissection for early gastric cancer with undifferentiated-type histology: a meta-analysis. *World J Gastroenterol*. 2015;**21**:6032–6043.
4. Cho BJ, Bang CS, Park SW, et al. Automated classification of gastric neoplasms in endoscopic images using a convolutional neural network. *Endoscopy*. 2019;**51**:1121–1129.

5. Kim H, Hwang Y, Sung H, et al. Effectiveness of gastric cancer screening on gastric cancer incidence and mortality in a community-based prospective cohort. *Cancer Res Treat.* 2018;**50**:582–589.
6. Bang CS, Baik GH. Using big data to see the forest and the trees: endoscopic submucosal dissection of early gastric cancer in Korea. *Korean J Intern Med.* 2019;**34**:772–774.
7. Gotoda T. Endoscopic resection of early gastric cancer. *Gastric Cancer.* 2007;**10**:1–11.
8. Soetikno R, Kaltenbach T, Yeh R, Gotoda T. Endoscopic mucosal resection for early cancers of the upper gastrointestinal tract. *J Clin Oncol.* 2005;**23**:4490–4498.
9. Gotoda T, Yamamoto H, Soetikno RM. Endoscopic submucosal dissection of early gastric cancer. *J Gastroenterol.* 2006;**41**:929–942.
10. Bang CS, Choi JH, Yang YJ, Lee JJ, Baik GH. Endoscopic submucosal dissection of early gastric cancer with mixed-type histology: protocol for a systematic review and meta-analysis. *Medicine.* 2018;**97**:e13838.
11. Zhu L, Qin J, Wang J, Guo T, Wang Z, Yang J. Early gastric cancer: current advances of endoscopic diagnosis and treatment. *Gastroenterol Res Pract.* 2016;**2016**:9638041.
12. Hirao M, Masuda K, Asanuma T, et al. Endoscopic resection of early gastric cancer and other tumors with local injection of hypertonic saline-epinephrine. *Gastrointest Endosc.* 1988;**34**:264–269.
13. Ono H, Yao K, Fujishiro M, et al. Guidelines for endoscopic submucosal dissection and endoscopic mucosal resection for early gastric cancer. *Dig Endosc.* 2016;**28**:3–15.
14. Choi J, Kim SG, Im JP, Kim JS, Jung HC, Song IS: Comparison of endoscopic ultrasonography and conventional endoscopy for prediction of depth of tumor invasion in early gastric cancer. *Endoscopy.* 2010;**42**:705–713.
15. Watari J, Ueyama S, Tomita T, et al. What types of early gastric cancer are indicated for endoscopic ultrasonography staging of invasion depth? *World J Gastrointest Endosc.* 2016;**8**:558–567.
16. Choi J, Kim SG, Im JP, Kim JS, Jung HC, Song IS. Endoscopic prediction of tumor invasion depth in early gastric cancer. *Gastrointest Endosc.* 2011;**73**:917–927.
17. Lee JH, Kim JG, Jung HK, et al. Clinical practice guidelines for gastric cancer in Korea: an evidence-based approach. *J Gastric Cancer.* 2014;**14**:87–104.
18. Numata N, Oka S, Tanaka S, et al. Useful condition of chromoendoscopy with indigo carmine and acetic acid for identifying a demarcation line prior to endoscopic submucosal dissection for early gastric cancer. *BMC Gastroenterol.* 2016;**16**:72.
19. Yoshimizu S, Yamamoto Y, Horiuchi Y, et al. A suitable marking method to achieve lateral margin negative in endoscopic submucosal dissection for undifferentiated-type early gastric cancer. *Endosc Int Open.* 2019;**7**:E274–E281.
20. Sawada S, Fujisaki J, Yamamoto N, et al. Expansion of indications for endoscopic treatment of undifferentiated mucosal gastric cancer: analysis of intramucosal spread in resected specimens. *Dig Dis Sci.* 2010;**55**:1376–1380.
21. Kim JH. Important considerations when contemplating endoscopic resection of undifferentiated-type early gastric cancer. *World J Gastroenterol.* 2016;**22**:1172–1178.
22. Kim H, Kim JH, Lee YC, et al. Growth patterns of signet ring cell carcinoma of the stomach for endoscopic resection. *Gut Liver.* 2015;**9**:720–726.
23. Bang CS, Baik GH. Pitfalls in the interpretation of publications about endoscopic submucosal dissection of early gastric cancer with undifferentiated-type histology. *Clin Endosc.* 2019;**52**:30–35.
24. Mehta N, Strong AT, Franco M, et al. Optimal injection solution for endoscopic submucosal dissection: a randomized controlled trial of Western solutions in a porcine model. *Dig Endosc.* 2018;**30**:347–353.
25. Wang H, Wang S. Effect of submucosal injection of normal saline and glycerol fructose on endoscopic polypectomy in patients with colorectal polyps. *Oncol Lett.* 2019;**17**:4449–4454.
26. Bang CS, Shin WG, Seo SI, et al. Effect of ilaprazole on the healing of endoscopic submucosal dissection-induced gastric ulcer: randomized-controlled, multicenter study. *Surg Endosc.* 2019;**33**:1376–1385.
27. Draganov PV, Wang AY, Othman MO, Fukami N. AGA Institute clinical practice update: endoscopic submucosal dissection in the United States. *Clin Gastroenterol Hepatol.* 2019;**17**:16–25.
28. Kim EH, Park SW, Nam E, Eun CS, Han DS, Park CH. Role of second-look endoscopy and prophylactic hemostasis after gastric endoscopic submucosal dissection: a systematic review and meta-analysis. *J Gastroenterol Hepatol.* 2017;**32**:756–768.
29. Kakushima N, Fujishiro M, Yahagi N, Kodashima S, Nakamura M, Omata M. Helicobacter pylori status and the extent of gastric atrophy do not affect ulcer healing after endoscopic submucosal dissection. *J Gastroenterol Hepatol.* 2006;**21**:1586–1589.
30. Kakushima N, Fujishiro M, Kodashima S, et al. Histopathologic characteristics of gastric ulcers created by endoscopic submucosal dissection. *Endoscopy.* 2006;**38**:412–415.
31. Uedo N, Takeuchi Y, Yamada T, et al. Effect of a proton pump inhibitor or an H2-receptor antagonist on prevention of bleeding from ulcer after endoscopic submucosal dissection of early gastric cancer: a prospective randomized controlled trial. *Am J Gastroenterol.* 2007;**102**:1610–1616.
32. Bang CS, Baik GH. Carbon dioxide insufflation in endoscopic submucosal dissection: is it an urgent need? *Clin Endosc.* 2017;**50**:407–409.
33. Choi IJ, Lee NR, Kim SG, et al. Short-term outcomes of endoscopic submucosal dissection in patients with early gastric cancer: a prospective multicenter cohort study. *Gut Liver.* 2016;**10**:739–748.
34. Lo SK, Fujii-Lau LL, Enestvedt BK, et al. The use of carbon dioxide in gastrointestinal endoscopy. *Gastrointest Endosc.* 2016;**83**:857–865.
35. Kawahara Y, Okada H, Yamamoto K. Prevention and management of ESD complications: two cases of air embolism during ESD procedures. *Gastroenterol Endosc.* 2009;**51**(Suppl 2):2086.
36. Green BT, Tendler DA. Cerebral air embolism during upper endoscopy: case report and review. *Gastrointest Endosc.* 2005;**61**:620–623.
37. Takeuchi H, Abe N, Sugiyama M. A case of air embolism during gastric ESD. *Gastroenterol Endosc.* 2012;**54**(Suppl 1):893.
38. Li X, Dong H, Zhang Y, Zhang G. CO2 insufflation versus air insufflation for endoscopic submucosal dissection: a meta-analysis of randomized controlled trials. *PLoS One.* 2017;**12**:e0177909.
39. Wang WL, Wu ZH, Sun Q, et al. Meta-analysis: the use of carbon dioxide insufflation vs. room air insufflation for gastrointestinal endoscopy. *Aliment Pharmacol Ther.* 2012;**35**:1145–1154.
40. Bang CS, Choi JH, Lee JJ, Baik GH. Endoscopic submucosal dissection of papillary adenocarcinoma of stomach; protocol for a systematic review and meta-analysis. *Medicine.* 2018;**97**:e13905.

41. Gotoda T, Yanagisawa A, Sasako M, et al. Incidence of lymph node metastasis from early gastric cancer: estimation with a large number of cases at two large centers. *Gastric Cancer*. 2000;**3**:219–225.
42. Japanese Gastric Cancer Association. Japanese gastric cancer treatment guidelines 2014 (ver. 4). *Gastric Cancer*. 2017;**20**:1–19.
43. Choi IJ, Lee JH, Kim YI, et al. Long-term outcome comparison of endoscopic resection and surgery in early gastric cancer meeting the absolute indication for endoscopic resection. *Gastrointest Endosc*. 2015;**81**:333–341.
44. Hirasawa T, Gotoda T, Miyata S, et al. Incidence of lymph node metastasis and the feasibility of endoscopic resection for undifferentiated-type early gastric cancer. *Gastric Cancer*. 2009;**12**:148–152.
45. Gotoda T, Iwasaki M, Kusano C, Seewald S, Oda I. Endoscopic resection of early gastric cancer treated by guideline and expanded National Cancer Centre criteria. *Br J Surg*. 2010;**97**:868–871.
46. Choi IJ. Exploring the evidence of expanded criteria for endoscopic resection of early gastric cancers. *Clin Endosc*. 2017;**50**:99–101.
47. Brunicardi FC, Schwartz SI. *Schwartz's Principles of Surgery*. New York: McGraw-Hill; 2018.
48. Jeon HK, Kim GH, Lee BE, et al. Long-term outcome of endoscopic submucosal dissection is comparable to that of surgery for early gastric cancer: a propensity-matched analysis. *Gastric Cancer*. 2018;**21**:133–143.
49. Suzuki H, Oda I, Abe S, et al. High rate of 5-year survival among patients with early gastric cancer undergoing curative endoscopic submucosal dissection. *Gastric Cancer*. 2016;**19**:198–205.
50. Hasuike N, Ono H, Boku N, et al. A non-randomized confirmatory trial of an expanded indication for endoscopic submucosal dissection for intestinal-type gastric cancer (cT1a): the Japan Clinical Oncology Group study (JCOG0607). *Gastric Cancer*. 2018;**21**:114–123.
51. Abdelfatah MM, Barakat M, Lee H, et al. The incidence of lymph node metastasis in early gastric cancer according to the expanded criteria in comparison with the absolute criteria of the Japanese Gastric Cancer Association: a systematic review of the literature and meta-analysis. *Gastrointest Endosc*. 2018;**87**:338–347.
52. Japanese Gastric Cancer Association. *Japanese gastric cancer treatment guidelines 2018 (ver. 5)*. Tokyo: Kanehara & Co.; 2018.
53. Guideline Committee of the Korean Gastric Cancer Association (KGCA), Development Working Group & Review Panel. Korean practice guideline for gastric cancer 2018: an evidence-based, multi-disciplinary approach. *J Gastric Cancer*. 2019;**19**:1–48.
54. Kim YI, Kim HS, Kook MC, et al. Discrepancy between clinical and final pathological evaluation findings in early gastric cancer patients treated with endoscopic submucosal dissection. *J Gastric Cancer*. 2016;**16**:34–42.
55. Lee H, Lee JH. Expanding indications of endoscopic submucosal dissection for early gastric cancer: hope or hype? *Gut Liver*. 2015;**9**:135–136.
56. Bang CS, Park JM, Baik GH, et al. Therapeutic outcomes of endoscopic resection of early gastric cancer with undifferentiated-type histology: a Korean ESD registry database analysis. *Clin Endosc*. 2017;**50**:569–577.
57. Horiuchi Y, Fujisaki J, Yamamoto N, et al. Undifferentiated-type component mixed with differentiated-type early gastric cancer is a significant risk factor for endoscopic non-curative resection. *Dig Endosc*. 2018;**30**:624–632.
58. Lee HH, Song KY, Park CH, Jeon HM. Undifferentiated-type gastric adenocarcinoma: prognostic impact of three histological types. *World J Surg Oncol*. 2012;**10**:254.
59. Hamilton SR, Aaltonen LA, eds. *WHO Classification of Tumours: Pathology and Genetics of Tumours of the Digestive System*. Lyon: IARC Press, 2000.
60. Lee JH, Min YW, Lee JH, et al. Diagnostic group classifications of gastric neoplasms by endoscopic resection criteria before and after treatment: real-world experience. *Surg Endosc*. 2016;**30**:3987–3993.
61. Min BH, Kang KJ, Lee JH, et al. Endoscopic resection for undifferentiated early gastric cancer: focusing on histologic discrepancies between forceps biopsy-based and endoscopic resection specimen-based diagnosis. *Dig Dis Sci*. 2014;**59**:2536–2543.
62. Lee JH, Kim JH, Rhee K, et al. Undifferentiated early gastric cancer diagnosed as differentiated histology based on forceps biopsy. *Pathol Res Pract*. 2013;**209**:314–318.
63. Yamamoto Y, Fujisaki J, Hirasawa T, et al. Therapeutic outcomes of endoscopic submucosal dissection of undifferentiated-type intramucosal gastric cancer without ulceration and preoperatively diagnosed as 20 millimetres or less in diameter. *Dig Endosc*. 2010;**22**:112–118.
64. Abe S, Oda I, Suzuki H, et al. Short- and long-term outcomes of endoscopic submucosal dissection for undifferentiated early gastric cancer. *Endoscopy*. 2013;**45**:703–707.
65. Mikami K, Hirano Y, Futami K, Maekawa T. Expansion of lymph node metastasis in mixed-type submucosal invasive gastric cancer. *Asian J Surg*. 2018;**41**:462–466.
66. Bang CS, Yang YJ, Lee JJ, Baik GH. Endoscopic submucosal dissection of early gastric cancer with mixed-type histology: a systematic review. *Dig Dis Sci*. 2019;**65**:276–291.
67. Komatsu S, Ichikawa D, Miyamae M, et al. Discrepancies in the histologic type between biopsy and resected specimens: a cautionary note for mixed-type gastric carcinoma. *World J Gastroenterol*. 2015;**21**:4673–4679.
68. Min BH, Kim KM, Park CK, et al. Outcomes of endoscopic submucosal dissection for differentiated-type early gastric cancer with histological heterogeneity. *Gastric Cancer*. 2015;**18**:618–626.
69. Hanaoka N, Tanabe S, Mikami T, Okayasu I, Saigenji K. Mixed-histologic-type submucosal invasive gastric cancer as a risk factor for lymph node metastasis: feasibility of endoscopic submucosal dissection. *Endoscopy*. 2009;**41**:427–432.
70. Takizawa K, Ono H, Kakushima N, et al. Risk of lymph node metastases from intramucosal gastric cancer in relation to histological types: how to manage the mixed histological type for endoscopic submucosal dissection. *Gastric Cancer*. 2013;**16**:531–536.
71. Zhong Q, Sun Q, Xu GF, et al. Differential analysis of lymph node metastasis in histological mixed-type early gastric carcinoma in the mucosa and submucosa. *World J Gastroenterol*. 2018;**24**:87–95.
72. Han JP, Hong SJ, Kim HK. Long-term outcomes of early gastric cancer diagnosed as mixed adenocarcinoma after endoscopic submucosal dissection. *J Gastroenterol Hepatol*. 2015;**30**:316–320.
73. Tanabe S, Ishido K, Matsumoto T, et al. Long-term outcomes of endoscopic submucosal dissection for early gastric cancer: a multicenter collaborative study. *Gastric Cancer*. 2017;**20**(Suppl 1):45–52.
74. Lauwers GY, Carneiro F, Graham DY, et al. Gastric carcinoma. In: Bowman FT, Carneiro F, Hruban RH, eds. *WHO Classification*

of *Tumours of the Digestive System*. Lyon: IARC Press; 2010:48–58.
75. Yu H, Fang C, Chen L, et al. Worse prognosis in papillary, compared to tubular, early gastric carcinoma. *J Cancer*. 2017;**8**:117–123.
76. Lee HJ, Kim GH, Park DY, et al. Is endoscopic submucosal dissection safe for papillary adenocarcinoma of the stomach? *World J Gastroenterol*. 2015;**21**:3944–3952.
77. Lee HJ, Kim GH, Park DY, et al. Endoscopic submucosal dissection for papillary adenocarcinoma of the stomach: is it really safe? *Gastric Cancer*. 2017;**20**:978–986.
78. Min BH, Byeon SJ, Lee JH, et al. Lymphovascular invasion and lymph node metastasis rates in papillary adenocarcinoma of the stomach: implications for endoscopic resection. *Gastric Cancer*. 2018;**21**:680–688.
79. Sekiguchi M, Sekine S, Oda I, et al. Risk factors for lymphatic and venous involvement in endoscopically resected gastric cancer. *J Gastroenterol*. 2013;**48**:706–712.
80. Kim TS, Min BH, Kim KM, Lee JH, Rhee PL, Kim JJ. Endoscopic submucosal dissection for papillary adenocarcinoma of the stomach: low curative resection rate but favorable long-term outcomes after curative resection. *Gastric Cancer*. 2019;**22**:363–368.
81. Chung IK, Lee JH, Lee SH, et al. Therapeutic outcomes in 1000 cases of endoscopic submucosal dissection for early gastric neoplasms: Korean ESD Study Group multicenter study. *Gastrointest Endosc*. 2009;**69**:1228–1235.
82. Kim JS, Kang SH, Moon HS, et al. Clinical outcome after endoscopic submucosal dissection for early gastric cancer of absolute and expanded indication. *Medicine*. 2017;**96**:e6710.
83. Kim SG, Park CM, Lee NR, et al. Long-term clinical outcomes of endoscopic submucosal dissection in patients with early gastric cancer: a prospective multicenter cohort study. *Gut Liver*. 2018;**12**:402–410.
84. Isomoto H, Shikuwa S, Yamaguchi N, et al. Endoscopic submucosal dissection for early gastric cancer: a large-scale feasibility study. *Gut*. 2009;**58**:331–336.
85. Ahn JY, Jung HY, Choi KD, et al. Endoscopic and oncologic outcomes after endoscopic resection for early gastric cancer: 1370 cases of absolute and extended indications. *Gastrointest Endosc*. 2011;**74**:485–493.
86. Shin KY, Jeon SW, Cho KB, et al. Clinical outcomes of the endoscopic submucosal dissection of early gastric cancer are comparable between absolute and new expanded criteria. *Gut Liver* 2015;**9**:181–187.
87. Han JP, Hong SJ, Kim HK, et al. Risk stratification and management of non-curative resection after endoscopic submucosal dissection for early gastric cancer. *Surgic Endosc*. 2016;**30**:184–189.
88. Gu L, Khadaroo PA, Chen L, et al. Comparison of long-term outcomes of endoscopic submucosal dissection and surgery for early gastric cancer: a systematic review and meta-analysis. *J Gastrointest Surg*. 2019;**23**:1493–1501.
89. Eom BW, Kim YI, Kim KH, et al. Survival benefit of additional surgery after noncurative endoscopic resection in patients with early gastric cancer. *Gastrointest Endosc*. 2017;**85**:155–163.
90. Tanabe S, Hirabayashi S, Oda I, et al. Gastric cancer treated by endoscopic submucosal dissection or endoscopic mucosal resection in Japan from 2004 through 2006: JGCA nationwide registry conducted in 2013. *Gastric Cancer*. 2017;**20**:834–842.
91. Bang CS, Baik GH, Shin IS, et al. Helicobacter pylori eradication for prevention of metachronous recurrence after endoscopic resection of early gastric cancer. *J Korean Med Sci*. 2015;**30**:749–756.
92. Mori G, Nakajima T, Asada K, et al. Incidence of and risk factors for metachronous gastric cancer after endoscopic resection and successful Helicobacter pylori eradication: results of a large-scale, multicenter cohort study in Japan. *Gastric Cancer*. 2016;**19**:911–918.
93. Nishida T, Tsujii M, Kato M, et al. Endoscopic surveillance strategy after endoscopic resection for early gastric cancer. *World J Gastrointest Pathophysiol*. 2014;**5**:100–106.
94. Choi IJ, Kook MC, Kim YI, et al. Helicobacter pylori therapy for the prevention of metachronous gastric cancer. *N Engl J Med*. 2018;**378**:1085–1095.

19

Gastric cancer
Surgery

Matthias Biebl, Dino Kröll, Sascha Chopra, and Johann Pratschke

Indications for resection in gastric cancer

Despite decreasing in incidence in the Western world, gastric cancer remains a common malignancy with a high mortality.[1] Early systemic spread occurs as soon as the tumour growth reaches the lymphatic or blood vessels within the gastric wall. As a consequence, only early T1a cancers limited to the gastric epithelium without reaching the vessels in the submucosa can be cured by local endoscopic excision.[2] However, in Europe, only 10–15% of gastric cancers are diagnosed as early carcinomas.[3] As for all gastrointestinal adenocarcinomas, chemotherapy alone, as well as chemoradiation, rarely results in cure. Data from second-line chemotherapy trials indicate a median overall survival of 5–9 months in patients in whom the tumour was not removed.[4] Therefore, in gastric cancer, curative treatment always includes a mechanical removal of the tumour-bearing sites of the gastrointestinal tract.

From an oncological point of view, partial clearance (debulking) is not helpful, as demonstrated by a randomized trial from Asia (REGATTA trial) comparing patients with gastric cancer and one additional non-curable factor (non-removable liver metastasis, peritoneal carcinomatosis, or para-aortic lymphatic involvement) undergoing chemotherapy with or without additional gastrectomy with similar progression-free and overall survival seen in both groups.[5] If complete macroscopic clearance of all the tumour sites (i.e. T4b tumours, tumours with extensive nodal spread, and/or non-resectable M1) cannot be obtained, surgical removal of the primary tumour is considered futile. Palliative resections should only be considered for alleviation of tumour-specific symptoms such as gastric outlet obstruction or refractory tumour bleeding, and, if performed, should be limited to the tumour-bearing segment with or without an en bloc omentectomy, but with no extensive lymphadenectomy.[6,7]

Aside from the early disease (T1aN0), curative treatment of gastric cancer in Europe involves a multidisciplinary approach which includes a perioperative systemic treatment whenever possible, followed by complete surgical resection of the tumour with clear oral, aboral, and circumferential margins, and removal of all regional lymph nodes within its draining area (Figure 19.1).[8]

Staging laparoscopy

A staging laparoscopy is part of the operative procedure in adenocarcinomas of the stomach (gastric cancer) and adenocarcinomas of the oesophagogastric junction (AOG tumours) and serves as an extended staging tool for determination of local resectability and for exclusion of occult peritoneal tumour spread. While radiological staging is weak in detecting early peritoneal carcinomatosis, staging laparoscopy reaches a sensitivity of close to 100%.[9] This staging accuracy not only prevents the patient from undergoing an unnecessary laparotomy in case of unresectable peritoneal spread, it can also alter treatment pathways owing to the advent of new intraperitoneal treatment options such as hyperthermic intraperitoneal chemotherapy for localized peritoneal carcinomatosis.[10] In order to decide this, the reporting of the extent of peritoneal carcinomatosis should be standardized using the peritoneal carcinomatosis index described by Sugarbaker.[11]

A staging laparoscopy should therefore be performed in all patients with advanced gastric cancer prior to the initiation of perioperative chemotherapy.

It is also recommended to include a standardized peritoneal lavage in any staging laparoscopy. Even without overt peritoneal carcinomatosis upon laparoscopy, tumour cells may be found in the peritoneal lavage fluid. Currently, the exact value of this finding is yet to be determined. However, newer investigations indicate that several histological features (i.e. presence of one or more signet cells, five or more cell clusters, or 50 or more single tumour cells in the lavage fluid) seem to indicate a dismal prognosis compared to patients with either no tumour cells in the lavage fluid, or with tumour cell numbers below the listed thresholds.[12] Consequently, determination of such high-risk patient collectives may result in altered treatment pathways, which are currently under investigation.

19 Gastric cancer: surgery

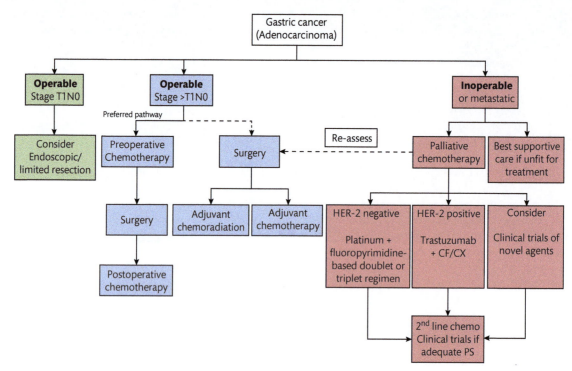

Figure 19.1 Treatment guidelines for gastric adenocarcinoma according to ESMO–ESSO–ESTRO guidelines. CF/CX, cisplatin and fluorouracil/cisplatin and capecitabine; PS, performance status.
Reproduced with permission from Waddell T, Verheij M, Allum W, Cunningham D, Cervantes A, Arnold D. Gastric cancer: ESMO-ESSO-ESTRO clinical practice guidelines for diagnosis, treatment and follow-up. *Eur J Surg Oncol.* 2014;40:584–591.

Types and definition of gastric resections according to the Japanese Gastric Cancer Association

Standard gastrectomy defines the principal surgical procedure that is performed with a curative intent for gastric cancer. It involves at least a subtotal gastrectomy (distal two-thirds of the stomach) with a D2 lymph node dissection.[13]

Several different surgical procedures have been described:

- Subtotal gastrectomy.
- Total gastrectomy.
- Transhiatal extended gastrectomy (for oesophagogastric junction tumours).

Non-standard gastrectomy encompasses all variations of the extent of gastric resection and/or lymphadenectomy required due to tumour or patient characteristics. This includes either modified surgery (the extent of resection of lymphadenectomy is reduced compared to the standard resection), or extended resection (gastrectomy with resection of adjacent involved organs or more-than-D2 lymphadenectomy).[13]

Non-curative surgery is offered to patients considered incurable. Depending on the intention, it can be divided into *palliative surgery* intended to relief tumour-specific local symptoms such as bleeding or obstruction, or *reduction surgery* aiming at prolonging survival or delaying the onset of symptoms by reducing tumour volume.[13] While reduction surgery is not recommended anymore, palliative surgery for obstruction can involve palliative gastrectomy or creation of a gastrojejunal anastomosis, depending on the individual patient's surgical risk. When performing a gastrojejunostomy, a stomach-partitioning gastrojejunostomy has been reported to be functionally superior compared to a simple gastrojejunostomy.[14]

Extent of resection in gastric cancer

The extent of resection is determined by the histological subtype of the cancer, the location of the tumour, and the TNM staging.

Histological differentiation and resection margins

Regarding the histological differentiation of the tumour, the classification of Laurén[15] is still relevant. There are two types of cancer growth, an intestinal and a diffuse type. The more common intestinal type of cancer is characterized by a mainly intraluminal growth pattern, and is more often localized to the distal part of the stomach. The diffuse type more often displays an intramural and discontinuous growth pattern in the submucosal and muscular layers of the gastric wall, which can extend over several centimetres. Consequently, the intramural extent of the tumour can vary substantially from the intraluminally definable borders of the visible lesion. The 'skip lesion' pattern has also to be considered when evaluating an intraoperative frozen section examination of the resection margin.

Resulting from these differences, a proximal resection margin of 5 cm for intestinal type cancers, and 8 cm for diffuse type cancers, is recommended. Of note, the recommendations for the resection margin only apply for the proximal resection margin, while the distal and circumferential margins are only required to be 'tumour free' (R0). These recommendations date back to data from Hermanek et al. from 1987,[16] where a low probability of a positive proximal margin was described when a 5–8 cm clearance was achieved. However, the accuracy of these recommendations has not been re-evaluated in another study. Using intraoperative frozen sections and confirmed negative margins, smaller proximal margins, especially for intestinal type cancers, have been recently discussed in the international literature. The Japanese gastric cancer treatment guidelines published in 2021 define as advisable an at least 3 cm proximal resection margin for intestinal type tumours greater than or equal to T2 and at least 5 cm for diffuse type tumours. However, if these margins cannot be achieved, a full-thickness frozen section confirming negative margins is considered sufficient rather than a conversion in surgical strategy. For tumours invading the oesophagus, a resection margin of 5 cm and confirmation of R0 status by frozen section histology is recommended.[13] Regarding the impact of the frozen section, a study from the US Gastric Cancer Collaborative evaluated the impact of the proximal resection margin status (R0 vs R1) on local recurrence and recurrence-free and overall survival.[17] They evaluated 520 proximal margins, of which 67 were initially positive (12.9%). By intraoperative re-resection if possible, they achieved 86% R0 resection, 9% R0-converted-from-initial-R1, and 5% R1 upon final histology. The risk of local recurrence was reduced from 32% in the R1 cohort to 10% in the R0-converted-from-initial-R1 cohort ($p = 0.01$); however, recurrence-free survival and overall survival were not different from the R1 cohort. By contrast, the initial R0 cohort displayed statistically improved recurrence-free and overall survival compared to the R1 group (20 vs 37 months ($p = 0.05$) and 26 vs 50 months ($p = 0.02$)), respectively. This may in part be explained by the prognostic relevance of other tumour-related factors such as T and N category, as well as tumour size or lymphatic and perineural infiltration, and the R1 situation may be more of a surrogate for a rather advanced tumour stage itself.

This oncological consideration seems relevant for the multidisciplinary board evaluation of the final histology. While generally the guidelines recommend a re-resection if technically possible for positive proximal and distal margins, a reoperation is discouraged in case of a circumferential margin involvement.[18] Additionally, the prognostic relevance of a positive resection margin seems to be balanced by the overall oncological prognosis if a lymphatic involvement with more than three lymph nodes is found upon final histology, as in such patients the tumour much more often recurs with distant or lymphatic disease, rather than locally.[18–20] Overall, current recommendations caution to balance the surgical risk of a re-resection with the expected oncological benefit of such a procedure, and rather recommend postoperative chemoradiation in case of a R+ situation upon final histology.[21]

Extent of resection according to tumour location and size

The different levels of resection for gastric cancer are defined according to the stomach volume to be resected[13]:

1. *Total gastrectomy*: resection of the stomach including the cardia and the pylorus. Reconstruction with small bowel (mostly Roux-en-Y reconstruction, alimentary limb length 50 cm).
2. *Distal gastrectomy*: gastric resection including the pylorus, while preserving the cardia. In the standard situation, the distal two-thirds of the stomach, including the left gastroepiploic artery and the left gastric vessels and the lesser curvature, are resected. The remnant is supplied by the short gastric vessels, reconstruction is with small bowel (mostly Roux-en-Y reconstruction, alimentary limb length 50 cm).
3. *Pylorus-preserving gastrectomy*: resection of the gastric corpus together with the left gastric vessels and the gastroepiploic arcade preserving the upper third of the stomach together with the pylorus and the distal portion of the antrum and direct anastomosis of both remnants.
4. *Proximal gastrectomy*: stomach resection including the cardia with preservation of the pylorus. Reconstruction with a small bowel segment, either as an interposition graft (Merendino procedure), or as a double-tract reconstruction with a Roux-en-Y oesophagojejunostomy and a side-to-side jejunogastrostomy 15 cm distal to the oesophagojejunostomy and 25 cm proximal to the lower anastomosis.
5. *Segmental gastrectomy*: circumferential resection of the stomach preserving both the cardia and the pylorus with direct anastomosis of both remnants.
6. *Local resection (wedge resection)*: non-circumferential resection of the stomach.
7. *Non-resectional surgery*: that is, bypass surgery, gastrostomy, jejunostomy.

For surgery of a previously operated gastric remnant, the following definitions apply:

8. *Completion gastrectomy*: total resection of the gastric remnant including the cardia and the pylorus, depending on the type of previous gastrectomy.
9. *Subtotal resection of the remnant stomach*: distal resection of a gastric remnant preserving the cardia.

Resections types 3–6 are not standard for gastric cancer surgery, as they do not address potential lymphatic spread. Therefore, only for limited cT1N0 tumours, a pylorus-preserving gastrectomy can be considered for tumours of the corpus with the distal tumour border at least 4 cm proximal to the pylorus, while a proximal gastrectomy can be performed for tumours of the cardia, which allows for preservation of at least the distal half of the stomach.

The standard resection for node-positive gastric cancer is either a subtotal or a total gastrectomy. A distal gastrectomy is selected for intestinal type tumours of the antrum, when a satisfactory proximal resection margin can be obtained. If this is not possible due to tumour location or histology (diffuse cancers usually mandate a total gastrectomy irrespective of the location), a total gastrectomy is chosen. T4 disease invading the left-sided pancreas mandates a total gastrectomy together with a distal pancreaticosplenectomy irrespective of the tumour location. Tumours located at the greater curvature should prompt a total gastrectomy due to potential lymphatic spread along the gastroepiploic arcade and the splenic hilum, even if tumour clearance at the level of the gastric wall could be obtained by distal gastrectomy. Japanese guidelines also mandate a splenectomy in such cases,[13] which is not generally recommended in such situations in Europe. This is based on findings that the difference in retrieved lymph nodes in patients undergoing oncological gastrectomy with or without splenectomy is about 5% (44 lymph nodes with gastrectomy vs 42 lymph nodes without gastrectomy; $p = 0.065$), and did not alter overall survival rates (p = not significant for all tumour stages).[22] Therefore, in Europe, an *en principe* splenectomy is not encouraged and should be reserved for patients with direct splenic tumour invasion.

For tumours arising within 5 cm of the oesophagogastric junction, a Siewert III tumour would routinely mandate a total gastrectomy with distal oesophageal resection (6 cm of distal oesophagus) with en bloc resection of the hiatal and retrocardial lymph nodes (stations 19, 20, 110, 111—see Figure 19.2). For AOG II tumours, both a transhiatal extended gastrectomy or a proximal gastrectomy with subtotal oesophageal resection (Ivor Lewis resection) is considered oncologically correct. From an oncological point of view, there are data indicating a higher percentage of mediastinal metastasis (>15%) in patients with tumours extending more than 2 cm above the oesophagogastric junction as compared to very rare mediastinal metastases in tumours below that level.[23] From a functional point of view, the two-cavity Ivor Lewis operation is more demanding for the patient and results in more postoperative pulmonary complications, while postoperative function and quality of life seems to be in favour of the Ivor Lewis operation in patients with normal oesophageal function. The maximum resection for cancers involving the oesophagogastric junction is a total gastrectomy and subtotal oesophagectomy with colon interposition graft and three-field lymphadenectomy (abdomen, chest, and neck). While there are long-term survivors of such an operation with histologically proven cervical lymph node involvement, a three-field lymphadenectomy is currently not recommended as routine practice. Table 19.1 outlines advantages and disadvantages of the respective procedures for oesophagogastric junction tumours as proposed by Hölscher.[23]

Lymph node dissection in curative gastric cancer surgery

Radical lymph node dissection is crucial in curative gastric cancer surgery owing to the early lymphatic spread of the carcinoma cells. The concept of lymphadenectomy here relies on the model of connected lymph nodes with a hierarchical architecture with local lymph nodes around the stomach and collecting regional lymph nodes along the main gastric arteries. The classification of the lymph node stations in the upper abdomen follows the Japanese system and is depicted in Figure 19.2. The lymph nodes are grouped in a local perigastric compartment D1 (stations 1–6), a regional compartment along the coeliac trunk and the hepatic hilum classified as compartment D2 (stations 7–12), and periaortic, peripancreatic, and mediastinal lymph nodes. According to the extent of lymph nodes removed, the lymphadenectomies are classified as D1, D1+, or D2. While a D1 and a D2 lymphadenectomy is clearly defined according to the nodal stations cleared, a D1+ lymphadenectomy is anything in between, that is, a lymphadenectomy aiming at D2 but leaving behind defined nodal stations that should have been resected to fulfil the criteria of a D2 resection.

According to the Japanese Gastric Cancer Association, the extent of systematic lymphadenectomy is defined according to the type of gastrectomy conducted[13]:

Total gastrectomy

See Figure 19.3.

- D0: lymphadenectomy less than D1.
- D1: No. 1–7.
- D1+: D1 plus No. 8a, 9, 11p.
- D2: D1 plus No. 8a, 9, 11p, 11d, 12a.

For tumours involving the distal oesophagus requiring a transhiatal extended gastrectomy, for a D1+ lymphadenectomy, nodal station 110 should be added, for a D2 lymphadenectomy, stations 19, 20, 110, and 111 should be added.

Subtotal gastrectomy

See Figure 19.4.

- D0: lymphadenectomy less than D1.
- D1: No. 1, 3, 4sb, 4d, 5, 6, 7.
- D1+: D1 plus No. 8a, 9.
- D2: D1 plus No. 8a, 9, 11p, 12a.

Following the criteria of the D system for lymphadenectomy, parenchyma-sparing resections such as a pylorus-preserving gastrectomy or a proximal gastrectomy, can only fulfil the criteria of a D1+ lymphadenectomy.

Due to a lack of data regarding the exact lymph node distribution in a Western population, a complete D2 lymphadenectomy has been defined as removal of at least 25 lymph nodes. This threshold was

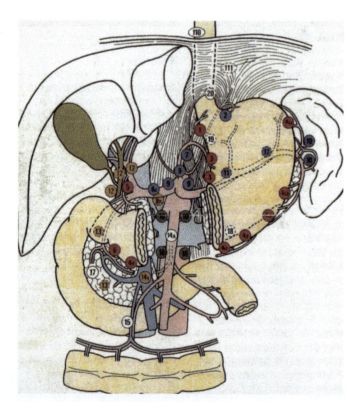

Figure 19.2 Upper abdominal lymph node station classification according to the Japanese Gastric Cancer Association.
Reproduced with permission from Japanese Gastric Cancer Association: Japanese classification of gastric carcinoma—2nd English edition. *Gastric Cancer*. 1998;1:10–24.

Table 19.1 Advantages and disadvantages of reconstruction after resection of oesophagogastric junction tumours

Oesophagectomy with gastric pull up	Extended gastrectomy with Roux-en-Y oesophagojejunostomy	Oesophagogastrectomy with colonic interposition
− 2 cavity operation (thorax/abdomen)	+ 1½ cavity operation (abdomen/transhiatal)	− 2 or 3 cavity operation (thorax/abdomen/neck)
− Safety margin distal (stomach)	− Safety margin proximal (oesophagus)	+ Wide safety margin (oesophagus/stomach)
+ Preservation of ¾, ⅔ of stomach	− Loss of stomach	− Loss of stomach
− Loss of ¾ of oesophagus	+ Preservation of ¾ of oesophagus	− Loss of stomach
+ Big reservoir	− Small reservoir	− Small reservoir
+ Pancreatocibal synchrony	− Pancreatocibal synchrony	− Pancreatocibal synchrony
− Incomplete D1 complete D2 lymphadenectomy	+ Complete D2 lymphadenectomy	+ Complete D2 lymphadenectomy
+ Radical mediastinal lymphadenectomy	− Only lower mediastinal lymphadenectomy	+ Radical mediastinal lymphadenectomy
+ Length of stomach	− Length of jejunum	+ Length of colon
− Danger of hiatal herniation of bowel	+ Low danger of hiatal herniation of bowel	− Danger of hiatal herniation of bowel
− Delayed gastric emptying	− Delayed jejunal emptying	− Delayed colonic emptying
− Pylorospasm	+ Not relevant	+ Not relevant
− Gastro-oesophageal reflux	+ Rare alkaline reflux	+ Rare alkaline reflux
− Necessity of PPI	− Necessity of B12	− Necessity of B12
+ Less dumping	− More dumping	− More dumping

+ advantage; − disadvantage.
Reproduced with permission from Hölscher AH, Law S. Esophagogastric junction adenocarcinomas: individualization of resection with special considerations for Siewert type II, and Nishi types EG, E = G and GE cancers. *Gastric Cancer*. 2020;23:3–9.

defined by anatomical studies describing a mean of 27 lymph nodes (range 17–44) in the compartments I and II.[24]

Indications for lymph node dissection

- In most Western national guidelines, the threshold of 25 lymph nodes is a required quality parameter for a complete D2 lymphadenectomy. In a curative setting, systematic *D2 lymphadenectomy* is indicated for greater than cT1 and/or cN+ tumours. Given the diagnostic weaknesses in adequate N staging, a D2 lymphadenectomy should always be performed whenever there is a possibility of nodal involvement.
- *D1 lymphadenectomy* is indicated for palliative resections and in a curative setting for either cT1a tumours that do not meet the criteria for endoscopic mucosal resection/endoscopic submucosal

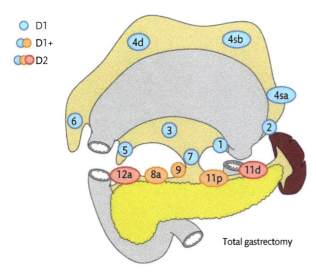

Figure 19.3 Levels of lymphadenectomy in total gastrectomy according to the Japanese Gastric Cancer Association. Blue stations indicate D1 lymphadenectomy; blue plus orange, D1+; blue plus orange plus red, D2 lymphadenectomy.
Reproduced from Japanese Gastric Cancer Association. Japanese gastric cancer treatment guidelines 2018 (5th edition). *Gastric Cancer*. 2021;24:1–21.; https://doi.org/10.1007/s10120-020-01042-y. Reproduced under a under a Creative Commons Attribution 4.0 International License (http://creativecommons.org/licenses/by/4.0/)

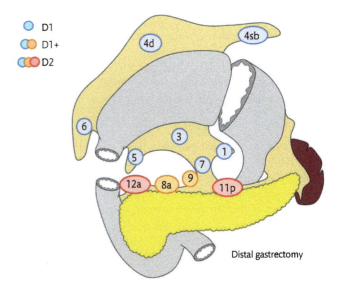

Figure 19.4 Levels of lymphadenectomy in subtotal gastrectomy according to the Japanese Gastric Cancer Association. Blue stations indicate D1 lymphadenectomy; blue plus orange, D1+; blue plus orange plus red, D2 lymphadenectomy.
Reproduced from Japanese Gastric Cancer Association. Japanese gastric cancer treatment guidelines 2018 (5th edition). *Gastric Cancer*. 2021;24:1–21.; https://doi.org/10.1007/s10120-020-01042-y. Reproduced under a under a Creative Commons Attribution 4.0 International License (http://creativecommons.org/licenses/by/4.0/)

dissection, or for intestinal type cT1bN0 tumours 1.5 cm or smaller in diameter (Japanese Gastric Cancer Association guideline[13]).
- *D1+ lymphadenectomy* is indicated for cT1N0 tumours other than the above.
- *D2+ lymphadenectomy* during total gastrectomy is considered an extended non-standard gastrectomy and involves removal of additional lymphatic nodal stations to a D2 lymphadenectomy. On the condition it can be conducted safely, this frequently includes:
  - Dissection of No. 10 (splenic hilar lymph nodes) with or without splenectomy for cancer of the upper stomach invading the greater curvature (D2 + No. 10).
  - Dissection of No. 14v (superior mesenteric venous lymph node) for cancer of the distal stomach with metastasis to the No. 6 lymph nodes (D2 + No. 14v).
  - Dissection of No. 13 (posterior pancreas head lymph node) for cancer invading the duodenum (D2 + No. 13). Metastases to the No. 13 nodes, which are not included in the regional lymph nodes for gastric cancer, should usually be classified as M1. However, since the No. 13 nodes are among the regional lymph nodes for cancer of the duodenum according to the TNM classification, these should be regarded as regional lymph nodes once gastric cancer invades the duodenum.
  - Dissection of No. 16 (abdominal aortic lymph node) after neoadjuvant chemotherapy for cancer with an extensive lymph node involvement (D2 + No. 16).

Miscellaneous procedures

Omentectomy and bursectomy for advanced gastric cancer

Omentectomy of the greater and lesser omentum is usually performed in resection for tumours greater than T2. In small T1/2 tumours, the omentum more than 3 cm distant to the gastroepiploic arcade may be preserved.[13] Bursectomy had been considered important for tumours at the dorsal aspect of the stomach; however, after the results of a randomized trial (JCOG1001), surgeons are advised not to perform this procedure any more on a routine basis, even for large posterior carcinomas.[13,25]

Reconstruction after gastrectomy

For each of the different resection types, several reconstruction methods are employed, each with a specific set of advantages and disadvantages. For total gastrectomy, a jejunal interposition, a Roux-en-Y oesophagojejunostomy, and a double tract reconstruction have been described. For reconstruction after subtotal gastrectomy, a Billroth I gastroduodenostomy, Billroth II gastrojejunostomy, a jejunal interposition, and a Roux-en-Y gastrojejunostomy have been used. While no explicit standard technique exists, the Roux-en-Y gastrojejunostomy is by far the most commonly used reconstruction technique for both resection types. The jejunal reconstruction can be performed creating a jejunal pouch or as an end-to-side oesophagogastrostomy. While current guidelines do not mandate a specific technique, the pouch seems to decrease the occurrence of dumping and weight loss in the early postoperative phase, and results in higher serum albumin levels 12–24 months after the resection.[26] Furthermore, a pouch reconstruction seems to be the most commonly applied technique worldwide.

Quality control and centralization in gastric cancer surgery

Oncological gastrectomy is defined as a complex visceral surgery in many healthcare systems and thus bound for centralization. Aside from surgical expertise during the surgical procedure, a main reason for this seems to be related to the capacity and expertise of the whole centre, and the avoidance of a failure to rescue after the procedure itself. Compelling data from a large national database from Japan, encompassing 145,523 distal stomach resections, revealed a 40% risk reduction from the baseline mortality achieved in low-volume centres with no more than ten procedures a year to 60% risk reduction in high-volume centres (51+ cases per year). In addition, operative parameters like intraoperative blood loss and operating time all significantly decreased with rising annual caseloads in the evaluated centres.[27]

REFERENCES

1. Siegel RL, Miller KD, Jemal A. Cancer statistics, 2016. *Cancer J Clin.* 2016;**66**:7–30.
2. Gotoda T, Iwasaki M, Kusano C, Seewald S, Oda I. Endoscopic resection of early gastric cancer treated by guideline and expanded National Cancer Centre criteria. *Br J Surg.* 2010;**97**:868–871.
3. Pimentel-Nunes P, Dinis-Ribeiro M, Ponchon T, et al. Endoscopic submucosal dissection: European Society of Gastrointestinal Endoscopy (ESGE) guideline. *Endoscopy.* 2015;**47**:829–854.
4. Harvey RC. Second-line treatments for advanced gastric cancer: a network meta-analysis of overall survival using parametric modelling methods. *Oncol Ther.* 2017;**5**:53–67.
5. Fujitani K, Yang HK, Mizusawa J, et al. Gastrectomy plus chemotherapy versus chemotherapy alone for advanced gastric cancer with a single non-curable factor (REGATTA): a phase 3, randomised controlled trial. *Lancet Oncol.* 2016;**17**:309–318.
6. Dittmar Y, Voigt R, Heise M, Rabsch A, Jandt K, Settmacher U. [Indications and results of palliative gastric resection in advanced gastric carcinoma]. *Zentralbl Chir.* 2009;**134**:77–82.
7. Lim S, Muhs BE, Marcus SG, Newman E, Berman RS, Hiotis SP. Results following resection for stage IV gastric cancer; are better outcomes observed in selected patient subgroups? *J Surg Oncol.* 2007;**95**:118–122.
8. Waddell T, Verheij M, Allum W, Cunningham D, Cervantes A, Arnold D. Gastric cancer: ESMO–ESSO–ESTRO clinical practice guidelines for diagnosis, treatment and follow-up. *Eur J Surg Oncol.* 2014;**40**:584–591.
9. Simon M, Mal F, Perniceni T, et al. Accuracy of staging laparoscopy in detecting peritoneal dissemination in patients with gastroesophageal adenocarcinoma. *Dis Esophagus.* 2016;**29**:236–240.
10. Rau B, Brandl A, Thuss-Patience P, et al. The efficacy of treatment options for patients with gastric cancer and peritoneal metastasis. *Gastric Cancer.* 2019;**22**:1226–1237.
11. Jacquet P, Sugarbaker PH. Clinical research methodologies in diagnosis and staging of patients with peritoneal carcinomatosis. *Cancer Treat Res.* 1996;**82**:359–374.

12. Higaki E, Yanagi S, Gotohda N, et al. Intraoperative peritoneal lavage cytology offers prognostic significance for gastric cancer patients with curative resection. *Cancer Sci.* 2017;**108**:978–986.
13. Japanese Gastric Cancer Association. Japanese gastric cancer treatment guidelines 2018 (5th edition). *Gastric Cancer.* 2021;**24**:1–21.
14. Kaminishi M, Yamaguchi H, Shimizu N, et al. Stomach-partitioning gastrojejunostomy for unresectable gastric carcinoma. *Arch Surg.* 1997;**132**:184–187.
15. Laurén P. The two histological main types of gastric carcinoma: diffuse and so-called intestinal type carcinoma. An attempt at a histo-clinical classification. *Acta Pathol Microbiol Scand.* 1965;**64**:31–49.
16. Hornig D, Hermanek P, Gall FP. The significance of the extent of proximal margins of clearance in gastric cancer surgery. *Scand J Gastroenterol.* 1987;**22**:69–71.
17. Squires MH 3rd, Kooby DA, Pawlik TM, et al. Utility of the proximal margin frozen section for resection of gastric adenocarcinoma: a 7-Institution Study of the US Gastric Cancer Collaborative. *Ann Surg Oncol.* 2014;**21**:4202–4210.
18. Lordick F, Ott K, Novotny A, Schuhmacher C, Siewert JR. R1 resection in the surgery of upper gastrointestinal tumors: relevance and therapeutic consequences. *Chirurg.* 2007;**78**:792–801.
19. Gertler P, Richter J, Stecher L, Nitsche U, Feith M. What to do after R1-resection of adenocarcinomas of the esophagogastric junction? *J Surg Oncol.* 2016;**114**:428–433.
20. Aurello P, Magistri P, Nigri G, et al. Surgical management of microscopic positive resection margin after gastrectomy for gastric cancer: a systematic review of gastric R1 management. *Anticancer Res.* 2014;**34**:6283–6288.
21. Stiekema J, Trip AK, Jansen EP, et al. Does adjuvant chemoradiotherapy improve the prognosis of gastric cancer after an R1 resection? Results from a Dutch cohort study. *Ann Surg Oncol.* 2015;**22**:581–588.
22. Lee KY, Noh SH, Hyung WJ, et al. Impact of splenectomy for lymph node dissection on long-term surgical outcome in gastric cancer. *Ann Surg Oncol.* 2001;**8**:402–406.
23. Hölscher AH, Law S. Esophagogastric junction adenocarcinomas: individualization of resection with special considerations for Siewert type II, and Nishi types EG, E=G and GE cancers. *Gastric Cancer.* 2020;**23**:3–9.
24. Wagner PK, Ramaswamy A, Ruschoff J, Schmitz-Moormann P, Rothmund M. Lymph node counts in the upper abdomen: anatomical basis for lymphadenectomy in gastric cancer. *Br J Surg.* 1991;**78**:825–827.
25. Kurokawa Y, Doki Y, Mizusawa J, et al. Bursectomy versus omentectomy alone for resectable gastric cancer (JCOG1001): a phase 3, open-label, randomised controlled trial. *Lancet Gastroenterol Hepatol.* 2018;**3**:460–468.
26. Syn NL, Wee I, Shabbir A, Kim G, So JB. Pouch versus no pouch following total gastrectomy: meta-analysis of randomized and non-randomized studies. *Ann Surg.* 2019;**269**:1041–1053.
27. Iwatsuki M, Yamamoto H, Miyata H, et al. Effect of hospital and surgeon volume on postoperative outcomes after distal gastrectomy for gastric cancer based on data from 145,523 Japanese patients collected from a nationwide web-based data entry system. *Gastric Cancer.* 2019;**22**:190–201.

20

Gastric cancer
Minimally invasive surgery and robotic surgery

Makoto Hikage and Masanori Terashima

Introduction

Laparoscopic surgery is gradually becoming common for several solid cancers, and its use has rapidly expanded in the field of gastric cancer treatment worldwide.[1] The incidence of gastric cancer in East Asian countries is high, and 75% of all gastric cancer cases are diagnosed in these countries.[2] This has made East Asian countries pioneers in studies on the disease state of gastric cancer and the understanding of the fine anatomy for gastric cancer surgery.[3] In Japan and Korea, early gastric cancer (EGC) is mainly diagnosed by screening, and endoscopic treatment and laparoscopic surgery was developed earlier in these countries than in other countries globally.[4,5] In recent years, robotic systems have been introduced to overcome the disadvantages of laparoscopic surgery, and the adoption of robot-assisted surgery is currently spreading.[6–11] This minimally invasive surgery is becoming increasingly common in Asian countries for various diseases, especially EGC.[12] Although this technique has a great influence on gastric cancer surgery, it has to be adopted carefully taking into consideration concerns regarding its safety and oncological feasibility.

In this review, we provide a histological outline and describe the development of laparoscopic surgery and robotic surgery for gastric cancer with existing evidence. Additionally, we comment on the future prospects of these techniques.

History

Laparoscopic gastrectomy for gastric cancer

In 1881, Theodor Billroth performed a distal gastrectomy in a 43-year-old woman at the University of Vienna, and this is considered to be the first successful gastric cancer surgery.[13] The patient recovered from the surgery with a favourable clinical course, and she was discharged from the hospital 22 days later. However, she died 4 months after the surgery owing to progression of pre-existing peritoneal dissemination. Surprisingly, although this surgery was performed more than 140 years ago, similar basic surgical techniques are still used today. The introduction of laparoscopy as a method of approaching the operating field marked a dramatic turning point in gastric cancer surgery (Table 20.1). Until the end of the 20th century, the iron-clad rule of abdominal surgery was to operate with a sufficiently large field of vision after making a large incision. However, Georg Kelling from Germany invented laparoscopic surgery with the aim of reducing invasiveness by minimizing injury to the body while obtaining a sufficient field of view. Kelling reported that he could observe many organs, including the stomach and intestine, by insufflating air into the abdominal cavity and inserting a laparoscope into the inflated space in animal experiments. The term 'laparoscopic' was first used by Hans Christian Jacobaeus, a Swedish researcher.[14] Thereafter, the use of this technique gradually spread to surgical procedures for treating benign diseases. Kurt Semm reported on laparoscopic appendectomy in 1980,[15] and Erich Mühe performed the first laparoscopic cholecystectomy in 1985.[16] With continuous advances in the knowledge and technique of laparoscopic surgery, laparoscopic gastrectomy (LG) for gastric cancer was first performed by Kitano et al. in 1991 (laparoscopy-assisted distal gastrectomy).[4] This was considered the first use of laparoscopy for the treatment of a malignant disease. Initially, as limited types of forceps were available and an operation under a pneumoperitoneum was not possible, the procedure was challenging. However, Kitano et al. continuously succeeded in performing partial resections, mucosal resections, and laparoscopy-assisted distal gastrectomies, which marked the beginning of minimally invasive surgery for gastric cancer.

Development of surgical robots

The development of 'telepresence robotic arms' was initiated around the 1950s, with the intention of using remotely controlled robots to handle hazardous substances or perform tasks under the sea or in outer space. The development of robotic arms made rapid progress with advances in computer technology in the late 1980s and early 1990s. A robotic system was first used in the clinical setting in 1985, when the Puma 200, an industrial robot, was used to perform neurological biopsy (Table 20.1).[6] In 1986, researchers at the IBM Thomas J. Watson Research Center and University of California completed the development of ROBODOC, a surgical robot for hip

Table 20.1 History of laparoscopy and laparoscopic/robotic gastrectomy

Year	Events
1901	Intraperitoneal observation with a laparoscope in animal (dog) experiments (Kelling)
1910	The term 'laparoscopy' was first used (Jacobaeus)
1980	Laparoscopic appendectomy (Semm)
1985	Laparoscopic cholecystectomy (Mouret) (use of a video camera with a laparoscope)
	Puma 200 was used for neurosurgical biopsy.
1986	ROBODOC was used for artificial joint replacement
1991	Laparoscopic gastrectomy for gastric cancer (Kitano)
1992	Laparoscopic partial hepatectomy (Gagner)
1994	AESOP (Computer Motion Inc.) was released and approved by the FDA
1998	ZEUS (Computer Motion Inc.) was released
1999	da Vinci Surgical System (Intuitive Surgical Inc.) was released
	Laparoscopic total gastrectomy, D2 lymphadenectomy (Uyama)
2000	da Vinci Surgical System was approved by the FDA
2001	First case of intercontinental telesurgery (US–France)
2002	Hashizume performed robot-assisted distal gastrectomy

FDA, Food and Drug Administration.

replacement, which became the first Food and Drug Administration (FDA)-approved surgery-assisting robot to be used in the clinical setting.[7] In 1994, Computer Motion Inc. (Goleta, CA, USA) developed the Automated Endoscopic System for Optimal Positioning (AESOP), which uses voice recognition to control the endoscope, and it could be adopted for solo endoscopic surgery.[17]

The development of medical robots with master–slave manipulators for telesurgery was initiated in the late 1980s, and this was largely led by the US Army. Initially, researchers intended to develop a robot that could be used by surgeons to perform telesurgery on wounded soldiers in the battlefield. Later, the usage setting shifted to the private sector with the founding of Intuitive Surgical Inc. (Sunnyvale, CA, USA) in 1995. Its da Vinci Surgical System (DVSS) was launched in 1999, and in 2000, the DVSS became the first robot-assisted surgical system to be approved by the FDA for general laparoscopic surgery. Computer Motion Inc., the developer of AESOP, developed ZEUS in 1998, adding a remote-control function to AESOP. Initially, both systems were used for cardiovascular surgery.[8,18] However, gradually, their use was expanded to digestive surgery, urology, and gynaecology.[10,19–21] In 2001, Jacques Marescaux performed a remote cholecystectomy between New York and Strasbourg in France using ZEUS, and this is the first reported case of telesurgery.[22] With regard to gastric cancer, Hashizume et al. reported the first robot-assisted case (robot-assisted distal gastrectomy (RDG)) in 2002.[23]

In 2003, Computer Motion Inc., the developer of ZEUS, was merged with Intuitive Surgical Inc., and since then, the DVSS has been the only FDA-approved surgery-assisting robot with a master–slave manipulator system, creating a near-perfect monopoly. In March 2015, the fourth generation of the DVSS (DaVinci Xi) was released, and as of March 2019, 5114 units of the DVSS had been installed worldwide, including 3283 in the US, 893 in Europe, and 661 in Asia.[24]

Robotic gastrectomy (RG) with the DVSS appears to have various advantages over LG, which is also a minimally invasive surgical procedure. As LG uses linear forceps, the range of motion is restricted, and RG overcomes this disadvantage by using forceps with seven degrees of freedom. Additionally, LG involves a two-dimensional field of view, which hinders depth perception, whereas RG involves a three-dimensional and tenfold magnified view of the operating field. Moreover, the motion scaling and tremor suppression functions in RG enable precise movement, which is believed to help reduce tissue damage and blood loss. Furthermore, the ergonomics-based surgeon console in RG can reduce fatigue among operators.[12] Initially, the surgical devices for RG were limited; however, ultrasonically activated scalpels (harmonic), vessel sealers, EndoWrist staplers, and various other instruments are now available for use in RG, and these have helped make RG non-inferior to LG.[25,26]

The challenges for operators performing RG include lack of tactile perception, which can lead to incomplete ligature; tissue damage due to excessive stress; and injury to other organs outside the field of view. The operator needs to judge the amount of force transmitted to the tissue by visual perception rather than tactile perception. Moreover, unlike conventional open surgery or laparoscopic surgery, the operator controls three arms in RG, and considerable training is required. As the DVSS involves a robot, it can potentially apply an unexpectedly strong force, which does not occur in conventional surgery; thus, even slight mishandling of the DVSS may lead to a fatal accident.

Laparoscopic gastrectomy for early gastric cancer

After LG was introduced by Kitano et al., its use rapidly spread. A survey conducted in Japan indicated that, as of 2004, LG with lymph node dissection had been performed in more than 4000 cases.[27] As the safety and efficacy of LG have not been established, it has been indicated only for EGC, which has a low risk of lymph node metastasis.[28] On the other hand, several retrospective case series comparing laparoscopic surgery and open surgery have reported that laparoscopic surgery is associated with favourable short-term outcomes, including reduced postoperative pain, faster recovery of intestinal peristalsis, shorter hospital stay, and shorter rehabilitation.[29,30] Additionally, a couple of retrospective comparable studies and small-scale single-institution randomized controlled trials (RCTs) conducted in Japan and Korea showed the superiority of laparoscopic surgery to open surgery with regard to short-term outcomes and postoperative quality of life.[31,32] Furthermore, the results of several meta-analyses indicated the advantages of LG in terms of the amount of intraoperative bleeding, time to the first flatus after surgery, length of postoperative hospital stay, and number of retrieved lymph nodes (Table 20.2).[33–36] These favourable outcomes motivated researchers to organize large-scale clinical studies to confirm the safety and oncological feasibility of laparoscopic surgery.

Table 20.3 provides a list of major multicentre clinical studies that were conducted in the past or are still ongoing. In Japan, a multicentre phase II trial (JCOG0703) was conducted by the Japan

Table 20.2 Summary of the meta-analyses comparing laparoscopic gastrectomy and open gastrectomy

First author	Year	Country	Subject	Number of studies/patients	Morbidity	Blood loss	Operative time	Retrieved LN	Hospital stay	Time to first flatus	5-year OS
Peng	2009	China	EGC	6/218	LG = OG	LG < OG	LG > OG	LG > OG	LG < OG	LG < OG	-
Zeng	2012	China	EGC	22/3411	LG < OG	LG < OG	LG > OG	LG = OG	LG < OG	LG < OG	-
Wang	2014	China	EGC	8/629	LG = OG	LG < OG	LG > OG	LG > OG	LG < OG	-	-
Deng	2015	China	EGC	7/390	LG < OG	LG < OG	LG > OG	LG = OG	LG < OG	LG < OG	-
Ramos	2011	Spain	AGC	7/452	-	LG = OG	LG > OG	LG = OG	LG < OG	-	LG = OG
Zou	2014	China	AGC	14/2596	LG = OG	LG < OG	LG = OG	LG = OG	LG < OG	LG < OG	LG = OG
Małczak	2018	Poland	AGC	8/1582	LG < OG	-	LG > OG	LG = OG	LG < OG	-	-
Li	2019	China	AGC	12/1651	LG < OG	LG < OG	LG = OG	LG = OG	LG < OG	LG < OG	LG = OG
Li	2019	China	AGC	15/4494	-	-	-	-	-	-	LG = OG
Beyer	2019	Germany	AGC	5/2157	LG = OG	LG = OG	LG > OG	LG = OG	LG = OG	LG = OG	-
Zeng	2020	China	EGC/AGC	17/5204	LG < OG	LG < OG	LG > OG	LG = OG	LG < OG	LG < OG	-
Shan	2020	China	EGC/AGC, elderly	13/4768	LG < OG	LG < OG	LG = OG	LG > OG	LG < OG	LG < OG	LG = OG
Zhu	2020	China	AGC	36/11,808	LG < OG	LG < OG	LG > OG	LG = OG	LG < OG	LG < OG	LG > OG
Chen	2020	China	AGC	30/16,029	LG < OG	LG < OG	LG > OG	LG = OG	LG < OG	LG < OG	LG = OG
Liao	2021	China	EGC/AGC, Siewert type II/III	7/1915	LG = OG	LG < OG	LG = OG	LG = OG	LG < OG	LG = OG	-
Aiolfi	2021	Italy	EGC/AGC	17/5768	LG = OG	LG < OG	LG > OG	LG = OG	LG < OG	LG < OG	LG = OG
Liao	2021	China	AGC, neoadjuvant	6/704	LG < OG	LG = OG	-	LG = OG	LG = OG	LG < OG	LG = OG
Zhang	2021	China	AGC	41/14,689	LG < OG	LG < OG	LG > OG	LG = OG	LG < OG	LG < OG	LG > OG
Song	2022	China	EGC/AGC	18/2102	LG < OG	LG < OG	LG = OG	LG = OG	LG < OG	LG < OG	-
Hakkenbrak	2022	Netherlands	EGC/AGC	22/5087	LG < OG	LG < OG	LG > OG	LG > OG	LG < OG	LG < OG	-
Otsuka	2022	Japan	AGC	23/13,698	LG < OG	LG < OG	LG > OG	LG = OG	LG < OG	-	LG = OG
Jiang	2022	China	AGC	12/4101	LG = OG	LG < OG	LG > OG	LG < OG	LG < OG	-	LG = OG
Lou	2022	China	EGC/AGC	28/7643	LG = OG	LG < OG	LG > OG	LG < OG	LG < OG	LG < OG	LG = OG
Argillander	2022	Netherlands	EGC/AGC, elderly	18/876	LG < OG	-	-	-	LG < OG	-	-
Garbarino	2022	Italy	EGC/AGC	34/24,098	LG < OG	LG < OG	LG > OG	LG = OG	LG < OG	LG < OG	LG = OG
Yang	2022	China	AGC	17/4742	LG < OG	LG < OG	LG > OG	LG = OG	LG < OG	LG < OG	LG = OG

AGC, advanced gastric cancer; EGC, early gastric cancer; LG, laparoscopic gastrectomy; LN, lymph node; OG, open gastrectomy; OS, overall survival.

Clinical Oncology Group (JCOG) to evaluate the safety of laparoscopic distal gastrectomy (LDG) for cStage I gastric cancer. The primary end point involved the proportion of patients who developed either anastomotic leakage or pancreatic fistula. The threshold value was set at 8%, and the expected value was set at 3%. This study enrolled 176 patients. The proportion of patients who developed anastomotic leakage or pancreatic fistula was 1.7% (80% confidence interval (CI) 0.6–3.8%). Thus, the null hypothesis was rejected, and the primary end point of the study was met.[37] According to this result, the JCOG performed a phase III trial (JCOG0912) in 2010 to evaluate the non-inferiority of LDG to open distal gastrectomy (ODG) in terms of relapse-free survival (RFS). The planned sample size was 920 patients, which was determined with a power of at least 80%, a one-sided alpha of 5%, and a non-inferiority margin for a hazard ratio (HR) of 1.54. A total of 921 patients were randomized (ODG 459, LDG 462) between March 2010 and November 2013.

Among the 921 patients, 912 (99%) underwent the assigned surgery. Conversion to ODG was needed for 16 patients (3.5%) in the LDG arm mainly because of advanced disease. In 2013, the short-term outcomes were published.[38] The results indicated that although the operative time was longer with LDG than with ODG, the amount of intraoperative bleeding was lower, the time to the first flatus after surgery was shorter, and pain was less severe with LDG than with ODG. According to these results, in 2014, the Japanese Gastric Cancer Treatment Guidelines recommended LG as a treatment option for cStage I gastric cancer indicated for distal gastrectomy.[39] The long-term outcomes were presented at the 2019 American Society of Clinical Oncology Annual Meeting.[40] In this study, before the first interim analysis, the primary end point was amended from overall survival (OS) to RFS in 2015 because the surrogacy of RFS for OS was demonstrated and the predicted number of OS events was lower than expected. The 5-year RFS rates were 94.0% (95% CI

20 Gastric cancer: minimally invasive surgery

Table 20.3 Multicentre prospective trials on laparoscopic gastrectomy

Study	Country	Type		Subject	Primary end point	Procedure	Sample size	Main results
JCOG0703	Japan	P-II		cStage I	Leak, PF	LDG	176	Leak: 1.1% (2/176); PF: 1.1% (2/176); 5-yr OS: 98.2%, 5-yr RFS: 98.2%
JCOG0912	Japan	P-III		cStage I	RFS	LDG vs ODG	921 (LDG462/ODG459)	5-yr RFS: 95.1% vs 94.0%, $p = 0.0075$; leak: 0.2% (1/457) vs 0.2% (1/455); PF: 0.4% (2/457) vs 0.4% (2/455); overall surgical complication: 3.3% (15/457) vs 3.7% (17/455)
KLASS-01	Korea	P-III		cStage I	5-yr OS	LDG vs ODG	1256 (LDG644/ODG612)	5-yr OS: 94.2% vs 93.3%, $p = 0.64$; 5-yr CSS: 97.1% vs 97.2%, $p = 0.91$; leak: 0.8% (5/644) vs 0.7% (4/612), $p = 1.000$; overall surgical complication: 13.0% (84/644) vs 19.9% (122/612), $p = 0.001$
JCOG1401	Japan	P-III		cStage I	Leak	LTG/LPG	245 (LTG195/LPG50)	Leak: 2.4% (6/245; 95% CI 0.9–5.3; one-sided $p = 0.0002$); in-hospital grade 3/4 adverse events: 29% (71/245)
KLASS-03	Korea	P-II		cStage I	Morbidity, mortality	LTG	160	Morbidity: 20.6% (33/160), mortality: 0.6% (1/160); Clavien–Dindo grade >3: 9.4%, re-operation: 1.9%
CLASS-02	China	P-III		cStage I	Morbidity and mortality	LTG vs OTG	227 (LTG113/OTG114)	Overall morbidity and mortality: 19.1% vs 20.2%, rate difference −1.1%
JLSSG0901	Japan	P-II/III	In progress	AGC	P-II: leak, PF; P-III: 5-yr RFS	LDG vs ODG	P-II: 176 (LDG86/ODG89), P-III: 500	Leak: 1.2% (1/86); PF: 3.5% (3/86); overall complication: 15% (13/86); CTCAE grade 3/4: 5.8% (5/86)
KLASS-02	Korea	P-III		AGC	3-yr RFS	LDG vs ODG	1050 (LDG526/ODG524)	3-yr RFS: 80.3% vs 81.3%, $p = 0.726$; early complication: 15.7% vs 23.4%, $p = 0.0027$; late complication: 2.0% vs 4.4%, $p = 0.0038$
CLASS-01	China	P-III		AGC	3-yr DFS	LDG vs ODG	1056 (LDG528/ODG528)	3-yr DFS: 76.5% vs 77.8%, $p = 0.59$; 3-yr OS: 83.1% vs 85.2%, $p = 0.33$; morbidity: 12.9% vs 15.2% (95% CI −1.9 to 6.6; $p = 0.285$); mortality: 0.0% vs 0.4% (95% CI −0.4 to 1.4; $p = 0.249$)
KLASS-06	Korea	P-II/III	In progress	AGC	3-yr RFS	LTG vs OTG	772 (LTG386/OTG386)	
LOGICA	Netherlands	P-III		cT1-4a, N0-3b, M0	Hospital stay	LG vs OG	227 (LG115/OG112)	Median hospital stay: 7 days (interquartile range, 5–9) in both groups ($p = 0.34$)
STOMACH	Netherlands	P-III		cT1-3, N0-1, M0 (after NAC)	Surgical radicality, retrieved LN	MITG vs OTG	96 (MITG47/OTG49)	Mean number of resected lymph nodes: 41.7 vs 43.4, $p = 0.612$; R0 resection: 44 vs 48 patients, $p = 0.617$
JCOG1809	Japan	P-II	In progress	Proximal AGC	PF	Splenic hilar dissection	85	
CLASS-04	China	P-II		Proximal AGC	Morbidity	Splenic hilar dissection	251	Overall postoperative complication: 13.6% (33/242)

AGC, advanced gastric cancer; CSS, cancer-specific survival; HR, hazard ratio; LDG, laparoscopic distal gastrectomy; LG, laparoscopic gastrectomy; LN, lymph node; LPG, laparoscopic proximal gastrectomy; LTG, laparoscopic total gastrectomy; MITG, minimally invasive total gastrectomy; NAC, neoadjuvant chemotherapy; ODG, open distal gastrectomy; OG, open gastrectomy; OS, overall survival; OTG, open total gastrectomy, PF, pancreatic fistula; P-II/III, phase II/III; RFS, recurrence-free survival.

91.4–95.9%) with ODG and 95.1% (95% CI 92.7–96.8%) with LDG. LDG was non-inferior to ODG in terms of RFS (HR 0.84, 90% CI 0.56–1.27 (<1.54); p for non-inferiority = 0.008). The 5-year OS rates were 95.2% (95% CI 92.7–96.8%) with ODG and 97.0% (95% CI 94.9–98.2%) with LDG (HR 0.83, 95% CI 0.49–1.40). Thus, the non-inferiority of LDG to ODG in terms of RFS was confirmed. LDG has been established as one of the standard treatments for cStage I gastric cancer in Japan.[41]

Additionally, in Korea, a phase III trial (KLASS-01) was conducted to evaluate the non-inferiority of LDG to ODG in terms of 5-year RFS among patients with cStage I gastric cancer.[42] The non-inferiority of LDG to ODG was confirmed (RFS rate: LDG 94.2% vs ODG 93.3%; p = 0.64).[43] These results indicate that LDG can be safely performed and may be oncologically acceptable for cStage I gastric cancer. In Korea, LDG is currently considered a standard treatment for cStage I gastric cancer.

Laparoscopic gastrectomy for proximal gastric cancer

The incidence of proximal gastric cancer has been increasing in recent years. Laparoscopic total gastrectomy (LTG) or laparoscopic proximal gastrectomy (LPG) is indicated for proximal gastric cancer. The anastomotic and reconstruction methods in these surgical procedures differ greatly from those in LDG. In particular, in oesophagojejunal anastomoses, the anastomotic site is located at the border between the mediastinum and the abdominal cavity, which makes surgery difficult. Because of this difficulty, the incidence of anastomotic leakage has been high, especially during the initial period.[44,45] Regarding the safety of LTG, a phase II trial (KLASS-03, Korea) was conducted with the incidence of postoperative complications as the primary end point. In this study, among 160 patients with EGC who underwent LTG, 20.6% (33/160) developed postoperative complications; however, this result was similar to that of a historical control (i.e. 18% incidence of complications after open surgery). Thus, the study concluded that LTG could be safely performed.[46] However, it is questionable whether the results are acceptable, because the researchers used data from Italian open gastrectomy (OG) as the historical control. The JCOG conducted a non-randomized confirmatory phase III trial (JCOG1401) with a clear clinical question.[47] In this study, LTG and LPG were evaluated, and the incidence of anastomotic leakage was the primary end point. As the clinical stage was the same as that in JCOG0912, the efficacy-related evidence obtained in JCOG0912 could be extrapolated on confirming the safety of LTG/LPG. Thus, this study was conducted as a single-arm confirmatory study. A total of 245 patients were enrolled. The incidence of anastomotic leakage at the site of the oesophagojejunal anastomosis was only 2.4% (6/245), which was significantly lower than the pre-set threshold value of 8% (one-sided p = 0.0002).[48] Overall, these results indicate that LTG/LPG can be safely performed by experienced surgeons. The CLASS-02 phase III study was also conducted in China to directly compare the safety of LTG with that of open total gastrectomy (OTG) for clinical stage I gastric cancer, and the morbidity and mortality within 30 days following surgeries was the primary outcome. The overall morbidity and mortality rates were not significantly different between the groups (LTG 19.1%, OTG 20.2%; rate difference, –1.1%; 95% CI –11.8% to 9.6%), and the study concluded the safety of LTG with lymphadenectomy by experienced surgeons was comparable to that of OTG as well.[49]

Laparoscopic gastrectomy for advanced gastric cancer

As the standard surgical approach for advanced gastric cancer (AGC) is gastrectomy with D2 lymph node dissection,[50] laparoscopic surgery should involve D2 lymph node dissection. Although the safety of LG had been demonstrated in patients with cStage I gastric cancer, the safety and efficacy of laparoscopic surgery in patients with AGC (cStage II or higher) were unclear. Regarding safety, as D2 lymph node dissection is somewhat technically demanding, there has been concern about an increase in morbidity (pancreatic fistula or intra-abdominal abscess). Furthermore, oncological issues, such as the risk of tumour cell dissemination into the abdominal cavity or bloodstream related to handling of a large tumour with laparoscopic forceps and the effects of pneumoperitoneum, should be considered.[51] With regard to the comparison of laparoscopic surgery and open surgery with D2 lymph node dissection in patients with AGC, retrospective studies, prospective small-scale RCTs, and multiple non-randomized control trials were possible around the year 2000. Collective data from these studies were reported as meta-analyses (Table 20.2).[52–73] The number of lymph nodes retrieved, rate of tumour recurrence/metastasis, and OS were not significantly different between laparoscopic surgery and open surgery. In addition, a Japanese large-scale multicentre retrospective case–control study using propensity score matching showed the non-inferiority of laparoscopic surgery to open surgery (5-year OS: OG 53.0% vs LG 54.2%, HR 1.01, 95% CI 0.80–1.29).[74]

Meanwhile, prospective RCTs to evaluate the non-inferiority of laparoscopic surgery to open surgery in patients with AGC have been conducted in Japan, Korea, and China. The JLSSG0901 study was conducted in Japan as a phase II/III trial to evaluate the technical safety and short-term and long-term outcomes of LDG with D2 lymph node dissection performed for cStage II/III gastric cancer. The incidence of pancreatic fistula or anastomotic leakage, which was the primary end point in the phase II part, was 4.7% (4/86) (pancreatic fistula, n = 3; anastomotic leakage, n = 1), and the incidence of postoperative grade 3 or greater complications was 5.8%, indicating the safety of LDG for AGC.[75] As the primary end point was met in the phase II part, the phase III part of the study was performed. The primary end point in the phase III part was 5-year recurrence-free survival. The non-inferiority margin was set as a HR of 1.31, and the sample size was calculated as 500 patients. Patient enrolment in the phase III part has been completed, and the results are expected to be published in 2023.

The KLASS-02 phase III study was conducted in Korea to evaluate the non-inferiority of LDG to ODG in patients with cT2–4a, Nx, M0 cancer, and 3-year RFS was the primary end point. The non-inferiority margin was set as a HR of 1.43, and the sample size was calculated as 1050 patients.[76] The short-term outcomes, which have already been published, indicated that although the operative time was longer with LDG that with ODG (227.1 min vs 165.0 min; p <0.001), the amount of blood loss was significantly lower (153.8

mL vs 230.1 mL; p <0.001) and the length of postoperative hospital stay was significantly shorter (8.1 days vs 9.3 days; p = 0.005) with LDG than with ODG. Furthermore, the incidence of postoperative complications was significantly lower with LDG than with ODG (16.6% vs 24.1%; p = 0.003); however, the reason for this is unclear.[77] The long-term outcomes were published in 2020. The 3-year RFS rates were 80.3% for the LDG group and 81.3% for the ODG group (p = 0.726). Cox regression analysis after stratification by the surgeon revealed a HR of 1.035 (95% CI 0.762–1.406, p = 0.827; p = 0.039 for non-inferiority), which confirmed the non-inferiority of the LDG in comparison with the ODG.[78] However, in a subgroup analysis, among patients with pStage I/II cancer, the 3-year OS rate was lower with LDG than with ODG despite favourable short-term outcomes.

The CLASS-01 phase III study was conducted in China to evaluate the non-inferiority of LDG to ODG in patients similar to those examined in KLASS-02, and 3-year disease-free survival was the end point. The non-inferiority margin was set at 10%, and the sample size was calculated as 1056 patients. The short-term outcomes indicated that although the operative time was significantly longer with LDG than with ODG (217.3 min vs 186.0 min; p <0.001), the amount of blood loss was significantly lower with LDG than with ODG (105.5 mL vs 117.3 mL; p = 0.001). Furthermore, the time to ambulation (p = 0.037), time to the first flatus (p = 0.011), time to the first liquid intake (p <0.001), and length of postoperative hospital stay (p <0.001) were significantly shorter with LDG than with ODG. Before other phase III studies, CLASS-01 confirmed the non-inferiority of LDG to ODG with regard to the long-term outcomes.[79] The non-inferiority of LDG to ODG in terms of the 3-year disease-free survival rate (LDG 76.5% vs ODG 77.8%; absolute difference −1.3%; one-sided 97.5% CI −6.5% to ∞, not crossing the pre-specified non-inferiority margin) was reported.[80] However, in a subgroup analysis, among patients with pStage III cancer, the 3-year OS rate was lower with LDG than with ODG (69.5% vs 73.2%). Although the results of these prospective randomized trials support the safety of LDG for AGC, the long-term outcomes of studies from Japan are awaited to confidently conclude the efficacy of LDG for AGC.

The role of laparoscopic gastrectomy in Western countries

Although LG for gastric cancer is an option in the clinical setting in Asian countries, it is questionable whether the evidence obtained from studies in Japan and Korea can be directly extrapolated to Western practice.[3] The incidence of gastric cancer is lower and gastric cancer is often detected at a more advanced stage in Western countries than in Eastern countries. Additionally, in Western countries, gastric cancer is located at the proximal portion of the stomach, and many of the tumours are of the diffuse type. Furthermore, in Western countries, many patients often have a different spectrum of comorbidities owing to a high overweight rate. Because of differences in pathophysiology and patient background, it is difficult to accumulate suitable patients for LG in Western countries, and previous studies are limited to small-scale prospective studies.

The LOGICA study was the first RCT comparing laparoscopic surgery to open surgery in the Western population.[81] This study was conducted in patients with resectable gastric cancer to evaluate the superiority of laparoscopic surgery to open surgery with regard to short-term outcomes, and the length of postoperative hospital stay was the primary end point. However, LG showed no difference in the duration of hospital stay (median hospital stay, 7 days in both group; p = 0.34), the incidence of postoperative complications (44% vs 42%; p = 0.91), and the oncological efficacy (1-year OS, 76% vs 78%; p = 0.74), compared with OG.[82] Similarly, the STOMACH study was an RCT being conducted in patients with gastric cancer after neoadjuvant chemotherapy to substantiate the non-inferiority of minimally invasive total gastrectomy (MITG) to OTG with regard to the quality of oncological resection, and the radicality of surgery and the number of retrieved lymph nodes are the primary end points.[83] Ninety-six patients were included in this trial, and 49 patients were randomized to OTG and 47 to MITG. The mean number of resected lymph nodes was 43.4 ± 17.3 in OTG and 41.7 ± 16.1 in MITG (p = 0.612). Forty-eight patients in the OTG group had a R0 resection and 44 patients in the MITG group (p = 0.617). One-year survival was 90.4% in OTG and 85.5% in MITG (p = 0.701). Thus, this trial provided evidence of non-inferiority regarding quality of the oncological resection in MITG compared to OTG in the treatment of AGC.[84] Successive RCTs following these trials conducted in Western countries will be creating new evidence for LG in the Western population.

Benefits and future prospects of laparoscopic gastrectomy

According to the results of previously conducted large-scale clinical studies, LG has been almost established as a standard treatment for cStage I gastric cancer. Moreover, the technical safety of LTG/LPG for proximal gastric cancer has been substantiated, and previous results indicate that LTG/LPG can be safely performed by experienced surgeons. From the perspective of minimizing surgical invasiveness, previously published reports have clearly show that LG has a substantial advantage. In recent years, as minimally invasive surgery has been further individualized, limited stomach resection and lymph node dissection combining laparoscopy and endoscopy cooperative surgery and the sentinel node concept are being assessed.[85–87] Additionally, a clinical study is currently being conducted to evaluate the oncological safety of individualized gastrectomy and functional preservation with individualized gastrectomy according to the sentinel node concept (UMIN000014401).[88] However, the RCT conducted in South Korea failed to show non-inferiority of laparoscopic sentinel node navigation surgery to LG for 3-year disease-free survival, with a 5% margin (91.8% vs 95.5%, difference 3.7%, 95% CI −0.6 to 8.1).[89] Easy application of functional organ preservation for gastric cancer should be cautious considering the survival.

Moreover, the favourable short-term outcomes of large-scale prospective clinical trials indicate that LG can be safely performed in patients with cStage II/III gastric cancer. If the long-term outcomes of these trials demonstrate the non-inferiority of LDG to ODG, the indication of LDG will be expanded to AGC. However, this is not the same in case of total gastrectomy. When total gastrectomy is performed for proximal AGC, a serious issue is splenectomy. According to the results of JCOG0110, D2 lymph node dissection with spleen preservation is recommended for advanced proximal gastric cancer without greater curvature invasion.[90] Considering that this surgical procedure does not differ much from LDG with D2 dissection, LTG is probably applicable for AGC in the proximal stomach. On the other hand, lymph node dissection with splenectomy is considered necessary for cancer with greater curvature invasion because complete dissection of the #10 lymph node is mandatory. However, laparoscopic #10 lymph node dissection with splenectomy is a very technically demanding procedure.[91] In recent years, several studies have reported the efficacy of spleen-preserving splenic hilar lymph node dissection.[92] This spleen-preserving procedure appears to take full advantage of laparoscopic surgery.[93] However, the safety and oncological feasibility of this procedure need to be validated in prospective clinical studies. The CLASS-04 phase II study was conducted in China to evaluate the safety of laparoscopic spleen-preserving total gastrectomy with #10 lymph node dissection for advanced upper-third gastric cancer, and the postoperative complication rate was the primary outcome. According to the preceding study, the complication rate of laparoscopic spleen-preserving total gastrectomy was 12.5% (expected value), whereas the incidence of complication of laparotomy was about 20.0% (target value). The non-inferiority value was set at 10%, and the sample size was calculated as 251 patients. In consequence, the overall complication rate was 13.6% (33/242). The major complication and mortality rates were 3.3% (8/242) and 0.4% (1/242), respectively. CLASS-04 concluded the feasibility of laparoscopic spleen-preserving total gastrectomy for advanced upper-third cancer by very experienced surgeons.[94,95] The JCOG is also currently conducting a prospective phase II trial to investigate the safety of spleen-preserving splenic hilar lymph node dissection (JCOG1809). If the safety of this procedure is confirmed, a phase III trial to examine its oncological validity will be planned.

According to the European Society for Medical Oncology–European Society of Surgical Oncology–European Society of Radiotherapy and Oncology Clinical Practice Guidelines, perioperative chemotherapy is recommended for resectable AGC.[96] In Japan, a prospective clinical trial is currently ongoing to evaluate the efficacy of neoadjuvant chemotherapy. If the efficacy of neoadjuvant chemotherapy is substantiated in the future, the feasibility of laparoscopic surgery after neoadjuvant chemotherapy should be evaluated.

Robotic gastrectomy

Many retrospective case–control studies comparing RG and LG have so far been conducted. Recently, several meta-analyses involving these studies have been performed, and the reported results were comparable (Table 20.4).[97–115] The results indicated that the amount of blood loss was lower with RG than with LG; however, the operation time was longer with RG than with LG. The duration of hospital stay, morbidity, and number of retrieved lymph nodes were comparable between RG and LG.

Very few prospective studies on RG have so far been conducted. We previously conducted a single-centre early/late phase II studies in patients with cStage I gastric cancer to evaluate the safety of RG.[116,117] We found that the incidence of intra-abdominal infectious complications of Clavien–Dindo grade II or greater was 0% in the early phase study and 3.3% in the late phase study; thus, the null hypothesis was rejected. The results indicate that RG can be safely performed for cStage I gastric cancer.

Table 20.4 Summary of the meta-analyses comparing RG and LG

Author	Year	Country	Number of studies	Number of patients	Morbidity	Blood loss	Operative time	Retrieved LN	Hospital stay	Time to first flatus	Medical cost	OS
Shen	2014	China	8	1875	RG = LG	RG < LG	RG > LG	RG = LG	RG = LG	-	-	-
Chuan	2015	China	5	1796	RG = LG	RG < LG	RG > LG	RG = LG	RG = LG	-	-	-
Hu	2016	China	12	3580	RG = LG	RG < LG	RG > LG	RG > LG	RG < LG	RG > LG	-	-
Wang	2017	China	3	562	RG = LG	RG < LG	RG > LG	RG = LG	RG = LG	-	-	-
Chen	2017	China	19	5953	RG = LG	RG < LG	RG > LG	RG = LG	RG = LG	RG = LG	RG > LG	-
Pan	2017	China	5	1614	-	-	-	-	-	-	-	RG = LG
Liao	2019	China	8	3410	RG = LG	-	-	-	RG = LG	-	-	RG = LG
Zheng	2019	China	16	4576	RG = LG	RG < LG	RG > LG	RG = LG	RG = LG	RG < LG	-	RG = LG
Qiu	2019	China	24	8413	RG = LG	RG < LG	RG > LG	RG = LG	RG = LG	RG = LG	RG > LG	RG = LG
Guerrini	2020	Italy	40	17712	RG < LG	RG < LG	RG > LG	RG > LG	RG = LG	RG = LG	RG > LG	-
Ma	2020	China	19	7275	RG = LG	RG < LG	RG > LG	RG = LG	RG = LG	RG < LG	-	RG = LG
Wu	2021	China	11	4142	-	-	-	-	-	-	-	RG = LG
Zhang	2021	China	15	3293	RG < LG	RG < LG	RG > LG	RG > LG	RG < LG	RG = LG	-	-
Zhang	2021	China	12	3176	RG < LG	RG < LG	RG > LG	RG = LG	RG = LG	RG < LG	-	-
Feng	2021	China	20	13446	RG < LG	RG < LG	RG > LG	RG > LG	RG < LG	RG < LG	RG > LG	RG = LG
Jin	2022	China	31	12401	RG < LG	RG < LG	RG > LG	RG > LG	RG = LG	RG < LG	RG > LG	RG = LG
Gong	2022	China	22	5386	RG = LG	RG < LG	RG > LG	RG = LG	RG = LG	RG < LG	RG = LG	RG = LG
Baral	2022	China	48	20151	RG = LG	RG < LG	RG > LG	RG = LG	RG = LG	RG = LG	-	RG = LG
Ali	2022	China	22	13585	RG < LG	RG < LG	-	RG > LG	-	-	-	-

LG—laparoscopic gastrectomy; LN—lymph node; OS—overall survival; RG—robotic gastrectomy

In a multicentre prospective phase II study conducted in Japan, the safety of RG was evaluated in patients with cStage I/II gastric cancer. Between October 2014 and January 2017, 330 patients were enrolled, and the relevant data were analysed. With regard to the primary end point, the incidence of postoperative complications of Clavien–Dindo grade III or greater was 2.45%, which was significantly lower than that in a historical control group (6.4%), confirming the safety of RG (95% CI 0.9755 (0.9522–0.9893) and $p = 0.0018$).[118] Based on these results, the use of RG for gastric cancer has been covered by national health insurance in Japan since April 2018.

In Korea, a multicentre prospective non-randomized controlled study was conducted with 434 patients undergoing RG or LG.[119] In this study, no significant difference was observed between RG ($n = 223$) and LG ($n = 211$) with regard to the incidence of postoperative complications (RG 11.9%, LG 10.3%), and the mortality rate was 0% in both groups. However, the operative time was approximately 40 minutes longer and the cost of surgery was approximately 5000 USD higher with RG than with LG. Thus, the authors concluded that RG has no advantages that counterbalance the time and cost disadvantages. In subsequent subgroup analysis, when D2 lymph node dissection was performed, the amount of blood loss was significantly lower with RG than with LG (98.9 mL vs 140.5 mL; $p = 0.021$).[120]

With regard to long-term outcomes, few retrospective case–control studies have been conducted in Japan and Korea. In a study conducted in Japan, data from 84 patients who underwent RG and 437 patients who underwent LG around the same time were retrospectively analysed. The 3-year OS rates with RG and LG were 86.9% and 88.8%, respectively, and the difference was not significant ($p = 0.636$).[121] A study conducted in Korea using propensity score matching found 5-year OS rates of 93.2% with RG and 94.2% with LG, and the difference was not significant ($p = 0.521$).[122] A study conducted in China also using propensity score matching found 3-year OS rates of 76.1% with RG and 81.7% with LG for AGC, and the difference was not significant ($p = 0.118$).[123]

Although these results indicate that the short- and long-term outcomes of RG appear to be at least non-inferior to those of LG, a prospective study should be conducted to verify the superiority of RG to LG. In China, the RCT with a non-inferiority design is currently running to evaluate the non-inferiority of RDG to LDG in terms of 3-year DFS among patients with cT1–4a and N0/+ gastric cancer. The safety data of RDG, which are secondary end points, has been published earlier. A total of 300 patients were randomly assigned to the RDG group ($n = 150$) or the LDG group ($n = 150$). After excluding non-eligible patients, 141 patients in the RDG group and 142 patients in the LDG group were included in the modified intention-to-treat analysis. Patients in the RDG group exhibited faster postoperative recovery, milder inflammatory responses, and reduced postoperative morbidity than patients in the LDG group (9.2% vs 17.6%, respectively; $p = 0.039$).[124] In Japan, phase III, prospective superiority randomized clinical trial of RG versus LG regarding reduction of complications with 241 patients with resectable gastric cancer (clinical stages I–III) was conducted. The primary end point was the incidence of postoperative intra-abdominal infectious complications. There was no significant difference in the incidence of intra-abdominal infectious complications (per-protocol population: 10 of 117 (8.5%) in the LG group vs 7 of 113 (6.2%) in the RG group). However, the overall incidence of postoperative complications of grade II or higher, which was defined as secondary end points, was significantly higher in the LG group than in the RG group (19.7% vs 8.8%; $p = 0.02$).[125] Regarding the safety, these two RCTs showed superiority of RG to LG, but these results derived in a limited number of facilities cannot be expected to be of high evidence level.

The JCOG is currently conducting a phase III trial to investigate the superiority of RG to LG in terms of the incidence of postoperative intra-abdominal infectious complications among patients with cT1–4a, N0–3 gastric cancer (Figure 20.1; MONA LISA study).[126] We hypothesize that a clinically meaningful difference will be observed if the incidence of intra-abdominal infectious complications decreases by half with RG (3.0%) when compared to that with LG (6.0%). To show this difference with a one-sided alpha of 0.05 at a power of 70%, the sample size of each group should be 503. Some patients might be lost, and thus, the estimated sample size for this study is 1040. The projected accrual period is 5 years. When our hypothesis is validated, we will consider that RG is more effective than LG.

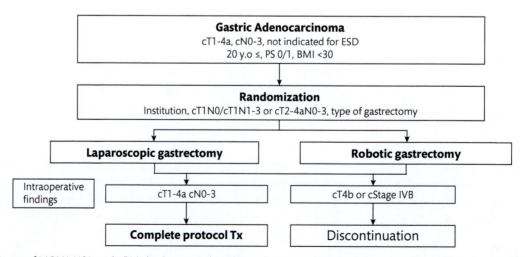

Figure 20.1 Schema of MONA LISA study. BMI, body mass index; ESD, endoscopic submucosal dissection; PS, performance status; Tx, treatment.

Advantages of robotic gastrectomy over laparoscopic gastrectomy

Ergonomics

Good ergonomics for the operator is one advantage of robot-assisted surgery. Unlike LG, during which the operator makes an incision in the standing position, RG can be performed while the operator is sitting in an ergonomically designed surgeon console, and this is expected to reduce operator fatigue. Although no study has been conducted solely on gastric cancer surgery, the results of a study involving 1215 surgeons from various fields suggested that robot-assisted surgery was associated with the least physical discomfort and physical symptoms on comparing it with open surgery and laparoscopic surgery.[127] Data breakdown indicated that although the incidence of neck, back, hip, knee, ankle, foot, shoulder, elbow, and wrist pain was low, the incidence of eye and finger pain was high with robot-assisted surgery. Another survey involving 432 surgeons from various fields reported that 56.1% complained of physical symptoms or discomfort during robot-assisted surgery, with the most frequent complaints being neck stiffness, finger pain, and eye fatigue.[128] Although robot-assisted surgery reduces physical symptoms and discomfort among surgeons when compared with open surgery and laparoscopic surgery, more than 50% of surgeons complain of a certain degree of physical stress, typically finger pain and eye strain.

Learning curve

With regard to the learning curve, 40–60 operations are considered to be required to achieve stability in LG,[129,130] whereas only 11–25 operations are considered to be required to achieve stability in RG.[131,132] With regard to RG, high-resolution three-dimensional imaging and instrument flexibility may help to make the learning curve less steep. Additionally, in many cases, RG is performed by an expert in LG. However, a recent study reported that the operation time stabilized after 25 operations, even among surgeons without prior LG experience, suggesting that prior LG experience might not be necessary.[132]

Disadvantages of robotic gastrectomy relative to laparoscopic gastrectomy

The operation time is longer with RG than with LG, which can be considered a disadvantage of RG. A detailed examination showed that 'junk time' is causing the prolongation, indicating that it takes considerable time to set up and place the DVSS or surgical instruments.[133] On the other hand, there was no significant difference between RG and LG with regard to the time required to complete the operative procedure. Although there was no difference in the number of instrument exchanges, the time required to exchange instruments was longer with RG than with LG. Moreover, we found that the operative time reduced by about 1 hour when ultrasonically activated devices were used.[134] In the future, we believe that the operative time can be further reduced by establishing an effective system set-up or by developing new devices, such as clips, which can be used consecutively.

With regard to RG, the future challenge is to establish evidence. Although RG has many theoretical advantages over LG, its usefulness has not been completely demonstrated. It has been 20 years since approval of the DVSS by the FDA; however, only a few prospective studies have been conducted. Moreover, no randomized controlled study has been conducted on RG. It cannot be denied that this is related to the high cost of RG. The results of meta-analyses and prospective studies conducted in Korea indicated that RG is 4000–5000 USD more expensive than LG.[119] However, since April 2018, RG has been covered by national health insurance in Japan; thus, patients can undergo RG without any extra cost. Although the economic burden on medical institutions remains, the groundwork to conduct randomized controlled studies has been completed. Currently, several companies, such as Verb Surgical (Verb Surgical Inc., Mountain View, CA, USA), Ethicon and Google's collaborative company, and Medtronic (Medtronic, Dublin, Ireland), are developing surgery-assisting robots, and we expect not only the development of new devices but also innovative advances, including miniaturization of machines, adoption of three-dimensional imaging, use of artificial intelligence, and application of virtual reality.[135]

Future perspectives of robotic gastrectomy

Robotic technology continues to advance with regard to self-optimized arm positioning, instrument reach, clamp stapling technology, ultra-fast vessel sealers, and expanded fluorescence techniques. Robots are now used for not only dissection but also more complete procedures, such as reconstruction, in gastric surgery. In the future, advances in robotics will become the driving force for revolutionary changes in surgical technology.

A criticism of robotic surgery is the lack of haptic feedback to the surgeon.[136] In minimally invasive surgery, haptic feedback is attenuated owing to the long shaft of the laparoscopic instrument. In robotic surgery, all haptic feedback is lost owing to the dissociation of the surgeon from the end effector in the robotic system. Studies have shown that absence of haptic feedback can result in the application of both excessive and inadequate forces to tissues during robotic surgery, which can lead to increased tissue injury and inappropriate suture handling. Haptic feedback is described as a combination of force/kinaesthetic feedback and tactile/cutaneous feedback. Force feedback is useful for assessing the tension or pressure across tissue or suture, whereas tactile feedback provides information on local tissue properties, such as compliance and viscosity. It appears that high sensory feedback is beneficial to surgeons.

Telesurgery, also called tele-robotics, combines the advantages of robotic surgery, including magnified view, augmented reality, and improved ergonomics and dexterity, and the provision of surgical care in remote areas and difficult-to-reach locations, such as spacecrafts and ships.[137] Telesurgery uses wireless networking and robotic technology to allow surgeons to operate on patients who are located far away. This technology not only helps overcome the current shortage of surgeons but also eliminates geographical barriers (preventing timely and high-quality surgical intervention), financial burden, and complications. This technology can also contribute to the achievement of consistent medical care everywhere.

Furthermore, the introduction of artificial intelligence is expected to help in the development of new surgical procedures.[138] Technologies, such as integrated imaging, preoperative and intraoperative simulation, and tissue recognition, will help in the growth and development of surgical robots, possibly resulting in the introduction of autonomous systems (true surgical robots). Although this appears distant at present, it may be closer than is actually believed.

Conclusion

Laparoscopic surgery and robot-assisted surgery for gastric cancer have been advancing rapidly owing to great efforts by surgeons, the establishment of education systems, and the development of medical instruments. In the future, these endoscopic approaches are expected to be used for complicated procedures, such as transhiatal surgery and post-chemotherapy surgery, and to improve patient prognosis by minimizing surgical invasiveness, even in highly advanced stages of gastric cancer. It can be said with some certainty that endoscopic surgery will play a leading role in gastric cancer therapy in the near future. Evidence based on clinical studies should be urgently established to facilitate advances in endoscopic surgery.

REFERENCES

1. Terashima M. The 140 years' journey of gastric cancer surgery: from the two hands of Billroth to the multiple hands of the robot. *Ann Gastroenterol Surg*. 2021;**5**:270–277.
2. Falk V, Diegeler A, Walther T, et al. Total endoscopic computer enhanced coronary artery bypass grafting. *Eur J Cardiothorac Surg*. 2000;**17**:38–45.
3. Griffin SM. Gastric cancer in the East: same disease, different patient. *Br J Surg*. 2005;**92**:1055–1056.
4. Kitano S, Iso Y, Moriyama M, et al. Laparoscopy-assisted Billroth I gastrectomy. *Surg Laparosc Endosc*. 1994;**4**:146–148.
5. Kitano S, Shimoda K, Miyahara M, et al. Laparoscopic approaches in the management of patients with early gastric carcinomas. *Surg Laparosc Endosc*. 1995;**5**:359–362.
6. Kwoh YS, Hou J, Jonckheere EA, et al. A robot with improved absolute positioning accuracy for CT guided stereotactic brain surgery. *IEEE Trans Biomed Eng*. 1988;**35**:153–160.
7. Paul HA, Bargar WL, Mittlestadt B, et al. Development of a surgical robot for cementless total hip arthroplasty. *Clin Orthop Relat Res*. 1992;**285**:57–66.
8. Reichenspurner H, Damiano RJ, Mack M, et al. Use of the voice-controlled and computer-assisted surgical system ZEUS for endoscopic coronary artery bypass grafting. *J Thorac Cardiovasc Surg*. 1999;**118**:11–16.
9. Falk V, Diegeler A, Walther T, et al. Total endoscopic computer enhanced coronary artery bypass grafting. *Eur J Cardiothorac Surg*. 2000;**17**:38–45.
10. Furukawa J, Miyake H, Tanaka K, et al. Console-integrated real-time three-dimensional image overlay navigation for robot-assisted partial nephrectomy with selective arterial clamping: early single-centre experience with 17 cases. *Int J Med Robot*. 2014;**10**:385–390.
11. Brodie A, Vasdev N. The future of robotic surgery. *Ann R Coll Surg Engl*. 2018;**100**:4–13.
12. Terashima M, Tokunaga M, Tanizawa Y, et al. Robotic surgery for gastric cancer. *Gastric Cancer*. 2015;**18**:449–457.
13. Billroth T. Offenes Schreiben an Herrn Dr. L. Wittelshöfer. *Wien Med Wschr*. 1881;**31**:S161–S165.
14. Litynski GS. Laparoscopy—the early attempts: spotlighting Georg Kelling and Hans Christian Jacobaeus. *J Society Laparoendoscopic Surg*. 1997;**1**:83–85.
15. Semm K. Endoscopic appendectomy. *Endoscopy*. 1983;**15**:59–64.
16. Muhe E. Interview by GS Litynski, tape recording, 4 December 1995. In Litynski GS. *Highlights in the History of Laparoscopy*. Frankfurt: Barbara Bernert Verlag; 1996:165–168.
17. Unger SW, Unger HM, Bass RT. AESOP robotic arm. *Surg Endosc*. 1994;**8**:1131.
18. Falk V, Walther T, Autschbach R, et al. Robot assisted minimally invasive solo mitral valve operation. *J Thorac Cardiovasc Surg*. 1998;**115**:470–471.
19. Cadiere GB, Himpens J, Germay O, et al. Feasibility of robotic laparoscopic surgery: 146 cases. *World J Surg*. 2001;**25**:1467–1477.
20. Marecik S, Kochar K, Park JJ. Current status and future of robotic colorectal surgery. *Dis Colon Rectum*. 2019;**62**:1025–1027.
21. Falcone T, Goldberg JM, Margossian H, et al. Robotic-assisted laparoscopic microsurgical tubal anastomosis: a human pilot study. *Fertil Steril*. 2000;**73**:1040–1042.
22. Marescaux J, Leroy J, Gagner M, et al. Transatlantic robot-assisted telesurgery. *Nature*. 2001;**413**:379–380.
23. Hashizume M, Shimada M, Tomikawa M, et al. Early experiences of endoscopic procedures in general surgery assisted by a computer-enhanced surgical system. *Surg Endosc*. 2002;**16**:1187–1191.
24. Intuitive Surgical, Inc. Investor Presentation Q2. 2019. https://isrg.gcs-web.com/static-files/880bf027-e866-4c32-b910-5332467cd8dc
25. D'Annibale A, Pende V, Pernazza G, et al. Full robotic gastrectomy with extended (D2) lymphadenectomy for gastric cancer: surgical technique and preliminary results. *J Surg Res*. 2011;**166**:e113–e120.
26. Uyama I, Kanaya S, Ishida Y, et al. Novel integrated robotic approach for suprapancreatic D2 nodal dissection for treating gastric cancer: technique and initial experience. *World J Surg*. 2012;**36**:331–337.
27. Japan Society for Endoscopic Survey. Nationwide survey on endoscopic surgery in Japan. *J Jpn Soc Endosc Surg*. 2004;**9**:491–499.
28. Mochiki E, Kamiyama Y, Aihara R, et al. Laparoscopic assisted distal gastrectomy for early gastric cancer: five years' experience. *Surgery*. 2005;**137**:317–322.
29. Dulucq JL, Wintringer P, Stabilini C, et al. Laparoscopic and open gastric resections for malignant lesions: a prospective comparative study. *Surg Endosc*. 2005;**19**:933–938.
30. Kim MC, Kim KH, Kim HH, et al. Comparison of laparoscopy-assisted by conventional open distal gastrectomy and extraperigastric lymph node dissection in early gastric cancer. *J Surg Oncol*. 2005;**91**:90–94.
31. Kitano S, Shiraishi N, Fujii K, et al. A randomized controlled trial comparing open vs laparoscopy-assisted distal gastrectomy for the treatment of early gastric cancer: an interim report. *Surgery*. 2002;**131**:S306–S311.
32. Hu Y, Huang C, Sun Y, et al. Morbidity and mortality of laparoscopic versus open D2 distal gastrectomy for advanced gastric cancer: a randomized controlled trial. *J Clin Oncol*. 2016;**34**:1350–1357.
33. Peng JS, Song H, Yang ZL, et al. Meta-analysis of laparoscopy-assisted distal gastrectomy and conventional open distal gastrectomy for early gastric cancer. *Chin J Cancer*. 2010;**29**:349–354.

34. Zeng YK, Yang ZL, Peng JS, et al. Laparoscopy-assisted versus open distal gastrectomy for early gastric cancer: evidence from randomized and nonrandomized clinical trials. *Ann Surg*. 2012;**256**:39–52.
35. Wang Y, Wang S, Huang ZQ, et al. Meta-analysis of laparoscopy assisted distal gastrectomy and conventional open distal gastrectomy for EGC. *Surgeon*. 2014;**12**:53–58.
36. Deng Y, Zhang Y, Guo TK. Laparoscopy-assisted versus open distal gastrectomy for early gastric cancer: a meta-analysis based on seven randomized controlled trials. *Surg Oncol*. 2015;**24**:71–77.
37. Katai H, Sasako M, Fukuda H, et al. Safety and feasibility of laparoscopy-assisted distal gastrectomy with suprapancreatic nodal dissection for clinical stage I gastric cancer: a multicenter phase II trial (JCOG 0703). *Gastric Cancer*. 2010;**13**:238–244.
38. Katai H, Mizusawa J, Katayama H, et al. Short-term surgical outcomes from a phase III study of laparoscopy-assisted versus open distal gastrectomy with nodal dissection for clinical stage IA/IB gastric cancer: Japan Clinical Oncology Group Study JCOG0912. *Gastric Cancer*. 2017;**20**:699–708.
39. Japanese Gastric Cancer Association. Japanese gastric cancer treatment guidelines 2014 (ver. 4). *Gastric Cancer*. 2017;**20**:1–19.
40. Katai H, Mizusawa J, Katayama H, et al. Randomized phase III trial of laparoscopy-assisted versus open distal gastrectomy with nodal dissection for clinical stage IA/IB gastric cancer (JCOG0912). *J Clin Oncol*. 2019;**37**(15 Suppl):4020.
41. Katai H, Mizusawa J, Katayama H, et al. Survival outcomes after laparoscopy-assisted distal gastrectomy versus open distal gastrectomy with nodal dissection for clinical stage IA or IB gastric cancer (JCOG0912): a multicentre, non-inferiority, phase 3 randomised controlled trial. *Lancet Gastroenterol Hepatol*. 2020;**5**:142–151.
42. Kim W, Kim HH, Han SU, et al. Decreased morbidity of laparoscopic distal gastrectomy compared with open distal gastrectomy for stage I gastric cancer: short-term outcomes from a multicenter randomized controlled trial (KLASS-01). *Ann Surg*. 2016;**263**:28–35.
43. Kim HH, Han SU, Kim MC, et al. Effect of laparoscopic distal gastrectomy vs open distal gastrectomy on long-term survival among patients with stage I gastric cancer: the KLASS-01 randomized clinical trial. *JAMA Oncol*. 2019;**5**:506–513.
44. Topal B, Leys E, Ectors N, et al. Determinants of complications and adequacy of surgical resection in laparoscopic versus open total gastrectomy for adenocarcinoma. *Surg Endosc*. 2008;**22**:980–984.
45. Jeong O, Ryu SY, Zhao XF, et al. Short-term surgical outcomes and operative risks of laparoscopic total gastrectomy (LTG) for gastric carcinoma: experience at a large-volume center. *Surg Endosc*. 2012;**26**:3418–3425.
46. Hyung WJ, Yang HK, Han SU, et al. A feasibility study of laparoscopic total gastrectomy for clinical stage I gastric cancer: a prospective multi-center phase II clinical trial, KLASS 03. *Gastric Cancer*. 2019;**22**:214–222.
47. Kataoka K, Katai H, Mizusawa J, et al. Non-randomized confirmatory trial of laparoscopy-assisted total gastrectomy and proximal gastrectomy with nodal dissection for clinical stage I gastric cancer: Japan Clinical Oncology Group Study JCOG1401. *J Gastric Cancer*. 2016;**16**:93–97.
48. Katai H, Mizusawa J, Katayama H, et al. Single-arm confirmatory trial of laparoscopy-assisted total or proximal gastrectomy with nodal dissection for clinical stage I gastric cancer: Japan Clinical Oncology Group study JCOG1401. *Gastric Cancer*. 2019;**22**:999–1008.
49. Liu F, Huang C, Xu Z, et al. Morbidity and mortality of laparoscopic vs open total gastrectomy for clinical stage I gastric cancer: the CLASS02 multicenter randomized clinical trial. *JAMA Oncol*. 2020;**6**:1590–1597.
50. Degiuli M, Sasako M, Ponti A. Morbidity and mortality in the Italian Gastric Cancer Study Group randomized clinical trial of D1 versus D2 resection for gastric cancer. *Br J Surg*. 2010;**97**:643–649.
51. Gutt CN, Kim ZG, Schmandra T, et al. Carbon dioxide pneumoperitoneum is associated with increased liver metastases in a rat model. *Surgery*. 2000;**127**:566–570.
52. Martinez-Ramos D, Miralles-Tena JM, Cuesta MA, et al. Laparoscopy versus open surgery for advanced and resectable gastric cancer: a meta-analysis. *Rev Esp Enferm Dig*. 2011;**103**:133–141.
53. Zou ZH, Zhao LY, Mou TY, et al. Laparoscopic vs open D2 gastrectomy for locally advanced gastric cancer: a meta-analysis. *World J Gastroenterol*. 2014;**20**:16750–16764.
54. Małczak P, Torbicz G, Rubinkiewicz M, et al. Comparison of totally laparoscopic and open approach in total gastrectomy with D2 lymphadenectomy—systematic review and meta-analysis. *Cancer Manag Res*. 2018;**10**:6705–6714.
55. Li Z, Zhao Y, Liu Y, et al. Laparoscopic versus open gastrectomy for high-risk patients with gastric cancer: a systematic review and meta-analysis. *Int J Surg*. 2019;**65**:52–60.
56. Li Z, Zhao Y, Lian B, et al. Long-term oncological outcomes in laparoscopic versus open gastrectomy for advanced gastric cancer: a meta-analysis of high-quality nonrandomized studies. *Am J Surg*. 2019;**218**:631–638.
57. Beyer K, Baukloh AK, Kamphues C, et al. Laparoscopic versus open gastrectomy for locally advanced gastric cancer: a systematic review and meta-analysis of randomized controlled studies. *World J Surg Oncol*. 2019;**17**:68.
58. Zeng F, Chen L, Liao M, et al. Laparoscopic versus open gastrectomy for gastric cancer. *World J Surg Oncol*. 2020;**18**:20.
59. Shan F, Gao C, Li XL, et al. Short- and long-term outcomes after laparoscopic versus open gastrectomy for elderly gastric cancer patients: a systematic review and meta-analysis. *J Laparoendosc Adv Surg Tech A*. 2020;**30**:713–722.
60. Zhu Z, Li L, Xu J, et al. Laparoscopic versus open approach in gastrectomy for advanced gastric cancer: a systematic review. *World J Surg Oncol*. 2020;**18**:126.
61. Chen X, Feng X, Wang M, et al. Laparoscopic versus open distal gastrectomy for advanced gastric cancer: a meta-analysis of randomized controlled trials and high-quality nonrandomized comparative studies. *Eur J Surg Oncol*. 2020;**46**:1998–2010.
62. Liao C, Feng Q, Xie S, et al. Laparoscopic versus open gastrectomy for Siewert type II/III adenocarcinoma of the esophagogastric junction: a meta-analysis. *Surg Endosc*. 2021;**35**:860–871.
63. Aiolfi A, Lombardo F, Matsushima K, et al. Systematic review and updated network meta-analysis of randomized controlled trials comparing open, laparoscopic-assisted, and robotic distal gastrectomy for early and locally advanced gastric cancer. *Surgery*. 2021;**170**:942–951.
64. Liao XL, Liang XW, Pang HY, et al. Safety and efficacy of laparoscopic versus open gastrectomy in patients with advanced gastric cancer following neoadjuvant chemotherapy: a meta-analysis. *Front Oncol*. 2021;**11**:704244.

65. Zhang W, Huang Z, Zhang J, et al. Long-term and short-term outcomes after laparoscopic versus open surgery for advanced gastric cancer: an updated meta-analysis. *J Minim Access Surg*. 2021;**17**:423–434.
66. Song Y, Du Y. Comparison of clinical efficacy between laparoscopic and open distal gastrectomy in the treatment of gastric carcinoma: a meta-analysis. *J Laparoendosc Adv Surg Tech A*. 2022;**32**:522–531.
67. Hakkenbrak NAG, Jansma EP, van der Wielen N, et al. Laparoscopic versus open distal gastrectomy for gastric cancer: a systematic review and meta-analysis. *Surgery*. 2022;**171**:1552–1561.
68. Otsuka R, Hayashi H, Uesato M, et al. Comparison of estimated treatment effects between randomized controlled trials, case-matched, and cohort studies on laparoscopic versus open distal gastrectomy for advanced gastric cancer: a systematic review and meta-analysis. *Langenbecks Arch Surg*. 2022;**407**:1381–1397.
69. Jiang J, Ye G, Wang J, et al. The comparison of short- and long-term outcomes for laparoscopic versus open gastrectomy for patients with advanced gastric cancer: a meta-analysis of randomized controlled trials. *Front Oncol*. 2022;**12**:844803.
70. Lou S, Yin X, Wang Y, et al. Laparoscopic versus open gastrectomy for gastric cancer: a systematic review and meta-analysis of randomized controlled trials. *Int J Surg*. 2022;**102**:106678.
71. Argillander TE, Festen S, van der Zaag-Loonen HJ, et al. Outcomes of surgical treatment of non-metastatic gastric cancer in patients aged 70 and older: a systematic review and meta-analysis. *Eur J Surg Oncol*. 2022;**48**:1882–1894.
72. Garbarino GM, Laracca GG, Lucarini A, et al. Laparoscopic versus open surgery for gastric cancer in western countries: a systematic review and meta-analysis of short- and long-term outcomes. *J Clin Med*. 2022;**11**:3590.
73. Yang Y, Chen Y, Hu Y, et al. Outcomes of laparoscopic versus open total gastrectomy with D2 lymphadenectomy for gastric cancer: a systematic review and meta-analysis. *Eur J Med Res*. 2022;**27**:124.
74. Kinoshita T, Uyama I, Terashima M, et al. Long-term outcomes of laparoscopic versus open surgery for clinical stage II/III gastric cancer: a multicenter cohort study in Japan (LOC-A study). *Ann Surg*. 2019;**269**:887–894.
75. Inaki N, Etoh T, Ohyama T, et al. A multi-institutional, prospective, phase II feasibility study of laparoscopy-assisted distal gastrectomy with D2 lymph node dissection for locally advanced gastric cancer (JLSSG0901). *World J Surg*. 2015;**39**:2734–2741.
76. Hur H, Lee HY, Lee HJ, et al. Efficacy of laparoscopic subtotal gastrectomy with D2 lymphadenectomy for locally advanced gastric cancer: the protocol of the KLASS-02 multicenter randomized controlled clinical trial. *BMC Cancer*. 2015;**15**:355.
77. Lee HJ, Hyung WJ, Yang HK, et al. Short-term outcomes of a multicenter randomized controlled trial comparing laparoscopic distal gastrectomy with D2 lymphadenectomy to open distal gastrectomy for locally advanced gastric cancer (KLASS-02-RCT). *Ann Surg*. 2019;**270**:983–991.
78. Hyung WJ, Yang HK, Park YK, et al. Long-term outcomes of laparoscopic distal gastrectomy for locally advanced gastric cancer: the KLASS-02-RCT randomized clinical trial. *J Clin Oncol*. 2020;**38**:3304–3313.
79. Li G. The current status of CLASS-01 trial: updated. KINGCA 2018; Abstract. http://2018.kingca.org/html/
80. Yu J, Huang C, Sun Y, et al. Effect of laparoscopic vs open distal gastrectomy on 3-year disease-free survival in patients with locally advanced gastric cancer: the CLASS-01 randomized clinical trial. *JAMA*. 2019;**321**:1983–1992.
81. Haverkamp L, Brenkman HJ, Seesing MF, et al. Laparoscopic versus open gastrectomy for gastric cancer, a multicenter prospectively randomized controlled trial (LOGICA-trial). *BMC Cancer*. 2015;**15**:556.
82. van der Veen A, Brenkman HJF, Seesing MFJ, et al. Laparoscopic Versus Open Gastrectomy for Gastric Cancer (LOGICA): a multicenter randomized clinical trial. *J Clin Oncol*. 2021;**39**:978–989.
83. Straatman J, van der Wielen N, Cuesta MA, et al. Surgical techniques, open versus minimally invasive gastrectomy after chemotherapy (STOMACH trial): study protocol for a randomized controlled trial. *Trials*. 2015;**16**:123.
84. van der Wielen N, Straatman J, Daams F, et al. Open versus minimally invasive total gastrectomy after neoadjuvant chemotherapy: results of a European randomized trial. *Gastric Cancer*. 2021;**24**:258–271.
85. Goto O, Takeuchi H, Kawakubo H, et al. First case of non-exposed endoscopic wall-inversion surgery with sentinel node basin dissection for early gastric cancer. *Gastric Cancer*. 2015;**18**:434–439.
86. Matsuda T, Nunobe S, Ohashi M, et al. Laparoscopic endoscopic cooperative surgery (LECS) for the upper gastrointestinal tract. *Transl Gastroenterol Hepatol*. 2017;**2**:40.
87. Takeuchi H, Goto O, Yahagi N, et al. Function-preserving gastrectomy based on the sentinel node concept in early gastric cancer. *Gastric Cancer*. 2017;**20**(Suppl 1):53–59.
88. Kitagawa Y, Takeuchi H, Takagi Y, et al. Sentinel node mapping for gastric cancer: a prospective multicenter trial in Japan. *J Clin Oncol*. 2013;**31**:3704–3710.
89. Kim YW, Min JS, Yoon HM, et al. Laparoscopic sentinel node navigation surgery for stomach preservation in patients with early gastric cancer: a randomized clinical trial. *J Clin Oncol*. 2022;**40**:2342–2351.
90. Sano T, Sasako M, Mizusawa J, et al. Randomized controlled trial to evaluate splenectomy in total gastrectomy for proximal gastric carcinoma. *Ann Surg*. 2017;**265**:277–283.
91. Uyama I, Sugioka A, Fujita J, et al. Laparoscopic total gastrectomy with distal pancreatosplenectomy and D2 lymphadenectomy for advanced gastric cancer. *Gastric Cancer*. 1999;**2**:230–234.
92. Hosogi H, Okabe H, Shinohara H, et al. Laparoscopic splenic hilar lymphadenectomy for advanced gastric cancer. *Transl Gastroenterol Hepatol*. 2016;**1**:30.
93. Son T, Lee JH, Kim YM, et al. Robotic spleen-preserving total gastrectomy for gastric cancer: comparison with conventional laparoscopic procedure. *Surg Endosc*. 2014;**28**:2606–2615.
94. Zheng CH, Xu YC, Zhao G, et al. Safety and feasibility of laparoscopic spleen-preserving No. 10 lymph node dissection for locally advanced upper third gastric cancer: a prospective, multicenter clinical trial. *Surg Endosc*. 2020;**34**:5062–5073.
95. Zheng C, Xu Y, Zhao G, et al. Outcomes of laparoscopic total gastrectomy combined with spleen-preserving hilar lymphadenectomy for locally advanced proximal gastric cancer: a nonrandomized clinical trial. *JAMA Netw Open*. 2021;**4**:e2139992.
96. Waddell T, Verheij M, Allum W, et al. Gastric cancer: ESMO-ESSO-ESTRO clinical practice guidelines for diagnosis, treatment and follow-up. *Eur J Surg Oncol*. 2014;**40**:584–591.

97. Shen WS, Xi HQ, Chen L, et al. A meta-analysis of robotic versus laparoscopic gastrectomy for gastric cancer. *Surg Endosc*. 2014;**28**:2795–2802.
98. Chuan L, Yan S, Pei-Wu Y. Meta-analysis of the short-term outcomes of robotic-assisted compared to laparoscopic gastrectomy. *Minim Invasive Ther Allied Technol*. 2015;**24**:127–134.
99. Hu LD, Li XF, Wang XY, et al. Robotic versus laparoscopic gastrectomy for gastric carcinoma: a meta-analysis of efficacy and safety. *Asian Pac J Cancer Prev*. 2016;**17**:4327–4333.
100. Wang Y, Zhao X, Song Y, et al. A systematic review and meta-analysis of robot-assisted versus laparoscopically assisted gastrectomy for gastric cancer. *Medicine (Baltimore)*. 2017;**96**:e8797.
101. Chen K, Pan Y, Zhang B, et al. Robotic versus laparoscopic gastrectomy for gastric cancer: a systematic review and updated meta-analysis. *BMC Surg*. 2017;**17**:93.
102. Pan JH, Zhou H, Zhao XX, et al. Long-term oncological outcomes in robotic gastrectomy versus laparoscopic gastrectomy for gastric cancer: a meta-analysis. *Surg Endosc*. 2017;**31**:4244–4251.
103. Liao G, Zhao Z, Khan M, et al. Comparative analysis of robotic gastrectomy and laparoscopic gastrectomy for gastric cancer in terms of their long-term oncological outcomes: a meta-analysis of 3410 gastric cancer patients. *World J Surg Oncol*. 2019;**17**:86.
104. Zheng B, Wang X, Li J, et al. Robotic gastrectomy versus laparoscopic gastrectomy for gastric cancer: meta-analysis and trial sequential analysis of prospective observational studies. *Surg Endosc*. 2019;**33**:1033–1048.
105. Qiu H, Ai JH, Shi J, et al. Effectiveness and safety of robotic versus traditional laparoscopic gastrectomy for gastric cancer: an updated systematic review and meta-analysis. *J Cancer Res Ther*. 2019;**15**:1450–1463.
106. Guerrini GP, Esposito G, Magistri P, et al. Robotic versus laparoscopic gastrectomy for gastric cancer: the largest meta-analysis. *Int J Surg*. 2020;**82**:210–228.
107. Ma J, Li X, Zhao S, et al. Robotic versus laparoscopic gastrectomy for gastric cancer: a systematic review and meta-analysis. *World J Surg Oncol*. 2020;**18**:306.
108. Wu HY, Lin XF, Yang P, et al. Pooled analysis of the oncological outcomes in robotic gastrectomy versus laparoscopic gastrectomy for gastric cancer. *J Minim Access Surg*. 2021;**17**:287–293.
109. Zhang Z, Zhang X, Liu Y, et al. Meta-analysis of the efficacy of Da Vinci robotic or laparoscopic distal subtotal gastrectomy in patients with gastric cancer. *Medicine (Baltimore)*. 2021;**100**:e27012.
110. Zhang X, Zhang W, Feng Z, et al. Comparison of short-term outcomes of robotic-assisted and laparoscopic-assisted D2 gastrectomy for gastric cancer: a meta-analysis. *Wideochir Inne Tech Maloinwazyjne*. 2021;**16**:443–454.
111. Feng Q, Ma H, Qiu J, et al. Comparison of long-term and perioperative outcomes of robotic versus conventional laparoscopic gastrectomy for gastric cancer: a systematic review and meta-analysis of PSM and RCT studies. *Front Oncol*. 2021;**11**:759509.
112. Jin T, Liu HD, Yang K, et al. Effectiveness and safety of robotic gastrectomy versus laparoscopic gastrectomy for gastric cancer: a meta-analysis of 12,401 gastric cancer patients. *Updates Surg*. 2022;**74**:267–281.
113. Gong S, Li X, Tian H, et al. Clinical efficacy and safety of robotic distal gastrectomy for gastric cancer: a systematic review and meta-analysis. *Surg Endosc*. 2022;**36**:2734–2748.
114. Baral S, Arawker MH, Sun Q, et al. Robotic versus laparoscopic gastrectomy for gastric cancer: a mega meta-analysis. *Front Surg*. 2022;**9**:895976.
115. Ali M, Wang Y, Ding J, et al. Postoperative outcomes in robotic gastric resection compared with laparoscopic gastric resection in gastric cancer: a meta-analysis and systemic review. *Health Sci Rep*. 2022;**5**:e746.
116. Tokunaga M, Sugisawa N, Kondo J, et al. Early phase II study of robot-assisted distal gastrectomy with nodal dissection for clinical stage IA gastric cancer. *Gastric Cancer*. 2014;**17**:542–547.
117. Tokunaga M, Makuuchi R, Miki Y, et al. Late phase II study of robot-assisted gastrectomy with nodal dissection for clinical stage I gastric cancer. *Surg Endosc*. 2016;**30**:3362–3367.
118. Uyama I, Nakauchi M, Suda K, et al. Clinical advantages of robotic gastrectomy for clinical stage I/II gastric cancer: a multi-institutional prospective single-arm study. *Gastric Cancer*. 2019;**22**:377–385.
119. Kim HI, Han SU, Yang HK, et al. Multicenter prospective comparative study of robotic versus laparoscopic gastrectomy for gastric adenocarcinoma. *Ann Surg*. 2016;**263**:103–109.
120. Park JM, Kim HI, Han SU, et al. Who may benefit from robotic gastrectomy? A subgroup analysis of multicenter prospective comparative study data on robotic versus laparoscopic gastrectomy. *Eur J Surg Oncol*. 2016;**42**:1944–1949.
121. Nakauchi M, Suda K, Susumu S, et al. Comparison of the long-term outcomes of robotic radical gastrectomy for gastric cancer and conventional laparoscopic approach: a single institutional retrospective cohort study. *Surg Endosc*. 2016;**30**:5444–5452.
122. Obama K, Kim YM, Kang DR, et al. Long-term oncologic outcomes of robotic gastrectomy for gastric cancer compared with laparoscopic gastrectomy. *Gastric Cancer*. 2018;**21**:285–295.
123. Gao Y, Xi H, Qiao Z, et al. Comparison of robotic- and laparoscopic-assisted gastrectomy in advanced gastric cancer: updated short- and long-term results. *Surg Endosc*. 2019;**33**:528–534.
124. Lu J, Zheng CH, Xu BB, et al. Assessment of robotic versus laparoscopic distal gastrectomy for gastric cancer: a randomized controlled trial. *Ann Surg*. 2021;**273**:858–867.
125. Ojima T, Nakamura M, Hayata K, et al. Short-term outcomes of robotic gastrectomy vs laparoscopic gastrectomy for patients with gastric cancer: a randomized clinical trial. *JAMA Surg*. 2021;**156**:954–963.
126. Terashima M. The 140 years' journey of gastric cancer surgery: from the two hands of Billroth to the multiple hands of the robot. *Ann Gastroenterol Surg*. 2021;**5**:270–277.
127. Plerhoples TA, Hernandez-Boussard T, Wren SM. The aching surgeon: a survey of physical discomfort and symptoms following open, laparoscopic, and robotic surgery. *J Robot Surg*. 2012;**6**:65–72.
128. Lee GI, Lee MR, Green I, et al. Surgeons' physical discomfort and symptoms during robotic surgery: a comprehensive ergonomic survey study. *Surg Endosc*. 2017;**31**:1697–1706.
129. Kim MC, Jung GJ, Kim HH. Learning curve of laparoscopy-assisted distal gastrectomy with systemic lymphadenectomy for early gastric cancer. *World J Gastroenterol*. 2005;**11**:7508–7511.

130. Jin SH, Kim DY, Kim H, et al. Multidimensional learning curve in laparoscopy-assisted gastrectomy for early gastric cancer. *Surg Endosc*. 2007;**21**:28–33.
131. Kang BH, Xuan Y, Hur H, et al. Comparison of surgical outcomes between robotic and laparoscopic gastrectomy for gastric cancer: the learning curve of robotic surgery. *J Gastric Cancer*. 2012;**12**:156–163.
132. An JY, Kim SM, Ahn S, et al. Successful robotic gastrectomy does not require extensive laparoscopic experience. *J Gastric Cancer*. 2018;**18**:90–98.
133. Liu H, Kinoshita T, Tonouchi A, et al. What are the reasons for a longer operation time in robotic gastrectomy than in laparoscopic gastrectomy for stomach cancer? *Surg Endosc*. 2019;**33**:192–198.
134. Hikage M, Tokunaga M, Makuuchi R, et al. Impact of an ultrasonically activated device in robot-assisted distal gastrectomy. *Innovations (Phila)*. 2017;**12**:453–458.
135. Iannessi A, Marcy PY, Clatz O, et al. A review of existing and potential computer user interfaces for modern radiology. *Insights Imaging*. 2018;**9**:599–609.
136. Abiri A, Pensa J, Tao A, et al. Multi-modal haptic feedback for grip force reduction in robotic surgery. *Sci Rep*. 2019;**9**:5016.
137. Choi PJ, Oskouian RJ, Tubbs RS. Telesurgery: past, present, and future. *Cureus*. 2018;**10**:e2716.
138. Han J, Davids J, Ashrafian H, et al. A systematic review of robotic surgery: from supervised paradigms to fully autonomous robotic approaches. *Int J Med Robot*. 2022;**18**:e2358.

21

Gastric cancer
Future aspects of treatment

Alexander B.J. Borgstein, Suzanne S. Gisbertz, and Mark I. van Berge Henegouwen

Current curative treatment of gastric cancer

The treatment of gastric cancer is influenced by the stage of the gastric tumour. Treatment options can be divided into those targeting early-stage gastric cancer and those used in advanced or metastatic disease. Early-stage gastric cancer is defined as a cT0–1N0 stage tumour, with invasion limited to the mucosa or submucosa. The prevalence of early-stage gastric cancer is higher in Asian countries compared to the Western world. This is mainly because of screening programmes for gastric cancer in Japan, which started in 1983.[1] Different endoscopic and surgical techniques have been developed to treat early-stage gastric cancer. Examples include endoscopic mucosal resection (EMR), endoscopic submucosal dissection (ESD) and function-preserving gastrectomy (FPG), which will be discussed in the 'Surgical treatment of early-stage gastric cancer' section.

Advanced gastric cancer is defined as an at least T2 or N+ stage tumour, according to the Japanese gastric cancer guidelines.[2] Traditionally, surgery has been the cornerstone of curative treatment for advanced gastric cancer. A (subtotal) gastrectomy with a D2 lymphadenectomy, usually in combination with neoadjuvant therapy, has formed the foundation for the curative treatment of advanced gastric cancer. An open gastrectomy has been the standard procedure; however, since the first minimally invasive gastrectomy in 1994, this approach has increasingly been implemented worldwide.[3] Different studies have indicated an advantage in short-term outcomes and similar oncological outcomes when comparing laparoscopic to open gastrectomy.[4–7] However, most of these studies have been conducted in Asian countries, where the prevalence of early-stage gastric cancer is much higher. Therefore, it is unclear whether these study findings can be translated to Western countries, in which gastric tumours are often diagnosed at a more advanced stage.[8] Newly developed surgical treatments for advanced gastric cancer will be discussed later in this chapter (see 'Surgical treatment of advanced gastric cancer').

Neoadjuvant therapy plays an important role alongside a gastrectomy in the curative treatment of advanced gastric cancer. Perioperative chemotherapy decreases tumour size and stage.[9] Additionally, it improves progression-free survival and overall survival rates compared to surgery alone.[9] Therefore, a combination of surgery with perioperative chemotherapy forms the standard curative treatment for advanced gastric cancer. However, different strategies exist for the application of neoadjuvant therapy in advanced gastric cancer. The newest developments of neoadjuvant therapy will be discussed later in this chapter (see 'Surgical treatment of advanced gastric cancer').

The final section in this chapter (see 'Non-surgical treatment of advanced gastric cancer and metastatic disease') will review the newest treatment options for metastatic disease, including palliative chemotherapy and immunotherapy.

Surgical treatment of early-stage gastric cancer

As mentioned in the first paragraph, gastric tumours in Asia are predominately detected at an early stage, which provides an opportunity to develop treatment specifically targeting them. However, there is a difference in the treatment of early-stage gastric cancer with N0 or N+ stage, which is indicated in the Japanese gastric cancer guidelines (Figure 21.1). A cT1N0 gastric tumour may be treated with an endoscopic or limited surgical resection. A cN+ tumour is an advanced cancer and needs to be treated with a standard (subtotal) gastrectomy with a D2 lymphadenectomy. Different types of limited surgical resections, also known as function-preserving gastrectomies, have been developed for cT1N0 gastric tumours. The type of resection that can be applied is determined by the tumour location. Endoscopic resections targeting early-stage gastric cancer are being increasingly used because of new developments.

Endoscopic mucosal resection and endoscopic submucosal dissection

An endoscopic resection can be considered for gastric tumours that have a very low chance of lymph node involvement and are suitable for piecemeal or en bloc resection.[2] With EMR, the tumour located

21 Gastric cancer: future treatments

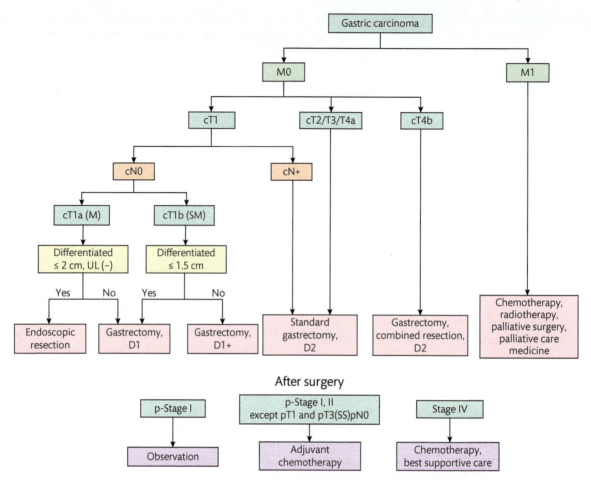

Figure 21.1 Algorithm of standard gastric cancer treatments according to the Japanese gastric cancer guidelines.
Reproduced from Kodera Y, Sano T. Japanese gastric cancer treatment guidelines 2014 (ver. 4) Japanese Gastric Cancer Association 1. Gastric Cancer. 2017;20(1):1–19. doi:10.1007/s10120-016-0622-4 under the Creative Commons Attribution 4.0 International License (http://creativecommons.org/licenses/by/4.0/)

in the mucosa is lifted with an injection of saline, followed by resection with a high-frequency steel snare. In ESD, a circumferential incision is made in the mucosa surrounding the tumour using a high-frequency electric knife and the submucosal layer is dissected from the muscle layer.

An endoscopic resection can only be considered for potentially node-negative early-stage gastric tumours, in which invasion is limited to the submucosal layer.[10]

Two indications have been established for the use of EMR/ESD: an absolute indication and an expanded indication for ESD, to be considered as investigational treatment.[2] The tumour characteristics of early-stage gastric cancer, for which the absolute indication to use EMR/ESD as standard treatment holds, are the following: differentiated-type adenocarcinoma, no ulceration, and depth of invasion clinically diagnosed as T1a and diameter less than or equal to 2 cm[2].

Tumour characteristics for which the investigational indications apply are the following:

1. T1a, differentiated-type adenocarcinoma, no ulceration, and diameter greater than 2 cm.
2. T1a, differentiated-type adenocarcinoma, ulceration, and diameter 3 cm or less.
3. T1a, undifferentiated-type adenocarcinoma, no ulceration, and diameter 2 cm or less.

The tumour characteristics described above have a very low chance of lymph node involvement, if the tumour is not associated with lymphovascular infiltration, making endoscopic resection possible. With the expanded criteria, the risk of lymph node metastases is equal to the risk of surgical mortality. ESD should be performed instead of EMR for the indication under investigation, in order to avoid incomplete dissection. Trials are in progress to investigate long-term outcomes in patients who have undergone ESD as an investigational indication for early-stage gastric cancer.[11]

An endoscopic resection is considered curative when the following post-resection conditions are met:

- En bloc resection.
- Tumour size 2 cm or less.
- Differentiated-type histology.
- pT1a.
- Negative horizontal and vertical margins.
- No lymphovascular infiltration.

Additional surgical treatments should be recommended if these criteria are not met. However, ESD accessories are being improved in order to increase the chance of realizing these postoperative conditions. These new accessories aim to increase the complete resection rate, reduce procedural times, and lower complication rates.[12] The improvement of the complete resection rate may increase the use of ESD as a curative treatment in early-stage gastric cancer.

New developments in ESD for early-stage gastric cancer

Upgrading the quality of the therapeutic endoscope used during ESD could improve treatment outcome. Currently used endoscopes provide standard-definition image quality. Implementation of high-definition image endoscopes could enable the endoscopist to determine the microvascular patterns and margins of the lesion more accurately.[12]

Additionally, the use of a laser system instead of an electric knife in ESD has been investigated.[13] A laser technique could improve surgical outcomes and reduce complications, including perforation. A study investigated the use of a thulium laser system.[13] This system emits a continuous 2 μm wavelength, with a penetration depth of 0.25 mm, reducing the risk of perforation. This study indicated the use of a laser system to be feasible[13]; however, if the wavelength of the laser could be controlled for incisions, dissections, and coagulation, performing ESD could become easier.[12]

Finally, several endoscopic robots are being developed to perform ESD in early-stage gastric cancer. ESD is technically more difficult to perform compared to other endoscopic methods (e.g. EMR), and has an increased risk of bleeding and perforation. This is partly due to the fact that using the standard flexible endoscopes employed in ESD it is difficult to perform advanced endosurgical procedures.[14] The endoscopes lack the ability to make basic manoeuvres, such as in-tissue manipulation.[14] The conduction of the force from the operator to the point of action is suboptimal because of the instability of the flexible endoscope.[14] Furthermore, the displayed field is determined by the direction of the endoscope, making visualization difficult when orientation is constantly changed with any movement.[14] Endoscopic robots provide the opportunity of bimanual handling and triangulation, resulting in improved precision. An example of an endoscopic robot is the MASTER system (EndoMASTER Pte, Singapore). This system contains a traction wire-controlled robotic arm, which has an integrated conventional double-channel endoscope. The safety and feasibility of the MASTER system has been established for early-stage gastric neoplasia in a multicentre prospective study.[15] The MASTER system, like other endoscopic robots, has great clinical potential; however, future trials are needed to provide evidence of improved surgical outcomes compared to current ESD techniques.

Limited surgical resection (function-preserving gastrectomy)

FPG can be applied to cT1N0 tumours, depending on the tumour location. FPG was originally derived from the treatment of gastroduodenal ulcers in the past. The first pylorus-preserving gastrectomy (PPG) was performed in 1967. FPG has been adapted for treatment of early-stage gastric cancer, for which it has been shown to improve patient outcomes compared to (subtotal) gastrectomy. In gastric cancer, FPG is characterized by the preservation of the oesophagogastric junction, pylorus, and capacity of the remnant stomach to maintain a functional reservoir.[16] Consequently, FPG maintains gastric function better compared to conventional gastrectomy. For this reason, FPG has been extensively studied as a possible surgical treatment in order to improve the quality of life in patients with early-stage gastric cancer. Different types of FPG have been developed, including PPG, proximal gastrectomy (PG), segmental gastrectomy, and local gastrectomy.

PPG, PG, and segmental/local gastrectomy

PPG preserves the upper third of the stomach combined with a 3–4 cm pyloric cuff. Additionally, PPG preserves the hepatic, pyloric, and coeliac branches of the vagal nerve as far as possible.[16] PPG is indicated for patients with cT1N0 early-stage gastric cancer located in the middle third of the stomach. The distance from the lesion to the pylorus should be at least 5 cm.[17]

PPG has been shown to improve quality of life in patients after treatment for early-stage gastric cancer. PPG results in a lower incidence of diarrhoea, dumping syndrome, duodenal juice reflux, and maintenance of body weight compared to conventional (subtotal) gastrectomy.[18–20] Studies have established PPG to be an oncological safe procedure with long-term outcomes comparable to standard gastrectomy. The 5-year survival rate after PPG in early-stage gastric cancer was found to range between 96% and 98%.[21] These findings are in line with long-term outcomes in patients after conventional gastrectomy, which range between 93% and 98%.[22] A multicentre randomized controlled trial (KLASS07) is in progress which compares the quality of life and long-term outcomes between patients with a laparoscopic PPG and laparoscopic distal gastrectomy in early-stage gastric cancer located in the middle of the body.[23]

In Japan, PG is recommended as a possible surgical option for the treatment of cT1N0 gastric cancer in the upper third of the stomach.[17] With an increase in the percentage of proximal gastric cancer in Asian countries,[24] the use of PG has increased in recent years.[25] The first laparoscopic PG was performed in 1995.[26] PG preserves more than half of the distal stomach, retaining its reservoir function. The pyloric ring function is preserved, which is associated with a lower rate of dumping syndrome and prevents duodenogastric reflux.[16] Furthermore, the hepatic branch, pyloric branch, and coeliac branches of the vagal nerve are preserved as much as possible.[27] PG uses different types of reconstruction methods, including oesophagogastrostomy, jejunal interposition, and double-tract reconstruction. These different methods have been developed to prevent gastro-oesophageal reflux after PG, which could result in reflux oesophagitis.

It is unclear which reconstructive method is optimal, different trials are in progress to compare these methods in order to find the best one after a PG.

Segmental gastrectomy and local/wedge gastrectomy are techniques that have been used for treatment of gastrointestinal stromal tumours, but are sometimes used to treat early-stage gastric cancer. Segmental gastrectomy is defined as a relatively small circumferential gastric resection, preserving the cardia and pylorus.[27] Local gastrectomy is characterized as a small non-circumferential gastric resection.[27]

The challenge for these two procedures is to achieve radicality, since an extended lymph node resection cannot be performed. Therefore, studies investigating the use of segmental gastrectomy and local gastrectomy in early-stage gastric cancer make use of sentinel node (SN) navigation.[28] SN navigation in gastric cancer is discussed later in this chapter (see 'Use of the sentinel node principle in gastric cancer').

New surgical techniques for early-stage gastric cancer

Endoscopic full-thickness resection (EFTR) is a newly developed technique combining endoscopic and laparoscopic surgery. This procedure includes the following steps: demarcation of the lesion and mucosal markings by endoscopic observation, followed by endoscopic circumferential submucosal injection and circumferential mucosal incision.[10] Afterwards, intentional perforation is performed on the exposed muscular layer and full-thickness resection is endoscopically performed with laparoscopic counteraction.[10] The tumour can be retrieved perorally or percutaneously. The intentional perforation is sutured laparoscopically. This procedure has been established to be feasible.[29] EFTR with laparoscopic assistance is related to organ preservation, avoidance of postoperative complications, and maintenance of quality of life. However, this technique is associated with iatrogenic tumour seeding. Tumour cells floating in the gastric juice may spread to the peritoneum, after the intentional perforation. A study indicated that 15% of all stomachs with early-stage gastric cancer contain tumour cells floating in the gastric juice.[30] Hence, EFTR with laparoscopic assistance is only indicated for subepithelial tumours, without exposure on the mucosal surface.

New methods, including non-exposure EFTR, have been developed to expand the indication of EFTR for early-stage gastric tumours without iatrogenic dissemination after the intentional perforation. One newly developed type of EFTR is non-exposed wall-inversion surgery (NEWS).[31] NEWS includes the following steps[31]: first, the resection area is endoscopically demarcated with mucosal markings, followed by laparoscopic serosal marking with endoscopic navigation. Second, a circumferential seromuscular incision is performed laparoscopically, followed by endoscopic submucosal injection. Next, the seromuscular layers are linearly sutured, with the lesion inverted towards the inside. This is followed by a muco-submucosal incision, which is done endoscopically. The lesion is trans-orally retrieved. This method is considered as an optimal surgical treatment for early-stage gastric cancer. However, NEWS needs to be combined with SN navigation in order to improve radicality.

Use of the sentinel node principle in gastric cancer

In recent years, researchers have tried to adopt the SN principle for gastric cancer treatment. The SN is thought to be the first lymph node(s) receiving lymphatic drainage from the primary tumour. Therefore, it is considered to be the first possible node of metastasis from the primary tumour.[32] If the SN is pathologically negative for metastasis, all regional lymph nodes may be considered to be negative as well.[33] Lymph node metastasis influences long-term outcomes in patients with gastric cancer, and so performing a complete lymphadenectomy is extremely important. However, around 20% of patients with early-stage gastric cancer have nodal metastases. Therefore, in nearly 80% of patients with early-stage gastric cancer, accurately identifying lymph node status could avoid unnecessary lymphatic dissection (and associated gastrectomy in cT1N1).[34] The SN principle could play a key role in minimizing the extent of gastric and lymphatic resection. In advanced gastric cancer, the SN principle could be used to limit unnecessary extensive lymphatic dissection and identify lymphatic drainage routes outside the standard dissection planes.[35] However, most studies investigate the use of the SN principle in early-stage gastric cancer. In advanced gastric cancer, the use of SN navigation is unreliable owing to lymphatic blockage by tumour cells and to neoadjuvant therapy in patients with advanced gastric cancer, which leads to fibrosis of lymph vessels where tumour cells were present.

Recent multicentre trials have indicated SN navigation to be an acceptable procedure in early-stage gastric cancer in terms of detection rate and accuracy of determination of lymph node status.[32,36] A Japanese trial found a SN detection rate of 98% and the accuracy of determination of metastatic status was 99%.[36] Until now, a dual-tracer method with radioactive colloids and blue dye has been considered the standard SN detection method to use in early-stage gastric cancer.[36,37] However, the blue dye deteriorates quickly and radioactive colloid shows a shine-through effect in the surgical field during gamma probe detection of hot lymph nodes.[34] An ideal tracer for SN procedures has to be easy to visualize, have good permeability, strong build-up in the SN, and little outflow to the secondary lymph nodes.

A newly developed SN procedure in gastric cancer uses indocyanine green (ICG) fluorescence. ICG fluorescence is an intraoperative imaging technology used in different surgical fields. It can be used for visualizing tumours, vascular structures, and lymph nodes or channels.[38] ICG binds to plasma proteins, after which it emits maximal fluorescence at an 840 nm wavelength. ICG fluorescence has multiple advantages compared to the standard SN procedure using blue dye and radioactive colloids. These include a lower frequency of allergic reaction, capability to detect bright nodes under adipose tissue, real-time visualization, high sensitivity to detect a minute concentration, and signal stability.[39–41] Studies have indicated ICG fluorescence to be a feasible procedure in both open and laparoscopic surgery in early-stage gastric cancer.[42] Different detection systems, using near-infrared technology,[43] have been developed to visualize ICG during open, laparoscopic, and robotic surgery.

The application of the SN principle in gastric cancer could make it possible to develop an individualized treatment for patients with early-stage gastric cancer, where the SN status plays a central role in deciding on the optimal treatment (Figure 21.2). Patients with an SN-negative status could be treated with FPG or endoscopic resection and sentinel basin dissection, whereas SN-positive

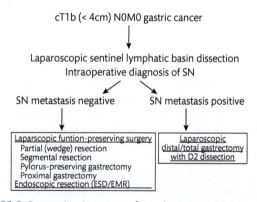

Figure 21.2 Personalized treatment for early-stage gastric cancer based on sentinel node mapping.

Reproduced with permission from Takeuchi H, Goto O, Yahagi N, Kitagawa Y. Function-preserving gastrectomy based on the sentinel node concept in early gastric cancer. *Gastric Cancer*. 2017;20:53–59. doi:10.1007/s10120-016-0649-6

status needs to be treated with a (subtotal) gastrectomy with D2 lymphadenectomy. A trial investigating long-term outcomes after FPG with SN mapping and basin dissection is in progress (UMIN000014401).

Surgical treatment of advanced gastric cancer

As described in the first paragraph, the curative treatment of advanced gastric cancer consists of a (subtotal) gastrectomy with a D2 lymphadenectomy, usually in combination with perioperative therapy. Open gastrectomy has been the standard approach; however, the number of minimally invasive gastrectomies is increasing worldwide. The following paragraphs will discuss new surgical techniques used in operable advanced gastric cancer.

Minimally invasive gastrectomy

The first laparoscopic gastrectomy was performed in 1994. In recent years, multiple studies have compared laparoscopic to open gastrectomy. Most of these studies have been performed in Asian countries.[44–48] In total, almost 4000 patients with early or advanced and subtotal/total gastrectomy were included in these studies. A recent systematic review concluded that laparoscopic gastrectomy with D2 lymphadenectomy had equivalent overall short-term morbidity and mortality compared to open gastrectomy for locally advanced gastric cancer.[49] However, further well-designed randomized controlled trials are needed to investigate long-term outcomes for laparoscopic versus open gastrectomy for locally advanced gastric cancer.

Conversely, all studies were performed in Asian countries where the percentage of early-stage gastric cancer is much higher compared to the Western world. Therefore, it is unclear whether these study findings can be translated to the treatment of advanced gastric cancer in the Western world.

Recently, two Dutch trials, STOMACH[50] and LOGICA,[51] investigated the use of laparoscopic gastrectomy in advanced gastric cancer. Both studies compared laparoscopic to open gastrectomy in order to establish the optimal surgical strategy for patients with advanced gastric cancer in the Western world. The results of these Dutch trials are awaited.

Omentectomy and bursectomy

Traditionally, complete omentectomy and bursectomy were simultaneously performed in patients undergoing a (subtotal) gastrectomy with D2 lymphadenectomy. Resection of the greater omentum was thought to be essential in order to eliminate micro-metastases in advanced gastric cancer.[52] Bursectomy includes resection of the anterior membrane of the transverse mesocolon and pancreatic capsule after total omentectomy, which is followed by complete resection of regional lymph nodes alongside blood vessels and beneath the peritoneum.[53] Additionally, it provides en bloc resection of the post-gastric cavity, where micro-metastases could be present, in order to reduce the incidence of cancer recurrence.[53] However, both procedures have a risk of postoperative complications, are technically challenging, and are time-consuming. Therefore, trials have been conducted in order to establish the exact survival benefit of omentectomy and bursectomy.

The OMEGA trial[54] found an incidence of 5% of metastases in the greater omentum, and when present associated with severely advanced disease and R1 resections. Thus, the trial indicated that omentectomy as part of gastrectomy may be omitted in patients with less than cT3 gastric cancer and limited to the stomach.[54]

A Japanese trial investigated the survival benefit of bursectomy combined with omentectomy in patients with resectable advanced gastric cancer.[53] No survival benefit was found in patients with additional bursectomy. Bursectomy is not recommended anymore as standard treatment for resectable advanced gastric cancer.

Robot-assisted gastrectomy

The use of robot-assisted surgery has increased over the last two decades in different surgical fields. In gastric cancer, the first robot-assisted gastrectomy was described in 2002.[55] Robot-assisted surgery makes use of the da Vinci Surgical System (Intuitive Surgical Inc., Sunnyvale, CA, USA), which has been on the market since 2000. Other systems are being developed as well, although the da Vinci System is currently the mostly used system worldwide.

The idea is that robot-assisted surgery has the same benefits as laparoscopic surgery compared to open procedures as discussed above. Additionally, robot-assisted surgery provides three-dimensional vision, high magnification, increased degree of freedom including endo-wristed instrumentation, stable optical platform, and tremor reduction technology.[56] This might result in enhanced surgical precision which could result in improved clinical outcomes compared to standard laparoscopic surgery.

Robot-assisted gastrectomy follows the same surgical principles as the established laparoscopic gastrectomy. Four robot ports and one assistant port are introduced, followed by the same oncological procedures as laparoscopic gastrectomy.

Although the use of robot-assisted gastrectomy seems promising, the rate of international implementation is rather slow. Only 4% of all gastrectomies in South Korea, a pioneer in the usage of robot-assisted gastrectomy, are performed with the use of a robot.[57] However, the incidence of gastric cancer and hospital volume in South Korea are much higher compared to other countries.[58]

High-level evidence indicating superior results compared to the existing treatment is needed in order to implement a newly developed procedure. In the case of robot-assisted gastrectomy, prospective randomized trials are missing. Studies comparing robot-assisted with laparoscopic gastrectomy mainly consist of case series and meta-analyses.[55,56,59–61] The available data indicate robot-assisted gastrectomy to be a safe procedure, with the same oncological outcomes (lymph node yield, R0 resections). However, the benefits are relatively minor compared to laparoscopic gastrectomy outcomes. Furthermore, the use of a robot system leads to increased operation time and costs. On average, the cost of a robot-assisted gastrectomy is around 5000 USD higher per patient.[62] Overall, it appears that high costs are the major hurdle for the international implementation of this new procedure. The use of robot-assisted surgery does provide the opportunity to use newly developed techniques such as fluorescence with ICG and augmented reality; however, these techniques can also be used in standard laparoscopic and open surgery. Trials are needed to show improved patient outcomes after robot-assisted gastrectomy compared to minimally invasive gastrectomy.

Image-guided gastrectomy

In minimally invasive surgery, detailed information about the patient's anatomy is important when planning and performing a resection. Due to a two-dimensional restricted field of view and absence of tactile feedback, laparoscopic surgery is more difficult to perform compared to open surgery. In contrast to laparoscopic surgery, robot-assisted surgery does provide a three-dimensional image. Image-guided surgery is developed as a guiding tool which can be used during laparoscopic or robot-assisted surgery. Computed tomography or magnetic resonance imaging provides high-quality structural information on a patient's anatomy, which can be used as a navigation tool to assist minimally invasive surgery.

Image guidance surgery was originally developed for the treatment of brain tumours and has now found its way into various types of surgery, including robot-assisted and laparoscopic gastrectomy.[61]

A pilot study developed a guiding system based on computed tomography images which assists in laparoscopic gastrectomy. This system provided accurate identification of vascular anatomy prior to partial gastrectomy.[63]

Another pilot study investigated the use of image guidance in robot-assisted gastrectomy; the findings indicated the use of the system to be feasible and safe.[61] The vascular anatomy around the stomach could be completely visualized during the operation from computed tomography images made preoperatively.[61]

Image-guided surgery provides tools for a surgeon that can be used during minimally invasive gastrectomy, which could make the procedure easier and safer. Additionally, image-guided surgery makes it possible to develop personalized operations, which are based on the patient's individual anatomy and tumour stage.

Non-surgical treatment of advanced gastric cancer and metastatic disease

As mentioned in the first paragraph, perioperative therapy plays an important role, besides a gastrectomy, in the curative treatment of advanced gastric cancer. The preferable treatment for patients with an operable greater than T1N0 gastric tumour consists of perioperative chemotherapy follow by a gastrectomy and postoperative chemotherapy.

Treatment options for patients with an inoperable gastric tumour or metastatic disease consist of palliative chemotherapy, which can be combined with immunotherapy.

Figure 21.3 provides a schematic overview of the different treatment options in gastric cancer. The following paragraphs will provide an overview of the newest developments of non-surgical treatment in gastric cancer.

Perioperative chemotherapy for advanced gastric cancer

The MAGIC trial was the first large trial indicating survival benefits of perioperative chemotherapy compared to surgery alone.[9] Patients in the MAGIC trials received three cycles of epirubicin, cisplatin, and fluorouracil (ECF) before and after surgery. Patients with perioperative chemotherapy had a significant improvement in overall survival compared to surgery alone.[9] The ECF protocol has formed the standard in recent years; however, outcomes for patients with gastric or gastro-oesophageal junction adenocarcinoma remained unsatisfactory. Therefore, new studies have been developed of which the FLOT trial showed improved outcomes compared to

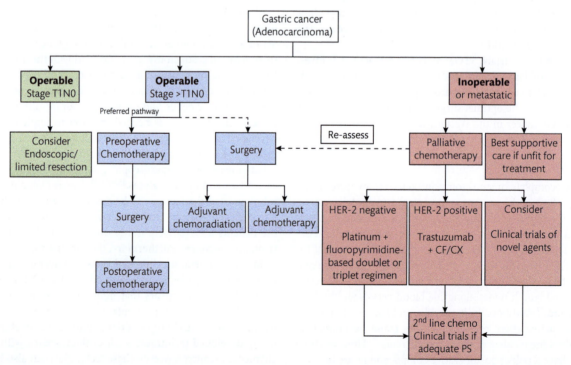

Figure 21.3 Algorithm for the management of gastric cancer in Europe. CF/CX, cisplatin and fluorouracil/cisplatin and capecitabine; PS, performance status.

Reproduced from Waddell T, Verheij M, Allum W, Cunningham D, Cervantes A, Arnold D. Gastric cancer: ESMO–ESSO–ESTRO Clinical Practice Guidelines for diagnosis, treatment and follow-up. Ann Oncol. 2013;24(Suppl 6):vi57–vi63. doi:10.1093/annonc/mdt344 under the Creative Commons Attribution 4.0 International License (http://creativecommons.org/licenses/by/4.0/)

the MAGIC trial in advanced gastric cancer.[64] This trial compared pre- and postoperative cycles of ECF or epirubicin, cisplatin, and capecitabine (ECX) with a fluorouracil/leucovorin, docetaxel, and oxaliplatin (FLOT) regimen. The FLOT group showed significantly improved overall survival, making the FLOT regimen the gold standard as perioperative chemotherapy for the treatment of locally advanced gastric cancer.[64]

Different trials are in progress to evaluate the effect of neoadjuvant chemoradiotherapy compared to neoadjuvant chemotherapy. These trials include TOPGEAR[65] and CRITICS-II,[66] which are both investigating the impact of additional preoperative radiotherapy. The aim of these studies is to establish the most effective neoadjuvant therapy in patients with resectable advanced gastric cancer.

Postoperative chemoradiotherapy for advanced gastric cancer

In 2001, the first study reported improved overall survival in patients with postoperative chemoradiotherapy compared to surgery alone in advanced gastric cancer.[67] After the result of the MAGIC trial in 2006,[9] it was questioned whether postoperative radiotherapy had additional benefits compared to postoperative chemotherapy alone. Recently, the CRITICS-I trial investigated whether postoperative chemoradiotherapy improves survival, as compared to postoperative chemotherapy, in patients who are treated with preoperative chemotherapy followed by surgery.[68] This trial failed to provide evidence for improved survival outcomes for patients receiving additional postoperative radiotherapy compared to chemotherapy alone,[68] indicating perioperative chemotherapy (FLOT regimen) to be the gold standard in treatment of resectable advanced gastric cancer.

Current treatment for metastatic gastric cancer

In the Western world, a large proportion of patients with gastric cancer present with inoperable advanced or metastatic disease for which curative surgery is not possible. Palliative chemotherapy is the standard treatment for these patients; however, a patient's performance status most be sufficient in order to receive chemotherapy. Palliative chemotherapy shows better results compared to best supportive care.[69]

Palliative chemotherapy for human epidermal growth factor receptor 2 (HER2)-negative gastric tumours consists of a combination of a platinum and fluoropyrimidine doublet regimen. Palliative treatment for HER2-positive gastric tumours includes addition of trastuzumab (immunotherapy) to cisplatin and fluoropyrimidine, which has been shown to increase overall survival (ToGA trial).[70]

For second-line chemotherapy, docetaxel, irinotecan, and paclitaxel have all demonstrated improved survival rates compared to best supportive care.[71] Two trials, RAINBOW[72] and REGARD,[73] have indicated a survival benefit of ramucirumab (vascular endothelial growth factor (VEGFR2) antagonist) as second-line treatment in palliative setting.

Molecular subtypes and targeted therapy for metastatic gastric

New treatment strategies focus on the development of immunotherapies. Recently, The Cancer Genome Atlas group identified four major molecular subtypes in gastric cancer[74]: Epstein–Barr virus-positive, microsatellite unstable, genomically stable, and chromosomal unstable tumours. Epstein–Barr virus-positive and microsatellite unstable gastric cancer are thought to have the most potential to respond to immunotherapy. Epstein–Barr virus-positive

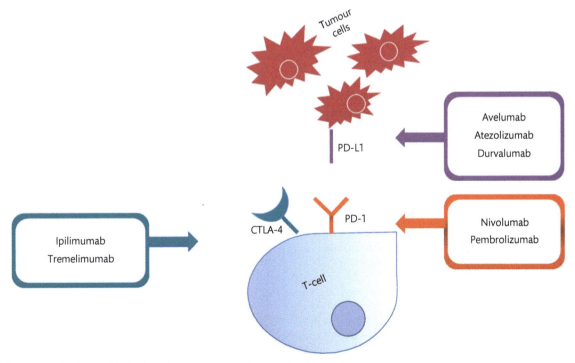

Figure 21.4 Immune checkpoint blockade with different monoclonal antibodies.
Reproduced from Magalhães H, Fontes-Sousa M, MacHado M. Immunotherapy in advanced gastric cancer: an overview of the emerging strategies. *Can J Gastroenterol Hepatol*. 2018;2018. doi:10.1155/2018/2732408 under the Creative Commons Attribution 4.0 International License (http://creativecommons.org/licenses/by/4.0/)

gastric cancer, representing around 9% of all gastric tumours, is associated with programmed cell death ligand 1 (PD-L1) gene amplification, suggesting higher immunogenicity.[71] Microsatellite unstable gastric tumours represent between 15% and 30% of all gastric tumours. This subtype is characterized by increased lymphocytic infiltration, which is the result of tumour antigens and genomic changes linked to PD-L1, indicating the potential role of immunotherapy.[75] Furthermore, microsatellite instability is associated with an adverse effect of chemotherapy on survival.

Cytotoxic T-lymphocyte-associated protein 4 (CTLA4) and programmed cell death protein 1 (PD-1) are located on T cells and inhibit T-cell response, thereby providing an escape mechanism for tumour cells from T-cell antitumour activity.[76] PD-L1 in gastric tumours cells interacts with the PD-1 receptor, which results in the inhibition of T-cell migration and proliferation. This results in an anti-apoptotic signal, preventing overactivation of the immune system towards the tumour cells.[71] Newly developed immunotherapies target CTLA4 and PD-1/PD-L1 in order to increase the immune response towards the gastric tumour cells. Figure 21.4 provides a schematic overview with different monoclonal antibodies binding CTLA4 or PD-1/PD-L1.

A phase III trial, ATTRACTION-2, showed survival benefit of nivolumab (PD-1 inhibitor) for heavily pretreated patients with advanced gastric cancer.[77] Another PD-1 inhibitor, pembrolizumab, showed improved patient survival as well.[78] Several trials are currently in progress to asses both nivolumab and pembrolizumab to be applied in earlier lines of therapy in advanced gastric cancer.

After a long period with only two molecular targets (trastuzumab and ramucirumab), which provided moderate results in overall survival, a new paradigm shift in the treatment of inoperable gastric cancer is occurring. Instead of targeting cancer cells, newly developed antibodies target the immune system, which stimulates a host immune response against its own cancer cells.[79]

In conclusion, new treatment options and strategies are being developed to target early-stage, advanced, or metastatic gastric cancer. In early-stage gastric cancer, FPG, in the form of EFTR, based on SN navigation may be the optimal treatment.

In advanced gastric cancer, future studies must provide insights on whether to use open, laparoscopic, or robot-assisted gastrectomy in the Western world.

For metastatic gastric cancer, targeted therapy based on immunotherapy could increase overall survival.

REFERENCES

1. Liu CY, Wu CY, Lin JT, Lee YC, Yen AMF, Chen THH. Multistate and multifactorial progression of gastric cancer: results from community-based mass screening for gastric cancer. *J Med Screen*. 2006;**13**(Suppl 1):S2–S5.
2. Japanese Gastric Cancer Association. Japanese gastric cancer treatment guidelines 2014 (ver. 4). *Gastric Cancer*. 2017;**20**:1–19.
3. Kitano S, Iso Y, Moriyama M, Sugimachi K. Laparoscopy-assisted Billroth I gastrectomy. *Surg Laparosc Endosc*. 1994;**4**:146–148.
4. Viñuela EF, Gonen M, Brennan MF, Coit DG, Strong VE. Laparoscopic versus open distal gastrectomy for gastric cancer: a meta-analysis of randomized controlled trials and high-quality nonrandomized studies. *Ann Surg*. 2012;**255**:446–456.
5. Xiong JJ, Nunes QM, Huang W, et al. Laparoscopic vs open total gastrectomy for gastric cancer: a meta-analysis. *World J Gastroenterol*. 2013;**19**:8114–8132.
6. Zeng YK, Yang ZL, Peng JS, Lin HS, Cai L. Laparoscopy-assisted versus open distal gastrectomy for early gastric cancer: evidence from randomized and nonrandomized clinical trials. *Ann Surg*. 2012;**256**:39–52.
7. Haverkamp L, Weijs TJ, van der Sluis PC, van der Tweel I, Ruurda JP, van Hillegersberg R. Laparoscopic total gastrectomy versus open total gastrectomy for cancer: a systematic review and meta-analysis. *Surg Endosc*. 2013;**27**:1509–1520.
8. Strong VE, Devaud N, Karpeh M. The role of laparoscopy for gastric surgery in the West. *Gastric Cancer*. 2009;**12**:127–131.
9. Cunningham D, Allum WH, Stenning SP, et al. Perioperative chemotherapy versus surgery alone for resectable gastroesophageal cancer. *N Engl J Med*. 2006;**355**:11–20.
10. Goto O, Takeuchi H, Kitagawa Y, Yahagi N. Hybrid surgery for early gastric cancer. *Transl Gastroenterol Hepatol*. 2016;**2016**:1–6.
11. Hasuike N, Ono H, Boku N, et al. A non-randomized confirmatory trial of an expanded indication for endoscopic submucosal dissection for intestinal-type gastric cancer (cT1a): the Japan Clinical Oncology Group study (JCOG0607). *Gastric Cancer*. 2018;**21**:114–123.
12. Jang JY. Future development of endoscopic accessories for endoscopic submucosal dissection. *Clin Endosc*. 2017;**50**:242–249.
13. Cho JH, Cho J, Kim MY, et al. Endoscopic submucosal dissection using a thulium laser: preliminary results of a new method for treatment of gastric epithelial neoplasia. *Endoscopy*. 2013;**45**:725–728.
14. Turiani Hourneaux de Moura D, Aihara H, Jirapinyo P, et al. Robot-assisted endoscopic submucosal dissection versus conventional ESD for colorectal lesions: outcomes of a randomized pilot study in endoscopists without prior ESD experience (with video). *Gastrointest Endosc*. 2019;**90**:290–298.
15. Phee SJ, Reddy N, Chiu PWY, et al. Robot-assisted endoscopic submucosal dissection is effective in treating patients with early-stage gastric neoplasia. *Clin Gastroenterol Hepatol*. 2012;**10**:1117–1121.
16. Nunobe S, Hiki N. Function-preserving surgery for gastric cancer: current status and future perspectives. *Transl Gastroenterol Hepatol*. 2017;**2**:77.
17. Sano T, Kodera Y. Japanese gastric cancer treatment guidelines 2010 (ver. 3). *Gastric Cancer*. 2011;**14**:113–123.
18. Fujita J, Takahashi M, Urushihara T, et al. Assessment of postoperative quality of life following pylorus-preserving gastrectomy and Billroth-I distal gastrectomy in gastric cancer patients: results of the nationwide postgastrectomy syndrome assessment study. *Gastric Cancer*. 2016;**19**:302–311.
19. Jiang X, Hiki N, Nunobe S, et al. Postoperative outcomes and complications after laparoscopy-assisted pylorus-preserving gastrectomy for early gastric cancer. *Ann Surg*. 2011;**253**:928–933.
20. Nunobe S, Sasako M, Saka M, Fukagawa T, Katai H, Sano T. Symptom evaluation of long-term postoperative outcomes after pylorus-preserving gastrectomy for early gastric cancer. *Gastric Cancer*. 2007;**10**:167–172.
21. Hiki N, Sano T, Fukunaga T, Ohyama S, Tokunaga M, Yamaguchi T. Survival benefit of pylorus-preserving gastrectomy in early gastric cancer. *J Am Coll Surg*. 2009;**209**:297–301.
22. Sano T, Sasako M, Kinoshita T, Maruyama K. Recurrence of early gastric cancer. Follow-up of 1475 patients and review of the Japanese literature. *Cancer*. 1993;**72**:3174–3178.

23. Lee CM, Park JH, In Choi C, et al. A multi-center prospective randomized controlled trial (phase III) comparing the quality of life between laparoscopy-assisted distal gastrectomy and totally laparoscopic distal gastrectomy for gastric Cancer (study protocol). *BMC Cancer*. 2019;**19**:206.
24. Isobe Y, Nashimoto A, Akazawa K, et al. Gastric cancer treatment in Japan: 2008 annual report of the JGCA nationwide registry. *Gastric Cancer*. 2011;**14**:301–316.
25. Harrison LE, Karpeh MS, Brennan MF. Total gastrectomy is not necessary for proximal gastric cancer. *Surgery*. 1998;**123**:127–130.
26. Uyama I, Ogiwara H, Takahara T, Kikuchi K, Iida S. Laparoscopic and minilaparotomy proximal gastrectomy and esophagogastrostomy: technique and case report. *Surg Laparosc Endosc*. 1995;**5**:487–491.
27. Nomura E, Okajima K. Function-preserving gastrectomy for gastric cancer in Japan. *World J Gastroenterol*. 2016;**22**:5888–5895.
28. Mitsumori N, Nimura H, Takahashi N, et al. Sentinel lymph node navigation surgery for early stage gastric cancer. *World J Gastroenterol*. 2014;**20**:5685–5693.
29. Park S, Chun HJ, Keum B, et al. Successful hybrid NOTES resection of early gastric cancer in a patient with concomitant advanced colon cancer. *Endoscopy*. 2010;**42**(Suppl 2):E1–E2.
30. Han TS, Kong SH, Lee HJ, et al. Dissemination of free cancer cells from the gastric lumen and from perigastric lymphovascular pedicles during radical gastric cancer surgery. *Ann Surg Oncol*. 2011;**18**:2818–2825.
31. Mitsui T, Niimi K, Yamashita H, et al. Non-exposed endoscopic wall-inversion surgery as a novel partial gastrectomy technique. *Gastric Cancer*. 2014;**17**:594–599.
32. Kitagawa Y, Fujii H, Mukai M, et al. The role of the sentinel lymph node in gastrointestinal cancer. *Surg Clin North Am*. 2000;**80**:1799–1809.
33. Hiramatsu Y, Takeuchi H, Goto O, Kikuchi H, Kitagawa Y. Minimally invasive function-preserving gastrectomy with sentinel node biopsy for early gastric cancer. *Digestion*. 2019;**99**:14–20.
34. Kinami S, Kosaka T. Laparoscopic sentinel node navigation surgery for early gastric cancer. *Transl Gastroenterol Hepatol*. 2017;**2**:42.
35. Tani T, Sonoda H, Tani M. Sentinel lymph node navigation surgery for gastric cancer: does it really benefit the patient? *World J Gastroenterol*. 2016;**22**:2894–2899.
36. Kitagawa Y, Takeuchi H, Takagi Y, et al. Sentinel node mapping for gastric cancer: a prospective multicenter trial in Japan. *J Clin Oncol*. 2013;**31**:3704–3710.
37. Takeuchi H, Kitagawa Y. New sentinel node mapping technologies for early gastric cancer. *Ann Surg Oncol*. 2013;**20**:522–532.
38. Bu L, Shen B, Cheng Z. Fluorescent imaging of cancerous tissues for targeted surgery. *Adv Drug Deliv Rev*. 2014;**76**:21–38.
39. Tajima Y, Murakami M, Yamazaki K, et al. Sentinel node mapping guided by indocyanine green fluorescence imaging during laparoscopic surgery in gastric cancer. *Ann Surg Oncol*. 2010;**17**:1787–1793.
40. Miyashiro I, Miyoshi N, Hiratsuka M, et al. Detection of sentinel node in gastric cancer surgery by indocyanine green fluorescence imaging: comparison with infrared imaging. *Ann Surg Oncol*. 2008;**15**:1640–1643.
41. Tajima Y, Yamazaki K, Masuda Y, et al. Sentinel node mapping guided by indocyanine green fluorescence imaging in gastric cancer. *Ann Surg*. 2009;**249**:58–62.
42. Kinami S, Oonishi T, Fujita J, et al. Optimal settings and accuracy of indocyanine green fluorescence imaging for sentinel node biopsy in early gastric cancer. *Oncol Lett*. 2016;**11**:4055–4062.
43. Herrera-Almario G, Patane M, Sarkaria I, Strong VE. Initial report of near-infrared fluorescence imaging as an intraoperative adjunct for lymph node harvesting during robot-assisted laparoscopic gastrectomy. *J Surg Oncol*. 2016;**113**:768–770.
44. Hyung WJ, Yang HK, Han SU, et al. A feasibility study of laparoscopic total gastrectomy for clinical stage I gastric cancer: a prospective multi-center phase II clinical trial, KLASS 03. *Gastric Cancer*. 2019;**22**:214–222.
45. Park YK, Yoon HM, Kim YW, et al. Laparoscopy-assisted versus open D2 distal gastrectomy for advanced gastric cancer. *Ann Surg*. 2018;**267**:638–645.
46. Katai H, Mizusawa J, Katayama H, et al. Short-term surgical outcomes from a phase III study of laparoscopy-assisted versus open distal gastrectomy with nodal dissection for clinical stage IA/IB gastric cancer: Japan Clinical Oncology Group Study JCOG0912. *Gastric Cancer*. 2017;**20**:699–708.
47. Hu Y, Huang C, Sun Y, et al. Morbidity and mortality of laparoscopic versus open D2 distal gastrectomy for advanced gastric cancer: a randomized controlled trial. *J Clin Oncol*. 2016;**34**:1350–1357.
48. Kim W, Kim HH, Han SU, et al. Decreased morbidity of laparoscopic distal gastrectomy compared with open distal gastrectomy for stage I gastric cancer: short-term outcomes from a multicenter randomized controlled trial (KLASS-01). *Ann Surg*. 2016;**263**:28–35.
49. Beyer K, Baukloh A-K, Kamphues C, et al. Laparoscopic versus open gastrectomy for locally advanced gastric cancer: a systematic review and meta-analysis of randomized controlled studies. *World J Surg Oncol*. 2019;**17**:68.
50. Straatman J, van der Wielen N, Cuesta MA, et al. Surgical techniques, open versus minimally invasive gastrectomy after chemotherapy (STOMACH trial): study protocol for a randomized controlled trial. *Trials*. 2015;**16**:123.
51. Haverkamp L, Brenkman HJF, Seesing MFJ, et al. Laparoscopic versus open gastrectomy for gastric cancer, a multicenter prospectively randomized controlled trial (LOGICA-trial). *BMC Cancer*. 2015;**15**:556.
52. Hagiwara A, Sawai K, Sakakura C, et al. Complete omentectomy and extensive lymphadenectomy with gastrectomy improves the survival of gastric cancer patients with metastases in the adjacent peritoneum. *Hepatogastroenterology*. 1998;**45**:1922–1929.
53. Kurokawa Y, Doki Y, Mizusawa J, et al. Bursectomy versus omentectomy alone for resectable gastric cancer (JCOG1001): a phase 3, open-label, randomised controlled trial. *Lancet Gastroenterol Hepatol*. 2018;**3**:460–468.
54. Jongerius EJ, Boerma D, Seldenrijk KA, et al. Role of omentectomy as part of radical surgery for gastric cancer. *Br J Surg*. 2016;**103**:1497–1503.
55. Hashizume M, Sugimachi K. Robot-assisted gastric surgery. *Surg Clin North Am*. 2003;**83**:1429–1444.
56. van Boxel GI, Ruurda JP, van Hillegersberg R. Robotic-assisted gastrectomy for gastric cancer: a European perspective. *Gastric Cancer*. 2019;**22**:909–919.
57. Lim SH, Lee HM, Son T, Hyung WJ, Kim HI. Robotic surgery for gastric tumor: current status and new approaches. *Transl Gastroenterol Hepatol*. 2016;**2**:28.
58. Kweon SS. Updates on cancer epidemiology in Korea, 2018. *Chonnam Med J*. 2018;**54**:90.

59. Quijano Y, Vicente E, Ielpo B, et al. Full robot-assisted gastrectomy: surgical technique and preliminary experience from a single center. *J Robot Surg*. 2016;**10**:297–306.
60. Barchi LC, Souza WP, Franciss MY, et al. Oncological robot-assisted gastrectomy: technical aspects and ongoing data. *J Laparoendosc Adv Surg Tech*. 2020;**30**:127–139.
61. Kim YM, Baek SE, Lim JS, Hyung WJ. Clinical application of image-enhanced minimally invasive robotic surgery for gastric cancer: a prospective observational study. *J Gastrointest Surg*. 2013;**17**:304–312.
62. Kim HI, Han SU, Yang HK, et al. Multicenter prospective comparative study of robotic versus laparoscopic gastrectomy for gastric adenocarcinoma. *Ann Surg*. 2016;**263**:103–109.
63. Hayashi Y, Misawa K, Oda M, Hawkes DJ, Mori K. Clinical application of a surgical navigation system based on virtual laparoscopy in laparoscopic gastrectomy for gastric cancer. *Int J Comput Assist Radiol Surg*. 2016;**11**:827–836.
64. Al-Batran SE, Homann N, Pauligk C, et al. Perioperative chemotherapy with fluorouracil plus leucovorin, oxaliplatin, and docetaxel versus fluorouracil or capecitabine plus cisplatin and epirubicin for locally advanced, resectable gastric or gastro-oesophageal junction adenocarcinoma (FLOT4): a randomised, phase 2/3 trial. *Lancet*. 2019;**393**:1948–1957.
65. Leong T, Smithers BM, Haustermans K, et al. TOPGEAR: a randomized, phase III trial of perioperative ECF chemotherapy with or without preoperative chemoradiation for resectable gastric cancer: interim results from an international, Intergroup Trial of the AGITG, TROG, EORTC and CCTG. *Ann Surg Oncol*. 2017;**24**:2252–2258.
66. Slagter AE, Jansen EPM, van Laarhoven HWM, et al. CRITICS-II: a multicentre randomised phase II trial of neo-adjuvant chemotherapy followed by surgery versus neo-adjuvant chemotherapy and subsequent chemoradiotherapy followed by surgery versus neo-adjuvant chemoradiotherapy followed by surgery in resectable gastric cancer. *BMC Cancer*. 2018;**18**:877.
67. Macdonald JS, Smalley SR, Benedetti J, et al. Chemoradiotherapy after surgery compared with surgery alone for adenocarcinoma of the stomach or gastroesophageal junction. *N Engl J Med*. 2001;**345**:725–730.
68. Cats A, Jansen EPM, van Grieken NCT, et al. Chemotherapy versus chemoradiotherapy after surgery and preoperative chemotherapy for resectable gastric cancer (CRITICS): an international, open-label, randomised phase 3 trial. *Lancet Oncol*. 2018;**19**:616–628.
69. Glimelius B, Ekström K, Hoffman K, et al. Randomized comparison between chemotherapy plus best supportive care with best supportive care in advanced gastric cancer. *Ann Oncol*. 1997;**8**:163–168.
70. Bang YJ, Van Cutsem E, Feyereislova A, et al. Trastuzumab in combination with chemotherapy versus chemotherapy alone for treatment of HER2-positive advanced gastric or gastro-oesophageal junction cancer (ToGA): a phase 3, open-label, randomised controlled trial. *Lancet*. 2010;**376**:687–697.
71. Magalhães H, Fontes-Sousa M, MacHado M. Immunotherapy in advanced gastric cancer: an overview of the emerging strategies. *Can J Gastroenterol Hepatol*. 2018;**2018**:2732408.
72. Wilke H, Muro K, Van Cutsem E, et al. Ramucirumab plus paclitaxel versus placebo plus paclitaxel in patients with previously treated advanced gastric or gastro-oesophageal junction adenocarcinoma (RAINBOW): a double-blind, randomised phase 3 trial. *Lancet Oncol*. 2014;**15**:1224–1235.
73. Fuchs CS, Tomasek J, Yong CJ, et al. Ramucirumab monotherapy for previously treated advanced gastric or gastro-oesophageal junction adenocarcinoma (REGARD): an international, randomised, multicentre, placebo-controlled, phase 3 trial. *Lancet*. 2014;**383**:31–39.
74. Bass AJ, Thorsson V, Shmulevich I, et al. Comprehensive molecular characterization of gastric adenocarcinoma. *Nature*. 2014;**513**:202–209.
75. Garattini SK, Basile D, Cattaneo M, et al. Molecular classifications of gastric cancers: novel insights and possible future applications. *World J Gastrointest Oncol*. 2017;**9**:194–208.
76. Lordick F, Shitara K, Janjigian YY. New agents on the horizon in gastric cancer. *Ann Oncol*. 2017;**28**:1767–1775.
77. Kang YK, Boku N, Satoh T, et al. Nivolumab in patients with advanced gastric or gastro-oesophageal junction cancer refractory to, or intolerant of, at least two previous chemotherapy regimens (ONO-4538-12, ATTRACTION-2): a randomised, double-blind, placebo-controlled, phase 3 trial. *Lancet*. 2017;**390**:2461–2471.
78. Fuchs CS, Doi T, Jang RW, et al. Safety and efficacy of pembrolizumab monotherapy in patients with previously treated advanced gastric and gastroesophageal junction cancer: phase 2 clinical KEYNOTE-059 trial. *JAMA Oncol*. 2018;**4**:e180013.
79. Shekarian T, Valsesia-Wittmann S, Caux C, Marabelle A. Paradigm shift in oncology: targeting the immune system rather than cancer cells. *Mutagenesis*. 2015;**30**:205–211.

Index

For the benefit of digital users, indexed terms that span two pages (e.g., 52–53) may, on occasion, appear on only one of those pages.
Tables and figures are indicated by *t* and *f* following the page number

acetic acid chromoendoscopy 15
achalasia 26–30
  aetiopathogenesis 26
  autoimmune associations 26
  botulinum toxin injection 28
  Chicago classification 17*t*, 27, 31*t*
  clinical symptoms 26–27
  definition 26
  diagnosis 27
  Eckardt score 26*t*
  epidemiology 26
  interdisciplinary treatment algorithm 30*f*
  laparoscopic Heller's cardiomyotomy 29–30
  oral drug therapy 27
  peroral endoscopic myotomy (POEM) 29
  pneumatic dilation 28–29
  redo myotomy 28
  robotic Heller's cardiomyotomy 29–30
  therapeutic options 27–30
acid exposure time 17–18
alcohol use 60, 178
Allgrove syndrome 26
aperistalsis 34
argon plasma coagulation 72
artificial intelligence 225–26
aspirin 120–22
Auerbach plexus 6–7, 9
autoimmune disease 26

baclofen 53
balloon-occluded retrograde transvenous obliteration 69
bariatric surgery 90–94
  biliopancreatic diversion with duodenal switch 92–93
  cholelithiasis 94
  complications 93–94
  deep vein thrombosis 93
  gastrointestinal leaks 93
  GORD 93
  internal hernias 93
  malnutrition 93–94
  marginal ulcers 93
  mechanism of weight loss 90
  oesophagitis 93
  one-anastomosis gastric bypass 92
  Roux-en-Y gastric bypass 90–91
  single-anastomosis duodeno-ileal bypass 93

  sleeve gastrectomy 91–92
  strictures 93
barium studies 19–21
Barrett's oesophagus 59–61
  chemoprevention 60
  definition 59
  endoscopic eradication therapy 60, 132
  epidemiology 59–60
  oesophagectomy 61
  Prague classification 14, 59
  risk factors 60
  screening 60
  tissue sampling 15
biliopancreatic diversion with duodenal switch 92–93
botulinum toxin injection
  achalasia 28
  oesophageal hypermotility disorders 33
Brombart classification 40*t*
bursectomy 214, 235

Chagas disease 26
checkpoint inhibitors 119–20, 172, 194, 238
Chicago classification 16–17, 17*t*, 25–26, 27, 31*t*
chief cells 10
cholecystokinin 10–11
chromoendoscopy 15
combined pH/impedance monitoring 17–19
contrast studies 19–21
corpus gastricus 8
cricopharyngeal bars 40
CTLA4 inhibitors 238

DeMeester score 18–19, 52
diet
  GORD 52
  weight loss 89–90
distal gastrectomy 211
distal oesophagus spasm 31–32
distal splenorenal shunt 70
Doppler endoscopic probe 73–74
dyspepsia 46

Eckardt score 26*t*
EGFR inhibitors 118–19
endoluminal functional lumen imaging probe (endoFLIP) 19

endoscopic adhesive application 66–68, 80
endoscopic band ligation 66–68
endoscopic full-thickness resection 234
endoscopic mucosal resection 129–36, 199, 231–33
endoscopic sclerotherapy 66–68
endoscopic submucosal dissection 129–36, 199–205, 231–33
  laser 233
  robot-assisted 233
endoscopic ultrasound 16
endoscopy, diagnostic 13
eosinophilic oesophagitis 15
epigastric pain syndrome 46
epinephrine injections 72
epiphrenic diverticulum 42–43
Epstein-Barr virus 178
Eso-Sponge 83–84
exercise, weight loss 90

fibrin plugs 80
Forrest classification 14, 14*t*, 71
functional dyspepsia 45–46
functional gut disorders, diagnosis 16–19
functional lumen imaging probe (FLIP) 19
function-preserving gastrectomy 233
fundoplication
  Nissen 54–55
  Toupet 55
fundus gastricus 8

gastrectomy
  completion 211
  distal 211
  function-preserving 233
  image-guided 236
  laparoscopic 217–23
  local 233
  minimally invasive 235
  non-standard 210
  proximal 211, 233
  pylorus-preserving 211, 233
  robot-assisted 217–18, 223–26, 235
  segmental 211, 233
  sleeve 91–92
  standard 210
  total 211

gastric cancer
  adjuvant (chemo) radiotherapy 192–93
  alcohol use 178
  barium swallow 179
  bursectomy 214, 235
  centralized surgery 214
  completion gastrectomy 211
  computed tomography 180–81
  CTLA4 inhibitors 238
  curative treatment 187–88, 231
  diagnosis 179–82
  distal gastrectomy 211
  endoscopic full-thickness resection 234
  endoscopic mucosal resection 199, 231–33
  endoscopic submucosal dissection 199–205, 231–33
  endoscopic ultrasound 180
  epidemiology 177–78
  Epstein-Barr virus 178
  ESMO–ESSO–ESTRO treatment algorithm 210*f*, 236*f*
  extent of resection 210–12
  FDG-PET 181–82
  function-preserving gastrectomy 233
  future aspects of treatment 231–40
  Helicobacter pylori 178
  HER2 inhibitors 193–94
  hyperthermic intraperitoneal chemotherapy 191–92
  image-guided gastrectomy 236
  immunotherapy 193–94, 237–38
  indications for resection 209
  JGCA treatment algorithm 232*f*
  laparoscopic gastrectomy 217–23
  laser ESD 233
  local gastrectomy 233
  local (wedge) resection 211
  lymph node dissection 212–14
  metastatic disease 191, 237–38
  minimally invasive gastrectomy 235
  monoclonal antibodies 193–94, 237–38
  multimodal treatment 187–97
  neoadjuvant (chemo) radiotherapy 193
  non-curative surgery 210
  non-exposed wall-inversion surgery (NEWS) 234

Index

gastric cancer (cont.)
  non-standard gastrectomy 210
  NSAID use 178
  obesity 178
  oesophagogastroduodenoscopy 179–80
  oligometastatic disease 188–89
  omentectomy 214, 235
  palliative therapy 193, 210, 237
  papillary adenocarcinoma 204
  PD-L1 inhibitors 194, 238
  perioperative chemotherapy 189–90, 236–37
  postoperative chemotherapy 190–91, 237
  prevention 177–78
  proximal gastrectomy 211, 233
  pylorus-preserving gastrectomy 211, 233
  quality control in surgery 214
  radiotherapy 192–93
  reconstruction after gastrectomy 213t, 214
  reduction surgery 210
  risk factors 177–78
  robot-assisted ESD (MASTER system) 233
  robot-assisted gastrectomy 217–18, 223–26, 235
  segmental gastrectomy 211, 233
  sentinel node principle 234–35
  socioeconomic status 178
  staging 182–84, 209
  staging-related treatment algorithm 188f
  standard gastrectomy 210
  subtotal resection of remnant stomach 211
  symptoms 178–79
  targeted therapy 193–94, 237–38
  tobacco smoking 178
  total gastrectomy 211
  types and definitions of resections 210
  vessel plus surface (VS) classification 179–80
gastric glands 10
gastric ulcer 46
gastric varices 67
gastrin 10
gastro-oesophageal junction 4
gastro-oesophageal reflux disease (GORD) 49–64
  acid exposure time 17–18
  antacid therapy 52
  baclofen trial 53
  bariatric surgery 93
  barium swallow 51
  Barrett's oesophagus 60
  clinical features and symptoms 49–50
  DeMeester score 18–19, 52
  diagnosis 50–52
  diet 52
  differential diagnosis 52
  endoscopic treatment 54
  epidemiology 49
  H2 receptor antagonists 53
  histology 50–51
  lifestyle modification 52
  LINX device 55–56
  metoclopramide 53

Nissen fundoplication 54–55
obesity link 49
oesophageal manometry 51
oesophageal pH monitoring 51–52
oesophagitis 50
proton pump inhibitors 53–54
recurrent symptoms 54
refractory 54
sodium alginate 52
surface agents (sucralfate) 52
surgical treatment 54–56
Toupet fundoplication 55
treatment approaches 52
upper gastrointestinal endoscopy 50
wireless pH monitoring 19
gastropexy 58
G cells 10
GLP-1 receptor antagonists 90
glucagon 11
greater omentum 8

H2 receptor antagonists 53
haemostatic forceps 72
Hassab's operation 70
Helicobacter pylori 15, 46, 178
Heller's cardiomyotomy 29–30, 34
Hemospray (TC-325) 74
HER2 inhibitors 119, 193–94
hiatal hernia 56–59
  classification 57
  diagnosis 57
  gastropexy 58
  indications for surgery 57–58
  recurrent 58–59
  surgical techniques 58
high-resolution manometry 16–17
hypercontractile oesophagus 32–33
hyperthermic intraperitoneal chemotherapy 191–92

image-guided gastrectomy 236
immunotherapy 193–94, 237–38
indocyanine green 156, 234
ineffective oesophageal motility 35
Ivor Lewis oesophagectomy 155–59

jackhammer oesophagus 32–33

Killian–Jamieson gap 40
Kocher manoeuvre 139

laparoscopic gastrectomy 217–23
laparoscopic Heller's cardiomyotomy 29–30, 34
laser endoscopic submucosal dissection 233
lesser omentum 8
limited resection of the GOJ with isoperistaltic jejunal interposition 151–53
LINX device 55–56
local gastrectomy 233
Los Angeles classification 14, 14t, 50t
lower oesophageal sphincter 4, 8
Lugol's solution 15
lymphatics 5, 8–9

MASTER system 233
McKeown oesophagectomy 155–59
mesentericoportal venous bypass 70

metoclopramide 53
minimally invasive gastrectomy 235
minimally invasive oesophagectomy 155–59
  robot-assisted 159–65
monoclonal antibodies 117–20, 172, 193–94, 237–38
mucosa 5
mucous cells 10

Nissen fundoplication 54–55
nitric oxide 33
non-exposed wall-inversion surgery (NEWS) 234
non-steroidal anti-inflammatory drugs (NSAIDs)
  gastric cancer 178
  peptic ulcer disease 46
non-variceal upper GI bleeding 70–75
  antithrombotic agents 71t
  argon plasma coagulation 72
  definitive surgery 74–75
  Doppler endoscopic probe 73–74
  early endoscopy 70–71
  endoscopic haemostasis 71–74
  epinephrine injections 72
  Forrest classification 14, 14t, 71
  haemostatic forceps 72
  Hemospray (TC-325) 74
  management algorithm 75f
  minimal surgical approach 74–75
  over-the-scope clips 72, 74
  pre-endoscopy pharmacotherapy 70
  pre-endoscopy risk stratification 70
  recurrent bleeding 73
  surgical management 74–75
  through-the-scope clips 72
  transcatheter arterial embolization 74
nutcracker oesophagus 32–33

obesity
  Barrett's oesophagus 60
  diet 89–90
  exercise 89–90
  gastric cancer link 178
  GLP-1 receptor antagonists 90
  GORD 49
  medical conditions related to 89t
  non-operative weight loss methods 89–90
  orlistat 90
  serotonin antagonists 90
  sympathomimetic therapy 90
  see also bariatric surgery
oesophageal anatomy 3–7
oesophageal blood supply 5
oesophageal cancer
  abdominothoracic en bloc oesophagectomy with high intrathoracic anastomosis 150–51
  active surveillance 123
  adenocarcinoma 100, 103f
  adjuvant chemotherapy 106–7, 111, 111t
  aspirin 120–22
  checkpoint inhibitors 119–20, 172
  chemotherapy agents 107

clinical response evaluation 122–23
definitive chemotherapy 115–17
diagnosis 100–1
EGFR inhibitors 118–19
endoscopic mucosal resection 129–36
endoscopic submucosal dissection 129–36
epidemiology 99–100
future aspects of treatment 169–73
HER2 inhibitors 119
limited resection of the GOJ with isoperistaltic jejunal interposition 151–53
minimally invasive oesophagectomy (Ivor Lewis/McKeown) 155–59
monoclonal antibody therapy 117–20, 172
multimodal treatment 105–27, 170
neoadjuvant chemoradiotherapy 112–15
neoadjuvant chemotherapy 106–7, 108, 109t, 114–15
organ preservation after neoadjuvant treatment 122–23
PD-1/PD-L1 inhibitors 119–20
perioperative chemotherapy 106–7, 108–11, 110t
radiotherapy 105–6
robot-assisted minimally invasive thoraco-laparoscopic oesophagectomy (RAMIO/RAMIE) 159–65
salvage surgery 117
squamous cell carcinoma 100, 103f
staging (AJCC) 101–2
subtotal en bloc oesophagectomy (abdominothoracic approach) 147–50
surgery as primary therapy 169–70
symptoms 100
targeted therapy 117
TAS-102 172
transhiatal blunt oesophageal dissection and gastric pull-up 138–46
VEGF inhibitors 118
oesophageal constrictions 4
oesophageal diverticula 39–44
  aetiology 39
  diagnostic workup 39–40
  epiphrenic diverticulum 42–43
  pathophysiology 39
  pharyngo-oesophageal (Zenker's) diverticulum 40t, 40–42
  pulsion diverticula 39, 42–43
  symptoms 39–40
  traction (true) diverticula 39
  tubular oesophagus 42–43
oesophageal hypermotility disorders 31–34
oesophageal innervation 5, 25
oesophageal lymphatics 5
oesophageal manometry 16–17
oesophageal motility disorders
  absent contractility 34
  Chicago classification 16–17, 17t, 25–26, 27, 31t

Index

distal oesophagus spasm 31–32
hypercontractile (jackhammer) oesophagus 32–33
hypermotility disorders 31–34
ineffective motility 35
oesophagogastric junction outflow obstruction 31
peristalsis disorders 31–35
secondary 26t
see also achalasia
oesophageal perforation 79–87
  causes 79
  combination therapies 82
  conservative approach 79–80
  diagnosis 79
  endoluminal vacuum therapy 83–84
  endoscopic suturing 82
  endoscopic therapy 80–84
  Eso-Sponge 83–84
  fibrin adhesives and plugs 80
  OverStitch system 82
  over-the-scope clips 80–82
  stenting 82–83
  surgical therapy 84
  therapy options 79–84
  through-the-scope clips 80–82
  T-tags 82
oesophageal peristalsis 7
  disorders 31–35
oesophageal pH and multichannel intraluminal impedance monitoring 17–19
oesophageal sections 4
oesophageal varices
  endoscopic treatment 66–67
  Paquet classification 14
oesophagectomy
  Barrett's oesophagus 61
  en bloc with high intrathoracic anastomosis 150–51
  minimally invasive (Ivor Lewis/McKeown) 155–59
  robot-assisted minimally invasive thoraco-laparoscopic (RAMIO/RAMIE) 159–65
  subtotal en bloc 147–50
oesophagitis
  bariatric surgery 93
  eosinophilic 15
  GORD 50
  Los Angeles classification 14, 14t, 50t
  Savary–Miller classification 51t
oesophagogastric junction outflow obstruction 31
  tumour definition 14, 101–2, 169
oesophagogastroduodenoscopy 179–80
omentectomy 214, 235
one-anastomosis gastric bypass 92
orlistat 90
OverStitch system 82
over-the-scope clips 72, 74, 80–82

Paquet classification 14
parietal cells 10
  PPI-associated hypertrophy 47
Paris classification 14
pars abdominalis 4, 5

pars cardiaca 7
pars cervicalis 4, 5
pars pylorica 8
pars thoracalis 4, 5
partial portocaval shunt 70
PD-1/PD-L1 inhibitors 119–20, 194, 238
pepsinogen 10
peptic ulcer disease 46–47
peristalsis 7
  disorders 31–35
peroral endoscopic myotomy (POEM) 29, 33–34
pharyngo-oesophageal (Zenker's) diverticulum 40t, 40–42
pneumatic dilation 28–29, 33
portocaval shunt 69–70
portosystemic shunt 69
postprandial distress syndrome 46
Prague classification 14, 59, 100, 100f
proton pump inhibitor therapy
  disorders linked to chronic use 47
  functional dyspepsia 46
  GORD 53–54
  metoclopramide and 53
  risks associated with 53–54
proximal gastrectomy 211, 233
pyloric sphincter 8
pylorus-preserving gastrectomy 211, 233

radiotherapy 105–6, 192–93
reflux hypersensitivity 17–18
Rex shunt 70
Rikkunshito 46
robot-assisted surgery
  endoscopic submucosal dissection 233
  gastrectomy 217–18, 223–26, 235
  Heller's cardiomyotomy 29–30, 34
  minimally invasive thoraco-laparoscopic oesophagectomy (RAMIO/RAMIE) 159–65
Rome IV criteria 46
Roux-en-Y gastric bypass 90–91

Savary–Miller classification 51t
Seattle protocol 15
secretin 11
segmental gastrectomy 211, 233
sentinel node principle 234–35
Siewert classification 14, 169
single-anastomosis duodeno-ileal bypass 93
sleeve gastrectomy 91–92
sodium alginate 52
splenectomy 70
stomach anatomy 7–10
strictures
  post-bariatric surgery 93
  post-endoresection 134
subtotal en bloc oesophagectomy 147–50
sucralfate 52
Sugiura procedure 70
swallowing 7
Sydney protocol 15

targeted therapy 117–14, 193–94, 237–38

TAS-102 172
tela submucosa 6, 9
telesurgery 225
through-the-scope clips 72, 80–82
timed barium oesophagogram 19–20
tissue sampling 15–16
tobacco smoking 60, 178
total gastrectomy 211
Toupet fundoplication 55
transcatheter arterial embolization 74
transhiatal blunt oesophageal dissection and gastric pull-up 138–46
transjugular intrahepatic portosystemic shunt (TIPSS) 68–69
trials
  ACCORD 108–11, 110t, 170, 189
  ACTS-GC 190–91
  ARTDECO 117
  ARTIST 192
  ATTRACTION 119, 172, 238
  CALGB 9781 113t, 113–14
  Checkmate 119–20
  CLASS 220t, 222–23
  CLASSIC 190–91
  CRITICS 192–93, 237
  CROSS 113t, 114, 120, 170, 171
  DANTE 172, 194
  EORTC 109t, 189–90
  ESOPEC 171
  ESOSTRATE 123
  FFCD 9901 113t, 114
  FLOT 108–11, 110t, 120, 170–71, 188–89, 190, 191, 236–37
  ICONIC 171
  INNOVATION 194
  JACCRO GC-07 191
  JACOB 194
  JCOG 111, 111t, 190, 218–21, 220t, 222–23
  JLSSG0901 221
  KEYNOTE 119–20, 172
  KLASS 220t, 221–22, 233
  LOGICA 220t, 222, 235
  MAGIC 108–11, 110t, 170, 189, 236–37
  MIRO 158
  MONA LISA 224
  Neo-AEGIS 171
  NEOCRTEC5010 113t, 114
  NeoFLOT 190
  OE02 108, 109t
  OE05 108, 109t
  OGSG1003 C11P11, C11T2t
  OMEGA 235
  PANDA 172
  PETRARCA 194
  POET 193
  RACE 171
  RAINBOW 237
  RAMIE 165
  RAMSES 194
  REGARD 118, 237
  REGATTA 188, 209
  REVATE 165
  ROBOT 160, 165
  RTOG 108, 109t, 117, 118–19

  SAKK 75/08 118–19
  SANO 123
  STO3 118
  STOMACH 220t, 222, 235
  TAGS 172
  TIME 158–59
  ToGA 194, 237
  TOPGEAR 171, 193, 237
tricyclic antidepressants, dyspepsia 46
triple A syndrome 26
T-tags 82
tunica adventitia 7
tunica mucosa 6, 9
tunica muscularis 6, 9
tunica serosa 9

upper gastrointestinal bleeding
  acid-related 75
  blood transfusion 66
  epidemiology 65
  fluid resuscitation 65–66
  initial management 65–66
  non-acid related 75
  see also non-variceal upper GI bleeding; variceal upper GI bleeding
upper gastrointestinal perforation *see* oesophageal perforation
upper oesophageal sphincter 4

variceal upper GI bleeding 65, 66–70
  balloon-occluded retrograde transvenous obliteration 69
  distal splenorenal shunt (selective or Warren shunt) 70
  endoscopic band ligation/sclerotherapy/tissue adhesive injection 66–68
  gastric varices 67
  Hassab's operation 70
  management options 67t
  mesentericoportal venous bypass 70
  non-shunt surgery 70
  oesophageal varices 66–67
  partial portocaval shunt 70
  pharmacological management 66
  portocaval shunt (total or non-selective shunt) 69–70
  portosystemic shunt 69
  re-bleeding prevention 67–68
  Rex shunt 70
  splenectomy 70
  Sugiura procedure 70
  surgical management 69–70
  transjugular intrahepatic portosystemic shunt (TIPSS) 68–69
VEGF inhibitors 118
vessel plus surface (VS) classification 179–80

Warren shunt 70
weight loss *see* obesity
wireless pH monitoring 19

Zenker's diverticulum 40t, 40–42
z-line 4